Type 2 Diabetes

Cardiovascular and Related Complications
and
Evidence-Based Complementary Treatments

Type 2 Diabetes

Cardiovascular and Related Complications
and
Evidence-Based Complementary Treatments

Robert Fried
Richard M. Carlton

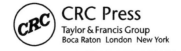

CRC Press
Taylor & Francis Group
Boca Raton London New York

CRC Press is an imprint of the
Taylor & Francis Group, an **informa** business

The authors thank wikipedia for permission to use the illustration, insulin molecule, in the cover design of our book.

CRC Press
Taylor & Francis Group
6000 Broken Sound Parkway NW, Suite 300
Boca Raton, FL 33487-2742

© 2019 by Taylor & Francis Group, LLC
CRC Press is an imprint of Taylor & Francis Group, an Informa business

No claim to original U.S. Government works

Printed on acid-free paper

International Standard Book Number-13: 978-1-138-58058-9 (Hardback); 978-1-138-58056-5 (Paperback)

Library of Congress Cataloging-in-Publication Data

Names: Fried, Robert, 1935- author. | Carlton, Richard M., author.
Title: Type 2 diabetes : cardiovascular and related complications and
evidence-based complementary treatments / Robert Fried and Richard M. Carlton.
Description: Boca Raton : CRC Press, 2018. | Includes bibliographical references.
Identifiers: LCCN 2018016357| ISBN 9781138580565 (pbk. : alk. paper) | ISBN
9781138580589 (hardback : alk. paper)
Subjects: | MESH: Diabetes Mellitus, Type 2--diet therapy | Diabetes
Mellitus, Type 2--complications | Hyperglycemia--physiopathology |
Complementary Therapies--methods | Evidence-Based Medicine--methods
Classification: LCC RC662.18 | NLM WK 815 | DDC 616.4/624--dc23
LC record available at https://lccn.loc.gov/2018016357

**Visit the Taylor & Francis Web site at
http://www.taylorandfrancis.com**

**and the CRC Press Web site at
http://www.crcpress.com**

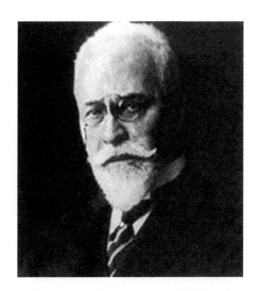

We dedicate this book to Oskar Minkowski (1858–1931) in recognition of his research on diabetes. In 1889, together with Josef von Mering, Professor Minkowski induced diabetes in dogs by removing their pancreas. It was Minkowski who performed the operation and made the crucial link to recognize that the symptoms of the treated dogs were due to diabetes: "After removal of the pancreas dogs get diabetes. It starts sometime after the operation and will persist for weeks continuously until their death...." (von Mering J, and O Minkowski. 1889)

von Mering J, and O Minkowski. 1889. Diabetes mellitus nach Pankreasextirpation. Archiv für experimentelle Patholgie und Pharmakologie (Leipzig), 26: 371.

Disclaimer

The information in this book is neither intended to diagnose nor treat any disease, nor is it a substitute for medical guidance. The authors do not propose that anyone who is undergoing treatment for any medical condition under the care of a physician, or any other qualified healthcare provider, should terminate such treatment in favor of any treatment or substance described here.

Rather, where it may seem helpful to adopt a nutrition strategy based on foods or supplements described here, the authors urge the reader to do so only with the advice and the supervision of his or her physician or other qualified healthcare provider.

The information provided here is intended only to educate the reader to what may be available and not to suggest self-treatment. The authors shall not be held liable or responsible for any misunderstanding or misuse of the information contained in this book or for any loss, damage, or injury caused or alleged to be caused directly or indirectly by any treatment, action, or application of any food or food source discussed in this book.

Contents

Preface

Medical science has made great strides in defining the pathophysiology of chronic hyperglycemia as Type 2 diabetes and in developing medications to treat this condition. There are now several classes of antidiabetic prescription medications, and most people with diabetes regularly take two or more of them in combination. Even so, good blood glucose control is hard to come by, and only about 30% of people on medications achieve it. Thirty percent—of 29 million sufferers—is rather a large number, actually.

There are also countless books that teach dietary means of lowering and regulating blood sugar by one food strategy, or another, and while these are often valid approaches, they do not help most diabetes sufferers for reasons related most often to inconvenience of implementation and noncompliance—sometimes they are costly. By the way, noncompliance is a problem with medications also.

This is a book about how cardiovascular and related functions are adversely affected by Type 2 diabetes, a complex disease entity and one that may entail more than simply chronic hyperglycemia. Although the *dependent variable* in most studies cited in medical and clinical research publications is serum glucose (often as HbA1c), and sometimes free radical assay values (FRAP), investigators invariably use the term "Type 2 Diabetes" when they should really stick to "blood glucose levels" because many things in diabetes do not change simply because blood glucose levels were lowered by the *independent variable(s)*. In fact, what we emphasize in this book is that by the time diabetes is diagnosed, most of the damage it caused is permanent.

Therefore, we often use the term "chronic hyperglycemia" to emphasize that we address the adverse—pathophysiological—impact of a specific metabolic condition on body function and not the effect of one disease on another one.

We live at a time when we have come to expect that we can solve most health problems (if they do not require surgery) with pills…. Would but that were so.

But there are now *integrative* approaches, based in sound clinical and biochemistry science, to help support blood sugar control, but they are not medical in the conventional sense that one might just acquire a prescription to the local pharmacy for them. We sometimes refer to these as "adjunctive." Still, there is a tendency to view these integrative approaches in the same vein as "herbals," that term now being pejorative—something perhaps not to be taken as seriously even as placebo treatment. Placebo treatment is, after all, thought to be benign, whereas herbals could even be hazardous.

What we have done in this book is first to catalog the pernicious and all-pervasive nature of Type 2 diabetes in cardiovascular and sensory body systems. Second, we describe some mostly botanical-based alternatives, "Functional Foods," and supplements that are upheld in their contribution to blood sugar control by valid scientific research evidence so as to bridge the gap between the conventional medications approach to blood glucose control and the integrative implementation of supports.

This book is not about "alternative" anything. It is about "integrative" and "complementary." It is about the addition of anything that has the backing of conventional, rigorous science to prove its efficacy in helping to control blood glucose in Type 2 diabetes. For that reason, this is not a self-help consumer "trade book."

Reading this book requires some basics in the sciences, and it is hoped that you will find it useful in your dealings with diabetes sufferers in whatever your capacity. In fact, in most instances, we have let the actual experiments speak for themselves, in a manner of speaking, to illustrate a given proposition so that it will be clear what science is saying, and also so that it will be clear when, in a few instances, we are speaking to the topic.

Please note the term "select" in some chapter titles. The botanicals, or other means of blood sugar control, or inflammation reduction, are not the only ones available to the average patient. But they were selected also to emphasize what few in the clinical setting still know about integrative and complementary treatment means: A vast number of such treatments were thoroughly studied in conventionally controlled clinical settings, and their outcome reports were published in mostly prestigious conventional journals. They serve as excellent models of what can be found in other instances as well. It takes little effort—one click on the keyboard—to access them on "NCBI," or PubMed, for instance.

Also, this is a book and not a medical journal, and we have taken a certain editorial license to edit the information presented here so as to make it a smoother "read." For instance:

Every single assertion in this book is referenced. That is what is meant by *evidence-based*. References are selected from a large number of invariably conventional science journal publications that come to the same or similar conclusions. Where there is serious controversy about a conclusion, at least one dissenting source is cited.

We have made it a point also to spell out the title of the journals that are cited in this book to make it easier for you to look up references, should you wish to do so. References are usually abbreviated in journals and all the readers of the journal know them. But this book aims to make science accessible to those of you who are not familiar with science journal-speak.

We only cite articles where we are satisfied that the sample size of participants is adequate to sustain the conclusions of a statistical analysis of the results. We are quite familiar with quantitative analysis methods (Fried 1964), and so we are comfortable with simply omitting the number of men and of women patients, or participants, in a given study. You can be sure that there are enough of them, and the actual numbers is just clutter here.

We only cite articles where we are satisfied about the "statistical significance" of the findings. Most often, this means the findings are not likely due to chance by stated probability criteria. For that reason we do not feel compelled, as we would for a journal article, to leave in P values, or confidence limits—science-babble. No study that does not meet such criteria appears in conventional science journals anyway. Editorial peer review has seen to that. And, so there is no purpose to that clutter either.

However, some investigators misuse statistical probability criteria to give unwarranted *oomph* to some of their findings. For instance, $P < 0.05$ does not lend less support to the *importance* of findings than $P < 0.0005$. The importance of findings is quite apart from the probability that the findings could occur by chance. Therefore, we omitted the use of different P criteria in the same study as used by naïve investigators to underscore that one finding is more valid (read "important") than another because of the P value. When the first author of this book taught quantitative methods, his students would not have been allowed that gaffe.

In a few cases, we have omitted description of the PROCEDURE altogether because it is conventional and well known; thus, describing it adds nothing and it "slows the flow," as it were.

However, you will always find the following:

- AIM of the study—what the researcher intended to accomplish with the treatment(s); a description of
- PARTICIPANTS in the treatment plan, including age, gender, health status, and so on, even species;
- METHOD, that is, protocols used in carrying out the treatment, including diagnostic laboratory and other test procedures used to evaluate pretrial to posttreatment changes; and the researcher's
- RESULTS and CONCLUSION(S) about statistically significant findings.

Background information providing context for the studies is conventionally found in the INTRODUCTION in journal articles. It has often been omitted here as the book itself provides that.

The information omitted is usually science or statistics jargon intended to convince the editors of a given medical science journal to which a study is submitted for publication that the research methodology is valid and sound and that the data and conclusions are reliable and valid. Having passed their accepted-for-publication test, there is, in most cases, no further need for that sort of information.

We have changed "subjects" to "participants" in all clinical studies including "control participant." "Subjects" is a vestige of nineteenth-century animal-model studies, and in any case, *subjects* sounds more appetizing than *rats*, or some other laboratory fauna. But this book is about people; in fact, people who mostly suffer from Type 2 diabetes, and not "subjects." Also, we refer to "diabetes patients" rather than to "diabetic patients" to conceptually separate the person from the disease because they are *persons* who suffer from diabetes and its adverse effects. "Diabetic" is a focus on the disease, not the person.

While it may seem tedious at times, we often cite the journal or book source of the support for a given finding or allegation—a journal, usually. That is how we can justify "evidence-based" in the title of this book.

Unlike scientific journal articles that adhere to certain reference citation conventions, we insist that at least three authors be cited in the text proper, and that *all authors* be cited in the references section at the end of each chapter, and that the name of the journal cited be spelled out rather than abbreviated. Abbreviating the number of authors credited is arbitrary, and it cannot be justified on the basis of the additional cost of paper and ink. All authors matter not just the first three… "et al." is not an author and does not deserve credit. Abbreviating the name of a journal makes the references useless to the average reader and that is actually the last thing that we would wish for.

REFERENCE

R Fried. 1964. *Introduction to Statistics for the Behavioral Sciences.* New York: Oxford University Press.

Acknowledgments

We wish to express our sincere appreciation to Ms. Randy Brehm, senior editor, CRC Press/Taylor & Francis Group LLC, for her enthusiastic support of this book project and for her patience.

Thanks are due to Jacqueline Perle, PhD, Tel Aviv, Israel, who assumed responsibility for making sure that we had permission from the primary source to reproduce figures or tables, and quotes—a nerve-wracking and merciless undertaking.

Our sincere thanks are due also to Naras Bhat, MD, Concord, California, and Nathan S. Bryan, PhD, Baylor College of Medicine, Houston, Texas, for their welcome support of this project.

Authors

Robert Fried, PhD, is Emeritus Professor, Doctoral Faculty in Behavioral Neuroscience, City University of New York (CUNY) and Emeritus member, American Physiological Society (APS–Cardiovascular and Respiration Divisions) and FASEB.

Formerly director, Rehabilitation Research Institute (RRI), ICD—International Center for the Disabled, New York, New York.

Richard M. Carlton, MD, is an integrative physician who includes complementary and alternative approaches in the treatment of numerous medical problems, including migraines, inflammatory bowel disease, and diabetes.

Formerly principal staff physician, Rehabilitation Research Institute (RRI), ICD—International Center for the Disabled, New York, New York.

1 Chronic Hyperglycemia— A Primer

It's Life that Should be Sweet, not Blood.

Anon

1.1 CHRONIC HYPERGLYCEMIA VERSUS TYPE 2 DIABETES MELLITUS

Following routine blood testing, it is often revealed by one's physician that the elevation in blood sugar indicates Type 2 diabetes. The addition of results from a hemoglobin A1c test further confirms that the condition is likely now chronic. "Type 2 diabetes" is a medical diagnosis of a complex disease and elevated blood sugar, hyperglycemia, on the face of it, is really only one indication. There are many others that emerge as the disease progresses. This book will show what they are in the cardiovascular and related systems and, after some time, that many of them are irreversible, lowering serum glucose notwithstanding.

Many of the clinical studies cited in this book are, traditionally, about levels of serum glucose, the *dependent variable*. While that tradition remains unchallenged, it is important to remember that simply lowering serum glucose levels is not exactly the same thing as "curing" diabetes: the body "stores information" about the disease and it takes more than glycemic control to alter many of the other elements.

This book describes the adverse impact of chronic hyperglycemia, the *dependent variable* in clinical studies, on cardiovascular and related functions—leaving the "treatment" of diabetes to medicine—and adjuvant/integrative treatment modalities as the *independent variable* in later chapters.

1.2 TIME MAY NOT BE ON YOUR SIDE

The diagnosis of diabetes may be followed by the admonishment that the fault lies most likely in diet—that it is probably nutrient poor and sugar rich—and lack of adequate exercise. What's more, prescription meds are needed to avert disaster.

All of that is true, of course, but what is rarely mentioned that is urgent is that these factors are actually aggravating the natural age-related decline in the ability of the body to utilize sugar to fuel life processes. It is important to understand that this makes it much more difficult to control diabetes simply with diet changes and more exercise, and it unjustly blames the sufferer who often falters while implementing diet change and exercise strategies.

Processing sugar as fuel calls on the body to produce an adequate supply of insulin to process glucose (derived from dietary intake of sugar and starch). That supply of insulin may decrease with age, but even if supplies of it are normal, it may not function as well as it had in the past (in other words, resistance to insulin may develop).

In fact, investigators aiming to determine how we develop insulin resistance reported, in the journal *Science*, a study of healthy, lean, elderly, and young participants matched for lean body mass and fat mass. They found that elderly participants were markedly insulin-resistant compared to young, healthy (control), participants (Petersen, Befroy, Dufour et al. 2003).

The availability of sugar—glucose to be precise, there are other forms—is tightly controlled in the body, mainly by insulin produced by the pancreas. Once glucose enters the cells, there are two phases by which the body breaks it down to extract the chemical energy stored in the molecules. The first phase is called glycolysis (meaning the *lysis* or breakdown of glucose). It takes place under anaerobic conditions (meaning that oxygen is not utilized), and it generates lactic acid along with a relatively small amount of adenosine triphosphate (ATP), a molecule that stores the energy that has just been generated.

In the second phase of glucose breakdown, the lactic acid that had been formed through glycolysis is converted to pyruvate and, in a process called *respiration*, the energy stored in pyruvate is extracted to generate considerable amounts of ATP. Somewhat akin to a battery, the molecules of ATP can be used to drive many types of reactions in the body.

Other factors being equal, the pancreas ages as we are aging, blood sugar levels will naturally rise as we get older. However, if our metabolic need for fuel does not rise accordingly, glucose levels will be chronically elevated in circulating blood and that will cause considerable mischief to the cardiovascular system and the heart, as well as many other organs including the brain.

To make matters worse, even as blood sugar levels rise, clinical studies have shown that the elderly show significant reduction in glucose tolerance because of decreased insulin activity. However, the degree of glucose intolerance and insulin insensitivity of elderly people who do not have Type 2 diabetes is still significantly less than that of comparable elderly who have Type 2 diabetes (Refaie, Sayed-Ahmed, Bakr. 2006). Glucose intolerance is a prediabetic state of elevated blood sugar that may precede Type 2 diabetes by many years.

As we age, our blood level of sugar rises anyway as, by the same token, we become less responsive to insulin. So the question is how rapidly, that is, how soon could we develop Type 2 diabetes and all that this augurs?

Figure 1.1 shows the steady increase in the prevalence of diabetes in the maturing to aging population. Many factors are embedded in this trend: impaired fasting glucose (IFG) and impaired glucose tolerance (IGT) are also increasingly prevalent with older age and some estimate that over the age of 80 years, the chance of having a fully normal glucose metabolism is about 30% (which intriguingly suggests that disordered glucose metabolism may be part of a normal aging process rather than a "disease," *per se*).

Type 2 diabetes is strongly associated with obesity, and as such, the major burden is now in the middle-income and developing countries where urbanization and recent affluence have rapidly changed lifestyles favoring "unhealthy food choices."

Figure 1.1 shows that the prevalence of diabetes is approximately the same in men and in women, but there are some indications that at the same level of obesity, men have a higher risk due to a more visceral adipose tissue distribution.

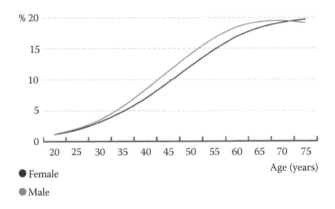

FIGURE 1.1 Prevalence of diabetes by age, as shown in the International Diabetes Federation (IDF) Diabetes Atlas 2013. [From Nijpels G. 2016. Epidemiology of type 2 diabetes [Internet]. Nov 23; *Diapedia*, 3104287123 rev. no. 18. With permission.]

Two out of every three diabetes patients live in urbanized areas, and those in the lower socio-economic classes are disproportionately affected. The reasons for this are still poorly understood, but unhealthier lifestyles may be an important mediating factor. Globally, it is the lower- to middle-income countries that contribute most to the prevalence of the disease, possible because these are the countries where recent urbanization and economic growth have most drastically changed life-style and longevity.

Physical activity has beneficial effects on glucose metabolism, and it can lower the risk of becoming obese. However, at the population level, sedentary behavior (i.e., the total lack of any physical activity) is probably more important as a risk factor than the lack of high-intensity physical activity. Particularly in children, clear associations are found between sedentary behaviors, such as TV viewing, and the risks of becoming obese.

Over the years, several dietary factors have been implicated as risk factors for diabetes. It is not surprising that, given the strong relationship between obesity and diabetes, some of the best evidence for prevention of diabetes comes from studies where dietary intervention (mainly caloric restriction) was coupled to increased physical activity. Apart from total caloric intake, certain dietary factors have been associated with the risk of diabetes. Of late, particularly sugar-sweetened beverages are thought to increase diabetes risk. Other factors, such as coffee and fiber intake, are associated with lower risks of getting diabetes. However, dietary studies are notoriously difficult to perform and prone to bias because people with healthy diets tend to exhibit other healthy behaviors as well (Whiting. 2011; Guariguata. 2013).

1.3 CHRONIC HYPERGLYCEMIA SERIOUSLY HARMS THE BODY

Three major metabolic defects contribute to hyperglycemia, leading to Type 2 diabetes: increased hepatic glucose production, impaired pancreatic insulin secretion, and peripheral tissue insulin resistance.

After eating a meal or ingesting glucose, insulin is secreted, hepatic glucose output is suppressed, and insulin-dependent glucose uptake by peripheral tissues is stimulated. In Type 2 diabetes, insulin resistance and impaired insulin secretion inhibit normal suppression of hepatic glucose output. As a consequence, the liver continues to release glucose into the circulation. Moreover, peripheral insulin resistance coupled with insufficient insulin results in decreased uptake of glucose by insulin-dependent target tissues, notably skeletal muscle and adipose tissue. These mechanisms contribute to postprandial (after meal) hyperglycemia in Type 2 diabetes.

In Type 2 diabetes, increased hepatic glucose production is the primary factor responsible for the fasting hyperglycemia. Moreover, in patients with Type 2 diabetes, fasting blood glucose levels correlate strongly with rates of hepatic glucose output. In the setting of peripheral insulin resistance, insulin-mediated glucose uptake cannot accommodate the increased hepatic glucose output and rise in fasting glucose levels (Kruszynska, and Olefsky. 1996; Henry. 1996).

The American Diabetes Association reports that of the approximately 30 million adults and children in the United States who have diabetes, nearly 95% have Type 2 diabetes (http://www.diabetes.org/diabetes-basics/statistics/infographics.html). This is a problem of epic proportions because Type 2 diabetes is a major cardiovascular and heart disease risk. It is a killer and, in fact, the incidence of death is directly proportional to the severity of the disease: HbA1C between 6% and 7.9% confers roughly double the incidence of cardiovascular mortality compared to HbA1C levels below 6% (Gerich. 2017).

A clinical study published in the journal *Diabetes* aimed to determine whether Type 2 diabetes predicts coronary heart disease in the elderly. The investigators reported that Type 2 diabetes and its medical control, and the duration of diabetes, are important predictors of cardiovascular and heart disease and mortality in the elderly particularly in women (Kuusisto, Mykkänen, Pyörälä et al. 1994). Thus, this was already common knowledge more than 20 years ago.

We cannot know exactly how many Americans die from this disease and its complications, but in 2010, for instance, diabetes was the seventh leading cause of death in the United States based on the death certificates where diabetes was listed as the underlying cause of death. In 2010 also, diabetes was mentioned as a cause of death in a total of more than 230,000 certificates. However, only about 35% to 40% of those with diabetes who died had diabetes listed anywhere on the death certificate, and about 10% to 15% had it listed as the underlying cause of death.

From 2003 to 2006, after adjusting for population age differences, rate of death from all causes was about 1.5 times higher among adults 18 years or older with diagnosed diabetes, than among adults without this diagnosis. Of course, we cannot discount hypertension, chronic elevated serum low-density lipoprotein (LDL) cholesterol, obesity, metabolic syndrome, sedentary lifestyle, smoking and alcohol abuse, air pollution, and, last but not least, heredity as possible contributors.

Nevertheless, despite constant warnings from health authorities concerning the increase in overweight, obesity, and Type 2 diabetes, the American public is in the throes of an epidemic with serious health and wealth consequences of ignoring those warnings.

In dollar terms, the American Diabetes Association tells us in a report dated March 6, 2013, that, in 2012, the estimated total cost of diagnosed diabetes has risen to $245 billion (http://www.diabetes .org/advocacy/news-events/cost-of-diabetes.html).

1.4   THE MORE SUGAR IN YOUR BLOOD, THE SHORTER YOUR LIFE

Figure 1.2 shows how blood sugar inevitably rises with age, and it also underscores how life span is affected by blood sugar levels. Notice how the subgroups that live longer have lower blood sugar—at the same age as their shorter-lived peers.

In men who live at least 70 years, death can be predicted more reliably from blood sugar level than from chronological age (Yashin, Ukraintseva, Arbeev et al. 2009).

The Yashin group, from the Duke University Center for Population Health and Aging, derived their data from the Framingham Heart Study (FHS) begun in the late 1940s, based on 5209 healthy participants. Roughly half were men and half were women between the ages of 28 and 62. The notation "LS" in the figures stands for life span.

Blood glucose levels rise with age in men and in women, albeit even for long-lived individuals. In women with the shortest life span, glucose levels are lower at the end of their life than it is in men with the same life span. Yet, women with the longest life span have higher glucose levels than men with the longest life span. However, in that life span range, women's glucose levels rose more slowly as they aged than it did in men in the same LS range. This could be an important lifesaving factor.

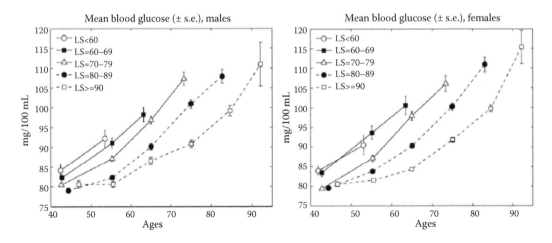

FIGURE 1.2   Four longevity ranges in men and in women compared to mean serum glucose levels-by-age. [Based on data in Yashin, Ukraintseva, Arbeev et al. 2009. With permission.]

The main difference in the blood glucose levels-by-age pattern is that it shows that in the long-lived people, blood glucose increases slowly with age up to 55 years of age, when it starts rising more rapidly. That, parenthetically, is reflected in the normal, nondiabetes, age-related rise in blood sugar.

1.4.1 THE LESSON

If we look only at serum blood sugar, the less of it, the longer one will likely live, the longer it takes for the level to rise as we age, the longer the life span.

Even in the face of the evidence that Type 2 diabetes may be more deadly, it would not be wise to overlook medical treatment for chronically elevated serum LDL cholesterol—hyperlipidemia. Here is why:

Figure 1.3a is based on data from the same FHS cohort, and it shows that serum cholesterol seems to paradoxically decline with age in both men and women, and so does diastolic blood pressure decline (Figure 1.3b).

1.4.2 SURVIVOR BIAS

Both Figure 1.3a and b show decline with age. What is missing from this picture is information needed to determine *survivor bias*. Survivor bias is the logical error of concentrating on the people who "survived" and inadvertently overlooking those who did not—they are not visible. This can lead to false conclusions in several different ways.

We cannot tell from the presentation of the graphed data whether the data points in the graph represent an equal number of observations. There could be 2000 observations at age 50, and 3 at age 90, and that would tell us only that the 3 individuals with the lowest cholesterol survived longest. This would apply to diastolic blood pressure as well: Those with the lowest blood pressure live longer, not that blood pressure declines with age.

Therefore, we cannot assume that cholesterol and blood pressure decline as we age whereas serum cholesterol rises. Such a conclusion would suggest that rising serum glucose lowers cholesterol and blood pressure. This is clearly an "alternate fact." Thus, what actually happens to serum cholesterol and to blood pressure as we age?

It was reported in the *International Journal of Epidemiology* that the level of serum cholesterol is known to rise with age. In that study, the authors investigated men and women whose serum cholesterol, habitual food intake, and body mass index (BMI) were measured between 1974 and 1979, and again in 1985. Serum cholesterol had increased by 14% in men and by 7% in women.

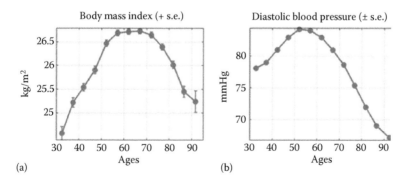

FIGURE 1.3 (a) Pattern of serum cholesterol by age. (b) Pattern of diastolic blood pressure by age. [With permission from Yashin, Arbeev, Wu et al. 2013 (http://journal.frontiersin.org/article/10.3389/fgene.2013.00003/full).] No changes were made to the figures.

In men, change in BMI partly explained the change in serum cholesterol, and in women, nothing could explain changes in serum cholesterol (Berns, de Vries, and Katan. 1988).

A report in the *Postgraduate Medical Journal* tells us that blood pressure rises with age, and this change is associated with structural changes in the arteries and especially with large artery stiffness (compliance) (Pinto. 2007). Hypertension and arterial stiffness are closely associated with age (Greenwald. 2007; Payne, Wilkinson, and Webb. 2010). In fact, the journal *Hypertension* explicitly links deteriorating glucose tolerance to increased arterial stiffness in connection with Type 2 diabetes, and increased cardiovascular and heart risk (Schram, Henry, van Dijk. 2004).

1.5   THE SUGAR IN BLOOD: BLOOD GLUCOSE

"Blood sugar" is a term in common usage, but it is misleading because what is meant is "glucose" and there are other sugars besides glucose that are always present in blood. The amount of glucose in the blood is known as the "blood glucose level."

Glucose is a simple sugar molecule that initiates metabolism and can be converted easily for energy. It is produced by digestion of carbohydrates or from protein or fat. Because it is a single molecule and doesn't need to be broken down like more complex sugars, it easily and quickly enters the bloodstream to be used for energy. The main function of sugar in its simplest form is to supply a ready source of energy to power cell functions.

The body does not store glucose, so it converts it to glycogen to be stored either in the liver or in muscle tissue. When the body has a sudden need for glucose, glycogen stored in the liver can be rapidly converted back to glucose for fuel.

There are many common sugars in our diet. The sugar in fruit is fructose. Lactose is the sugar found in cow milk. Table sugar is sucrose, a type of sugar called a disaccharide, which means it is composed of two simpler sugars, fructose and glucose, that can be refined from either sugarcane or beet sugar. There are industrial sweeteners such as high-fructose corn syrup also called glucose–fructose; isoglucose and glucose–fructose syrup made from corn starch, and food additives including sorbitol and maltose, but these are not subject to control by insulin.

We have unquestionably developed a very strong fondness for sugar, and we are drawn to its taste. Perhaps to our Paleolithic ancestors, the taste of sugar signaled something desirable. In fact, naturally occurring sugar is typically nutritious and contains fiber as it occurs in sugarcane, beets, fruit, and certain sweet vegetables.

Glucose is typically the main source of fuel that supplies the energy of cells, while blood lipids such as fats and oils are the main way we store energy. The bloodstream transports glucose from the intestines, or the liver, to body cells where it is absorbed with the help of insulin. The diet is one source of circulating glucose, and it also provides carbon and energy sources for liver gluconeogenesis, the way that the liver generates glucose from non-carbohydrate substances including lactate, glycerol, and certain amino acids.

The liver is the major glucose metabolic regulatory organ. About 90% of all circulating glucose not derived directly from the diet comes from the liver. The liver contains significant amounts of stored glycogen available for rapid release into circulation. In addition to controlling plasma glucose, the liver is responsible for synthesis and release of the lipoproteins that adipose and other tissues use as the source of cholesterol. Adipose tissue is connective tissue that can store energy in the form of fat.

1.6   DIURNAL CYCLE OF BLOOD GLUCOSE

"Tell me what you eat, and I will tell you what you are" is a phrase attributed to Jean Anthelme Brillat-Savarin (1755–1826), a French lawyer and politician who gained fame as an epicure and gastronome. It is often rudely paraphrased "You are what you eat." But Halberg, Haus, Cornelissen et al. (1955) put it this way: "You are when you eat." Could well be: Glucose level is typically lowest in the morning, before the first meal of the day—the fasting level—and it rises after meals for an hour or two.

As reported in the *British Medical Journal*, oral glucose tolerance tests (OGTTs) were performed in the morning and afternoon of separate days on 31 people with normal blood glucose levels. It was found that blood sugar levels were higher in the afternoon, 60 min after the glucose "load." The degree of diurnal variation was similar in men and in women, but greater in the older half of the group.

Glucose tolerance was inversely related to obesity. The plasma insulin response was lower in the afternoon, but significantly greater than the morning values at 120 and 150 min after the glucose load (Zimmet, Wall, Rome et al. 1974).

1.6.1 CAVEAT

Researchers from the National Institute of Diabetes and Digestive and Kidney Diseases, in Bethesda, Maryland, reporting in the *Journal of the American Medical Association*, tell us that current diagnostic criteria for diabetes indicate diabetes based on plasma glucose levels in blood samples with a value of 126 mg/dL or more, obtained from patients in the morning after an overnight fast. However, many patients are seen by their physicians in the afternoon. Because plasma glucose levels are higher in the morning, it is unclear whether these diagnostic criteria can be applied to patients tested for diabetes in the afternoon.

The researchers therefore undertook to document diurnal variation in fasting plasma glucose levels in adults not known to have diabetes and to examine the applicability of the findings to afternoon-examined patients. The data were obtained from the US population–based Third National Health and Nutrition Examination Survey (1988–1994) on participants aged 20 years or older, who had no previously diagnosed diabetes, who were randomly assigned to morning or afternoon examinations, and who fasted before blood sampling.

The morning and afternoon groups did not differ in age, BMI, waist-to-hip ratio, physical activity index, HbA1C level, and other factors. Average fasting plasma glucose levels were higher in the "morning" group (97.4 mg/dL) than in the "afternoon" group (92.4 mg/dL).

The prevalence of participants with fasting plasma glucose levels of 126 mg/dL or greater examined in the morning was twice that of participants examined in the afternoon. The diagnostic fasting plasma glucose value for participants examined in the afternoon that resulted in the same prevalence of diabetes found in morning-examined participants was 114 mg/dL or more.

The rather startling conclusion drawn from this study was that if current diabetes diagnostic criteria are applied to patients seen in the afternoon, approximately half of all cases of undiagnosed diabetes in these patients would be missed (Troisi, Cowie, and Harris. 2000).

1.7 METABOLISM: FUELING THE MACHINERY OF LIFE

Glucose is the basic fuel that energizes metabolism, the sum of all the chemical reactions that take place in our body cells that are required to sustain life. These reactions transform and convert food into a fuel form, providing the energy that powers cellular processes.

The transformation consists largely of the conversion of food by digestion to building blocks for proteins, lipids, nucleic acids, and some carbohydrates, and the elimination of nitrogen wastes. As previously noted, in the first phase of glucose metabolism, the glucose is broken down anaerobically by glycolysis to form lactate, along with a small amount of ATP. In the more efficient second phase, respiration, lactate is converted to pyruvate, which is then broken down to generate large amounts of ATP.

There are two types of metabolism: *Catabolism* is the "breaking down" of organic matter by cellular respiration. *Anabolism* is the "building up" of components of cells such as proteins and nucleic acids. Whereas "breaking down" releases energy, "building up" consumes energy.

Energy is required for the normal functioning of the organs in the body. Many tissues can also metabolize fat, or protein, as an energy source, but others, such as the brain and red blood cells, can only utilize glucose.

The chemical reactions of metabolism are organized (conceptually) into metabolic *pathways*, where transformation is facilitated by enzymes. Enzymes act as catalysts that allow the reactions to proceed more rapidly. Enzymes also allow the regulation of metabolic pathways in response to changes in the environment of cells or to signals from other cells.

Two different pathways are involved in the metabolism of glucose: one anaerobic and one aerobic. The anaerobic process occurs in the cytoplasm and is only moderately efficient. The aerobic cycle takes place in the mitochondria and results in the greatest release of energy. As the name implies, though, it requires oxygen.

Glucose is the body's main fuel. Without glucose, or without being able to convert it into energy rapidly and efficiently, we could not survive in good health. Hence, it's very important that our energy-metabolism system works efficiently. Here is a very simple explanation of how we convert glucose into energy:

Following a meal, the pancreas releases insulin, which takes up the glucose and transports it into cells that need extra energy. The glucose enters the cell via "glucose transporter" molecules. The cells that need glucose have specific insulin receptors on their surface so that insulin can bind to them, facilitating glucose entry and utilization in the cells.

The cell metabolizes glucose, thereby producing ATP, a molecule that stores and releases energy as required by the cell, and heat as a by-product.

The metabolism of glucose into energy may occur either in combination with oxygen (aerobic metabolism) or without it (anaerobic metabolism). The mitochondria—small cells within the cells—use oxygen to burn glucose. However, red blood cells do not have mitochondria, so they change glucose into energy without the use of oxygen.

Glucose is also converted to energy in muscle cells—which are probably the most important energy "customers." Muscle cells contain mitochondria, so they can process glucose with oxygen. But even if the oxygen level in muscle cell mitochondria falls too low, the cells can derive energy from glucose without oxygen.

1.8   THE PANCREAS PRODUCES THE HORMONE INSULIN

The pancreas is an endocrine (hormone producing) glandular organ about 6 inches long. The "head" of the pancreas is on the right side of the abdomen and is connected to the duodenum, the first section of the small intestine, through the pancreatic duct. The narrow end of the pancreas, called the "tail," extends to the left side of the body.

The pancreas secretes hormones, including insulin, glucagon, and others, into circulating blood. The pancreas is also a digestive organ secreting a juice containing digestive enzymes and buffers that assist digestion and the absorption of nutrients in the small intestine. The pancreatic enzymes help to further break down the carbohydrates, proteins, and lipids in the chyme, the semi-fluid mass of partly digested food that is expelled by the stomach into the duodenum, the beginning of the small intestine.

1.9   THE LIVER

The liver is the main site of action of the pancreatic hormones. Because blood flow from the pancreas proceeds directly to the liver, and because the liver is the major site of inactivation of most peptide hormones, the liver is exposed to higher levels of pancreatic hormones than any other tissue.

In the liver, insulin stimulates glycogen synthesis and inhibits glycogen breakdown. It also stimulates glycolysis and inhibits gluconeogenesis. In addition to its effects on glucose metabolism, insulin has a variety of anabolic actions in the liver, stimulating lipid synthesis and release and protein synthesis, and inhibiting the breakdown of these compounds.

The liver has some ability to respond directly to high levels of plasma glucose by increasing glucose uptake and glycogen synthesis in an insulin-independent manner. However, the majority of liver glucose regulatory functions require insulin action.

The liver has about 300,000 insulin receptors per cell (a very large number), but experiences maximal response to insulin when a small fraction of the receptors are occupied; this allows the organ to respond to insulin even when the plasma insulin concentration is less than the K_d for the receptor (K_d is the drug concentration at which half of the receptors are bound).

The rate of storage and release of carbohydrate by the liver is regulated by the plasma concentrations of glucose, and of the hormones insulin and glucagon.

"Simulation" studies reported in the journal *Federation Proceedings* have led to the conclusion that glucose exerts a rapid moment-to-moment influence on the rate of uptake of glucose by the liver. Insulin, however, by exerting a lesser influence on the sensitivity of the liver to glucose, is very effective in "optimizing" the amount of glycogen that the liver stores during food intake (Bergman. 1977).

The liver is exposed to higher nutrient levels than are other body tissues because it has first access to most ingested nutrients since they are absorbed into the hepatic portal vein. It can store and release glucose to minimize changes in glycemia between the fed and fasting states.

In the normal individual, the intake of a mixed meal results in modest hyperglycemia, accompanied by substantial storage of glycogen (see below) in the liver. After the meal (postprandial), there are carefully adjusted changes in hormone secretion as well as changes in nonglucose substrates, which combine to direct the partitioning of the glucose load among the various tissues.

In persons with poorly controlled Type 2 diabetes, however, there is significant postprandial hyperglycemia and impaired hepatic glycogen accumulation (Krssak, Brehm, Bernroider et al. 2004). It is estimated that the human liver disposes of approximately 25% to 35% of an oral glucose load (Ferrannini, Bjorkman, Reichard et al. 1985; Mari, Wahren, DeFronzo et al. 1994).

After a moderately sized oral glucose load, the liver extracts approximately one-third of the glucose; together, the muscles and fat take up approximately one-third; and the committed noninsulin-sensitive glucose–using tissues dispose of the remaining one-third. Thus, the liver takes up glucose and also curtails its release of glucose postprandially.

Thus, these proportions underestimate the role of the liver in glycemic control because the glucose consumed by the committed glucose-requiring tissues has to be derived from the absorbed glucose, as a result of the end of hepatic glucose production. Consequently, the liver is actually responsible for the disposal of the equivalent of approximately 60% to 65% of an oral glucose load. Any impairment in its function, therefore, can lead to excessive postprandial glycemia. For a detailed description of liver function, see Moore, Coate, Winnick et al. (2012).

1.10 DIABETIC KETOACIDOSIS

Ketone bodies are three water-soluble molecules, acetoacetate (AcAc), beta-hydroxybutyrate, and their spontaneous breakdown product, acetone, produced by the liver from fatty acids during periods of low food intake including fasting, carbohydrate restrictive diets, starvation, prolonged intense exercise, or in untreated or poorly treated Type 1 diabetes. These ketone bodies are readily picked up by the tissues and converted into a form that is then oxidized for energy in the mitochondria.

Thus, ketone bodies are always present in the blood but their levels rise during fasting and prolonged exercise. Diabetes is the most common cause of elevated blood ketones. In diabetic ketoacidosis (DKA), high levels of ketones are produced in response to low insulin levels and high levels of counter-regulatory hormones. In acute DKA, the ketone body concentration can sometimes rise 10-fold.

In response to insulin therapy, levels of 3HB (3-beta-hydroxybutyrate—one of the ketone types produced) commonly decrease long before levels of AcAc—one of the other of the three types of ketone produced. The frequently employed nitroprusside test only detects AcAc in blood and urine. This test is inconvenient, does not assess the best indicator of ketone body levels (3HB), provides only a semiquantitative assessment of ketone levels, and is associated with false-positive results.

Inexpensive quantitative tests of 3HB levels have recently become available for use with small blood samples (5–25 μmoL). These tests offer new options for monitoring and treating diabetes and other states characterized by the abnormal metabolism of ketone bodies (Laffel. 1999).

1.11 INSULIN

Insulin is a hormone produced by the *beta*-cells (β-cells) of the pancreatic islets (of Langerhans). It regulates the metabolism of carbohydrates, fats, and protein by promoting the absorption of glucose from the blood. In the liver and skeletal muscles, it is converted to glycogen, a form for energy storage. Glucose production and excretion into the blood by the liver is reduced by high concentrations of insulin in the blood (Sonksen, and Sonksen. 2000).

To understand how insulin works in the body, it may help to know what hormones are, where in the body they are made, and what they do.

A hormone is any one of a class of signaling molecules produced by glands in our body and transported by the circulatory system to distant organs, where they regulate the activity of the target organs. "Signaling molecule" is a generic term applied to any substance that communicates information from cells A, in order to instigate a biological activity or process in cells or organ B.

There are many different hormones with diverse chemical structures in human physiology. They regulate physiological and behavioral activities including digestion, metabolism, respiration, tissue function, sensory perception, sleep, excretion, lactation, stress, growth and development, movement, reproduction, and mood and sexuality (https://medline plus.gov/hormones.html).

Hormones bind to specific receptor proteins in the target cell(s) by the activation of a signal transduction pathway causing change in cell function. The first of these is called gene transcription, the increased gene direction of some given target cell outcome. For instance, serum glucose concentration affects insulin production. The control of enzyme levels in cells is a result of regulation of transcription (replication) of DNA sequences. All proteins are produced in some way from DNA genetic code, and this step forms a key control point.

A "signal transduction pathway" means a set of chemical reactions in a cell that occurs when a molecule, such as a hormone, attaches to a receptor on the cell membrane. The pathway is not a "pathway," per se, but a metaphor for a cascade of biochemical events inside the cell that eventually result in a reaction in the target cell.

1.11.1 INCRETINS

Incretins are hormones that stimulate insulin secretion in response to meals. The two most important incretin hormones are glucagon-like peptide-1 (GLP-1), and glucose-dependent insulinotropic polypeptide (GIP). The incretin hormones are released during meals from gut endocrine cells. They potentiate glucose-induced insulin secretion and may be responsible for up to 70% of postprandial insulin secretion.

The incretin hormones may also promote proliferation/neogenesis of β-cells and prevent their decay (apoptosis). Both hormones contribute to insulin secretion from the beginning of a meal and their effects increased progressively as plasma glucose concentrations rise.

The effect of incretins is diminished, even absent, in patients with Type 2 diabetes. In addition, there is hyperglucagonemia, which is not suppressible by glucose.

It is reported that in such patients, the secretion of GIP is near normal, but its effect on insulin secretion, particularly the late phase, is severely impaired. The loss of GIP action is probably a consequence of diabetes, since it is also observed in patients with diabetes secondary to chronic pancreatitis, in whom the incretin effect is also lost. GLP-1 secretion, on the other hand, is also impaired, but its insulinotropic and glucagon-suppressive actions are preserved, although the potency of glucose-dependent insulinotropic polypeptide (GLP) is decreased compared to levels in healthy people.

The impaired action of GLP-1 and GIP in Type 2 diabetes may be at least partly restored by improved glycemic control, as shown in studies involving 4 weeks of intensive insulin therapy (Holst, Vilsbøll, and Deacon. 2009). The reduced incretin effect is believed to contribute to impaired regulation of insulin and glucagon secretion in Type 2 diabetes, and exogenous GLP-1 administration may restore blood glucose regulation to near-normal levels. Thus, the pathogenesis of Type 2 diabetes seems to involve a dysfunction of both incretins.

1.12 THE ISLET OF LANGERHANS

One important regulator of pancreatic hormone release is the paracrine signaling that occurs within the islets of Langerhans in the pancreas. Insulin inhibits its own release, and also inhibits the release of glucagon (see below). Glucagon inhibits its own release, and stimulates insulin release. Somatostatin (see below) inhibits the release of both insulin and glucagon. The local changes in hormone levels act as a primary negative feedback mechanism to prevent excessive changes in pancreatic hormone levels.

This feedback mechanism is illustrated by the effects of untreated Type 1 diabetes, where the loss of insulin inhibition of glucagon secretion results in overproduction of glucagon—the high levels of glucagon in the absence of insulin action throughout the body result in the severe metabolic changes of DKA.

1.12.1 β-CELLS SECRETE INSULIN

β-Cells in the islets of Langerhans primarily store and release insulin. When glucose levels in the blood are high, the pancreatic β-cells secrete insulin into the blood, and when glucose levels in the blood are low, there is less secretion of insulin (Koeslag, Saunders, and Terblanche. 2003). β-Cells can respond quickly to spikes in blood glucose concentrations by secreting some of their stored insulin while simultaneously producing more. But prolonged elevation of glucose may exhaust the β-cell stores of insulin and exceed their ability to synthesize more, resulting in hyperglycemia.

1.12.2 DIABETES AND β-CELL DYSFUNCTION

Some investigators point specifically to β-cell mitochondria dysfunction as a causal factor in Type 2 diabetes (Ma, Zhao, and Turk. 2012). Mitochondria are the power generators of the cell, converting oxygen and nutrients into ATP. ATP is the chemical energy "currency" of the cell that powers the metabolic activities of cells.

Investigators reported pancreatic tissue studies from autopsies of obese individuals (BMI greater than 27 kg/m^2) in the journal *Diabetes*; some with Type 2 diabetes, some with IFG; some non-diabetic, and lean cases (BMI less than 25 kg/m^2); some Type 2 diabetic, and some nondiabetic participants.

They found that the frequency of β-cell self-destruction (apoptosis) was increased 10-fold in lean and 3-fold in obese cases of Type 2 diabetes, compared with their respective nondiabetic control group, and they concluded that β-cell mass is decreased in Type 2 diabetes, and that the mechanism underlying this is increased β-cell apoptosis.

The investigators concluded that since the major defect leading to a decrease in β-cell mass in Type 2 diabetes is increased apoptosis, while new islet formation and β-cell replication are normal, therapeutic approaches designed to arrest apoptosis could be a significant new development in the management of Type 2 diabetes, because this approach might actually reverse the disease to a degree, rather than just palliate glycemia (Butler, Janson, Bonner-Weir et al. 2003).

1.12.3 Diabetes and Mitochondrial β-Cell Dysfunction—Mitochondrial Diabetes

Researchers from the Department of Molecular Cell Biology, Leiden University Medical Centre, Leiden, the Netherlands, report mitochondrial (mtDNA) mutations strongly associated with diabetes, the most common being the A3243G mutation in the mitochondrial DNA-encoded tRNA(Leu,UUR) gene: The main feature of this form is a gradual development of pancreatic β-cell dysfunction with aging, rather than insulin resistance (Maassen, 'T Hart, Van Essen et al. 2004).

1.12.4 α-Cells Secrete Glucagon

α-cells (alpha-cells) are likewise endocrine cells in the pancreatic islets of Langerhans. They produce and secrete the hormone glucagon that elevates the glucose levels in the blood. Glucagon has the opposite effect of insulin by stimulating the liver to release glucose.

The secretion of insulin and glucagon into the blood in response to the blood glucose level is the primary mechanism responsible for keeping the glucose levels in the extracellular fluids within very narrow limits at rest, after meals, and during exercise and starvation.

The pancreas releases glucagon when the concentration of glucose in the bloodstream falls too low, by causing the liver to convert stored glycogen into glucose, which is then released into the bloodstream. Thus, glucagon and insulin are part of a feedback system that keeps blood glucose levels stable.

Release of glucagon from the α-cells is stimulated by low plasma glucose and by catecholamines and glucocorticoids. Release of glucagon is inhibited by insulin and somatostatin. Release of glucagon is also inhibited by glucose; it is not known whether this is a direct effect of glucose on the α-cells, or an indirect consequence of elevated insulin levels.

Because glucagon has actions opposite to those of insulin, it therefore functions to maintain plasma glucose levels between meals. However, unlike insulin, glucagon action is probably mostly in the liver, with limited effects in other tissues. It stimulates liver amino acid uptake, gluconeogenesis, and glucose release, and inhibits glycolysis and fatty acid synthesis.

The glucagon receptor is coupled to adenylyl cyclase, and glucagon actions are mediated by elevation in cAMP levels. In general, actions of glucagon are mediated by increased phosphorylation of existing enzymes. Prolonged stimulation by glucagon may have some effects on gene transcription, usually in the opposite direction from that of insulin. If the insulin:glucagon ratio is low for a prolonged period (i.e., several days), an alteration in liver enzyme levels occurs, which causes increased production of ketone bodies.

1.12.5 δ-Cells Secrete Somatostatin

Somatostatin is a hormone that inhibits the secretion of growth hormone by the pituitary gland. It is released from the δ-cells (delta-cells) under control of the same stimuli that result in insulin release and that act primarily as a regulator of insulin release, preventing insulin levels from rising too rapidly. It may also have an endocrine role as an inhibitor of nutrient absorption in the gut.

1.13 INSULIN AND GLUCAGON: THE YIN AND YANG OF IT

We know that serum glucose is controlled in the body principally by the pancreas, releasing certain hormones that control its concentration in blood. Principal among these is insulin and glucagon. These work in a sort of reciprocal, yin/yang, fashion. As one rises, it inhibits the release of the other, and vice versa: Simply put, glucagon promotes serum glucose, whereas insulin inhibits it. What happens to these two as we age?

First, our pancreas produces less insulin as we age: The journal *Seminars in Nephrology* reported the following (*we paraphrase*):

As we age, we experience increased incidence of hypertension, Type 2 diabetes, and coronary heart disease. These conditions tend to cluster in the same individuals, and therefore, it has been thought that they have a common basis: Many authorities have proposed a causal link between glucose intolerance, high plasma triglyceride and low high-density lipoprotein (HDL) levels (dyslipidemia), higher systolic and diastolic blood pressures, and insulin resistance syndrome (metabolic syndrome).

The elderly are more glucose intolerant and insulin resistant. However, it is not known whether this dysfunction is an inevitable consequence of "biological aging," or the result of environmental or lifestyle variables such as obesity, or physical inactivity common in the aging. All of these modifiable factors have been shown to cause increased insulin resistance, and they are risk factors for development of metabolic syndrome.

Insulin secretion, on the other hand, declines with age even after adjustments for differences in adiposity, fat distribution, and physical activity. This may be responsible for the glucose intolerance in the aging even after improvements have been made in their lifestyle factors (Muller, Elahi, Tobin et al. 1996).

1.13.1 THE DISPOSITION INDEX

Given that insulin secretion decreases with age, what happens to insulin sensitivity now becomes of prime importance: Type 2 diabetes results from both decreased secretion and decreased sensitivity to insulin. The ratio of insulin secretion to insulin resistance is termed the *disposition index*.

Insulin response is estimated as the change in insulin divided by the change in glucose from 0 to 30 min: It is a measure of the sensitivity to glucose of the β-cells in the pancreas (Lorenzo, Wagenknecht, Rewers et al. 2010). The relation between β-cell responsivity and insulin sensitivity is assumed to be constant (Cobelli, Toffolo, Man et al. 2007). In fact, oral disposition index (DI_O) predicts the development of diabetes in the future more reliably than fasting and 2-h glucose levels (Utzschneider, Prigeon, Faulenbach et al. 2009).

Oral glucose insulin sensitivity (OGIS) is a method for the assessment of insulin sensitivity from the OGTT. The OGIS provides an index that correlates with the index of insulin sensitivity obtained from the hyperinsulinemic–euglycemic clamp (described in Chapter 9).

In a normal individual, impaired insulin sensitivity increases pancreatic β-cell responsivity, whereas in someone with impaired tolerance, this does not occur.

The *American Journal of Physiology—Endocrinology and Metabolism* reported on the insulin sensitivity response in IGT—as in Type 2 Diabetes—and normal glucose tolerance: In normal circumstances, when insulin sensitivity decreases, insulin secretion increases to maintain normal blood glucose, but when insulin secretion fails to compensate, we develop abnormal tolerance to blood sugar.

This tells us that in Type 2 diabetes, insulin secretion cannot keep up with declining insulin sensitivity (Cobelli, Toffolo, Man et al. 2007), and it gives us a pretty good idea that we can expect IGT as we age, since insulin sensitivity declines with age, but does this mean that we can expect glucagon to increase as insulin decreases—as it did when we were younger?

Actually, there is a disconnect: A report in the journal *Diabetologia* informs us that glucagon suppression by both elevated blood sugar and elevated serum insulin is not different in young and older people; the metabolic clearance rate of glucagon is similar in young and older individuals or participants, but liver sensitivity to increments in plasma glucagon is increased in older people (Gosmanov, Adair Gosmanov, Gerich 2011; Simonson, and DeFronzo. 1983; Alford, Bloom, and Nabarro. 1976).

1.14   DIABETES: "THE WASTING AND THIRST DISEASE" (消渴)

The term "diabetes" is the shortened version of the full name of the disease, diabetes mellitus (DM). The term "diabetes" is said to be derived from the Greek word *diabainein* meaning siphon, or "to pass through," attributed to the Greek physician, Aretus of Cappadocia (central Turkey), in the first century BCE.

Diabetes has long been known to affect our lives: Ancient Egyptian manuscripts dating to 1550 BCE also cited an ailment that today we suspect to be diabetes. In India—circa 600 BCE—a test for the condition that they called "sweet urine disease" consisted of determining whether ants were attracted to a person's urine. In earlier times, a diagnosis of diabetes was likely a death sentence.

So far as can be determined, the term "pancreas" first appears in the works of Rufus of Ephesus, a first-century Greek doctor, who was probably the first to use this term to refer to this organ. However, no function was attributed to the pancreas, and he believed that the pancreas was only an extension of the digestive system.

In 1674, the English physician Thomas Willis (1621–1675) was the first in modern medical literature to observe sugar in urine, stating that the urine he tasted was *wonderfully sweet as if it were imbued with honey or sugar.* His taste test led him to add the term "mellitus" (from the Latin word for honey) to this form of diabetes. In pre-Elizabethan English, "wonderful" was akin to "surprising" rather than "enjoyable."

History Footnote 1: Oskar Minkowski

Together with Josef von Mering, Oskar Minkowski studied diabetes at the University of Strasbourg. In 1889, they surgically removed the pancreas of dogs and discovered serendipitously that they had induced the body wasting process of diabetes. It was Minkowski who performed the operation and made the crucial link to recognize that the symptoms of the treated dogs were due to diabetes. Thus, they were able to conclude that the pancreas contained regulators of blood sugar.

The disease, diabetes mellitus, results from a failure of the body to produce or to respond properly to the hormone insulin, thus resulting in abnormal metabolism of carbohydrates, and elevated levels of glucose in the blood and in urine.

Type 1 diabetes mellitus, previously referred to as "insulin-dependent diabetes mellitus" (IDDM) or "juvenile diabetes," results from the failure of the pancreas to produce sufficient insulin. Type 2 diabetes begins with insulin resistance, a condition where body cells fail to respond properly to insulin. With the progress of the diseases, there may eventually also be a lack of insulin. This form was previously referred to as "non–insulin-dependent diabetes mellitus" (NIDDM) or "adult-onset diabetes."

Type 1 diabetes results from an autoimmune reaction that destroys pancreatic β-cells so that they can no longer produce insulin and secrete it into the bloodstream. This results in abnormally high blood glucose concentrations, and generalized body wasting. Type 2 diabetes is not due to an autoimmune process. The destruction of β-cells is less pronounced than in Type 1 diabetes and, instead, there is an accumulation of aggregates of certain proteins, amyloid, in the pancreatic islets that become folded into a shape that allows many to stick together, forming fibrils.

Type 2 diabetes is characterized by high rates of secretion of glucagon into the blood, the rates unaffected by, and unresponsive to, the concentration of glucose in the blood. Glucagon is a hormone, produced by α-cells of the pancreas that raises the concentration of glucose in the bloodstream. Therefore, insulin is still secreted into the blood in response to the blood glucose, and thus, the insulin levels, even when the blood sugar level is normal, are much higher than they are in healthy persons (https://en. wikipedia.org/wiki/Insulin#cite_note-pmid 23222785-10).

History Footnote 2: Paul Langerhans, Frederick Grant Banting, and Charles Herbert Best

In 1869, Paul Langerhans published "Contributions to microscopic anatomy of the pancreas." He had noted small polygonal cells in the functional tissue of the pancreas that appeared in pairs or small clusters that seemingly formed islets. The function of these islet cells remained unknown until

1893 when Gustav Édouard Laguesse, a French histologist, first referred to the pancreatic islets as the "islets of Langerhans," and suggested that they might be endocrine in function.

Oskar Minkowski and Josef von Mering had shown that removing the pancreas of a dog caused it to develop diabetes. Subsequently, Eugene Lindsay Opie found that there were morphological changes in pancreatic islet cells of patients who died of diabetes. He suspected that pancreatic islets are the source of a hormone that prevents diabetes. Edward Albert Sharpey-Schafer, a British physiologist, called this hormone insulin.

In 1921, Frederick Grant Banting and Charles Herbert Best began experiments that led to the discovery of the function of insulin: They initially extracted it from dog and other animal pancreas and found that the extract lowered glucose levels in dogs that had induced diabetes. Its impurities however made it unsuitable for clinical use.

Eventually, a successful method of extraction was developed that enabled large amounts of highly purified insulin to be obtained from ox pancreas, and this made it possible for a clinical study to commence in January 1922. The study was a great success and confirmed the effectiveness of insulin in treating diabetes.

In 1922, Banting, Best, and Collip, the latter purified the extract, were granted patent rights for producing insulin, and they sold those rights to the University of Toronto for one dollar. In 1923, Frederick Grant Banting and John James Rickard Macleod, in whose laboratory insulin was first extracted, were awarded the Nobel Prize and Banting gave half of his prize money to Best, while Macleod gave half of his to Collip.

1.15 SYMPTOMS OF DIABETES

Early signs and symptoms of chronically elevated serum glucose (hyperglycemia) include the following:

- Excessive thirst
- Increased hunger
- Headaches
- Trouble concentrating
- Blurred vision
- Frequent urination
- Fatigue (weak, tired feeling)
- Weight loss
- Frequent infections and slow to heal wounds
- Blood sugar more than 180 mg/dL
- Erectile dysfunction

1.16 EFFECT OF MEALS ON PANCREATIC HORMONE RELEASE

Eating foods, as noted above, causes the pancreas to adjust the release of insulin and glucagon in response to changes in plasma glucose and other circulating nutrients. The response to a meal depends on the composition of the food consumed. In fact, intravenous infusion of glucose would elicit a smaller rise in insulin release than would oral administration of an equivalent amount of glucose.

The increase in insulin levels caused by actually eating food is thought to be due to gastrointestinal peptide hormones released in response to food absorption and they potentiate the glucose effect on insulin release. Consuming a meal rich in carbohydrate causes insulin levels to rise and glucagon levels to fall. The decrease of glucagon is due to inhibition of its release by insulin and to the elevation in plasma glucose.

Consuming a meal rich in protein causes insulin levels to rise, because insulin secretion is also stimulated by the amino acids into which proteins are broken down. Glucagon levels also rise because glucagon release is likewise stimulated by amino acids. Were the release of insulin caused by amino acids unopposed by a corresponding increase in release of glucagon, it would result in hypoglycemia because little glucose is being made available.

Because the pancreas has intestinal peptide hormones that respond to the types of nutrients in the meal, it can regulate the disposal of the nutrients without an undue change in plasma glucose. It would be difficult to attain this adjustment in pancreatic hormone release by the injections of insulin, and that is part of the problem faced by individuals with Type 1 diabetes. Hence, insulin and glucagon work synergistically to keep blood glucose concentrations normal. Once consumed, glucose is absorbed by the intestines and into the blood. Extra glucose is stored in the muscles and liver as glycogen. When needed, it is hydrolyzed to glucose and released into the blood.

1.17   THE ROLE OF INSULIN IN MUSCLE

In muscle, insulin stimulates amino acid uptake and protein synthesis, and glucose uptake and incorporation into glycogen. The muscle plays an important role in absorbing about 80% to 95% of sudden increases in plasma glucose levels, such as those observed during a rich carbohydrate meal.

During exercise, the muscle becomes more sensitive to insulin action and therefore retains the ability to import glucose from circulation despite the exercise-induced reduction in insulin levels.

1.18   BLOOD GLUCOSE AFTER EXERCISE

Food intake affects blood glucose levels, but there are other reasons why they may rise or decline, including infection or either physical or psychological stress. Exercise will affect it as well.

It is reported that barely 39% of adults with diabetes are physically active compared with 58% of nondiabetic American adults (Morrato, Hill, Wyatt et al. 2003). Thus, for most people with Type 2 diabetes, exercise is recommended for diabetes management and can be undertaken safely and effectively. Structured interventions combining physical activity and modest weight loss have been shown to lower the risk of Type 2 diabetes by up to 58% in high-risk populations. Most benefits of physical activity for diabetes management are realized through acute and long-term improvements in insulin action accomplished with both aerobic and resistance training (Colberg, Sigal, and Fernhall. 2010).

1.19   DIABETES AND BMI

The *International Journal of Clinical Practice* reported a study aimed at determining the relation between BMI and the prevalence of diabetes, hypertension, and elevation of plasma cholesterol, triglycerides, or both, or a low HDL level (dyslipidemia) in two population databases: the National Health and Nutrition Examination Survey–CDC (NHANES) and the Study to Help Improve Early evaluation and management of risk factors Leading to Diabetes (SHIELD).

It was found that increased BMI was associated with increased prevalence of diabetes, hypertension, and dyslipidemia. For each condition, more than 75% of patients had BMI greater than or equal to 25 kg/m^2. Estimated prevalence of diabetes and hypertension was similar in both the NHANES and the SHIELD studies, while dyslipidemia was substantially higher in NHANES than in SHIELD.

In both studies, prevalence of diabetes, hypertension, and dyslipidemia occurred across all ranges of BMI, but increased with higher BMI. However, not all overweight or obese patients had these metabolic diseases, and not all with these conditions were overweight or obese (Bays, Chapman, and Grandy. 2007).

Investigators from The George Institute for Global Health, University of Oxford, Oxford, UK, and the Cardiovascular Research Group, Institute of Cardiovascular Sciences, University of Manchester, Manchester, UK, reported the association between usual blood pressure and the risk of diabetes in a cohort of 4.1 million adults, free of diabetes and cardiovascular disease in the *Journal of the American College of Cardiology*. Here is what they found among the overall cohort:

- A 10 mmHg higher diastolic blood pressure (DBP) was associated with a 52% higher risk of new-onset diabetes.
- A 20 mmHg higher systolic blood pressure (SBP) was associated with a 58% higher risk of new-onset diabetes.

The strength of the association declined with age per 20 mmHg higher SBP and with increasing BMI. Estimates were similar even after excluding individuals prescribed antihypertensive or lipid-lowering medication therapies (Emdin, Anderson, Woodward et al. 2015).

Diabetes is clearly linked to BMI (Bays, Chapman, and Grandy. 2007; Gray, Picone, Sloan et al. 2015; Feller, Boeing, and Pischon. 2010), and BMI was also shown to be related to atherosclerosis (Oren, Vos, Uiterwaal et al. 2003) and coronary heart disease (Flint, Rexrode, Hu et al. 2010), and, as shown in a meta-analysis, it does not discriminate on the basis of gender (Mongraw-Chaffin, Peters, Huxley et al. 2015), hypertension (Ganz, Wintfeld, Li et al. 2014), and metabolic syndrome (Gierach, Gierac, Ewertowska et al. 2014).

REFERENCES

Alford FP, Bloom SR, and JD Nabarro. 1976. Glucagon metabolism in man, studies on the metabolic clearance rate and the plasma acute disappearance time of glucagon in normal and diabetic subjects. *Journal of Clinical Endocrinology and Metabolism*, May; 42(5): 830–838. DOI: 10.1210/jcem-42-5-830.

Bays HE, Chapman RH, and S Grandy. 2007. The relationship of Body Mass Index to diabetes mellitus, hypertension and dyslipidaemia: Comparison of data from two national surveys. *International Journal of Clinical Practice*, 61: 737–747.

Bergman RN. 1977. Integrated control of hepatic glucose metabolism. *Federation Proceedings*, Feb; 36(2): 265–270. PMID: 190047.

Berns MA, de Vries JH, and MB Katan. 1988. Determinants of the increase of serum cholesterol with age: A longitudinal study. *International Journal of Epidemiology*, Dec; 17(4): 789–796. PMID: 3225086.

Butler AE, Janson J, Bonner-Weir S, Ritzel R, Rizza RA, and PC Butler. 2003. β-cell deficit and increased β-cell apoptosis in humans with Type 2 diabetes. *Diabetes*, Jan; 52: 102–110. PMID: 12502499.

Cobelli C, Toffolo GM, Man CD, Campioni M, Denti P, Caumo A, Butler P, and R Rizza. 2007. Assessment of β-cell function in humans, simultaneously with insulin sensitivity and hepatic extraction, from intravenous and oral glucose tests. *American Journal of Physiology - Endocrinology and Metabolism*, 6 Jul; 293(1): E1–E15. DOI: 10.1152/ajpendo.00421.2006.

Colberg SR, Sigal RJ, Fernhall B, Regensteiner JG, Blissmer BJ, Rubin RR, Chasan-Taber L, Albright AL, and B Braun. 2010. Exercise and type 2 diabetes. The American College of Sports Medicine and the American Diabetes Association: Joint position statement. *Diabetes Care*, Dec; 33(12): e147–e167. DOI: 10.2337/dc10-9990.

Emdin CA, Anderson SG, Woodward M, and K Rahimi. 2015. Usual blood pressure and risk of new-onset diabetes: Evidence from 4.1 million adults and a meta-analysis of prospective studies. *Journal of the American College of Cardiology*, 66(14): 1332–1562.

Feller S, Boeing H, and T Pischon. 2010. Body mass index, waist circumference, and the risk of Type 2 diabetes mellitus. Implications for routine clinical practice. *Deutsches Arztenblatt International* (German Medical Journal International), Jul; 107(26): 470–476. DOI: 10.3238/arztebl.2010.0470.

Ferrannini E, Bjorkman O, Reichard GA Jr, Pilo A, Olsson M, Wahren J, and RA DeFronzo. 1985. The disposal of an oral glucose load in healthy subjects. A quantitative study. *Diabetes*, Jun; 34(6): 580–588. PMID: 3891471.

Flint AJ, Rexrode KM, Hu FB, Glynn RJ, Caspard H, Manson JE, Willett WC, and EB Rimm. 2010. Body mass index, waist circumference, and risk of coronary heart disease: A prospective study among men and women. *Obesity Research in Clinical Practice*, Jul–Sept; 4(3): e171–e181. DOI: 10.1016/j.orcp.2010.01.001.

Ganz ML, Wintfeld N, Li Q, Alas V, Langer J, and M Hammer. 2014. The association of body mass index with the risk of type 2 diabetes: A case-control study nested in an electronic health records system in the United States. *Diabetology and Metabolic Syndrome*, 6(1): 50. http://www.dmsjournal.com /content/6/1/50.

Gerich JE. 2017. Getting to goal in Type 2 diabetes: Role of postprandial glycemic control. *Medscape*, Wed. April 19. http://www.medscape.org/viewarticle/473744.

Gierach M, Gierac J, Ewertowska M, Arndt A, and R Junik. 2014. Correlation between body mass index and waist circumference in patients with metabolic syndrome. *International Scholarly Research Notices. Endocrinology*, Vol 2014, Article ID 514589, 6 pages. http://dx.doi.org/10.1155/2014/514589.

Gosmanov NR, Gosmanov AR, and JE Gerich. 2011. Glucagon Physiology, NCBI Endotext National Center for Biotechnology Information, U.S. National Library of Medicine 8600 Rockville Pike, Bethesda MD, 20894 USA. https://www.ncbi. nlm.nih.gov/books/NBK279127/.

Gray N, Picone G, Sloan F, and A Yashkin. 2015. The relationship between BMI and onset of diabetes mellitus and its complications. *The Southern Medical Journal*, Jan; 108(1): 29–36. DOI: 10.14423/SMJ .0000000000000214.

Greenwald SE. 2007. Ageing of the conduit arteries. *Journal of Pathology*, Jan; 211(2): 157–172. DOI: 10.1002 /path.2101.

Guariguata L. 2013. Global estimates of diabetes prevalence for 2013 and projections for 2035. *Diabetes Research and Clinical Practice*. Elsevier BV; 103(2): 137–149. Available from: http://dx.doi.org/10.1016 /j.diabres.2013.11.002.

Halberg F, Haus E, and G Cornelissen. 1995. From biologic rhythms to chromomes relevant for nutrition. In Marriott BM (ed.): Not Eating Enough: Overcoming Underconsumption of Military Operational Rations. National Academy Press, Washington DC 1995, pp. 361–372.

Henry RR. 1996. Glucose control and insulin resistance in non-insulin-dependent diabetes mellitus. *Annals of Internal Medicine*, Jan; 124(1 Pt 2): 97–103. PMID: 8554221.

Holst JJ, Vilsbøll T, and CF Deacon. 2009. The incretin system and its role in type 2 diabetes mellitus. *Molecular and Cell Endocrinology*, Jan; 297(1–2): 127–136. DOI: 10.1016/j.mce.2008.08.012.

Koeslag JH, Saunders PT, and E Terblanche. 2003. A reappraisal of the blood glucose homeostat which comprehensively explains the type 2 diabetes mellitus-syndrome X complex. *The Journal of Physiology*, Jun; 549 (Pt 2): 333–346. DOI: 10.1113/ jphysiol. 2002.037895.

Krssak M, Brehm A, Bernroider E, Anderwald C, Nowotny P, Dalla Man C, Cobelli C, Cline GW, Shulman GI, Waldhäusl W, and M Roden. 2004. Alterations in postprandial hepatic glycogen metabolism in type 2 diabetes. *Diabetes*, Dec; 53(12): 3048–3056. PMID: 15561933.

Kruszynska YT, and JM Olefsky. 1996. Cellular and molecular mechanisms of non-insulin dependent diabetes mellitus. *Journal of Investigative Medicine*, Oct; 44(8): 413–428. PMID: 8952222.

Kuusisto J, Mykkänen L, Pyörälä K, and M Laakso. 1994. NIDDM and its metabolic control predict coronary heart disease in elderly subjects. *Diabetes*, 1994 Aug; 43(8): 960–967. PMID: 8039603.

Laffel L. 1999. Ketone bodies: A review of physiology, pathophysiology and application of monitoring to diabetes. *Diabetes/Metabolism Research and Review*, Nov–Dec; 15(6): 412–426. PMID: 10634967.

Lorenzo C, Wagenknecht LE, Rewers MJ, Karter AJ, Bergman RN, Hanley AJ, and SM Haffner. 2010. Disposition index, glucose effectiveness, and conversion to type 2 diabetes: The Insulin Resistance Atherosclerosis Study (IRAS). *Diabetes Care*, Sep; 33(9): 2098–2103. DOI: 10.2337/dc10-0165.

Ma ZA, Zhao Z, and J Turk. 2012. Mitochondrial dysfunction and β-cell failure in Type 2 diabetes mellitus. *Experimental Diabetes Research*, Vol 2012, Article ID 703538, 11 pages. http://dx.doi.org/10.1155 /2012/703538.

Maassen JA, 'T Hart LM, Van Essen E, Heine RJ, Nijpels G, Jahangir Tafrechi RS, Raap AK, Janssen GM, and HH Lemkes. 2004. Mitochondrial diabetes: Molecular mechanisms and clinical presentation. *Diabetes*, Feb; 53 Suppl 1: S103–S109. PMID: 14749274.

Mari A, Wahren J, DeFronzo RA, and E Ferrannini. 1994. Glucose absorption and production following oral glucose: Comparison of compartmental and arteriovenous-difference methods. *Metabolism*, Nov; 43(11): 1419–1425. PMID: 7968597.

Mongraw-Chaffin ML, Peters SA, Huxley RR, and M Woodward. 2015. The sex-specific association between BMI and coronary heart disease: A systematic review and meta-analysis of 95 cohorts with 1.2 million participants. *Lancet, Diabetes and Endocrinology*, Jun; 3(6): 437–349. DOI: 10.1016/S2213 -8587(15)00086-8.

Moore MC, Coate KC, Winnick JJ, An X, and AD Cherrington. 2012. Regulation of hepatic glucose uptake and storage in vivo. *Advances in Nutrition*, May; 3(3): 286–294.

Morrato EH, Hill JO, Wyatt HR, Ghushchyan V, and PW Sullivan. 2003. Physical activity in U.S. adults with diabetes and at risk for developing diabetes, *Diabetes Care*, Feb; 30(2): 203–209. DOI: 10.2337 /dc06-1128.

Muller DC, Elahi D, Tobin JD, and R Andres. 1996. The effect of age on insulin resistance and secretion: A review. *Seminars in Nephrology*, Jul; 16(4): 289–298. PMID: 8829267.

Nijpels G. 2016. Epidemiology of type 2 diabetes [internet]. Nov 23; *Diapedia*, 3104287123 rev. no. 18 https:// doi.org/10.14496/dia.3104287123.18.

Oren A, Vos LE, Uiterwaal CSPM, Gorissen WHM, Grobbee DE, and ML Bots. 2003. Change in body mass index from adolescence to young adulthood and increased carotid intima-media thickness at 28 years of age: The Atherosclerosis Risk in Young Adults study. *International Journal of Obesity*, 27: 1383–1390. DOI: 10. 1038/sj.ijo.0802404.

Payne RA, Wilkinson IB, and DJ Webb. 2010. Arterial stiffness and hypertension. Emerging concepts. *Hypertension*, 55: 9–14. https://doi.org/10.1161/HYPERTENSIONAHA.107.090464.

Petersen KF, Befroy D, Dufour S, Dziura J, Ariyan C, Rothman DL, DiPietro L, Cline GW, and GI Shulman. 2003. Mitochondrial dysfunction in the elderly: Possible role in insulin resistance. *Science*, May 16; 300(5622): 1140–1142. DOI: 10.1126/science.1082889.

Pinto E. 2007. Blood pressure and ageing. *Postgraduate Medical Journal*, Feb; 83(976): 109–114. DOI: 10.1136 /pgmj.2006.048371.

Refaie MR, Sayed-Ahmed NA, Bakr AM, Aziz MYA, El Kannishi MH, and SS Abdel-Gawad. 2006. Aging is an inevitable risk factor for insulin resistance. *Journal of Taibah University Medical Sciences*, 1(1): 30–41. http://doi.org/10.1016/S1658-3612(06)70005-1.

Schram MT, Henry RMA, van Dijk RAJM, Kostense PJ, Dekker JM, Nijpels G, Heine RJ, Bouter LM, Westerhof N, and CDA Stehouwer. 2004. Increased central artery stiffness in impaired glucose. Metabolism and Type 2 Diabetes. The Hoorn Study. *Hypertension*, 43: 176–181. DOI: 10.1161/01.HYP .0000111829.46090.92.

Simonson DC, and RA DeFronzo. 1983. Glucagon physiology and aging: Evidence for enhanced hepatic sensitivity. *Diabetologia*, 25(1): 1–7. DOI: 10.1007/BF00251887.

Sonksen P, and J Sonksen. 2000. Insulin: Understanding its action in health and disease. *British Journal of Anaesthesia*, 85(1): 69–79. DOI: 10.1093/bja/85.1.69.

Troisi RJ, Cowie CC, and MI Harris. 2000. Diurnal variation in fasting plasma glucose: Implications for diagnosis of diabetes in patients examined in the afternoon. *Journal of the American Medical Association*, Dec; 284(24): 3157–3159. PMID: 11135780.

Utzschneider KM, Prigeon RL, Faulenbach MV, Tong J, Carr DB, Boyko EJ, Leonetti DL, McNeely MJ, Fujimoto WY, and SE Kahn. 2009. Oral disposition index predicts the development of future diabetes above and beyond fasting and 2-h glucose levels. *Diabetes Care*, Feb; 32(2): 335–341. DOI: 10.2337/dc0.

Whiting DR. 2011. IDF Diabetes Atlas: Global estimates of the prevalence of diabetes for 2011 and 2030. *Diabetes Research and Clinical Practice*. Elsevier BV; 94(3): 311–321. Available from: http://dx.doi.org /10.1016/j.diabres.2011.10.029.

Yashin AY, Arbeev KG, Wu D, Arbeeva LS, Kulminski A, Akushevich I, Culminskaya I, Stallard E, and SV Ukraintseva. 2013. How lifespan associated genes modulate aging changes: Lessons from analysis of longitudinal data. *Frontiers in Genetics*, Jan; 22: 2013 https://doi.org/10.3389/fgene.2013.00003.

Yashin IA, Ukraintseva VS, Arbeev GK, Akushevich I, Arbeeva SL, and MA Kulminski. 2009. Maintaining physiological state for exceptional survival: What is the normal level of blood glucose and does it change with age? *Mechanisms of Ageing and Development*, 130(9): 611–618.

Zimmet PZ, Wall JR, Rome R, Stimmler L, and RJ Jarrett. 1974. Diurnal variation in glucose tolerance: Associated changes in plasma insulin, growth hormone, and non-esterified. *British Medical Journal*, Mar 16; 1(5906): 485–488. PMCID: PMC1633483.

2 Hyperglycemia Impairs Blood Vessel Function

In formal logic, a contradiction is the signal of defeat, but in the evolution of real knowledge it marks the first step in progress toward a victory.

Alfred North Whitehead

2.1 ON A LIMB

It is generally held that Type 2 diabetes is a distinct disease entity separate from, but linked to chronic systemic inflammation, atherosclerosis, and cardiovascular and heart disease, as well as other related disorders—even diabetes-related blindness. However, the clinical and research pathophysiology literature compels a somewhat different interpretation: Chronic systemic inflammation, atherosclerosis, and cardiovascular and heart disease, as well as other related disorders—even diabetes-related blindness—might well be consequences of Type 2 diabetes rather than conditions aggravated by it as conventionally thought.

This hypothesis will be explained in this chapter, and the next one, and its basis will be carefully documented with references from conventional medical laboratory and clinic reports in refereed medical journals.

We know that hyperglycemia damages the *endothelium* lining of blood vessels, thus impairing its ability to synthesize nitric oxide (NO). The 1998 Nobel Prize in Medicine was awarded to three US scientists for discovering the biological role of NO: one of its most important roles is to control blood flow throughout the body and the brain.

2.1.1 NO FROM L-ARGININE

NO activates cytosolic guanylate cyclase and stimulates cyclic guanosine monophosphate (cGMP) formation in mammalian cells. It causes vascular smooth muscle relaxation and inhibition of platelet aggregation by mechanisms involving cGMP and has led to development of clinically useful nitrovasodilators. NO is synthesized by various mammalian tissues including vascular endothelium, macrophages, neutrophils, hepatic Kupffer cells, adrenal tissue, cerebellum, and other tissues. NO is synthesized from endogenous L-arginine by a NO synthase (NOS) system that possesses different cofactor requirements in different cell types.

There are three isoforms of NOS identified according to their activity or the tissue type in which they were first described. They are endothelial NOS (or eNOS), neuronal NOS (or nNOS), and inducible NOS (or iNOS). iNOS mediates nonspecific host defense central in the clearance of bacterial, viral, fungal, and parasitic infections.

The NO formed diffuses out of its cells of origin and into nearby target cells, where it binds to the heme group of cytosolic guanylate cyclase and thereby causes enzyme activation. This interaction represents a novel and widespread signal transduction mechanism that links extracellular stimuli to the biosynthesis of cGMP in nearby target cells. The small molecular size and the lipophilic nature of NO enable communication with nearby cells containing cytosolic guanylate cyclase. The extent of transcellular communication is limited by the short half-life of NO, thereby ensuring a localized response (Ignarro. 1990).

It is dogma that impaired NO formation, one of the principal bases of cardiovascular and heart disease, attributed to endothelium dysfunction, is commonly blamed mainly on atherosclerosis.

But we now have reason to believe that, in the presence of Type 2 diabetes, atherosclerosis, contrary to common belief, does not impair the ability of the endothelium to form NO. On the contrary, the preponderance of the scientific evidence now is that the inability of the endothelium to form NO results in a failure to prevent atherosclerosis. In fact, restoration of endothelium viability and therefore restoring NO formation have even been shown to prevent formation of atheromas and reverse arterial plaque accumulation.

The Journal of Clinical Investigation confirmed this in an animal model (Cooke, Singer, Tsao et al. 1992), and so did the journal *Molecular and Cellular Biochemistry* (Dhawan, Handu, Nain et al. 2005), and so also did the *Lancet* in hypercholesterolemic patients (Drexler, Zeiher, and Meinzer. 1991).

Restoring NO prevents—even reverses—atherosclerosis and diabetes impairs NO formation by damaging the endothelium that forms it. The rest of this chapter aims to document how it does that, and the rest of the book, how to prevent it.

Corollary: In the presence of Type 2 diabetes, treatment of cardiovascular and heart disorders ranging from atherosclerosis to coronary artery disease, even diabetes-related vision loss, must address endothelium impairment and relieve it. In most cases, this could begin with glycemic control possibly supplemented with an oral L-arginine or citrulline nutraceutical, or a combination to enhance endothelial NO formation as recommended in a report in the *Journal of Cardiovascular Pharmacology and Therapeutics* (Heffernan, Fahs, Ranadive et al. 2010) and also in the *Cardiology Journal* (Orea-Tejeda, Orozco-Gutiérrez, Castillo-Martínez et al. 2010).

It would also be very helpful; to implement a diet rich in nitrates as described in *Nitrite and Nitrate in Human Health and Disease* (Brian, and Loscalzo. 2017).

2.2 THE FOCUS ON ARTERIAL BLOOD VESSELS

A report in the journal *Reviews in Endocrine and Metabolic Disorders* supports the contention that insulin resistance directly affects the vascular endothelium and contributes to systemic insulin resistance, thus impairing the actions of insulin to redistribute blood flow as part of its normal actions driving muscle glucose uptake.

Exposing endothelium to hyperglycemia promotes cell dysfunction. In diabetic patients, exposing coronary circulation to increasing amounts of acetylcholine actually causes *paradoxical* constriction instead of vasodilation (Nitenberg, Valensi, Sachs et al. 1993). This response suggests that endothelial cells exposed to hyperglycemia may face increased *apoptosis*, the death of cells that otherwise occurs as normal and controlled growth or development.

The consequence of increased apoptosis is detachment of endothelial cells that are released into the bloodstream and can be recognized and measured as circulating endothelial cells. It has been shown that circulating endothelial cell levels are more frequent in Type 2 diabetic patients as represented by glycated hemoglobin (HbA1c) levels, irrespective of glucose control (McClung, Naseer, Saleem et al. 2005).

Besides circulating endothelial cells, there are powerful pro-coagulant micro-particles (endothelial micro-particles) that are released from intact cells that may also play a role in the normal process of keeping blood within a damaged vessel (hemostasis). A report in the journal *Current Diabetes Reviews* tells us that elevated endothelial cell-derived endothelial micro-particle levels are predictive of the presence of coronary artery lesions, and this is a more significant independent risk factor than duration of diabetes, lipid levels, or presence of hypertension (Nomura. 2009).

The journal *Diabetes Care* reports that the consequence of the apoptosis results in the so-called arterial denudation, which triggers important pro-atherosclerotic processes such as smooth muscle cell proliferation, migration, and matrix secretion (Avogaro, Albiero, Menegazzo et al. 2011).

To wit: in Type 2 diabetes, at least, endothelium damage *precedes* atherosclerosis. Impaired vascular function is a component of the insulin resistance syndrome and is a feature of Type 2 diabetes.

The reason that endothelium damage precedes atherosclerosis may be due to the adverse effect of hyperglycemia on the *vasa vasorum* (see Section 2.2.1) and that this damage favors formation of atheromas.

On this basis, the vascular endothelium has emerged as a therapeutic target with the intent to improve systemic metabolic state by improving vascular function. Therapies that improve systemic insulin resistance improve vascular function (Mather. 2013).

This chapter and the next one will document the argument with references to conventional medical clinical and research publications that support it.

2.2.1 DIABETES AND BLOOD VESSELS OF THE BLOOD VESSELS: VASA VASORUM

With the exception of peripheral artery disease, and retinal blood vessel damage, the focus on the pathophysiology of diabetes is generally on more "popular" organs such as the heart and the kidneys—"popular" in the sense that these are what is mostly talked about; hence, "cardiovascular" and not "vasculocardiac." In fact, even the endothelium is now finally granted well deserved status as an organ, and attention to its function is currently much in vogue.

And so, we examine the effect of hyperglycemia on the coronary arteries that deliver blood to the heart muscles, for instance, but we tend to overlook the blood vessels that supply blood to the blood vessels, that is, the *vasa vasorum*, which also parenthetically deliver blood to the coronary arteries.

Few seem to even know that the *vasa vasorum* exists, and most anatomical renderings on blood vessels don't show them. One of the few that show *vasa* is Frank Netter's *Structure of Coronary Arteries* (https://www.netterimages.com/structure-of-coronary-arteries-unlabeled-cardiology-hypertension -frank-h-netter-2461.html Srteeius; accessed 5/29/17), and it is anatomically problematic, if not outright incorrect.

The wall of an artery consists of three layers: The tunica externa or tunica adventitia is the outermost layer, which attaches the vessel to the surrounding tissue. This layer is mostly connective tissue with varying amounts of elastic and collagenous fibers. The connective tissue in this layer is quite dense where it is adjacent to the tunica media, but it is loose connective tissue near the periphery of the vessel.

The middle layer, the tunica media, is primarily smooth muscle and is usually the thickest layer. It not only provides support for the vessel but also changes vessel diameter to regulate blood flow and blood pressure.

The innermost layer, the tunica intima (also called tunica interna), is simple squamous epithelium surrounded by a connective tissue basement membrane with elastic fibers. The endothelium is the thin cell layer that lines the interior surface of blood vessels (and lymphatic vessels). It forms an interface between circulating blood in the lumen and the rest of the vessel wall.

The *vasa vasorum* (Figure 2.1) is a network of microvessels that supply oxygen and nutrients to the outer layers of the arterial wall.

The function of *vasa vasorum* is both to deliver nutrients and oxygen to arterial and venous walls and to remove "waste" products, either produced by cells in the wall or introduced by diffusion through the endothelium of the artery or vein (Ritman, and Lerman. 2007; see also Mulligan-Kehoe. 2010).

Figure 2.1 shows an isolated pig coronary artery and the associated *vasa vasorum*. Figure 2.2 shows the cross section of a blood vessel and the location of the *vasa* in the *tunica adventitia*.

Having established the nature of *vasa*, its location on and in blood vessels, and having summarized its basic function, we can turn our attention to the impact of diabetes on this vascular structure.

The authors of a study published in the journal *Atherosclerosis* contended that although the relationship between blood glucose levels and the microvascular complications of diabetes is well established, the effects of hyperglycemia on *vasa vasorum* are not known. Therefore, the aim of their study was to determine the effects of hyperglycemia on the *vasa vasorum* and to examine the consequences of these effects on the development of atherosclerosis in an animal (mouse) model.

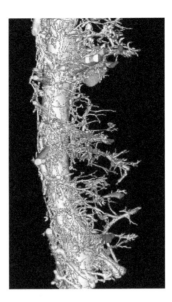

FIGURE 2.1   Micro-CT images of a normal left anterior descending coronary artery (LAD) of a pig showing vasa vasorum. [From Gössl, Malyar, Rosol et al. 2003. *American Journal of Physiology - Heart and
Circulatory Physiology*, Nov; 285(5): H2019–H2026. With permission.]

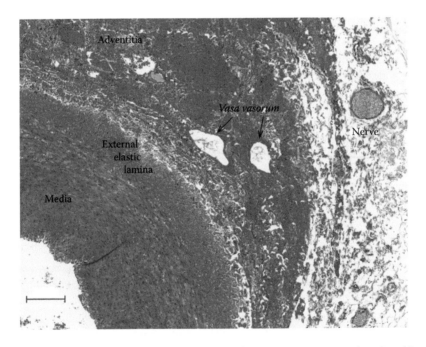

FIGURE 2.2   Porcine carotid artery. The black arrows point to vasa vasorum at the adventitia. Scale bar
represents 200 μm. [From Cheng, Sun, Vuong et al. 2012. Endovascular optical coherence intensity kurtosis:
visualization of vasa vasorum in porcine carotid artery. *Biomedical Optics Express*, Jan; 3(3): 388–399. With
permission.]

They examined the micro- and macrovascular effects of hyperglycemia in streptozotocin-injected apolipoprotein-E-deficient [ApoE(−/−)] mice on retina and aortic sinus in hyperglycemic and normo-glycemic control animals. ApoE is essential for the normal catabolism of triglyceride-rich lipoprotein constituents.

Retinal and *vasa vasorum* microvessel densities were assessed and evaluated against athero-sclerotic lesion development. The expression levels of pro-angiogenic factors including vascular endothelial growth factor (VEGF) and VEGF receptor 2 were determined.

It was found that in normoglycemic ApoE(−/−) mice, atherogenesis is associated with *vasa vaso-rum* expansion, whereas in hyperglycemic ApoE(−/−) mice, there is no significant neovasculariza-tion of the *vasa vasorum*, despite the fact that lesions are significantly larger. These findings are the first evidence that hyperglycemia alters the structure of the *vasa vasorum*. Such microvascular changes directly correlate and may contribute to the development and progression of atherosclerosis in hyperglycemic ApoE-deficient mice (Veerman, Venegas-Pino, Shi et al. 2013).

The aim of a study published in the *European Journal of Vascular and Endovascular Surgery* was to determine whether *vasa vasorum* (vv) neoangiogenesis is altered with increased arterial damage in diabetic patients with peripheral artery obstructive disease (PAOD). Neoangiogenesis is the mechanism responsible for the formation of blood vessels throughout the human body.

In patients with PAOD and critical lower limb ischemia, a number of them with Type 2 diabetes, the study examined endothelial cell markers (CD34 and von Willebrand factor); real-time reverse transcription polymerase chain reaction (RT-PCR) was used to evaluate arterial wall expression of VEGF, enzyme-linked immunosorbent assay (ELISA) was employed to assess blood VEGF, and flow cytometry was used to detect circulating endothelial cells (CECs).

Patients with PAOD and diabetes have a higher frequency (60% vs. 45%) of advanced atheroscle-rotic lesions and a significant reduction in CD34(+) capillaries in the arterial media. Adventitial neo-angiogenesis was increased equally [CD34(+) and vWF(+)] in all patients. Likewise, all patients have increased CEC and VEGF concentration in the blood as well as in situ VEGF transcript expression.

The authors concluded that patients with PAOD have considerable arterial damage despite increased *in situ* and circulating expression of the pro-angiogenic VEGF; a dysfunctional *vasa vaso-rum* angiogenesis was seen in diabetics, which also showed a higher frequency of parietal damage.

It was concluded that in diabetic arterial wall, injury is worsened by *vasa vasorum* inability to final-ize an effective VEGF-driven arterial wall neoangiogenesis (Orrico, Pasquinelli, Foroni et al. 2010).

Investigators who have examined the *vasa vasorum* in occluded vessels of nondiseased experi-mental animals find that damaged *vasa vasorum* increases the probability of animals developing atheromas. There is increasing evidence that adverse changes in *vasa vasorum* enhance the disease process and diabetes causes adverse changes in *vasa vasorum* (Mulligan-Kehoe. 2010).

In brief, chronic hyperglycemia damages the *vasa vasorum*, a network of microvessels that tend to the needs of macrovessels.

2.3   ADDICTION TO SUGAR IS MORE DAMAGING IN AGING

"Sugar gave rise to the slave trade, now sugar has enslaved us." So said Jeff O'Connell, author of *Sugar Nation: The Hidden Truth behind America's Deadliest Habit and the Simple Way to Beat It* (O'Connell 2011).

The problem is not sugar *per se*, but chronic elevated blood sugar, glucose to be exact. And, coupled with increased insulin resistance as we age, our levels of blood sugar will rise because most of us consume more sugar and carbohydrates than the body can ordinarily manage, and so it remains to circulate at high levels in our blood where it causes damage to many organs and tissues.

A clinical study reported in *The Journal of Clinical Investigation* aimed to find out how abnor-mal carbohydrate tolerance occurs in aging in elderly and nonelderly, nonobese patients. It was found that serum glucose and insulin levels were significantly elevated in the elderly compared to the nonelderly participants during a 75-g oral glucose tolerance test (GTT), suggesting an insulin-resistant state.

Peripheral insulin sensitivity was assessed in both groups during an insulin infusion rate of 40 mU/m^2 per minute. Similar steady-state serum insulin levels led to a peripheral glucose disposal rate of 151 ± 17 mg/m^2 per minute in the elderly compared to 247 ± 12 mg/m^2 per minute in the nonelderly, documenting the presence of insulin resistance in the elderly participants.

Insulin binding to isolated adipocytes (fat cells) and monocytes (phagocytic white blood cell) was similar in the elderly and nonelderly groups, indicating that insulin resistance in the presence of normal insulin binding suggests a postreceptor defect in insulin action. The results confirm the presence of a postreceptor defect as well as a rightward shift in the dose–response curve (Kolterman, Gray, Griffin et al. 1981).

The ability of insulin to suppress hepatic glucose output was lesser in the elderly during the 15 mU/m^2 per minute insulin infusion, but hepatic glucose output was fully and equally suppressed in both groups during the 40 and 1200 mU/m^2 per minute infusion.

There was a significant inverse relationship between the degree of glucose intolerance in the individual elderly, as reflected by the 2-h serum glucose level during the oral GTT and the degree of peripheral insulin resistance as assessed by the glucose disposal rate during the 40 mU/m^2 per minute insulin infusion.

The investigators concluded that carbohydrate intolerance develops as part of the aging process, and it appears to be the consequence of peripheral insulin resistance caused by a postreceptor defect in target tissue insulin action, which causes both a decrease in the maximal rate of peripheral glucose disposal and a rightward shift in the insulin action dose–response curve.

In elderly participants, the severity of the abnormality in carbohydrate tolerance was found to be directly correlated to the degree of peripheral insulin resistance (Fink, Kolterman, Griffin et al. 1983).

A report in the *American Journal of Physiology, Endocrinology and Metabolism* confirms that glucose tolerance progressively declines with age and that there is a high prevalence of Type 2 diabetes, and post-challenge hyperglycemia, in the older population. Furthermore, age-related glucose intolerance is often accompanied by insulin resistance, but, paradoxically, circulating insulin levels are similar to those of younger people.

Under some conditions of hyperglycemic challenge, insulin levels are lower in older people, suggesting beta-cell (β-cell) dysfunction. When controlling for insulin sensitivity, insulin secretion defects have been consistently demonstrated in the aging. Impaired β-cell compensation in age-related insulin resistance may predispose older people to develop post-challenge hyperglycemia and Type 2 diabetes (Chang, and Halter. 2003).

So, as we age, we produce less insulin, and simultaneously, our body cells become increasingly "resistant" to it, that is, less sensitive to insulin.

Indeed, chronic elevated blood sugar (hyperglycemia) is more dangerous than most people realize and there is a tendency to think that all one needs to do, if given this diagnosis by a physician, is to take the prescribed meds and all will be fine. Sadly, that is not exactly the case.

Investigators from the Department of Internal Medicine, Valley Hospital Medical Center, Las Vegas, Nevada, tell us that "Diabetes is a deadly and costly disease." The number of adults in the United States with newly diagnosed diabetes has nearly tripled from 1980 to 2011. At the current pace, one in three US adults will have diabetes in his/her lifetime.

Fourteen classes of prescription drugs are currently available to treat Type 2 diabetes, but *"only 36% of patients with type 2 diabetes achieve glycemic control with the currently available therapies. Therefore, new treatment options are desperately needed"* (Miller, Nguyen, Hu et al. 2014) (our italics for emphasis).

In 2013, Dr. Banerji, Director of the Diabetes Treatment Center, State University of New York Downstate Medical Center, Brooklyn, New York, wrote that the incidence and prevalence of Type 2 diabetes continue to grow in the United States and worldwide, along with the growing prevalence of obesity. Patients with Type 2 diabetes are at greater risk for cardiovascular disease, which dramatically affects overall healthcare costs. Not to mention the cost in suffering.

Dr. Banerji and a colleague, Dr. Dunn, examined the impact of the control of blood sugar level and medication adherence on rate of disease, mortality, and healthcare costs of patients with Type 2 diabetes, and highlighted the need for new drug therapies to improve outcomes in this patient population. They reported that despite improvements in the management of cardiovascular risk factors in these patients, the outcome remains poor. The costs of the management of Type 2 diabetes increase dramatically, yet the prevalence of the disease rises. Medication adherence to long-term drug therapy remains poor in these patients and it contributes to inadequate control of levels of blood sugar increasing healthcare resource utilization and costs, as well as increased rates of disease and mortality.

The investigators concluded that "drug therapies are needed that enhance patient adherence and persistence levels far above levels reported with currently available drugs. Improvements in adherence to treatment guidelines and greater rates of lifestyle modifications are also needed. Thus, there is a serious unmet need for better patient outcome, more effective and more tolerable drugs, as well as marked improvements in adherence to treatment guidelines and drug therapy to reduce healthcare costs and resource use" (Banerji, and Dunn. 2013).

There are many more such reports in the medical journals that address the issues concerning rising incidence of Type 2 diabetes, patient noncompliance with treatment, and failure to reach treatment goals, the failure often being attributed to the medication regimen.

Clearly, this is a serious problem and it is growing. The potential disaster of treatment failure can be gauged from the causal impact of chronic hyperglycemia on the often coexisting medical conditions.

2.4   METABOLIC MEMORY

Early intensive control of blood glucose reduces the risk of diabetic complications. However, research data suggest that there is a persistent long-term influence of early metabolic control on later clinical outcomes. This phenomenon, termed "Metabolic Memory," was first hypothesized and described by M. Brownlee in the journal *Nature* (Brownlee. 2001).

It has since been shown by many researchers that overproduction of free radicals forms the unifying link between hyperglycemia and the complications of diabetes. It has also been shown that antioxidants can at least partially reverse these complications both clinically and in the laboratory. A study published in the journal *Endocrine Abstract* reports confirming in three different models, that is, human endothelial cells, retinal cells, and retina from diabetic animals, that even when normalizing blood sugar, a persistent activation of diabetic complications remains.

Furthermore, even normalizing glycemia does not eliminate overproduction of free radicals, but that inhibiting their production, particularly at the mitochondrial level, can switch off the effect of the "memory" of hyperglycemia (Ceriello. 2009).

The authors of a study reported in *Frontiers in Physiology* also noted that it was unknown why vascular damage still occurs in diabetes patients even in the presence of intensive glycemic control. They averred that hyperglycemic memory may explain why intensive glucose control failed to improve cardiovascular outcomes in patients with diabetes and wondered why hyperglycemia promotes vascular dysfunction even after glucose normalization. Accumulating observations support the conclusion that ROS-driven hyperglycemic stress is "remembered" in the vasculature (Tang, Luo, Chen et al. 2014).

A mitochondrial adaptor protein is critical in the hyperglycemic memory in vascular endothelial cells, in human aortic endothelial cells exposed to high glucose, and in aortas of diabetic mice. Activation of this adaptor protein persists after returning to normoglycemia. Persistent adaptor protein upregulation is associated with continued ROS production, reduced NO bioavailability, and apoptosis (Paneni, Mocharla, Akhmedov et al. 2012).

It would be easy to believe that correcting Type 2 diabetes would promptly normalize endothelial function, but this is clearly not the case. The Diabetes Control and Complications Trial and the United Kingdom Prospective Diabetes Study follow-up trials gave strength to the so-called "metabolic memory" theory where the effects of either prolonged or transient changes in glycemia persist long after these have been re-adjusted (Roy, Sala, Cagliero et al. 1990; Chan, Kanwar, and Kowluru. 2010).

2.5 DIABETES AND ENDOTHELIUM (DYS)FUNCTION

If one were asked, what is the damage caused by hyperglycemia? The answer would certainly be, well, it seems to cause hypertension, atherosclerosis, cardiovascular and heart disease, metabolic syndrome, kidney disease, peripheral artery disease, male erectile dysfunction, blindness, and more. That would of course be right, in a way, but it overlooks the fact that damage to the cells forming the *endothelium* of our blood vessels—termed *endocardium* in the heart—lies at the very core of each one of those disorders and many more. What's more, it is now increasingly clear that it may be a unifying causal factor.

In fact, an article in the journal *Biochimica et Biophysica Acta (BBA) - Molecular Basis of Disease* reports that endothelial dysfunction is central to pathophysiological conditions including atherosclerosis, hypertension, and diabetes. Patients with diabetes invariably show an impairment of endothelium-dependent vasodilation. Therefore, understanding and treating endothelial dysfunction should be a major aim of the prevention of blood vessel complications associated with all forms of diabetes.

The mechanisms of endothelial dysfunction in diabetes includes altered glucose metabolism, impaired insulin signaling, low-grade inflammatory state, and increased unopposed generation of free radicals and reactive oxygen species (ROS).

The article further emphasizes the importance of developing new pharmacological approaches aimed at raising endothelium-derived NO synthesis (Sena, Pereira, and Seiça. 2013).

The following publications further detail the role of Type 2 diabetes in degrading the function of blood vessels.

2.5.1 THE ENDOTHELIUM

The arterial blood vessels that carry oxygenated blood from the lungs to body tissues range in size from large arteries down to smaller *arterioles* and finally to *capillaries*. The latter feed deoxygenated blood to *venules* and then back to the lungs via veins.

As previously noted, arteries are made up of three major wall layers encircled by muscle rings. From the outside in, the *tunica adventitia* is made entirely of collagen; the middle layer, the *tunica media*, has an extra layer of smooth muscle that allows the vessel to increase or decrease in size; the *tunica intima* is the inner cell layer.

The interior channel through which blood flows is called the *lumen*. The inner cell layer lying on the intima is the *endothelium*, and it determines how the vessels control blood flow by its ability to expand or to constrict.

Figure 2.3 shows the scanning electron micrograph of a cross section of a small arterial blood vessel with red blood cells shown in the lumen. The endothelium, the fluted structure resembling the folds of an accordion, is surrounded by the three cell layers and the outer muscle cell layer shown in pink. The "fluting" of the endothelium allows the blood vessel to dilate and to constrict to accommodate needed changes in blood flow and pressure as dictated by arousal and physical activity level.

Blood vessels respond to action hormones termed "neurotransmitters," for instance, noradrenaline, which may constrict them in some cases, or acetylcholine, which may relax or dilate them in other cases to adjust blood flow as required. But most important, it is the endothelium that forms the gas NO, triggering the intrinsic vasodilator cGMP, to relax the blood vessels and increase blood flow to organs ranging from the heart to the brain.

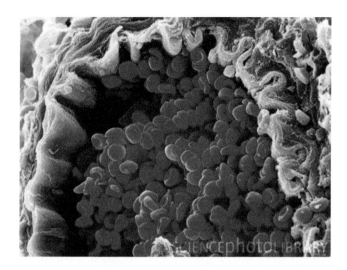

FIGURE 2.3   Colorized scanning electron micrograph of blood cells in an artery showing a layer of endothelial cells surrounded by outer blood vessel wall muscle. With permission from Science Source Library.

The endothelium can be considered to be *the business end* of the blood vessels and its control by NO is the discovery that resulted in the 1998 Nobel Prize awarded to three American scientists, Drs. Robert F. Furchgott, Louis J. Ignarro, and Ferid Murad.

No one knew before their discovery of the biological role of NO that the endothelium was anything but a sort of lining not unlike a bed sheet, inside blood vessels. No one thought that it served any biological purpose, much less that it actually controls the blood vessel inner diameter (caliber) and therefore the volume of blood flow.

To the point here: It so happens that our typical American diet, the so-called Western Diet, or the Standard American Diet, loaded with lots of sugar and carbs, is particularly damaging to the endothelium and the consequent cumulative effect of impaired blood flow is thought to be the principal culprit in cardiovascular and heart catastrophe.

The Journal of Nutrition reported a study of postprandial elevated blood glucose. Healthy men were given 75 g of glucose, or fructose, after an overnight fast. Brachial artery flow-mediated dilation (FMD), plasma glucose and insulin, antioxidants, malondialdehyde (MDA), inflammatory proteins, arginine, and ADMA were measured at regular intervals during the 3-h postprandial period.

Brachial artery FMD is an ultrasound method used to measure arterial diameter and blood flow in response to an increase in shear stress. Shear stress is induced by first blocking (with a tourniquet on the arm, usually) and then releasing blood to flow through the vessel. The resulting dilation and increased blood flow after it has been briefly blocked, and then released, result from the action of NO on the vessel smooth muscle.

MDA is a marker of oxidative stress, essentially an imbalance between free radicals and the ability of the body to neutralize their harmful effects by antioxidants.

Postprandial FMD was reduced following the ingestion of glucose only. Postprandial MDA concentrations rose more in response to consuming glucose than it did to consuming fructose.

Postprandial brachial artery FMD and MDA were inversely related, suggesting that hyperglycemia-induced lipid peroxidation (lipids oxidized by free radical) suppresses postprandial arterial blood vessel vascular function.

Lipid peroxidation is the oxidative degradation of lipids where free radicals "steal" electrons from the lipids in cell membranes causing cell damage and in turn causing them to become ROS.

Collectively, these findings suggest that postprandial hyperglycemia in healthy men reduces endothelium (NO)-dependent vasodilation by increasing lipid peroxidation independent of inflammation (Mah, Noh, Ballard et al. 2011).

According to a report in the journal *Diabetes and Metabolism*, in nondiabetic individuals, blood concentrations of glucose, lipids, and insulin rise after each meal, and postprandial changes last a long time after the meals. Transient increase of blood concentrations of glucose, triglycerides and fatty acids, and insulin is able to depress endothelium (NO)-dependent vasodilation in healthy persons, and hyperglycemia, hypertriglyceridemia, and hyperinsulinemia are generators of free radicals (Nitenberg, Cosson, and Pham. 2006).

In other words, damage to the endothelium may result from the ROS generated by free radicals formed by elevated levels of blood glucose, triglycerides, and insulin. And, damaging the endothelium is a very bad idea:

The endothelium is a single semipermeable layer of cells that forms an interface between the blood and surrounding tissues. It facilitates transport of substances such as nutrients and leukocytes across the vessel wall and it secretes numerous mediators necessary for normal vascular functioning, including those that regulate blood vessel tone, coagulation, immune responses, and vascular cell growth (Roberts, and Porter. 2013).

As noted above, a key function of the endothelium is the synthesis of NO produced by the action of the enzyme, endothelial NO synthase (eNOS). NO diffuses into neighboring vascular smooth muscle producing cGMP triggering blood vessel relaxation.

Conversely, the endothelium is also able to secrete the potent vasoconstrictor endothelin (ET-1), which magnifies the manner of development (pathogenesis) of cardiovascular and heart disease via pro-inflammatory effects (Böhm and Pernow. 2007). The endothelium maintains a fine balance between anti- and pro-thrombotic states.

In terms of cardiovascular health, endothelial dysfunction boils down to the inability to synthesize NO as needed to regulate vascular homeostasis leading to altering the physiological balance toward vasoconstriction, inflammation, and platelet aggregation (Xu, and Zou. 2009).

A number of other crucial points are made in the publication by Roberts and Porter titled "Cellular and molecular mechanisms of endothelial dysfunction in diabetes" appearing in the journal *Diabetes and Vascular Disease Research* in 2013. These emphasize the crucial impact of diabetes on the endothelium and its cardiovascular and other regulatory functions (Roberts, and Porter. 2013).

They point out that although hyperglycemia is clearly linked to endothelial dysfunction, the actual process that results in that dysfunction is largely left to speculation because diabetes patients usually display multiple physiological imbalances alongside the hyperglycemia. These disturbances are also known to induce endothelial dysfunction independent of the presence of diabetes, indicating a multifactor etiology rather than just hyperglycemia per se (Pasimeni, Ribaudo, and Capoccia. 2006; Steinberg, Chaker, and Leaming. 1996).

2.5.2 Oxidative Stress

One of the common factors in Type 2 diabetes is oxidative stress, the accumulation of ROS when production exceeds the ability of cellular antioxidant systems to eliminate them (Förstermann. 2008). Oxidative stress diminishes NO bioavailability putatively by damaging the endothelium.

Consistent unchallenged free radical attacks on the endothelium promote endothelial dysfunction characterized by altered endothelium (NO)-mediated vasodilation, rising blood pressure and heart rate (vascular reactivity), platelet aggregation, and clot (thrombus) formation. Decreased NO bioavailability and increased generation of ROS are among the major molecular changes associated with endothelial dysfunction (Montezano, and Touyz. 2012).

A study published in the journal *Diabetes Metabolism. Research and Reviews* also concludes that hyperglycemia, either stable or oscillating, increases oxidative stress and endothelial cell death (apoptosis) through excess ROS production (Piconi, Quagliaro, Assaloni et al. 2006).

A report in the journal *Vascular Health and Risk Management* suggests that both diabetes and insulin resistance cause endothelial dysfunction, which may impair the ability of the endothelium to prevent atherosclerosis. Both insulin resistance and endothelial dysfunction appear to precede the development of overt hyperglycemia in patients with Type 2 diabetes.

The authors note that although antioxidants provide short-term improvement of endothelial function, all studies of the effectiveness of preventive antioxidant therapy have been disappointing. Control of hyperglycemia thus remains the best way to improve endothelial function and to prevent atherosclerosis and other cardiovascular complications of diabetes (Hadi, and Al Suwaidi. 2007).

A report in the journal *Endocrine Reviews* tells us that the commonest cause of death and disease is atherosclerosis and that the main cause of atherosclerosis is endothelial dysfunction. Endothelial dysfunction has been documented in patients with diabetes and in individuals with insulin resistance, or those at high risk for developing Type 2 diabetes.

Several interventions have been tested in clinical trials aimed at improving endothelial function in patients with diabetes. Insulin sensitizers such as thiazolidinediones may have a beneficial effect in the short term, but the virtual absence of trials with cardiovascular end points precludes any definitive conclusion.

In a study published in the journal *Diabetes/Metabolism Research and Reviews*, the investigators exposed cultures of human endothelial cells to intermittent high glucose, thus partly mimicking what really happens *in vivo* in diabetic patients. It was found that stable high glucose produced an increase in apoptosis and in oxidative stress generation, and confirmed that intermittent glucose worsens the pro-apoptotic effects of high glucose, thereby enhancing oxidative stress generation.

Apoptosis was accompanied by an increase of both nitrotyrosine and 8-OHdG and was reversed by both superoxide dismutase (SOD) and the SOD mimetic manganese (III) tetrakis(4-benzoic acid) porphyrin chloride (MnTBAP). MnTBAP is a cell-permeable SOD mimetic and peroxynitrite scavenger.

It was shown for the first time that inhibiting the mitochondrial electron transport complex II preserves endothelial cells from apoptosis induced by hyperglycemia, both stable and fluctuating. The effect of thenoyltrifluoroacetone, a specific antioxidant, active at the mitochondrial level in normalizing apoptosis, as well as nitrotyrosine and 8-OHdG, was equivalent to those of both SOD and MnTBAP, suggesting therefore that an overproduction of free radicals at the mitochondrial level is the mediator of the pro-apoptotic effect of hyperglycemia, stable or oscillating.

The fact that a specific mitochondrial oxidative stress inhibitor achieves the same results suggests that the major source of ROS inside the cell, due to high glucose exposure, is the mitochondrial electron transport chain. To be specific, thenoyltrifluoroacetone selectively inhibits mitochondrial complex II activity (Piconi, Quagliaro, Assaloni et al. 2006).

The overproduction of superoxide at the mitochondrial level emerges as a unifying explanation of the hyperglycemia-related diabetic complications, and there is confirmation that this pathway damages the retina (Du, Miller, and Kern. 2003) and β-cells (Krauss, Zhang, Scorrano et al. 2003) when exposed to high glucose.

2.5.3 SHOULD MINIMAL BLOOD GLUCOSE VARIABILITY BECOME THE GOLD STANDARD OF GLYCEMIC CONTROL?

There is considerable evidence that in diabetes, the major source of damage is the rapid variation of blood glucose linked to the postprandial state (Hirsch, and Brownlee. 2005), and the authors concluded that hyperglycemia stimulates antioxidant enzyme synthesis (Ceriello, Morocutti, Mercuri et al. 2000) and that the decreased capacity of diabetic patients to respond to those repeated insults is tightly related to the onset of diabetic complications (Kesavulu, Giri, Kameswara Rao et al. 2000; Carmeli, Coleman, and Berner. 2004).

The authors concluded that exposing endothelial and retinal cells to high oscillating glucose levels jeopardizes the antioxidant response of the cells and increases levels of oxidative stress markers, leading to higher cell damage and apoptosis than exposure to high constant glucose: hyperglycemia, both stable and oscillating, increases endothelial cell apoptosis through ROS overproduction at the mitochondrial electron transport chain. Endothelial cell damage plays an important role in the pathogenesis of diabetic complication. Therefore, the prevention of mitochondrial oxidative damage seems to be a future important therapeutic strategy in diabetes (Piconi, Quagliaro, Assaloni et al. 2006).

2.5.4 STATINS IMPROVE ENDOTHELIUM FUNCTION INDEPENDENT OF LOWERING CHOLESTEROL

The effect of lipid-lowering agents on endothelial function in diabetes is still not clear (Calles-Escandon, and Cipolla. 2001). However, there is ample evidence that statins are anti-inflammatory and that they are beneficial in preventing plaque formation (Antonopoulos, Margaritis, Lee et al. 2012). Furthermore, as reported in the journal *Vascular Pharmacology*, for instance, there is also substantial evidence that the vascular effects of statins are independent of cholesterol lowering and that they appear to involve directly restoring or improving endothelial function by increasing NO production, promoting restoration of endothelium after arterial blood vessel injury, and inhibiting inflammatory responses within the vessel wall (Ii, and Losordo. 2007).

It was reported also in the journal *Current Vascular Pharmacology* that the preventive aspect of statins is not solely attributed to cholesterol lowering, but also to various effects on the vascular wall, which include improved endothelial function. Improvement in arterial stiffness (see below) by the antioxidant and anti-inflammatory effects of statin therapy has been demonstrated in patients with or without hypercholesterolemia (Dilaveris, Giannopoulos, Riga et al. 2007).

2.5.5 GLUCAGON-LIKE PEPTIDE-1

A study published in the *American Journal of Physiology - Endocrinology and Metabolism* aimed to determine the effects of another approach to treatment of Type 2 diabetes, glucagon-like peptide-1 (GLP-1), on endothelial function and insulin sensitivity in two groups: Type 2 diabetes patients with stable coronary artery disease and healthy participants with normal endothelial function and insulin sensitivity. GLP-1 enhances the secretion of insulin. It is a product of a polypeptide that splits to produce many hormones including glucagon.

Patients underwent infusion of recombinant GLP-1, and healthy participants received saline. Endothelial function was measured by FMD ultrasonography of the brachial artery.

In Type 2 diabetic patients, GLP-1 infusion significantly increased relative changes in brachial artery diameter from baseline FMD, with no significant effects on insulin sensitivity. In healthy participants, GLP-1 infusion affected neither FMD nor insulin sensitivity.

The authors concluded that GLP-1 reduces endothelial dysfunction but not insulin resistance in Type 2 diabetic patients with coronary heart disease (Nyström, Gutniak, Zhang et al. 2004).

The small sample of clinical and research publications cited above merely reflects the considerable number of such reports now that support the contention that Type 2 diabetes causes endothelial dysfunction *via* cellular damage caused by ROS. If that is correct, then the next question concerns the cellular target of the ROS generated by the diabetes.

One clue comes from a report in the journal *Experimental Diabetes Research*. The authors contend that there is evidence that endoplasmic reticulum stress in the endothelium cells caused by free radicals might be an important contributor to diabetes-related vascular complications (Basha, Samuel, Triggle et al. 2012).

2.5.6 ENDOTHELIAL DYSFUNCTION VIA STRESSED ENDOPLASMIC RETICULUM

The endoplasmic reticulum is an organelle in the cell nucleus—there are two actually, one smooth, and the other one, rough. The rough endoplasmic reticulum, depending on the cell type in a given organ tissue, is involved in the production (termed folding) and quality control of some proteins including hemoglobin. The smooth endoplasmic reticulum is involved in the production of lipids, steroid hormones, and detoxification, as well as the release of calcium ions.

Alterations in protein-folding in the endoplasmic reticulum cause accumulation of improperly structured (misfolded) proteins that profoundly affect cellular signaling processes, including reduction–oxidation (redox) homeostasis, energy production, inflammation, differentiation, and apoptosis. The *unfolded protein response* is a set of signaling pathways that resolve protein misfolding and restore an efficient protein-folding environment.

Production of ROS has been linked to endoplasmic reticulum stress that is thought to play a critical role in many cellular processes and can be produced in the aqueous component of the cytoplasm of a cell where organelles and particles are suspended (cytosol) as well as the endoplasmic reticulum and mitochondria. It is suggested that altered redox homeostasis in the endoplasmic reticulum is sufficient to cause stress, which could, in turn, induce the production of ROS in the endoplasmic reticulum and mitochondria.

However, it is unclear how changes in the protein-folding environment in the endoplasmic reticulum cause oxidative stress or how ROS production and protein misfolding cause apoptosis of the cell, or how this process contributes to various degenerative diseases (Cao, and Kaufman. 2014).

A report in the journal *Diabetes Care* tells us that Type 2 diabetes is characterized by a two- to fourfold increased risk of cardiovascular disease generally attributed to the adverse effects of hyperglycemia causing oxidative stress in blood vessels. It has also been shown that even patients with prediabetic conditions, including impaired fasting glucose and impaired glucose tolerance, are at increased risk of cardiovascular disease as well (Kirpichnikov, and Sowers. 2001). This suggests that abnormalities in carbohydrate metabolism progressively worsen cardiovascular health.

The first step of the adverse events in plaque formation is endothelial dysfunction (Avogaro, Fadini, Gallo et al. 2006). Endothelial cells form mediators that can alternatively effect either vasoconstriction (via endothelin-1 and thromboxane A2) or vasodilation (NO). In patients with diabetes, endothelial dysfunction is a consistent finding and it seems that hyperglycemia and diabetes lead to an impairment of NO production and activity.

2.5.7 Diabetes Impairs Endothelium Self-Repair

The endothelium has a limited ability to self-repair because it consists of terminally differentiated cells with a low potential for proliferation. That is why endothelial repair is accomplished through the contribution of circulating cells termed "endothelial progenitor cells" (EPCs). Diabetes impairs all the steps of EPC mobilization and function.

This process is graphically detailed in Fadini, Sartore, Agostini et al. (2007) in their Figure 1, *The contribution of EPCs in the setting of endothelial damage and angiogenesis*, and their Figure 2, *Diabetes impairs all the steps of EPC mobilization and function*, that can be accessed at http://care.diabetesjournals.org/content/30/5/1305.

2.6 ANTIDIABETIC TREATMENT (METFORMIN) IMPROVES ENDOTHELIAL WOUND HEALING

A number of studies have proposed that treatment of diabetes may hinge on targeting EPCs. A study published in *PLoS ONE* found that mobilization of EPCs is impaired in mice with induced diabetes (Westerweel, Teraa, Rafii et al. 2013). But a study, also employing mice, published in the journal *Cardiovascular Diabetology*, determined that metformin could accelerate wound healing by improving their impaired EPC functions.

The study reported that metformin accelerated wound closure and stimulated formation of new blood vessels (angiogenesis), and the number of circulating progenitor cells increased significantly in the metformin-treated diabetic mice.

Metformin enhanced NO production in the progenitor cells of the diabetic mice, and *in vitro*, it also improved impaired cell functions and increased NO production (Yu, Deng, Han et al. 2016).

It has been suggested that metformin works by improving hyperglycemia by suppressing hepatic glucose production and increasing glucose uptake in muscle. However, recent studies have suggested that it also has a direct anti-inflammatory action in addition to improving chronic inflammation through the improvement of metabolic parameters such as hyperglycemia, insulin resistance, and atherogenic dyslipidemia (Saisho. 2015).

2.7   DIABETES AND MITOCHONDRIA DYSFUNCTION

The journal *Frontiers in Physiology* reported that mitochondrial dysfunction in vascular endothelial cells is an important aspect of hyperglycemic damage (Kizhakekuttu, Wang, Dharmashankar et al. 2012). Mitochondria are organelles that function as the power generators of the cell, converting oxygen and nutrients into adenosine triphosphate, the chemical energy that powers cell metabolism.

In Type 2 diabetes patients, mitochondrial function is impaired as evidenced by lower mitochondrial O_2 consumption and higher ROS production (Hernandez-Mijares, Rocha, Rovira-Llopis et al. 2013). Hyperglycemia-induced increase in the production of ROS in endothelial cells has been implicated in glucose-mediated vascular damage (Nishikawa, Edelstein, Du et al. 2000; Brownlee. 2001; Du, Matsumura, Edelstein et al. 2003).

In addition, elevated glucose concentration leads to oxidative stress that favors apoptosis in several endothelial cell types, and metformin actually prevents this cell death. So say the investigators of a study published in the journal *Diabetes* who proposed that metformin improves diabetes-associated vascular disease by lowering blood glucose (Detaille, Guigas, Chauvin et al. 2005).

There is strong evidence that mitochondria are intimately involved in hyperglycemia-induced endothelial dysfunction in at least three different ways: ROS production, apoptosis, and damage memory.

Hyperglycemia upregulates the production of ROS and inhibits activity of the endothelial ROS buffering system, which leads to damage of DNA and other mitochondrial components that are important for normal endothelial function. In addition, the balance between anti- and pro-apoptotic pathways is altered. However, it is still not known how mitochondria-mediated endothelial dysfunction contributes to secondary vascular diseases, such as atherosclerosis (Tang, Luo, Chen et al. 2014).

This conclusion is also supported by a report in the *Journal of Smooth Muscle Research* that there is increasing evidence that mitochondrial morphological and functional changes are implicated in vascular endothelial dysfunction. Abnormal mitochondrial biogenesis and disturbance of mitochondrial autophagy (controlled self-digestion) increase the accumulation of damaged mitochondria, such as irreversibly depolarized or leaky mitochondria, and facilitate cell death.

Augmented mitochondrial ROS production and Ca^{2+} overload in mitochondria not only cause the maladaptive effect on the endothelial function but also are potentially detrimental to cell survival (Pangare, and Makino. 2012).

2.7.1   "OBESITY AND INACTIVITY" THEORY OF MITOCHONDRIAL DYSFUNCTION IN DIABETES

Mitochondria play a major role in fuel utilization and energy production; therefore, their disordered function at the cellular level can affect whole-body metabolic homeostasis. A report in the journal *Endocrine Reviews* proposes that the association of diabetes with obesity and inactivity indicates an important and potentially pathogenic link between fuel and energy homeostasis and the emergence of metabolic disease.

The authors propose a hypothesis that defective mitochondrial function might play a potentially pathogenic role in mediating risk of Type 2 diabetes. They review previous studies on metabolic phenotypes of existing animal models of impaired mitochondrial function and conclude that genetically determined and/or inactivity-mediated alterations in mitochondrial oxidative activity may directly affect adaptive responses to overnutrition, causing an imbalance between oxidative activity and nutrient load. This imbalance may lead in turn to chronic accumulation of lipid oxidative metabolites that can mediate insulin resistance and secretory dysfunction (Patti, and Corvera. 2010).

2.7.2 AN AGING MITOCHONDRION IS A FAT MITOCHONDRION

A report in the journal *Science* attributes insulin resistance in Type 2 diabetes to aging. The investigators studied healthy, lean, elderly, and young participants matched for lean body mass and fat mass and found that elderly participants were markedly insulin-resistant, as compared to young control participants, and this resistance was found to be attributable to reduced insulin-stimulated muscle glucose metabolism.

It was also found that these changes were associated with increased fat accumulation in muscle and liver tissue and with an approximately 40% reduction in mitochondrial oxidative activity (Petersen, Befroy, Dufour et al. 2003).

2.8 WHAT KIND OF "VESSELS" ARE BLOOD VESSELS?

The term "vessel" conjures images of hollow containers, perhaps jugs that hold fixed quantities of material, usually liquid, in a fixed volume, or it could mean a tubular shape that conducts fluids. These can be considered *passive* because neither type can alter its shape to accomplish any end. Of course, some are flexible and can be made to alter shape by increasing or decreasing the inside pressure on its walls, but even in this case, the vessel is passive. In any event, it is not intended in the fabrication of such vessels that they be *active* and be able to alter their shape. It is rather intended that, if all goes well, their shape remains unchanged.

By that definition of "vessels" then, blood vessels are not vessels. They are conduits, of course, but they are conduits contrived in such a manner that they participate actively in conducting fluid that courses through them, and their participation is not simply a matter of expanding or constricting to alter blood flow and pressure. They appear to have active pulsatile, wave-like, rhythmic forward motion—something like *peristalsis*—that propels forward the fluid that is being conducted, quite separate from the blood expelled by the heart in bursts.

The complex of blood vessels in the body functions, metaphorically, as a second heart also actively propelling blood in circulation. It is inconceivable that the force of the blood expelled by the left heart into what would be close to 60,000 miles of blood vessels were they stretched out—some with a "resting" lumen diameter less than that of a red blood cell (ca. 6 to 8 μm)—could account for circulation with the typical systolic blood pressure (SBP).

This motion of blood can be observed in the early-stage development of the chick embryo, for instance, when blood flow can be clearly seen to be a pulsating flow in the chorioallantoic membrane surrounding the embryo—absent any evidence of anything resembling a heart (first author personal observation). The pulsating electrochemical signals, source unknown, that produces this wave motion may well be the precursors of heart "action," but they are quite distinct from conventional adult arterial electrophysiology, which also has an amplitude modulated spectrum (first author personal observation).

A principle of cardiovascular function that is generally underestimated is that the way that blood circulates is as important to heart function as heart function is to the way that blood circulates. Therefore, it stands to reason that the adverse effect of diabetes on blood vessels would also alter the basic function of the heart proper.

The journal *Biomechanics and Modeling in Mechanobiology* reports that "[the] Function of the heart is essential for embryo survival, and thus the heart starts beating and pumping blood early in embryogenesis when it is still a linear tube with no valves or chambers. As such, key morphogenetic changes which transform the heart from a straight tube into a complex, multichambered structure all occur under blood flow conditions. Constant interactions between cardiac tissue motion and blood flow dynamics shape the development of the heart. In the absence of blood flow the heart does not develop properly [Hove, Köster, Forouhar et al. 2003] and deviations from normal hemo-dynamic conditions lead to cardiac malformations" (Goenezen, Rennie, and Rugonyi. 2012).

A "straight tube" is not a heart, and this simply misses the point that blood can circulate without a heart, as we understand a heart to be composed of one or more muscle chambers whose sequential contractions propel blood into circulation.

A number of physiological indices of blood vessel function suggest that the "primitive" functions of blood vessels, before the emergence of a heart, are still in some ways functioning in circulation to propel blood through the vascular conduits, and that they are essential to circulation, and that, most importantly, diabetes may adversely affect them.

It should be noted that diabetes affects not only blood vessels but also the heart muscle proper (Boudina and Abel. 2010). However, the means by which diabetes directly affects heart muscle, that is, diabetic cardiomyopathy, is not known (Guha, Harmancey, Taegtmeyer. 2008) and at least one authority attributes it to mitochondrial dysfunction (Duncan. 2011).

2.9 ARTERIAL PULSE WAVE ANALYSIS IN DIABETES

Pulse strength, pulse rate, and temporal pulse pattern are hardly new tools in medical science. Yet, medicine is rediscovering the value of arterial pulse analysis beyond pulse strength, rate, and temporal pattern. In simple terms, the "pulse" is commonly observed as a momentary distention in a segment of an artery wall due to transient blood pressure change consequent on the contraction of the left ventricle of the heart as it ejects blood into the ascending aorta.

This distention is caused by the sudden increase in volume and pressure in the vessel segment that already contained blood, but to which the blood ejected is now added. This momentary distention pulse is then propagated along the circulatory system.

Arterial pulse analysis has long been known as a vital aspect of medical diagnosis in numerous ancient cultures: It is recorded that "Abu Ali placed his hand on the patient's pulse...." Abu Ali Ibn Sina is now better known as Avicenna, a Persian scholar and a prominent physician of the Middle Ages (Niz. 2017). Pulse was studied in China about 2500 years ago. It was first mentioned in the "Internal Medicine Classics, *Nei Ching*," reportedly written by the Yellow Emperor, Huang Ti (698–598 BCE).

The principal means of diagnosis employed in the Nei Ching is the physical examination of the arterial pulse. The theory of the pulse is based on the various stages of interaction between Yin (disease) and Yang (health).

The ancient Chinese physicians developed the ability to judge the state of disease—its cause, duration, and prognosis—by the volume, strength, weakness, regularity, or interruption of the four main varieties of pulse beats (superficial, deep, slow, and quick). The examination was performed on both wrists, and the best time for examination was thought to be early in the morning because that is when Yin and Yang were believed to be in balance.

The physician would judge the pulse rate based on the ratio between the beating pulse and respiration, four beats to one respiration being considered to be normal.

The arterial pulse in ancient China was divided into three parts: inch (the one closest to the hand), cubit (the one further up in the arm), and bar (the one in between). Each of the pulse locations in each arm would represent the condition of two different organs of the body (Ghasemzadeh, and Zafari. 2011).

We can now analyze the pressure-change-induced arterial distention with a device that can measure changes in blood volume in the artery—a plethysmograph—that shows a characteristic pattern of pulse distention that is not readily observable by simply holding fingers above an artery in the wrist, as is common practice: the degree, timing, and temporal pattern of the distention are said to reflect the degree of rigidity or stiffness of the blood vessel as it resists distention by rising pulse pressure. The rise in that degree of stiffness is age-related, and it also indicates cardiovascular and heart health.

Pressure changes, in any readily accessible location, are converted from an analog electric signal emitted by the plethysmograph transducer that rises and falls as it follows pressure changes in the blood vessel at that location. The pattern of blood pressure changes in the pulse is the arterial pulse wave. Unlike the electrocardiograph, the electrical activity of contracting heart muscles, arterial pulse wave (Figure 2.4), is not the electrical activity of the blood vessel proper but an analog of changes in blood volume in the vessel reflecting changes in blood pressure for the duration of the pulse.

Systolic and diastolic pressures are the peak and trough of the waveform. The *augmentation pressure* is the additional pressure added to the forward wave by the reflected wave. *Augmentation index* (AIx) is defined as the augmentation pressure as a percentage of pulse pressure. The *dicrotic notch* represents closing of the aortic valve and is used to calculate ejection duration. Time to reflection is calculated as the time at the onset of the ejected pulse waveform to the onset of the reflected wave (Stoner, Young, and Fryer. 2012).

Systolic pressure and pulse pressure differ between central and peripheral arteries, but there is little regional variation in diastolic pressures within large arteries and conduit arteries. Central augmentation pressure is the height above the first systolic shoulder of the aortic waveform and central AIx is the ratio of augmentation pressure to central pulse pressure. Augmentation pressure is thought to relate to pressure wave reflection (Chowienczyk. 2011).

Arterial pulse waveform analysis is cited here to support understanding its contribution to establishing the effect of diabetes on blood vessels. Of particular interest in connection with hyperglycemia is that ingestion of food, even just a glucose drink, can reduce wave reflection from the splanchnic (visceral) bed and thus alter the contour of the arterial pressure wave, particularly the degree of late systolic augmentation. It is attributed to the action of insulin (Westerbacka, Wilkinson, Cockcroft et al. 1999).

Here are some parameters in connection with this technology:

Pulse wave velocity (PWV) is the speed with which the arterial pulse travels through the circulatory system. It is used clinically as a measure of arterial stiffness. Presumably, arterial stiffness reflects at least the extent of atherosclerosis.

The *augmentation index* is a ratio calculated from the blood pressure waveform; it is a measure of wave reflection and therefore also of arterial stiffness. AIx is commonly accepted as a measure of the enhancement (augmentation) of central aortic pressure by a reflected pulse wave (see Figure 2.5).

In this context, a thorough review of research on blood vessel stiffness can be found in Catalano, Scandale, and Dimitrov et al. (2013).

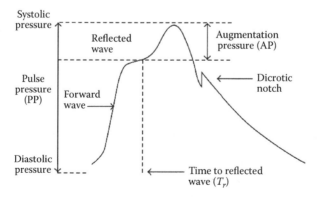

FIGURE 2.4 Arterial pulse pressure waveform. [From Stoner, Young, and Fryer. 2012. *International Journal of Vascular Medicine*, 2012: 903107. With permission.]

2.9.1 Arterial PWV Analysis Improves Observation of Vasodilation

PWV is the speed of the arterial pulse traveling through the circulatory system. Measurement in the past used pressure sensors placed precisely over the carotid artery in the neck and the femoral artery in the groin to measure the speed at which pulse waves travel down the aorta by the duration of the event, given the length it must traverse. Doppler-based methods are now mostly used instead.

2.9.1.1 Quantification and Norms Values of the Arterial PWV

The *European Heart Journal* published a study aimed to determine the PWV parameters in healthy people and in those with cardiovascular risk factors so as to establish *normal* and *reference* values.

The authors report that carotid artery to femoral artery PWV is a "direct" measure of aortic stiffness and is therefore important for total cardiovascular risk estimation. However, they point out that its application as a routine diagnostic tool has been hampered by the lack of reference values. The aim of their study therefore was to establish reference and normal values for PWV based on a large European population.

To that end, they gathered data on PWV and basic clinical parameters from nearly 17,000 volunteer participants and patients from 13 different centers in eight European countries. The reference values population, of which the subset with optimal/normal blood pressures was the normal value population, consisted of ca. 11,000 individuals who were free of overt cardiovascular disease, were nondiabetic, and were not treated by either antihypertensive or lipid-lowering drugs.

Participants were classified by age decade and further subdivided according to blood pressure categories: For normal and reference values, the population was classified according to the following:

- Age decade: <30, 30–39, 40–49, 50–59, 60–69, and ≥70 years
- Blood pressure category reference population only: optimal, that is, <120/80
- Normal blood pressure: ≥120/80
- High normal blood pressure: <130/85
- High normal: ≥130/85 and <140/90
- Grade I hypertension: ≥140/90 and <160/100
- Grade II/III hypertension: ≥160/100 mmHg

Here follows the authors' description of the data compilation and analysis: Transit times were assessed as the time difference between two characteristic points on carotid and femoral waveforms. The characteristic points chosen were dependent on the type of waveform (flow, pressure, or diameter distension) and the algorithm used for detection.

The two most popular algorithms are the intersecting tangent algorithm (SphygmoCor system and for manual identification) and the point of maximal upstroke during systole (as used in the Complior system). However, different algorithms applied on the same waveforms can lead to differences in measured PWV values of 5% to 15%. Since the point of maximal upstroke was shown to underestimate PWV, especially when the rise time of the waveform is low, transit time on the intersecting tangent algorithm was chosen for standardization.

To convert maximal upstroke transit times into the intersecting tangent algorithm, the relationship previously found by Millasseau, Stewart, Patel et al. (2005) was used.

PWV values are also markedly dependent on the carotid–femoral pathway measurement. This pathway can be either the direct distance measured between the carotid and femoral measurement sites or the distance obtained by subtracting the carotid measurement site to sternal notch distance from the sternal notch to femoral measurement site distance. However, differences in path length alone can lead to differences in PWV values of up to 30%. Equations to convert between these path length definitions with good precision were recently published (see Vermeersch, Rietzschel, De Buyzere et al. 2009).

The bulk of the data in the reference value database consists of pulse wave velocities calculated by the direct path length. Subtracted path lengths were therefore standardized into direct path lengths. However, as the use of direct distance (i.e., measured over the body surface) leads to overestimation of real PWV [using magnetic resonance imaging (MRI) or invasive measurements], a scaling factor of 0.8 derived from Sugawara, Hayashi, Yokoi et al. (2008) and Weber, Ammer, Rammer et al. (2009) was used to convert PWV obtained using direct distances to "real" PWV. In the tables, PWV is calculated using the intersecting tangent algorithm and the direct carotid to femoral path length, and then rescaled to "real" PWV.

Their Table 1 is a description of general clinical parameters of the reference value and normal value populations. Their Table 2 shows the number of participants included in each of the age and blood pressure categories in the reference values population.

Their Table 3 is the influence of gender and major cardiovascular risk factors on PWV, before and after adjustment on quadratic age and mean blood pressure.

Diabetic participants and participants treated for hypertension and dyslipidemia had significantly elevated PWV values, compared with untreated participants, even after correction for age and MBP.

Mean blood pressure (MBP) was calculated from SBP and diastolic BP (DBP) as MBP = DBP + 0.4 (SBP − DBP).

Gender, smoking, and lipid status have no independent influence on PWV after correction for quadratic age and BP differences. Therefore, the reference value population was defined as including all untreated (i.e., with no antihypertensive or lipid-lowering agents) nondiabetic participants.

Their Table 4 (Table 2.1) is the distribution of PWV (m/s) according to the age category in the normal values population.

Their Table 5 (Table 2.2) is the distribution of PWV values (m/s) in the reference value population according to age and blood pressure category. PWV increased with increasing age and with blood pressure levels in the reference value population. The increase in PWV with age was more pronounced when blood pressure increased; likewise, the increase in PWV was more pronounced in older participants.

This is the first study to establish reference and normal values for the distribution of PWV changes with age and blood pressure category. Normal values are proposed based on the PWV values observed in the nonhypertensive subpopulation who had no additional cardiovascular risk factors (Mattace-Raso, Hofman, Verwoert et al. 2010; doi: 10.1093/eurheartj/ehq165 PMCID: PMC2948201).

TABLE 2.1

Distribution of Pulse Wave Velocity (m/s) According to the Age Category in the Normal Values Population

Age Category (years)	Mean (±2 SD)	Median (10–90 pc)
<30	6.2 (4.7–7.6)	6.1 (5.3–7.1)
30–90	6.5 (3.8–9.2)	6.4 (5.2–8.0)
40–49	7.2 (4.6–9.8)	6.9 (5.9–8.6)
50–59	8.3 (4.5–9.8)	8.1 (6.3–10.0)
60–69	10.3 (5.5–15.0)	9.7 (7.9–13.1)
≥70	10.9 (5.5–16.3)	10.6 (8.0–14.6)

Source: From Mattace-Raso, Hofman, Verwoert et al. 2010. *European Heart Journal*, Oct; 31(19): 2338–2350. With permission.

TABLE 2.2
Distribution of Pulse Wave Velocity (m/s) According to the Age and Blood Pressure Categories

Age Category (years)	Blood Pressure Category				
PWV as Means (±2 SD)	Optimal	Normal	High Normal	Grade I HT	Grade II/III HT
<30	6.1 (4.6–7.5)	6.6 (4.9–8.2)	6.8 (5.1–8.5)	7.4 (4.6–10.1)	7.7 (4.4–11.0)
30–90	6.6 (4.4–8.9)	6.8 (4.2–9.4)	7.1 (4.5–9.7)	7.3 (4.0–10.7)	8.2 (3.3–13.0)
40–49	7.0 (4.5–9.6)	7.5 (5.1–10.0)	7.9 (5.2–10.7)	8.6 (5.1–12.0)	9.8 (3.8–15.7)
50–59	7.6 (4.8–10.5)	8.4 (5.1–11.7)	8.8 (4.8–12.8)	9.6 (4.9–14.3)	10.5 (4.1–16.8)
60–69	9.1 (5.2–12.9)	9.7 (5.7–13.6)	10.3 (5.5–15.1)	11.1 (6.1–16.2)	12.2 (5.7–18.6)
≥70	10.4 (5.2–15.6)	11.7 (6.0–17.9)	11.8 (5.7–17.9)	12.9 (6.9–18.9)	14.0 (7.4–20.6)

Source: From Mattace-Raso, Hofman, Verwoert et al. 2010. *European Heart Journal*, Oct; 31(19): 2338–2350. With permission.

2.9.2 Characteristics of the Pulse Waveform and PWV in Diabetes

Although there is a considerable amount of clinical and research data on the difference in pulse waveform and PWV between diabetes sufferers and nonsufferers, these indices are rarely featured in common descriptions of signs and symptoms of Type 2 diabetes—even in connection with atherosclerosis. Yet, it is well known that persons with Type 2 diabetes show increased carotid–radial pulse wave velocity (crPWV) and carotid–ankle pulse wave velocity (caPWV) and lower AIx than persons not so afflicted (Zhang, Bai, Ye et al. 2011). This means that persons with Type 2 diabetes have increased stiffness of central elastic arteries, and this signifies the presence of atherosclerosis, and it is actually a health hazard because cardiovascular disease is the primary cause of death in diabetic patients.

Arterial stiffness assessment using pulse wave analysis predicts cardiovascular "events," and for that reason, a systematic review of the current knowledge of links between diabetes and pulse wave analysis was conducted, and it was published in the *Biomedical Papers of the Medical Faculty of the University of Palacky Olomouc, Czech Republic*. It was based largely on a MEDLINE search to retrieve both original and review articles addressing the relations and influences on arterial stiffness in diabetics.

The authors concluded that pulse wave analysis is to be considered a "gold standard" in cardiovascular risk evaluation for patients at risk, especially diabetics. They proposed that arterial stiffness assessment may be helpful for choosing more aggressive diagnostic and therapeutic strategies, particularly in younger patients to reduce the incidence of cardiovascular disease in these patients (Gajdova, Karasek, Goldmannova et al. 2017).

2.9.2.1 The Augmentation Index

The AIx is a ratio calculated from the blood pressure waveform; it is a measure of wave reflection and arterial stiffness. AIx is commonly accepted as a measure of the enhancement (augmentation) of central aortic pressure by a reflected pulse wave, and it is a sensitive marker of arterial status.

AIx has been shown to be a predictor of adverse cardiovascular events in a variety of patient populations: higher AIx is associated with target organ damage (Shimizu, and Kario. 2008), and it can also distinguish between the effects of different vasoactive medications, whereas upper arm blood pressure and PWV do not (Boutouyrie, Achouba, Trunet et al. 2010).

Conventionally, the assessments of endothelial function and arterial stiffness require different sets of equipment, making the inclusion of both tests impractical for clinical and epidemiological studies. Pulse wave analysis provides useful information regarding the mechanical properties of the *arterial tree* and can also be used to assess endothelial function. It is a simple, valid, reliable, and

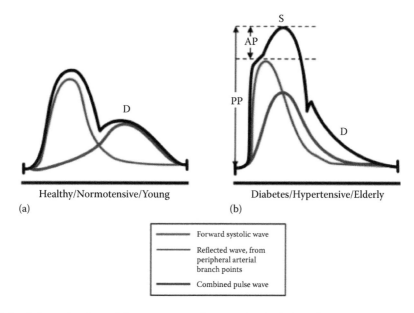

FIGURE 2.5 Schematic of arterial pressure waveforms and calculation of augmentation index. (a) Pulse waveforms in healthy compliant vasculature, timing of rebound wave reflection occurs during diastole (D). (b) Pulse wave reflection is faster and earlier in stiffer arteries, thus amplifying the measured systolic BP peak (S), and reducing diastolic pressures (D), hence pulse pressure (PP) is increased (total height of combined pulse wave peak). AP, augmentation pressure. [From Kum, and Karalliedde. 2010. *Integrated Blood Pressure Control*, Jun; 3: 63–71. With permission.]

inexpensive technique, offering great clinical and epidemiological potential (Stoner, Young, and Fryer. 2012).

A stylized version of arterial pressure waveforms is shown in Figure 2.5, illustrating a sample of waveforms reflecting health or disease.

2.9.3 Diabetes and NO Regulation of Blood Vessels

In studies cited above, there was considerable support for linking abnormal pulse waveform and velocity to attenuated blood vessel flexibility thought to be due to atherosclerosis. Since atherosclerosis has also previously been shown to impair endothelium-derived NO formation, the evidence points again to the conclusion that diabetes affects blood vessel distensibility by promoting atherosclerosis. Thus, we may see diabetes in those who show abnormal blood vessel distensibility presenting as atherosclerosis, without attributing the latter to the former... but the former to the latter.

In a report published in the journal *Circulation*, the investigators first reiterated the hypothesis that NO acting locally regulates arterial distensibility *in vivo*, and the aim of this experiment was to test this hypothesis in an animal model (sheep).

PWV was calculated by the foot-to-foot methodology in anesthetized subjects. Intra-arterial infusion of NG-monomethyl-L-arginine (L-NMMA) increased iliac PWV significantly. L-NMMA is a NOS inhibitor. Infusion of acetylcholine and glyceryl trinitrate reduced PWV significantly; glyceryl trinitrate is nitroglycerin and it promotes vasodilation via NO formation. Only the effect of acetylcholine, however, was significantly inhibited during co-infusion of NG-monomethyl-L-arginine. There was no change in systemic arterial pressure throughout the studies.

The investigators concluded that basal NO production influences large-artery distensibility. In addition, exogenous acetylcholine and glyceryl trinitrate both increase arterial distensibility, the former mainly through NO production. This may help explain why conditions that exhibit endothelial dysfunction are also associated with increased arterial stiffness (Wilkinson, Qasem, McEniery et al. 2002).

It stands to reason therefore that pulse waveform and velocity reflect endothelial function and, thus, NO formation and availability, and it is therefore also not surprising to find abnormal pulse waveform and velocity in diabetes and atherosclerosis.

A study published in the *British Journal of Clinical Pharmacology* reported that incremental doses of the NOS inhibitor L-NG-monomethyl arginine or placebo were infused in eight healthy men. Arterial stiffness was assessed noninvasively by pulse wave analysis.

It was shown that infusion of L-NMMA led to a dose-dependent increase in mean arterial pressure, peripheral vascular resistance, and aortic and systemic arterial stiffness compared to placebo. There was an accompanying reduction in heart rate and cardiac index.

Of note is that the highest dose of L-NMMA resulted in an increase of 25% in AIx compared with infusion of saline (Wilkinson, MacCallum, Cockcroft et al. 2002). Similarly, a study in the journal *Hypertension* the following year aimed to determine the effects of the same NOS inhibitor, NG-monomethyl-L-arginine, on carotid–femoral PWV (cfPWV) and aortic AIx as an indirect measure of arterial stiffness.

The authors reported that L-NMMA and norepinephrine increased mean arterial blood pressure by 7.8 ± 1.7 mm Hg and 9.7 ± 2.1 mm Hg, respectively, and increased PWV by 0.7 ± 0.2 ms and 1.0 ± 0.3 ms. Dobutamine, at doses that produced a similar increase in mean arterial blood pressure (9.6 ± 2.9 mm Hg), increased mean PWV by 0.8 ± 0.2 ms. Changes in PWV caused by the three pressor agents were closely correlated with changes in mean arterial blood pressure. L-NMMA and norepinephrine increased AIx, but dobutamine decreased it. Dobutamine increases the strength of muscle contraction.

The investigators concluded that the effects of inhibition of basal NO release on cfPWV were explained by the change in mean arterial blood pressure that this causes, rather than any specific effect of NO inhibition within the aorta (Stewart, Millasseau, Kearney et al. 2003).

The authors of a report in the journal *Clinical Science* (London) pointed out that, traditionally, NO endothelium-mediated alteration in blood vessel tone has been inferred from changes in flow, in response to physical and pharmacological interventions using plethysmographic or ultrasonic techniques. However, alteration in pulsatile arterial function may represent a more sensitive measure to detect and monitor NO-mediated modulation of arterial smooth muscle tone, as noted above.

To test this hypothesis, male volunteers had radial artery pressure pulse waveforms recorded using a calibrated tonometer device. A tonometer measures pressure, and it was originally developed to measure intra-ocular pressure. A computer-based assessment of the diastolic pressure decay quantified the changes in arterial waveform morphology of altered pulsatile (arterial compliance) and steady-state (peripheral resistance) hemodynamics.

The volunteers were infused intravenously with N(G)-nitro-L-arginine methyl ester (L-NAME), a stereo-specific inhibitor of NO synthesis, in incrementally increasing doses for 8 min each. The volunteers then received either L-arginine or D-arginine intravenously in a "blind" control fashion.

On a separate day, radial artery pressure pulse waveforms were recorded before and after the sublingual administration of glyceryl trinitrate, an exogenous NO donor.

It was found that cardiac output and heart rate decreased and mean arterial blood pressure increased significantly in response to the incremental intravenous infusion of L-NAME, a nonselective inhibitor of NOS. Small artery compliance decreased, whereas systemic vascular resistance increased in response to NO synthesis inhibition.

The intravenous infusion of L-arginine restored the pulsatile and steady-state hemodynamic parameters to pretreatment values, whereas D-arginine had no effect. Sublingual glyceryl trinitrate, a NO donor, decreased systemic vascular resistance, whereas large artery and small artery compliance increased.

The authors concluded that pressure pulse contour analysis represents a sensitive and convenient technique capable of tracking changes in the pulsatile function of arteries accompanying NO-mediated alteration in arterial smooth muscle tone (McVeigh, Allen, Morgan et al. 2001).

Since these studies established the validity of arterial pulse wave analysis in observing NO endothelium-mediated vasodilation, it therefore supports its use in evaluating the effects of hyperglycemia on endothelial function since Type 2 diabetes is shown to impair endothelial NO formation.

2.9.4 Clinical Correlates of Arterial Pulse Waveform and Velocity in Type 2 Diabetes

Clinical application of pulse wave analysis in diabetes yields some rather striking findings. For instance, a study published in the journal *Circulation* aimed to determine whether aortic PWV (AoPWV) predicts cardiovascular and all-cause mortality in Type 2 diabetes and glucose-tolerance-tested multiethnic population samples.

A multiethnic sample of participants from a Type 2 diabetes outpatient clinic and nondiabetic control participants from primary care registers were given a GGT.

Brachial blood pressures and Doppler-derived AoPWV were measured. Mortality data over a 10-year follow-up were obtained.

At any level of SBP, AoPWV was greater in participants with diabetes than in controls. Mortality risk doubled in participants with diabetes (hazard ratio = 2.34) and in those with glucose intolerance (hazard ratio = 2.12) compared to controls.

For all groups combined, age, sex, and SBP predicted mortality; the addition of PWV independently predicted all-cause and cardiovascular mortality (hazard ratio = 1.08 to 1.14 for each 1 m/s increase) but displaced SBP. Glucose tolerance status and smoking were other independent contributors, with African-Caribbeans experiencing reduced mortality risk (hazard ratio = 0.41 to 0.69).

It was concluded that AoPWV is a powerful independent predictor of mortality in both diabetes and GTT populations. In displacing SBP as a prognostic factor, AoPWV is probably further along the causal pathway for arterial disease and may represent a useful integrated index of vascular status and hence cardiovascular risk (Cruickshank, Riste, Anderson et al. 2002).

Aortic stiffness reflects vascular aging and it may predict outcome in diabetes as well. In this study published in the journal *Diabetologia*, the investigators relied on cfPWV to determine the association between fasting glucose, post-challenge glucose, and derived insulin resistance (HOMA-IR) with aortic stiffness. HOMA-IR, the homeostatic model assessment (HOMA) is a method for assessing β-cell function and insulin resistance (IR) from basal (fasting) glucose and insulin or C-peptide concentrations.

cfPWV was measured with a Doppler ultrasound probe in groups; half were men and the other half were women, with newly identified age- and sex-matched normal glucose metabolism (NGM), impaired glucose regulation (IGR) and diabetes populations. Their average age was ca. 59.

It was found that IGR and diabetes were associated with significant aortic stiffening compared with NGM (adjusted cfPWV: NGM = 9.15 m/s; IGR = 9.76 m/s; diabetes = 9.89 m/s).

IGR stratification indicated that the cfPWV in people with impaired fasting glucose (IFG = PWV 9.71 m/s) was similar to that of people with post-challenge impaired glucose tolerance (PWV = 9.82 m/s). Modeled predictors of cfPWV were used to assess independent metabolic associations with arterial stiffness.

Fasting glucose concentration, 2-h post-challenge glucose, and HOMA-IR were independently related to cfPWV after adjustment for age, sex, mean arterial pressure, heart rate, body mass index, renal function, and antihypertensive medication.

The authors concluded that IGR characterized by fasting or post-challenge hyperglycemia is associated with significant vascular stiffening. Post-challenge glucose and HOMA-IR were the most powerful metabolic predictors of arterial stiffness, implying that hyperglycemic excursion and insulin resistance play important roles in the pathogenesis of arteriosclerosis (Webb, Khunti, Silverman et al. 2010).

The journal *Cardiovascular Diabetology* reported a study that concluded that evaluation of brachial–ankle PWV (baPWV), in addition to carotid intima-media thickness and conventional risk factors, improved the ability to identify the diabetic individuals with high risk for cardiovascular events (Katakami, Osonoi, Takahara et al. 2014).

The *Journal of the American Society of Nephrology* reported a study concerned with the fact that development of microalbuminuria raises the risk for cardiovascular disease in Type 2 diabetes. It is not known why, but it is thought that it may involve arterial stiffness, an independent risk marker for cardiovascular disease mortality.

To determine the nature of this confluence, AoPWV and albumin/creatinine ratio were measured in patients with Type 2 diabetes without overt renal impairment (serum creatinine less than 150 μmol/L). Albumin/creatinine ratio ranged from 0.2 to 153 mg/mmol.

Patients with higher albumin/creatinine ratio (greater than or equal to 3 mg/mmol) had higher AoPWV, poorer diabetic control, and higher pulse pressure and SBP than those with normal albumin/creatinine ratio.

The closest associations of AoPWV were with rising age, duration of diabetes, SBP, higher pulse pressure, albumin/creatinine ratio, and insulin treatment, and it was inversely associated with glomerular filtration rate and weight.

The significant predictors of AoPWV were age, SBP or higher pulse pressure, duration of diabetes, gender, number of antihypertensive medications, and use of angiotensin-converting enzyme inhibitors or angiotensin receptor blockers, which together explained 55% of the "variance" of AoPWV.

When albumin/creatinine ratio was substituted for arterial pressure in a separate model, it became a significant predictor of AoPWV. After age adjustment, patients with lower, below median glomerular filtration rate had higher AoPWV than those with glomerular filtration rate above the median.

In patients with Type 2 diabetes without overt renal impairment, raised albumin/creatinine ratio is associated with higher AoPWV, a relationship most likely mediated by raised blood pressure. The authors concluded that the observed link of AoPWV to reduced glomerular filtration rate suggests that even modest renal dysfunction may affect the viscoelastic properties of large arteries (Smith, Karalliedde, De Angelis et al. 2005).

The journal *Cardiovascular Diabetology* reported a study that aimed to determine the clinical difference between PWV and AIx in diabetic retinopathy. Patients with Type 2 diabetes were tested for both AIx and baPWV.

It was found that baPWV was significantly higher in patients with diabetic retinopathy than in individuals without the disease (20.13 ± 3.66 m/s vs.17.14 ± 3.60 m/s). However, AIx was not significantly higher in patients with diabetic retinopathy (19.5 ± 15.2 vs. 14.8 ± 20). The association between AIx and diabetic retinopathy was not found to be statistically significant.

The authors concluded that baPWV is associated with diabetic retinopathy, whereas AIx is not. There appears to be a difference between PWV and AIx in patients with diabetes (Ogawa, Hiraoka, Watanabe et al. 2008). Neither the pathophysiology underlying that difference nor the clinical significance of that difference was explained.

2.9.4.1 Windkessel and Diabetes

The Windkessel (air chamber) effect is an elastic reservoir model of the shape of arterial blood pressure waveform as an interaction between stroke volume and the compliance of the aorta and large elastic arteries. The walls of large elastic arteries contain elastic fibers that distend when the blood pressure rises during systole and recoil when the blood pressure falls during diastole. Since the rate of blood entering these elastic arteries exceeds that leaving them due to the peripheral resistance, there is a net storage of blood during systole that discharges during diastole.

The Windkessel effect is the damping of the fluctuation in blood pressure over the cardiac cycle and the maintenance of organ perfusion during diastole when cardiac ejection ceases.

The Windkessel effect diminishes with age as the elastic arteries become less compliant due most often to atherosclerosis. The reduction in the Windkessel effect results in increased pulse pressure and elevated systolic pressure for a given stroke volume.

The Windkessel model was featured in a study of "Vascular abnormalities in non-insulin-dependent diabetes mellitus identified by arterial waveform analysis" appearing in the *American Journal of Medicine*.

Intra-arterial branchial artery waveforms were analyzed in patients with non-insulin-dependent diabetes and in control participants matched for age and gender. The investigators employed a computer-based assessment of the diastolic pressure decay and a modified Windkessel model of the circulation to quantify changes in arterial waveform focused on large-artery compliance (C1), the oscillatory diastolic waveform (C2), inertance, and systemic resistance. *Inertance* is a measure of the pressure difference in a fluid required to cause a unit change in the rate of change of volumetric flow rate with time.

It was found that there was no difference in heart rate, mean arterial blood pressure, cardiac output, or stroke volume between the two groups. However, the mean oscillatory arterial compliance estimate was significantly reduced in diabetic patients as compared to the control participants. Oscillatory compliance values were uniformly reduced in the diabetic patients regardless of the presence or absence of physical complications of the disease. The AIx and the "oscillatory" compliance (C2) are wave contour analysis parameters for the central aorta (Pao) and radial artery pressure wave (Prad), respectively. Both are sensitive to cardiovascular risk factors such as aging, hypertension, and diabetes and have been proposed as prognostic markers for cardiovascular disease (Segers, Qasem, De Backer et al. 2001).

No differences in large-artery compliance, inertance, or systemic resistance were found between groups. No positive correlations were found between indices of glycemic control, the known duration of diabetes, and any of the hemodynamic variables.

It was concluded that quantitative changes in the arterial pressure pulse waveform, reflected by a reduced oscillatory compliance estimate, were found in patients with Type 2 diabetes. This estimate may be an early marker for the vascular abnormalities associated with diabetes before complications of the disease become clinically apparent. By contrast, no changes in large-artery compliance were found in this patient population free from clinically obvious macrovascular disease (McVeigh, Brennan, Hayes et al. 1993).

2.9.5 DIABETES AND THE RISK OF STROKE

From 1965 to 1968, the Honolulu Heart Program followed a cohort of men in a prospective study of cardiovascular disease. From 1965 to 1968, the Honolulu Heart Program followed a cohort of men in a prospective study of cardiovascular disease. The investigators reported examining the 12-year risk of stroke in a sample of diabetic and nondiabetic participants free of coronary heart disease or stroke when the study began.

In 12 years of follow-up, 62.3 per 1000 diabetic men and 32.7 per 1000 nondiabetic men experienced a stroke. The relative risk of thromboembolic stroke for those with diabetes compared with those without diabetes was $\simeq 2.0$.

Although diabetes was usually associated with an atherogenic risk profile, control of hypertension, complicating myocardial infarction, other risk factors failed to diminish the effect of diabetes on stroke: Among those without diabetes, the relative risk of thromboembolic stroke for those at the 80th percentile of serum glucose level compared with those at the 20th percentile was 1.4. In the nondiabetic sample, the relative risk of thromboembolic stroke for those with glucosuria compared with those without glucosuria was 2.7. There was no statistical association between diabetes, or measures of glucose intolerance, and hemorrhagic stroke.

The authors concluded that diabetes, even in a possibly undiagnosed subset of hyperglycemic individuals, confers an additional independent risk of stroke unexplained by clinically measured risk factors (Abbott, Donahue, MacMahon et al. 1987).

Cerebral white matter lesions (WMLs) are associated with an increased risk of stroke.

It is thought that arterial stiffness in patients with Type 2 diabetes may be associated with WMLs.

A study in the journal *Diabetes* reports that cerebral white matter hyperintensities are common in older people and they correlate with cognitive decline and vascular risk factors. Their presence can be identified by MRI and graded qualitatively with the Breteler scale (Wardlaw, Ferguson, and Graham. 2004). In patients with well-controlled Type 2 diabetes, PWV was found to be higher than that in control participants and was independently associated with WMLs.

PWV may represent a clinically relevant parameter in the evaluation of cerebrovascular disease risk in Type 2 diabetes (Schmidt, Launer, Nilsson 2004; Laugesen, Hoyem, Stausbol-Gron et al. 2013).

2.9.6 ADVANCED GLYCATION END PRODUCTS AND BLOOD VESSEL STIFFNESS IN DIABETES

Advanced glycation end products (AGEs) are proteins or lipids that become glycated with exposure to sugars. They can be a factor in aging and in the development of chronic inflammation and the worsening of many diseases, such as diabetes, atherosclerosis, cardiovascular and heart disease, and chronic kidney disease.

Some foods in the common diet have a high potential for resulting in AGEs while other foods have a low potential. For instance:

- Protein-rich foods such as red meat and cheese tend to have the most. In descending order, chicken, fish, eggs, and legumes have less.
- Grains such as boiled grains (e.g., rice and oatmeal) and sandwich breads are low in AGEs. When grains are processed into crispy brown crackers or fatty cookies and sweetened with sugars, however, their AGE content can soar.
- Dairy including milk and yogurt are low in AGEs, but when moisture is removed and fat is concentrated (as in cream, butter, and cheese), the AGE content rises dramatically.
- Vegetable fats tend to have fewer AGEs than animal fats.

According to a report in the *Korean Journal of Physiology and Pharmacology*, protein glycation and formation of AGEs play an important role in diabetic complications like retinopathy, nephropathy, neuropathy, cardiomyopathy, osteoporosis, and aging. AGEs contribute to the development of diabetic complications by their release of pro-inflammatory free radicals (Singh, Bali, Singh et al. 2014).

The *American Journal of Hypertension* reported a study aimed to determine whether elevated serum AGEs are associated with increased arterial stiffness in relatively healthy, community-dwelling adults. The investigators observed AoPWV, an index of aortic stiffness, and serum AGEs, as represented by the specific AGE serum carboxymethyl-lysine, in adults aged 26 to 93 years old.

They reported that elevated AGEs are associated with increased arterial stiffness, a known predictor of adverse cardiovascular outcomes, among relatively healthy community-dwelling adults (Semba, Najjar, Sun et al. 2009).

AGEs is described in greater detail in Chapter 7.

2.9.6.1 Arterial Pulse Waveform, AIx, and Diabetes

The AIx is a measure of the enhancement (augmentation) of central aortic blood pressure by a reflected pulse wave (see Figure 2.5). According to the *Journal of the American College of Cardiology*, it represents degree of arterial stiffness, and it rises with degree of atherosclerosis and diabetes and with age (Wilhelm, Klein, Friedrich et al. 2007).

Arterial augmentation and the AIx reflect arterial stiffness and are commonly used as predictors of cardiovascular risk. Investigators reported in the *Journal of the American College of Cardiology* that arterial augmentation increases in patients with diabetes and in those with cardiovascular disease without diabetes, but not in healthy control participants. Moreover, AIx was higher in cardiovascular patients than in healthy controls participants. This is an outline of their study:

The aim of their study was to compare parameters in diabetic patients and nondiabetic cardiovascular risk patients to those in healthy control participants. There were nonsmoking participants between 35 and 70 years old, including those with cardiovascular disease but not diabetes, those with Type 2 diabetes, and healthy control participants.

Arterial stiffness was measured by the difference between the second and the first systolic peak of the central pressure waveform, and the arterial AIx was calculated as the percentage of AIx from pulse pressure (Wilkinson, Prasad, Hall et al. 2002).

Pulse wave velocity is the speed of the blood pressure wave traveling a given distance between two sites of the arterial system. It is a function of vessel wall elasticity, wall thickness, and blood density. Pulse wave velocity correlates with arterial distensibility and stiffness and is a useful non-invasive index to assess atherosclerosis.

Arterial endothelial dysfunction is one of the early events in atherogenesis, preceding structural atherosclerotic changes. This study reported in the *Indian Heart Journal* aimed to determine the coincidence between noninvasive estimation of arterial wall stiffness by pulse wave velocity, and degree of endothelial dysfunction in participants at high risk of atherosclerosis.

Men and women participants, 51 years old on average, included those with hypertension, Type 2 diabetes, concomitant Type 2 diabetes and hypertension, and primary dyslipidemia with neither diabetes nor hypertension.

Pulse wave velocity was measured by the Vascular Profiler 1000 (VP-1000: https://omronhealthcare .com.au/pdf2/17588_VP1000_Brochure_d.pdf) waveform analysis and vascular evaluation system, an automated, noninvasive, screening device. Endothelial function was assessed by FMD of the brachial artery.

It was found that increased pulse wave velocity indicating arterial stiffness correlated with reduced brachial artery FMD. These findings suggested that noninvasive estimation of the pulse wave velocity and endothelial function estimation by FMD of the brachial artery are useful in the clinical assessment of preclinical atherosclerosis (Jadhav, and Kadam. 2005).

2.9.7 Mechanisms of Arterial Dysfunction in Diabetes Involve Glucose and Insulin

The authors of a report in the journal *Clinical and Experimental Pharmacology and Physiology* compared measures of blood vessel stiffness in diabetes. It is reproduced here:

1. This commentary reviews and discusses the association between increased arterial stiffness and indices of glucose and insulin metabolism and diabetes mellitus (DM).
2. Diabetes mellitus is associated with increased cardiovascular events, is an established major independent risk factor for cardiovascular disease and is included in current risk assessment algorithms. Based on Framingham risk assessment, the incremental risk due to DM, at a given level of baseline risk in non-diabetics, is approximately equivalent to 10 years and, at any given level of other major risk factors, DM increases risk three- to fourfold.
3. Increased aortic stiffness has been shown to be an independent risk factor for both cardiovascular and overall mortality in high-risk groups and recently in the general population. Both DM1 and DM2 are associated with accelerated stiffening of the elastic arteries, over and above that associated with normal ageing, and DM can be considered as imparting added biological age and, thus, added cardiovascular risk.
4. Aortic stiffness provides a plausible mechanism relating diabetes to increase cardiovascular disease.
5. A proportion of the increased risk of cardiovascular events in DM is a sequel of stiff arteries. Direct measures of arterial stiffness, such as aortic pulse wave velocity, are likely to be better candidates than pulse wave analysis for refining interventions to improve outcomes in diabetes. (From Cameron and Cruickshank. 2007. With permission.)

2.10   ASSESSING ENDOTHELIAL DYSFUNCTION IN DIABETES BY REACTIVE HYPEREMIA

Reactive hyperemia is the transient increase in blood flow that follows a brief period of arterial occlusion. The aim of a study reported in the *International Journal of Cardiology* was to assess endothelial function in Type 2 diabetic patients with angiographically normal coronary arteries compared to diabetic patients with obstructive coronary artery disease, and to nondiabetic patients, with and without coronary artery disease.

Patients undergoing coronary angiography were assigned to the following groups: group 1, those with diabetes and coronary artery disease; group 2, those with diabetes without coronary artery disease; group 3, those with coronary artery disease but without diabetes; and group 4, those without coronary artery disease and diabetes.

Endothelial function in these patients was assessed by the reactive hyperemia index using fingertip peripheral arterial tonometry and compared to values obtained in 20 healthy volunteers.

It was reported that reactive hyperemia was significantly lower in patients with diabetes than in those without diabetes. Diabetes and coronary artery disease were found to be significant predictors of endothelial dysfunction; coronary artery disease and HbA1c in diabetic patients were significant independent predictors of endothelial dysfunction. Diabetic patients with endothelial dysfunction had higher levels of HbA1c than diabetic patients with normal endothelial function, and reactive hyperemia measures correlated inversely with HbA1c.

The authors concluded that diabetic patients with and without coronary artery disease show significantly impaired peripheral vascular function compared to nondiabetic patients without coronary artery disease. Endothelial function in diabetic patients without coronary artery disease is comparable to that of patients with coronary artery disease but without diabetes. HbA1c was found to be a weak independent predictor of endothelial dysfunction (Gargiulo, Marciano, Savarese et al. 2013).

REFERENCES

Abbott RD, Donahue RP, MacMahon SW, Reed DM, and K Yano. 1987. Diabetes and the risk of stroke. The Honolulu Heart Program. *Journal of the American Medical Association* (JAMA), Feb; 257(7): 949–952. DOI:10.1001/jama.1987.033900700 69025.

Antonopoulos AS, Margaritis M, Lee R, Channon K, and C Antoniades. 2012. Statins as anti-inflammatory agents in atherogenesis: molecular mechanisms and lessons from the recent clinical trials. *Current Pharmaceutical Design*, Apr; 18(11): 1519–1530. Published online 2012 Apr. Doi: 10.2174/1381 61212799504803.

Avogaro A, Albiero M, Menegazzo L, de Kreutzenberg S, and GP Fadini. 2011. Endothelial dysfunction in diabetes. The role of reparatory mechanisms. *Diabetes Care*, May; 34(Supplement 2): S285–S290. https://doi.org/10.2337/dc11-s239.

Avogaro A, Fadini GP, Gallo A, Pagnin E, and S de Kreutzenberg. 2006. Endothelial dysfunction in type 2 diabetes mellitus. *Nutrition, Metabolism and Cardiovascular Diseases*, Mar; 16 Suppl 1: S39–45. DOI: 10.1016/j.numecd.2005.10.015.

Banerji MA, and JD Dunn. 2013. Impact of glycemic control on healthcare resource utilization and costs of type 2 diabetes: current and future pharmacologic approaches to improving outcomes. *American Health and Drug Benefits*, Sep; 6(7): 382–392. PMCID: PMC4031727.

Basha B, Samuel SM, Triggle CR, and H Ding. 2012. Endothelial dysfunction in diabetes mellitus: possible involvement of endoplasmic reticulum stress? *Experimental Diabetes Research*, Jun; 2012 (Article ID 481840): 14 pages. http://dx.doi.org/10.1155/2012/481840.

Böhm F, and J Pernow. 2007. The importance of endothelin-1 for vascular dysfunction in cardiovascular disease. *Cardiovascular Research*, Oct 1; 76(1): 8–18. DOI: 10. 1016/j.cardiores.2007.06.004.

Boudina S, and ED Abel. 2010. Diabetic cardiomyopathy, causes and effects. *Reviews in Endocrine and Metabolic Disorders*, Mar; 11(1): 31–39. DOI: 10.1007/s11154-010-9131-7.

Boutouyrie P, Achouba A, Trunet P, S. Laurent and the EXPLOR Trialist Group. Collaborators: Gosse P, London G, Pannier B, Poncelet P, Lantelme P, Legedz L, Fesler P, Levy B, Thuillez C, Joannides R, Stephan D, Laurent P, Doll G. 2010. Amlodipine–valsartan combination decreases central systolic blood pressure more effectively than the amlodipine–atenolol combination: the EXPLOR study. *Hypertension*, Jun; 55(6): 1314–1322. DOI: 10.1161/HYPERTENSIONAHA.109.148999.

Brownlee M. 2001. Biochemistry and molecular cell biology of diabetic complications. *Nature*, Dec; 414, 813–820. DOI: 10.1038/414813a.

Bryan N, and J Loscalzo (Eds.). 2017. *Nitrite and Nitrate in Human Health and Disease*. Springer.

Calles-Escandon J, and M Cipolla. 2001. Diabetes and endothelial dysfunction: A clinical perspective. *Endocrine Reviews*, 22(1): 36–52. DOI: https://doi.org/10.1210/edrv.22.1.0417.

Cameron JD, and JK Cruickshank. 2007. Glucose, insulin, diabetes and mechanisms of arterial dysfunction. *Clinical and Experimental Pharmacology and Physiology*, Jul; 34(7): 677–682. DOI: 10.1111/j.1440-1681.2007.04659.x.

Cao SS, and RJ Kaufman. 2014. Endoplasmic reticulum stress and oxidative stress in cell fate decision and human disease. *Antioxidants and Redox Signaling*, Jul 20; 21(3): 396–413. DOI: 10.1089/ars.2014.5851.

Carmeli E, Coleman R, and YN Berner. 2004. Activities of antioxidant scavenger enzymes (superoxide dismutase and glutathione peroxidase) in erythrocytes in adult women with and without type II diabetes. *Experimental Diabesity Research*, Apr–Jun; 5(2):171–175. DOI: 10.1080/15438600490451659.

Catalano M, Scandale G, and G Dimitrov. 2013. Chapter 6. Arterial stiffness: A review in Type 2 diabetes. In K Masuo (Ed.), *Type 2 Diabetes*. ISBN 978-953-51-1171-9 DOI: 10.5772/56582.

Ceriello A, Morocutti A, Mercuri F, Quagliaro L, Moro M, Damante G, and GC Viberti. 2000. Defective intracellular antioxidant enzyme production in type 1 diabetic patients with nephropathy. *Diabetes*, Dec; 49(12): 2170–2177. PMID: 11118022.

Ceriello A. 2009. The metabolic memory. *Endocrine Abstract*, 20 S15.2.

Chan PS, Kanwar M, and RA Kowluru. 2010. Resistance of retinal inflammatory mediators to suppress after reinstitution of good glycemic control: novel mechanism for metabolic memory. *Journal of Diabetes and Its Complications*, 2010 Jan–Feb; 24(1): 55–63. DOI: 10.1016/j.jdiacomp.2008.10.002.

Chang AM, and JB Halter. 2003. Aging and insulin secretion. *American Journal of Physiology, Endocrinology and Metabolism*, Jan; 284(1): E7–E12. DOI: 10.1152/ajpendo.00366.2002.

Cheng KHY, Sun C, Vuong B, Lee KKC, Mariampillai A, Marotta TR, Spears J, Montanera WJ, Herman PR, Kiehl T-R, Standish BA, and VXD Yang. 2012. Endovascular optical coherence tomography intensity kurtosis: visualization of vasa vasorum in porcine carotid artery. *Biomedical Optics Express*, Jan; 3(3): 388–399.

Chowienczyk P. 2011. What do the numbers mean? *Hypertension*, 57: 1051–1052. https://doi.org/10.1161/HYPERTENSIONAHA.111.171504 http://hyper.aha journals.org/content/57/6/1051Pulse Wave Analysis.

Cooke JP, Singer AH, Tsao P, Zera P, Rowan RA, and ME Billingham. 1992. Antiatherogenic effects of L-arginine in the hypercholesterolemic rabbit. *The Journal of Clinical Investigation*, Sep; 90(3): 1168–1172. DOI: 10.1172/JCI115937.

Cruickshank K, Riste L, Anderson SG, Wright JS, Dunn G, and RG Gosling. 2002. Aortic pulse-wave velocity and its relationship to mortality in diabetes and glucose intolerance. An integrated index of vascular function? *Circulation*, Oct; (16): 106: 2085–2090. PMID: 12379578.

Detaille D, Guigas B, Chauvin C, Batandier C, Fontaine E, Wiernsperger N, and X Leverve. 2005. Metformin prevents high-glucose-induced endothelial cell death through a mitochondrial permeability transition-dependent process. *Diabetes*, Jul; 54(7): 2179–2187. PMID: 15983220.

Dhawan V, Handu SS, Nain CK, and NK Ganguly. 2005. Chronic L-arginine supplementation improves endothelial cell vasoactive functions in hypercholesterolemic and atherosclerotic monkeys. *Molecular and Cellular Biochemistry*, Jan; 269(1–2): 1–11. PMID: 15786711.

Dilaveris P, Giannopoulos G, Riga M, Synetos A, and C Stefanadis. 2007. Beneficial effects of statins on endothelial dysfunction and vascular stiffness. *Current Vascular Pharmacology*, Jul; 5(3): 227–237. PMID: 17627566.

Drexler H, Zeiher AM, and MDK Meinzer. 1991. Correction of endothelial dysfunction in coronary microcirculation of hypercholesterolaemic patients by L-arginine. *Lancet*, Dec; 38(8782–8783): 1546–1550. https://doi.org/10.1016/0140-6736(91) 92372-9.

Du X, Matsumura T, Edelstein D, Rossetti L, Zsengellér Z, Szabó C, and M Brownlee. 2003. Inhibition of GAPDH activity by poly(ADP-ribose) polymerase activates three major pathways of hyperglycemic damage in endothelial cells. *Journal of Clinical Investigation*, Oct; 112(7): 1049–1057. DOI: 10.1172/JCI18127.

Du Y, Miller CM, and TS Kern. 2003. Hyperglycemia increases mitochondrial superoxide in retina and retinal cells. *Free Radical Biology and Medicine*, Dec; 35(11): 1491–1499. PMID: 14642397.

Duncan JG. 2011. Mitochondrial dysfunction in diabetic cardiomyopathy. *Biochimica et Biophysica Acta*, Jul; 1813(7): 1351–1359. DOI: 10.1016/j.bbamcr.2011.01.014.

Fadini CP, Sartore S, Agostini C, and A Avogaro. 2007 – *Diabetes Care*, May; 30(5): 1305–1313. https://doi .org/10.2337/dc06-2305.

Fink RI, Kolterman OG, Griffin J, and JM Olefsky. 1983. Mechanisms of insulin resistance in aging. *The Journal of Clinical Investigation*, Jun; 71(6): 1523–1535. DOI: 10.1172/JCI110908.

Förstermann U. 2008. Oxidative stress in vascular disease: causes, defense mechanisms and potential therapies. *Nature Clinical Practice. Cardiovascular Medicine*, Jun; 5(6): 338–349. DOI: 10.1038/ncpcardio1211.

Gajdova J, Karasek D, Goldmannova D, Krystynik O, Schovanek J, Vaverkova H, and J Zadrazil. 2017. Pulse wave analysis and diabetes mellitus: A systematic review. *Biomedical Papers of the Medical Faculty of the University Palacky Olomouc, Czech Republic*, Jun 5. DOI: 10.5507/bp.2017.028.

Gargiulo P, Marciano C, Savarese G, D'Amore C, Paolillo S, Esposito G, Santomauro M, Marsico F, Ruggiero D, Scala O, Marzano A, Cecere M, Casaretti L, and P Perrone Filardi. 2013. Endothelial dysfunction in type 2 diabetic patients with normal coronary arteries: a digital reactive hyperemia study. *International Journal of Cardiology*, Apr 30; 165(1): 67–71. DOI: 10.1016/j.ijcard.2011.07.076.

Ghasemzadeh N, and AM Zafari. 2011. Review article. A brief journey into the history of the arterial pulse. *Cardiology Research and Practice*, Volume 2011, Article ID 164832, 14 pages. http://dx.doi.org/10.4061 /2011/164832.

Goenezen S, Rennie MY, and S Rugonyi. 2012. Biomechanics of early cardiac development. *Biomechics and Modeling in Mechanobiology*, Nov; 11(8): 1187–1204. Published online 2012 Jul 4. DOI: 10.1007 /s10237-012-0414-7.

Gössl M, Malyar NM, Rosol M, Beighley PE, and EL Ritman. 2003. Impact of coronary vasa vasorum functional structure on coronary vessel wall perfusion distribution. *American Journal of Physiology - Heart and Circulatory Physiology*, Nov; 285(5): H2019–H2026. DOI: 10.1152/ajpheart .00399.2003.

Guha A, Harmancey R, and H Taegtmeyer. 2008. Nonischemic heart failure in diabetes mellitus. *Current Opinion in Cardiology*, May; 23(3): 241–248. DOI: 10.1097/HCO.0b013e3282fcc2fa.

Hadi HAR, and J Al Suwaidi. 2007. Endothelial dysfunction in diabetes mellitus. *Vascular Health and Risk Management*, Dec; 3(6): 853–876. PMCID: PMC2350146.

Heffernan KS, Fahs CA, Ranadive SM, and EA Patvardhan. 2010. L-Arginine as a nutritional prophylaxis against vascular endothelial dysfunction with aging. *Journal of Cardiovascular Pharmacology and Therapeutics*, Mar; 15(1): 17–23. PMCID: PMC 2922760 NIHMSID: NIHMS216215 DOI: 10.1177 /1074248409354 599248409354599.

Hernandez-Mijares A, Rocha M, Rovira-Llopis S, Bañuls C, Bellod L, de Pablo C, Alvarez A, Roldan-Torres I, Sola-Izquierdo E, and VM Victor. 2013. Human leukocyte/endothelial cell interactions and mitochondrial dysfunction in type 2 diabetic patients and their association with silent myocardial ischemia. *Diabetes Care*, Jun; 36(6): 1695–1702. DOI: 10.2337/dc12-1224.

Hirsch IB, and M Brownlee. 2005. Should minimal blood glucose variability become the gold standard of glycemic control? *Journal of Diabetes and its Complications*, May–Jun; 19(3): 178–181. PMID: 15866065 DOI: 10.1016/j.jdiacomp.2004.10.001.

Hove JR, Köster RW, Forouhar AS, Acevedo-Bolton G, Fraser SE, and M Gharib. 2003. Intracardiac fluid forces are an essential epigenetic factor for embryonic cardiogenesis. *Nature*, Jan 9; 421(6919): 172–177. DOI: 10.1038/nature01282.

Ignarro LJ. 1990. Nitric oxide. A novel signal transduction mechanism for transcellular communication. *Hypertension*, Nov; 16(5):477–483. PMID: 1977698.

Ii M, and DW Losordo. 2007. Statins and the endothelium. *Vascular Pharmacology*, Jan; 46(1):1–9. Epub 2006 Jun 21. DOI: 10.1016/j.vph.2006.06.012.

Jadhav UM, and NN Kadam. 2005. Non-invasive assessment of arterial stiffness by pulse-wave velocity correlates with endothelial dysfunction. *Indian Heart Journal*, May; 57(3): 226–232. https://www.ncbi.nlm .nih.gov/labs/articles/16196179/1.

Katakami N, Osonoi T, Takahara M, Saitou M, Matsuoka T-a, Yamasaki Y, and I Shimomura. 2014. Clinical utility of brachial-ankle pulse wave velocity in the prediction of cardiovascular events in diabetic patients. *Cardiovascular Diabetology*, 201413: 128. DOI: 10.1186/s12933-014-0128-5.

Kesavulu MM, Giri R, Kameswara Rao B, and C Apparao. 2000. Lipid peroxidation and antioxidant enzyme levels in type 2 diabetics with microvascular complications. *Diabetes and Metabolism*, Nov; 26(5): 387–392. PMID: 11119018.

Kirpichnikov D, and JR Sowers. 2001. Diabetes mellitus and diabetes-associated vascular disease. *Trends in Endocrinology and Metabolism*, Jul; 12(5): 2252–2230. PMID: 11397648.

Kizhakekuttu TJ, Wang J, Dharmashankar K, Ying R, Gutterman DD, Vita JA, and ME Widlansky. 2012. Adverse alterations in mitochondrial function contribute to type 2 diabetes mellitus-related endothelial dysfunction in humans. *Arteriosclerosis, Thrombosis, and Vascular Biology*, Oct; 32(10): 2531–2539. doi: 10.1161/ATVBAHA. 112.256024. DOI: 10.1161/ATVBAHA.112.256024.

Kolterman OG, Gray RS, Griffin J, Burstein P, Insel J, Scarlett JA, and JM Olefsky. 1981. Receptor and post-receptor defects contribute to the insulin resistance in noninsulin-dependent diabetes mellitus. *Journal of Clinical Investigation*, Oct; 68(4): 957–969. DOI: 10.1172/JCI110350.

Krauss S, Zhang CY, Scorrano L, Dalgaard LT, St-Pierre J, Grey ST, and BB Lowell. 2003. Superoxide-mediated activation of uncoupling protein 2 causes pancreatic beta cell dysfunction. *Journal of Clinical Investigation*, Dec; 112(12): 1831–1842. DOI: 10.1172/JCI19774.

Kum F, and J Karalliedde. 2010. Critical appraisal of the differential effects of antihypertensive agents on arterial stiffness. *Integrated Blood Pressure Control*, Jun; 3: 63–71. PMCID: PMC3172069.

Laugesen E, Hoyem P, Stausbol-Gron B, Mikkelsen A, Thrysoe S, Erlandsen M, Christiansen JS, Knudsen ST, Hansen KW, Kim WY, Hansen TK, and PL Poulsen. 2013. Carotid-femoral pulse wave velocity is associated with cerebral white matter lesions in Type 2 diabetes. *Diabetes Care*, Mar; 36(3): 722–728. DOI: 10.2337/dc12-0942.

Mah E, Noh SK, Ballard KD, Matos ME, Volek JS, and RS Bruno. 2011. Postprandial hyperglycemia impairs vascular endothelial function in healthy men by inducing lipid peroxidation and increasing asymmetric dimethylarginine: arginine. *The Journal of Nutrition*, Nov; 141(11): 1961–1968. DOI: 10.3945/jn.111.144592.

Mather KJ. 2013. The vascular endothelium in diabetes—a therapeutic target? *Reviews in Endocrine and Metabolic Disorders*, Mar; 14(1): 87–99. DOI: 10.1007/s11154-013-9237-9.

Mattace-Raso F, Hofman A, Verwoert GC, Witteman JCM, Mattace-Raso F, Hofman A, Verwoert GC, Witteman JCM, Laurent S, Boutouyrie P, Bozec E, Hansen TW, Torp-Pedersen C, Ibsen H, and J Jeppesen. 2010. Determinants of pulse wave velocity in healthy people and in the presence of cardiovascular risk factors: establishing normal and reference values. *European Heart Journal*, Oct; 31(19): 2338–2350. DOI: 10.1093/eurheartj/ehq165.

McClung JA, Naseer N, Saleem M, Rossi GP, Weiss MB, Abraham NG, and A Kappas. 2005. Circulating endothelial cells are elevated in patients with type 2 diabetes mellitus independently of HbA(1)c. *Diabetologia*, Feb; 48(2): 345–350. Epub 2005 Jan 20. DOI: 10.1007/s00125-004-1647-5.

McVeigh G, Brennan G, Hayes R, Cohn J, Finkelstein S, and D Johnston. 1993. Vascular abnormalities in non-insulin-dependent diabetes mellitus identified by arterial waveform analysis. *The American Journal of Medicine*, Oct; 95(4): 424–430. https://doi.org/10.1016/0002-9343(93)90313-E.

McVeigh GE, Allen PB, Morgan DR, Hanratty CG, and B Silke. 2001. Nitric oxide modulation of blood vessel tone identified by arterial waveform analysis. *Clinical Science (Lond)*. Apr; 100(4): 387–393. PMID: 11256976.

Millasseau SC, Stewart AD, Patel SJ, Redwood SR, and PJ Chowienczyk. 2005. Evaluation of carotid-femoral pulse wave velocity: influence of timing algorithm and heart rate. *Hypertension*, Feb; 45(2): 222–226. DOI: 10.1161/01.HYP.0000154229.97341.d2.

Miller BR, Nguyen H, Jia-Haur Hu C, Lin C, and QT Nguyen. 2014. New and emerging drugs and targets for Type 2 diabetes: Reviewing the evidence. *American Health and Drug Benefits*, Nov; 7(8): 452–463. PMCID: PMC4280522.

Montezano AC, and RM Touyz. 2012. Reactive oxygen species and endothelial function—role of nitric oxide synthase uncoupling and Nox family nicotinamide adenine dinucleotide phosphate oxidases. *Basic and Clinical Pharmacology and Toxicology*, Jan; 110(1): 87–94. DOI: 10.1111/j.1742-7843.2011.00785.x.

Mulligan-Kehoe MJ. 2010. The vasa vasorum in diseased and nondiseased arteries. *American Journal of Physiology - Heart and Circulatory Physiology*, Feb; 298(2): H295–H305. DOI: 10.1152/ajpheart.00884.2009 http://ajpheart.physiology.org/content/298/2/H295.

Nishikawa T, Edelstein D, Du XL, Yamagishi S, Matsumura T, Kaneda Y, Yorek MA, Beebe D, Oates PJ, Hammes HP, Giardino I, and M Brownlee. 2000. Normalizing mitochondrial superoxide production blocks three pathways of hyperglycaemic damage. *Nature*, Apr 13; 404(6779): 787–790. DOI: 10.1038/35008121.

Nitenberg A, Cosson E, and I Pham. 2006. Postprandial endothelial dysfunction: role of glucose, lipids and insulin. *Diabetes and Metabolism*, Sep; 32 Spec No 2: 2S28–33. PMID: 17375404.

Nitenberg A, Valensi P, Sachs R, Dali M, Aptecar E, and J-R Attali. 1993. Impairment of coronary vascular reserve and ACh-induced coronary vasodilation in diabetic patients with angiographically normal coronary arteries and normal left ventricular systolic function. *Diabetes*, Jul; 42(7): 1017–1025. https://doi.org/10.2337/diab.42.7.1017.

Niz, MA. 2017. *The Chahar Maqala of Nidhami-i-'Arudi-i-Samarqandi.* Palala Press.

Nomura S. 2009. Dynamic role of microparticles in type 2 diabetes mellitus. *Current Diabetes Reviews,* Nov; 5(4): 245–2451. PMID: 19531024.

Nyström T, Gutniak MK, Zhang Q, Zhang F, Holst JJ, Ahrén B, and Å Sjöholm. 2004. Effects of glucagon-like peptide-1 on endothelial function in type 2 diabetes patients with stable coronary artery disease. *American Journal of Physiology - Endocrinology and Metabolism,* Nov; 287(6): E1209–E1215. DOI: 10.1152/ajpendo.00237.2004.

O'Connell J, 2011. *Sugar Nation: The Hidden Truth Behind America's Deadliest Habit and the Simple Way to Beat It.* New York: Hachette Books.

Ogawa O, Hiraoka K, Watanabe T, Kinoshita J, Kawasumi M, Yoshii H, and R Kawamori. 2008. Diabetic retinopathy is associated with pulse wave velocity, not with the augmentation index of pulse waveform. *Cardiovascular Diabetology,* Apr; 7: 11. Published online 2008 Apr 25. DOI: 10.1186/1475-2840-7-11.

Orea-Tejeda A, Orozco-Gutiérrez JJ, Castillo-Martínez L, Keirns-Davies C, Montano-Hernández P, Vázquez-Díaz O, Valdespino-Trejo A, Infante O, and R Martínez-Memije. 2010. The effect of L-arginine and citrulline on endothelial function in patients in heart failure with preserved ejection fraction. *Cardiology Journal,* 17(5): 464–470. PMID: 20865676.

Orrico C, Pasquinelli G, Foroni L, Muscarà D, Tazzari PL, Ricci F, Buzzi M, Baldi E, Muccini N, Gargiulo M, and A Stella. 2010. Dysfunctional vasa vasorum in diabetic peripheral artery obstructive disease with critical lower limb ischaemia. *European Journal of Vascular and Endovascular Surgery,* Sep; 40(3): 365–374. DOI: 10.1016/j. ejvs.2010.04.011.

Paneni F, Mocharla P, Akhmedov A, Costantino S, Osto E, Volpe M, Lüscher TF, and F Cosentino. 2012. Gene silencing of the mitochondrial adaptor p66(Shc) suppresses vascular hyperglycemic memory in diabetes. *Circulation* Research, Jul 20; 111(3): 278–289. DOI: 10.1161/CIRCRESAHA.112.266593.

Pangare M, and A Makino. 2012. Mitochondrial function in vascular endothelial cell in diabetes. *Journal of Smooth Muscle Research,* 48(1): 1–26. PMCID: PMC3655204.

Pasimeni G, Ribaudo MC, and D Capoccia. 2006. Non-invasive evaluation of endothelial dysfunction in uncomplicated obesity: relationship with insulin resistance. *Microvascular Rese*arch, 71: 115–120.

Patti ME, and S Corvera. 2010. The role of mitochondria in the pathogenesis of type 2 diabetes. *Endocrine Reviews,* Jun; 31(3): 364–395. DOI: 10.1210/er.2009-0027. PMCID: PMC3365846.

Petersen KF, Befroy D, Dufour S, Dziura J, Ariyan C, Rothman DL, DiPietro L, Cline GW, and GI Shulman. 2003. Mitochondrial dysfunction in the elderly: Possible role in insulin resistance. *Science,* May 16; 300(5622): 1140–1142. DOI: 10.1126/science.1082889.

Piconi L, Quagliaro L, Assaloni R, Da Ros R, Maier A, Zuodar G, and A Ceriello. 2006. Constant and intermittent high glucose enhances endothelial cell apoptosis through mitochondrial superoxide overproduction. *Diabetes Metabolism. Research and Reviews,* May/June; 22(3): 198–203.

Ritman EL, and A Lerman. 2007. The dynamic vasa vasorum. *Cardiovascular Research,* Sep; 75(4): 649–658. DOI: 10.1016/j.cardiores.06.020.

Roberts AC, and KE Porter. 2013. Cellular and molecular mechanisms of endothelial dysfunction in diabetes. *Diabetes and Vascular Disease Research,* Sept; 10(6): 472–482. DOI: 10.1177/1479164113500680.

Roy S, Sala R, Cagliero E, and M Lorenzi. 1990. Overexpression of fibronectin induced by diabetes or high glucose: phenomenon with a memory. *Proceedings of the National Academy of Sciences U S A.* Jan; 87(1): 404–408. PMCID: PMC53272.

Saisho Y. 2015. Metformin and inflammation: its potential beyond glucose-lowering effect. *Endocrine, Metabolic and Immune Disorders Drug Targets,* 15(3): 196–205. PMID: 25772174.

Schmidt R, Launer LJ, Nilsson L-G, Pajak A, Sans S, Berger K, Breteler MM, de Ridder M, Dufouil C, Rebecca Fuhrer R, Giampaoli S, and A Hofman, for the CASCADE Consortium. 2004. Magnetic resonance imaging of the brain in diabetes. The cardiovascular determinants of dementia (CASCADE) study. *Diabetes,* 53: 687–692.

Segers P, Qasem A, De Backer T, Carlier S, Verdonck P, and A Avolio. 2001. Peripheral "oscillatory" compliance is associated with aortic augmentation index. *Hypertension.* Jun; 37: 1434–1439. https://doi.org/10.1161/01.HYP.37.6.1434.

Semba RD, Najjar SS, Sun K, Lakatta EG, and L Ferrucci. 2009. Serum carboxymethyl-lysine, an advanced glycation end product, is associated with increased aortic pulse wave velocity in adults. *American Journal of Hypertension,* Jan; 22(1): 74–79. DOI: 10.1038/ajh.2008.320.

Sena CM, Pereira AM, and R Seiça. 2013. Endothelial dysfunction—a major mediator of diabetic vascular disease. *Biochimica et Biophysica Acta (BBA) - Molecular Basis of Disease,* Dec: 1832(12): 2216–2231. https://doi.org/10.1016/j.bbadis.2013.08.006.

Shimizu M, and K Kario. 2008. Role of the augmentation index in hypertension. *Therapeutic Advances in Cardiovascular Diseases*, Feb; 2(1): 25–35. DOI: 10.1177/1753944707086935.

Singh VP, Bali A, Singh N, and AS Jaggi. 2014. Advanced glycation end products and diabetic complications. *Korean Journal of Physiology and Pharmacology*, Feb; 18(1): 1–14. DOI: 10.4196/kjpp.2014.18.1.1.

Smith A, Karalliedde J, De Angelis L, Goldsmith D, and G Viberti, 2005. Aortic pulse wave velocity and albuminuria in patients with Type 2 diabetes. *Journal of the American Society of Nephrology*, Apr; 16(4): 1069–1075. Published online before print March 2, 2005 DOI: 10.1681/ASN.2004090769 JASN April.

Steinberg H, Chaker H, and R Leaming. 1996. Obesity/insulin resistance is associated with endothelial dysfunction. Implications for the syndrome of insulin resistance. *Journal of Clinical Investigation*, 97: 2601–2610.

Stewart AD, Millasseau SC, Kearney MT, Ritter JA, and PJ Chowienczyk. 2003. Effects of inhibition of basal nitric oxide synthesis on carotid-femoral pulse wave velocity and augmentation index in humans. *Hypertension*, Nov; 42: 915–918. http://dx.doi.org/10.1161/01.HYP.0000092882.65699.19.

Stoner L, Young JM, and S Fryer. 2012. Assessments of arterial stiffness and endothelial function using pulse wave analysis. *International Journal of Vascular Medicine*, 2012: 903107. DOI: 10.1155/2012/903107.

Sugawara J, Hayashi K, Yokoi T, and H Tanaka. 2008. Age-associated elongation of the ascending aorta in adults. *Journal of the American College of Cardiology. Cardiovascular Imaging*, Nov; 1(6): 739–748. DOI: 10.1016/j.jcmg.2008.06.010. PMID: 19356510.

Tang X, Luo Y-X, Chen H-Z, and D-P Liu. 2014. Mitochondria, endothelial cell function, and vascular diseases. *Frontiers in Physiology*, May 6; 5: 175. DOI: 10.3389/fphys.2014.00175.

Veerman KJ, Venegas-Pino DE, Shi Y, Khan MI, Gerstein HC, and GH Werstuck. 2013. Hyperglycaemia is associated with impaired vasa vasorum neovascularization and accelerated atherosclerosis in apolipoprotein-E deficient mice. *Atherosclerosis*, Jan; 227(2): 250–258. DOI: 10.1016/j.atherosclerosis .2013.01.018.

Vermeersch SJ, Rietzschel ER, De Buyzere ML, Van Bortel LM, Gillebert TC, Verdonck PR, Laurent S, Segers P, and P Boutouyrie. 2009. Distance measurements for the assessment of carotid to femoral pulse wave velocity. *Journal of Hypertension*, Dec; 27(12): 2377–2385. DOI: 10.1097/HJH.0b013e3283313a8a.

Wardlaw JM, Ferguson KJ, and C Graham. 2004. White matter hyperintensities and rating scales—observer reliability varies with lesion load. *Journal of Neurology*, May; 251(5): 584–590. DOI: 10.1007/s00415 -004-0371-x.

Webb DR, Khunti K, Silverman R, Gray LJ, Srinivasan B, Lacy PS, Williams B, and MJ Davies. 2010. Impact of metabolic indices on central artery stiffness: independent association of insulin resistance and glucose with aortic pulse wave velocity. *Diabetologia*, Jun; 53(6): 1190–1198. DOI: 10.1007/s00125-010-1689-9.

Weber T, Ammer M, Rammer M, Adji A, O'Rourke MF, Wassertheurer S, Rosenkranz S, and B Eber. 2009. Noninvasive determination of carotid-femoral pulse wave velocity depends critically on assessment of travel distance: a comparison with invasive measurement. *Journal of Hypertension*, Aug; 27(8): 1624– 1630. DOI: 10.1097/HJH.0b013e32832cb04e.

Westerbacka J, Wilkinson I, Cockcroft J, Utriainen T, Vehkavaara S, and H Yki-Järvinen. 1999. Diminished wave reflection in the aorta. A novel physiological action of insulin on large blood vessels. *Hypertension*, May; 33(5): 1118–1122. PMID: 10334797.

Westerweel PE, Teraa M, Rafii S, Jaspers JE, White IA, Hooper AT, Doevendans PA, and MC Verhaar. 2013. Impaired endothelial progenitor cell mobilization and dysfunctional bone marrow stroma in diabetes mellitus. *PLoS ONE*, https://doi.org/10.1371/journal.pone.0060357 PLOS Published: March 28, 2013.

Wilhelm B, Klein J, Friedrich C, Forst S, Pfützner A, Kann PH, Weber MM, and T Forst. 2007. Increased arterial augmentation and augmentation index as surrogate parameters for arteriosclerosis in subjects with diabetes mellitus and nondiabetic subjects with cardiovascular disease. *Journal of Diabetes Science and Technology*, 2007 Mar; 1(2): 260–263. DOI: 10.1177/193229680700100217.

Wilkinson IB, MacCallum H, Cockcroft JR, and DJ Webb. 2002. Inhibition of basal nitric oxide synthesis increases aortic augmentation index and pulse wave velocity in vivo. *British Journal of Clinical Pharmacology*, Feb; 53(2): 189–192. DOI: 10.1046/j.1365-2125.2002.1528adoc.x.

Wilkinson IB, Prasad K, Hall IR, Thomas A, MacCallum H, Webb DJ, Frenneaux MP, and JR Cockcroft. 2002. Increased central pulse pressure and augmentation index in subjects with hypercholesterolemia. *Journal of the American College of Cardiology*, Mar: 39(6): DOI: 10.1016/S0735-1097(02)01723-0.

Wilkinson IB, Qasem A, McEniery CM, Webb DJ, Avolio AP, and JR Cockcroft. 2002. Nitric oxide regulates local arterial distensibility in vivo. *Circulation*, Jan; 105(2): 213–217. PMID: 11790703.

Xu J, and M-H Zou. 2009. Molecular insights and therapeutic targets for diabetic endothelial dysfunction. *Circulation*, Sep 29; 120(13): 1266–1286. DOI: 10.1161/CIRCULATIONAHA.108.835223.

Yu JW, Deng YP, Han X, Ren GF, Cai J, and GJ Jiang GJ. 2016. Metformin improves the angiogenic functions
     of endothelial progenitor cells via activating AMPK/eNOS pathway in diabetic mice. *Cardiovascular
     Diabetology*, Jun 18; 15:88. DOI: 10. 1186/s12933-016-0408-3.
Zhang M, Bai Y, Ye P, Luo L, Xiao W, Wu H, and D Liu. 2011. Type 2 diabetes is associated with increased
     pulse wave velocity measured at different sites of the arterial system but not augmentation index in a
     Chinese population. *Clinical Cardiology*, Oct; 34(10): 622–627. DOI: 10.1002/clc.20956.

3 Cardiovascular and Related Complications of Diabetes

Above all else, guard your heart, for everything you do flows from it.

Proverbs 4:23

3.1 INTRODUCTION

The previous chapter of this book explained that a principal way that diabetes mellitus causes us harm is by impairing the ability of the endothelium to form nitric oxide (NO), and that this impairment may be the basis of conventional cardiovascular and heart diseases, and diabetes-related vision loss. Distilling the essence of the many reports, of which those cited were only a very small sample, gave support to the contention that the damage done by diabetes is the outcome of hyperglycemia surges that result in significant free radical and reactive oxygen species (ROS) assaults on all the tissues in the body, but principally on the endothelium. Research supports this conclusion.

This chapter takes key elements of cardiovascular and heart diseases as well as selected other complications of diabetes and details their connection, in that context, to Type 2 diabetes as explained in contemporary medical clinical and research reports.

3.2 HYPERGLYCEMIA AND HYPERTENSION

When someone has diabetes and hypertension, which came first, diabetes or hypertension? It may well turn out that both are caused by a common—perhaps more than one in common—factor. In either case, most authorities now agree that both are linked to the adverse impact of ROS on endothelial NO formation.

A study published in the journal *BMC Public Health* conducted in Cameroon (Central Africa) aimed to determine the rate of coincident diabetes and hypertension and assess the levels of co-awareness, treatment, and control in a semi-urban population. The study included adult men and women "self-selected" from the community. Existing diabetes and hypertension and treatment data were collected in addition to blood pressure and fasting blood glucose.

Age-standardized prevalence rates of men versus those in women were 40.4% and 23.8% for hypertension alone, 3.3% and 5.6% for diabetes alone, and 3.9% and 5.0% for hypertension and diabetes.

The age-standardized awareness, treatment, and control rates for hypertension alone were 6.5%, 86.4%, and 37.2% for men and 24.3%, 52.1% and 51.6% for women. Equivalent figures for diabetes alone were 35.4%, 65.6%, and 23.1% for men and 26.4%, 75.5%, and 33.7% for women; those for hypertension and diabetes were 86.6%, 3.3%, and 0 in men and 74.7%, 22.6%, and 0 in women.

Gender, age, and adiposity were said to be the main determinants of the three conditions.

The investigators concluded that coincident diabetes and hypertension is as high as diabetes alone in this population, and it is related to gender, age, and adiposity (Katte, Dzudie, Sobngwi et al. 2014).

Another study, conducted in India, found that during 2009 to 2010, diabetes was prevalent in 34.7% of patients, and 46.0% of patients had hypertension. Diabetes and hypertension were coexistent in 20.6% of patients. Among those whose disease status was not known at enrollment, 7.2% and 22.2% of patients were newly diagnosed with diabetes and hypertension, respectively. An additional

18.4% of patients were classified as having prediabetes and 60.1% were classified as having pre-hypertension (Joshi, Saboo, Vadivale et al. 2012).

There is a considerable research and clinical literature relating either diabetes to hypertension or hypertension to diabetes, but it is difficult to ferret out causality. Depending on whether the researchers are looking at hypertension, then diabetes is viewed to be a causative factor; on the other hand, if the investigators are looking at diabetes, then hypertension is the villain. The one thing on which more recent investigators agree is that in either case, impaired endothelium function is a central factor, and this conclusion clearly makes sense because unopposed free radicals and ROS targeting the endothelium can account for both conditions.

Hence, since this book is about diabetes and not hypertension, it begins with the assumption that diabetes somehow contributes to hypertension, and let the research and clinical publications point us one way or the other.

In an article titled "Type 2 diabetes mellitus and hypertension: an update" appearing in the journal *Endocrinology and Metabolism Clinics of North America*, the investigators report that we can expect to find hypertension in more than 50% of patients with diabetes in whom it can cause significant blood vessel problems (Lastra, Syed, Kurukulasuriya. 2014; see also Sowers. 2013; and Stamler, Vaccaro, Neaton et al. 1993).

In fact, the risk for cardiovascular disease is four times higher in patients with both diabetes and hypertension than it is in those free of diabetes and who have normal blood pressure (Hu, Jousilahti, and Tuomilehto. 2007).

It was reported in the journal *Trends in Cardiovascular Medicine* that the well-known Framingham Heart Study found that diabetes is likely to cause a two- to fourfold increased risk of heart attack and myocardial infarction, congestive heart failure, peripheral arterial disease, stroke, and death (Fox. 2010). However, a more recent analysis of the Framingham data showed that those with hypertension at the time of the diagnosis of diabetes had a one-third higher rate of mortality for all causes, that is, 32 per 1000 per year, versus 20 per 1000 person-years, and a higher incidence of cardiovascular events, that is, 52 per 1000 person-years, versus 31 per 1000 person-years, compared to those with normal blood pressure with diabetes.

The authors concluded that the increased risk is likely due to coexistent hypertension (Chen, McAlister, Walker et al. 2010).

Another article, published in the journal *Current Atherosclerosis Reports*, asks whether there is a "common metabolic pathway" between diabetes and hypertension, because diabetes and hypertension occur so frequently together and there appears to be a substantial overlap between these disorders in terms of both etiology and disease mechanisms including obesity, inflammation, oxidative stress, and insulin resistance (Cheung, and Li. 2012).

The journal *The Cardiometabolic Syndrome* also reports that diabetes and hypertension frequently coexist and additively increase the risk of life-threatening cardiovascular events: Hypertension occurs in 75% of patients with the more prevalent form of Type 2 diabetes. Hypertension often precedes Type 2 diabetes, and it also plays an important role in the development of kidney damage, and in the small blood vessel complications of diabetes (Schutta. 2007).

So far, it seems generally agreed that diabetes at the very least may aggravate hypertension, which seems mostly to precede it.

A "Brief review. Diabetes mellitus and hypertension," in the journal *Hypertension*, summarizes basic facts about the relationship between diabetes and hypertension—from the perspective of diabetologists. Here first is the abstract of the review:

> Diabetes mellitus and hypertension are common diseases that coexist at a greater frequency than chance alone would predict. Hypertension in the diabetic individual markedly increases the risk and accelerates the course of cardiac disease, peripheral vascular disease, stroke, retinopathy, and nephropathy. Our understanding of the factors that markedly increase the frequency of hypertension in the diabetic

individual remains incomplete. Diabetic nephropathy is an important factor involved in the development of hypertension in diabetics, particularly type I patients. However, the etiology of hypertension in the majority of diabetic patients cannot be explained by underlying renal disease and remains 'essential' in nature. The hallmark of hypertension in type I and type II diabetics appears to be increased peripheral vascular resistance. Increased exchangeable sodium may also play a role in the pathogenesis of blood pressure in diabetics. There is increasing evidence that insulin resistance/hyperinsulinemia may play a key role in the pathogenesis of hypertension in both subtle and overt abnormalities of carbohydrate metabolism. Population studies suggest that elevated insulin levels, which often occurs in type II diabetes mellitus, is an independent risk factor for cardiovascular disease. Other cardiovascular risk factors in diabetic individuals include abnormalities of lipid metabolism, platelet function, and clotting factors. The goal of antihypertensive therapy in the patient with coexistent diabetes is to reduce the inordinate cardiovascular risk as well as lowering blood pressure (Epstein, and Sowers. 1992). With permission.

The "hallmark" of hypertension in diabetes is increased vascular resistance, a function of the caliber of the arterial lumen: If an arterial blood vessel is narrowed by vasoconstriction, vascular resistance rises and so does blood pressure. In other words, in diabetes, hypertension is caused by elevated blood pressure.

Then, they say that "... the hyper-insulinemia existing in disorders of carbohydrate tolerance, such as that in hypertension associated with Type 2 diabetes and obesity, could accelerate atherosclerosis both directly and secondarily by promoting hypertension." This is, of course, a description and not an explanation. Their Table 3 (Table 3.1) summarizes some basics that show the overlap between individuals with essential hypertension who also have diabetes, and the degree of coincidence makes it difficult to differentiate between these groups.

It seems that, for the most part, the authors are drawn—and logically so—to the role played by insulin, that is, lack of, or resistance to, in both hypertension and diabetes, but there is no clear suggestion about what comes first, or what might be causal. Although the finding that endothelium-derived NO regulates endothelium-derived vasodilation and, therefore, the caliber of blood vessels, the role of NO would not likely have been a feature in diabetes research and treatment reports in 1992.

TABLE 3.1
Typical Profile of Blood Pressure Regulatory Mechanisms in the Hypertensive Individual

Factor	Typical Findings in Hypertensive Diabetes
Total exchangeable sodium	Typically increased
Plasma rennin activity	Low normal to low
Plasma norepinephrine	Usually normal in nanozotemic nonketotic patients
Plasma aldosterone	Low to normal low
Baroreceptor sensitivity	Typically decreased
Vascular compliance	Typically decreased
Peripheral vascular resistance	Typically increased
Vascular pressor responses	Typically increased
Evidence of renal dysfunction	Typically present in type I patients
Central adiposity	Often increased in type II patients
Insulin resistance	Typically increased in type II patients
Abnormal cation transport mechanisms	Often present in both type I and II diabetic states

Source: Epstein, and Sowers. 1992. *Hypertension*, 19:403–418. With permission.

3.2.1   Hyperglycemia, Hypertension, and Insulin Deficiency

A report in the journal *Molecular and Cell Endocrinology* tells us that a common mechanism in the development of hypertension in both Type 1 and Type 2 diabetes is cellular-level insulin deficiency: impaired cellular response to insulin rather than excess insulin production (hyperinsulinemia) predisposes to increased blood vessel partial contraction known as "muscle tone," the hallmark of hypertension in the diabetic state (Sowers. 1990).

It has been shown that insulin normally reduces small blood vessel tone and contractile response to vaso-stimulants. Abnormal small blood vessel cellular calcium (Ca^{2+}) homeostasis may be the connection between insulin resistance and increased blood vessel tone (Sowers, Khoury, Standley et al. 1991).

Skeletal muscle insulin resistance is a feature in essential hypertension but it is not known if it also affects heart glucose uptake. In this study published in *The Journal of Clinical Investigation*, the authors measured whole body, heart, and skeletal glucose uptake rates in middle-aged mildly essential hypertensive and in normotensive participants. Left ventricular mass was similar in the hypertensive and the normotensive participants.

It was found that in those with hypertension, both whole body and femoral glucose uptake rates were decreased compared to the normotensive controls. In contrast, heart glucose uptake was 33% higher in the hypertensives and correlated with systolic blood pressure.

It was concluded that insulin-stimulated glucose uptake decreased in skeletal muscle but increased in proportion to cardiac work in essential hypertension. The increase in heart glucose uptake in mild essential hypertensives with a normal left ventricular mass may reflect increased oxygen consumption and represents an early signal that precedes the development of left ventricular hypertrophy (Nuutila, Mäki, Laine et al. 1995).

3.2.1.1   Implication of the Recommended Treatment Guidelines for Chronic Hyperglycemia with Hypertension

The *Journal of Hypertension* addressed the issue of the treatment of hypertension in individuals with Type 2 diabetes: The authors tell us that although the optimal blood pressure in persons with diabetes has not been established, there are indications that it should be lower than the 130/85 mmHg systolic/diastolic pressure recommended by current guidelines. Furthermore, where there may be multiple associated risk factors, most guidelines suggest a threshold for intervention when blood pressure is 140/90 mmHg or more. In particular, in hypertensive diabetic patients, "intervention should be early and aggressive" (Ruilope, and García-Robles. 1997).

Because of the close association of diabetes and hypertension, regular monitoring and record-keeping of blood pressure is also recommended in the next chapter.

3.2.2   Hyperglycemia, Hypertension, and Endothelial Dysfunction

A clearer picture of hypertension in diabetes emerged when the research and clinical applications of NO science became better known. This study reported in the journal *Kardiologiia* aimed to determine the impact of combined antihypertensive therapy with enalapril + indapamide on endothelial dysfunction in patients with arterial hypertension and Type 2 diabetes.

Enalapril is an angiotensin-converting enzyme inhibitor used to treat hypertension and congestive heart failure. Indapamide is used to treat high blood pressure by reducing fluid retention (edema).

Patients 40 to 65 years old, with stage II–III hypertension and Type 2 diabetes, were given the combined antihypertensive therapy for 12 weeks. Endothelial function was determined by the concentration of NO metabolites and endothelin-1 in serum and urine, the results of occlusion test. Endothelin-1 is a vasoconstrictor.

After the 12 weeks of treatment, all the patients achieved blood pressure goals. No impairment of carbohydrate metabolism was noted and endothelial function was improved in hypertensive patients with Type 2 diabetes: both serum and urinary NO production marker rose and urinary endothelin-1 secretion declined. The number of patients with normal microcirculation increased from 13.3% to 53.3%.

The investigators concluded that the treatment with the combined antihypertensive medications was highly effective and safe for recovering endothelial function in hypertensive patients with Type 2 diabetes (Statsenko, and Derevianchenko. 2015).

The authors of a report published in the *Journal of the American Society of Nephrology* tell us that endothelial dysfunction reduces vasodilation, promotes a proinflammatory state, and has prothrombic properties. It is associated with most forms of cardiovascular disease, such as hypertension, coronary artery disease, chronic heart failure, peripheral artery disease, diabetes, and chronic renal failure. The mechanisms involved in reduced vasodilation in endothelial dysfunction include reduced NO formation and excess free radical formation.

The proinflammatory response consists of the upregulation of adhesion molecules, the generation of chemokines such as macrophage chemo-attractant peptide-1, and the production of plasminogen activator inhibitor-1. These responses create a prothrombic state. Furthermore, vasoactive peptides such as angiotensin II and endothelin-1, combined with the accumulation of asymmetric dimethylarginine (ADMA, an endogenous NO inhibitor), hypercholesterolemia, hyperhomocysteinemia, altered insulin signaling, and hyperglycemia, also contribute to these different mechanisms. Detachment and apoptosis of endothelial cells (anoikis) is an associated phenomenon.

3.2.3 ENDOTHELIUM DYSFUNCTION AS THE "LINK" BETWEEN HYPERGLYCEMIA AND HYPERTENSION

Investigators propose in *Current Hypertension Reports* that impairment of the endothelium may be the link between diabetes and cardiovascular disease. They cite evidence that suggests that the pathogenesis of hypertensive and diabetic vascular disease may involve a reduced bioavailability of endothelium-derived NO. Furthermore, they propose that inactivation of NO by ROS targeting the endothelium is an important common mechanism by which endothelial dysfunction may occur (Cosentino and Lüscher. 2001).

3.3 CHRONIC HYPERGLYCEMIA AND ATHEROSCLEROSIS

Endothelial dysfunction is an important early occurrence in the pathogenesis of atherosclerosis, contributing to plaque initiation and progression. Reductions in circulating endothelial progenitor cells that participate in regeneration of the endothelium contribute to endothelial pathophysiology.

Since the discovery in the 1970s that acetylcholine requires the presence of endothelial cells to elicit vasodilation (Furchgott, and Zawadzki. 1980), the importance of the endothelial cell layer for vascular homeostasis has been increasingly appreciated. Endothelial dysfunction has been implicated in the pathophysiology of hypertension, coronary artery disease, chronic heart failure, peripheral artery disease, diabetes, and chronic renal failure (Endemann, and Schiffrin. 2004).

3.3.1 HYPERGLYCEMIA, VASA VASORUM, AND ATHEROSCLEROSIS

The *vasa vasorum*, the blood vessel of blood vessels (see Chapter 2), unlike other blood vessels in the body, depends exclusively on endothelium-derived vasorelaxation. In a study titled "On the regulation of tone in vasa vasorum" published in *Cardiovascular Research*, it was shown that *vasa vasorum* relaxation was solely endothelium-dependent, that is, NO-dependent, whereas the arterial vessel responded to both endothelium-dependent and endothelium-independent relaxation signals (Scotland, Vallance, and Ahluwalia. 1999). In brief, the damage done by atherosclerosis to the endothelium intimately involves first changes in the *vasa vasorum*.

Writing in the journal *Medical Hypotheses* in 2009, researchers contended that known risk factors for atherosclerosis, such as high blood pressure and nicotine, reduce blood flow in the end branches of the *vasa vasorum*. Local impaired blood flow affects the cells of the endothelium causing local inflammation. This makes the endothelium permeable to large particles such as various bacteria, low-density lipoproteins (LDLs), and other fatty acids, which macrophages engulf, transforming them into foam cells (Järvilehto, and Tuohimaa. 2009). Damage to the endothelium is caused by damage to the *vasa vasorum* that then deprives it of oxygen, thus allowing sludge to infiltrate the blood vessel walls (Fried. 2014).

The *vasa vasorum*, as previously noted, is gaining recognition for its role in atherogenesis. It would be only a matter of time before diabetes would be implicated at the very least as a complication. In fact, investigators reported in the journal *Hypertension* that in normoglycemic ApoE(−/−) mice, atherogenesis is associated with *vasa vasorum* expansion, probably corresponding to the increasing blood supply demands of the thickening artery wall. In similar hyperglycemic animals, there is no significant neovascularization of the *vasa vasorum*, despite the fact that lesions are significantly larger. This defect may result from a localized deficiency in vascular endothelial growth factor (VEGF), a signal protein that stimulates vasculogenesis and angiogenesis.

These findings are said to be the first evidence that hyperglycemia alters the structure of the *vasa vasorum*. Such microvascular changes directly correlate and may contribute to the development and progression of atherosclerosis in hyperglycemic ApoE-deficient mice (Veerman, Venegas-Pino, Shi et al. 2013).

The authors of a publication titled "Microvasular and macrovascular complications in diabetes mellitus: distinct or continuum?" published in the *Indian Journal of Endocrinology and Metabolism* contend that diabetes and related complications are linked to long-term damage and failure of various organ systems. However, the line of demarcation between the pathogenic mechanisms of microvascular and macrovascular complications of diabetes and differing responses to therapeutic interventions is blurred.

Diabetes induces changes in the microvasculature, causing extracellular matrix protein synthesis and capillary basement membrane thickening, which are among the features of diabetic microangiopathy. These changes in conjunction with advanced glycation end products (AGEs), oxidative stress, low-grade inflammation, and neovascularization of *vasa vasorum* can lead to macrovascular complications.

Hyperglycemia is the principal cause of microvasculopathy, but it also appears to play an important role in causation of macrovasculopathy. The investigators hold that macrovascular complications seem to be strongly interconnected with microvascular diseases promoting atherosclerosis through processes such as hypoxia and changes in *vasa vasorum*. It is not clear whether microvascular complications distinctly precede macrovascular complications, or whether both progress simultaneously (Chawla, Chawla, and Jaggi. 2016).

Clinical studies of peripheral artery disease have shown that the degree of atherosclerosis in limbs tends to reflect the degree of atherosclerosis in other blood vessels throughout the body (Newman. 2000; Muller, Reed, Leuenberger et al. 2013). However, the obverse does not hold: It has been noted that even in the presence of relatively low levels of atherosclerosis throughout the body, there can be significant plaque formation in coronary arteries.

The journal *Atherosclerosis* published an interesting study titled "Microangiopathy of large artery wall: a neglected complication of diabetes mellitus." The authors aimed to show that diabetic patients with microangiopathy of the retinal microcirculation would also show impaired carotid adventitial microcirculation.

Using contrast-enhanced ultrasound imaging, they quantified the signal of the *vasa vasorum* of the common carotid artery in two subgroups of Type 2 diabetic patients who did not have previous cardiovascular disease: one group with retinopathy and the other group without retinopathy. There was also a reference *vasa vasorum* signal that was measured in a group of healthy volunteers to establish the ratio of the contrast agent signal of the *vasa vasorum* to that of the lumen of the artery.

Patients with diabetic retinopathy showed a higher mean adventitial *vasa vasorum* signal than those without retinopathy. This difference remained highly significant after adjusting for cardiovascular risk factors. Common carotid intima–media thickness (IMT) and carotid plaque prevalence were not different between diabetic subgroups.

It was concluded that Type 2 diabetes patients with retinopathy show increased angiogenesis of the *vasa vasorum* of the common carotid artery, suggesting the existence of a diabetic microangiopathic complication affecting the wall of the large arteries that may be an important contributor to the cardiovascular disease burden in diabetes (Arcidiacono, Traveset, Rubinat et al. 2013).

3.3.2 INTERPRANDIAL AND POSTPRANDIAL GLUCOSE SWINGS PROMOTE ATHEROSCLEROSIS

Chronic hyperglycemia, usually assessed from hemoglobin A1c (HbA1c) determinations, results in excessive glycation and generation of oxidative stress. Consequently, chronic hyperglycemia has been identified as a risk factor for diabetes complications leading to accelerated atherosclerosis. Both fasting and postprandial hyperglycemia contribute to this process. However the acute glucose fluctuations that occur in diabetes have been recently described as an additional factor that activates oxidative stress.

Because of acute glucose swings, including upward (postprandial) and downward (interprandial) fluctuations can be considered as risk factors for cardiovascular events and should be included in the "dysglycemia" of diabetes in combination with fasting and postprandial hyperglycemia.

Since postprandial glucose is a contributor of both acute glucose fluctuations and chronic sustained hyperglycemia, it remains difficult to know whether these mechanisms are equivalent or not equivalent risk factors for cardiovascular disease (Colette, and Monnier. 2007).

3.3.3 HYPERGLYCEMIA AND ENDOPLASMIC RETICULUM STRESS

The issue of causality concerning diabetes and atherosclerosis seems somewhat less obscure. A report in the journal *Cardiovascular and Hematological Disorders Drug Targets* points to endoplasmic reticulum stress and the unfolded protein response pathways as a possible factor. Endoplasmic reticulum stress was previously noted in connection with the impact of diabetes on blood vessel function in Chapter 2.

Endoplasmic reticulum stress has been directly implicated in complications that are associated with diabetes, including pancreatic beta-cell dysfunction and insulin resistance (McAlpine, Bowes, and Werstuck. 2010).

3.3.4 ADVANCED GLYCATION END PRODUCT RECEPTOR

A report in the *Canadian Journal of Diabetes* proposed to link the receptor for advanced glycation end products (RAGEs) to the pathogenesis of complications in diabetes. Because modern diets are largely heat-processed, they contain high levels of AGEs, proteins, or lipids that become glycated as a result of exposure to sugars. See also Chapter 7 for more detail.

Dietary advanced glycation end products (dAGEs) are known to increase oxidant stress and inflammation, factors linked to the recent epidemics of diabetes and cardiovascular disease. Animal-derived foods that are high in fat and protein are generally AGE-rich and prone to new AGE formation during cooking. In contrast, carbohydrate-rich foods such as vegetables, fruits, whole grains, and milk contain relatively few AGEs, even after cooking.

The formation of new AGEs during cooking can be significantly reduced by cooking with moist heat, using shorter cooking times, cooking at lower temperatures, and by use of acidic ingredients such as lemon juice or vinegar (Uribarri, Woodruff, Goodman et al. 2010).

The nature of the AGE receptor has led to the explanation that hyperglycemia-stimulated cellular activation results from the formation of AGEs, which signal through RAGE, as well as the recruitment and activation of inflammatory cells to AGE-laden tissues in diabetes. Such activated inflammatory cells may release proinflammatory ligands of RAGE, thereby contributing to the initiation and amplification of perturbation in both micro- and macrovascular tissues in diabetes.

Strong support for the role of RAGE in the pathogenesis of diabetes-related complications has been shown by antagonizing the ligand-RAGE in animal models, and also by testing the impact of RAGE deletion in diabetic mice.

The authors suggest that RAGE antagonism may offer a viable approach to treatment of diabetic complications (Ramasamy, Yan, and Schmidt. 2006). See Chapter 7 for more details.

3.3.5 ALTERNATE HYPOTHESIS

The preponderance of the evidence presented in this book supports the theory that microvascular complications of diabetes are due predominantly to hyperglycemia. It should be noted, however, that there is an alternate hypothesis that makes a sufficient amount of sense to be worth reporting here. Both the hyperglycemia theory and the alternate theory have ROS as the effect endpoint.

The authors of a study largely paraphrased here, titled "AGEs, rather than hyperglycemia, are responsible for microvascular complications in diabetes: a 'glycoxidation-centric' theory," published in the journal *Nutrition, Metabolism and Cardiovascular Diseases*, propose that excessive AGEs is one of the most important mechanisms involved in the pathophysiology of chronic diabetic complications. Their review summarizes the role these compounds play in microvascular pathogenesis, particularly in the light of recently proposed biochemical mechanisms for diabetic retinopathy, nephropathy, and neuropathy.

Then, they focus on the relationship between AGEs and metabolic memory, trying to clarify the role of metabolic memory in the link between micro- and macrovascular complications. They hold that an excessive AGE formation has been demonstrated in the newly disclosed biochemical pathways involved in the microvascular pathobiology of Type 2 diabetes, confirming the central role of AGEs in the progression of diabetic neuropathy, retinopathy, and nephropathy.

As shown by recent studies, AGEs seem to be not "actors," but "directors" of processes leading to these complications for at least two main reasons: first, AGEs have several intra- and extracellular targets, so they can be seen as a "bridge" between intracellular and extracellular damage; second, whatever the level of hyperglycemia, AGE-related intracellular glycation of the mitochondrial respiratory chain proteins has been found to produce more ROS, triggering a vicious cycle that amplifies AGE formation. This may help to explain the clinical link between micro- and macrovascular disease in diabetes, contributing to clarify the mechanisms behind metabolic memory (Chilelli, Burlina, and Lapolla. 2013).

3.4 HYPERGLYCEMIA, CARDIOVASCULAR DISEASE, AND HEART DISEASE

The British medical journal *Lancet* reported that diabetes is responsible for an approximately twofold increased risk for coronary heart disease, stroke, and deaths from cardiovascular causes, including heart failure, cardiac arrhythmia, sudden death, hypertensive disease, and aortic aneurysms (Sarwar, Gao, Seshasai. 2010). Similarly, other reports of the link between diabetes and cardiovascular and heart disease have looked at different aspects each to determine its role in the pathophysiological outcome.

The Russian journal of clinical medicine *Klinicheskaia meditsina* (*Mosk*) reported a study aimed to determine the role of postprandial hyperglycemia, and high glucose level, 2 h after glucose load in the development of cardiovascular disorders, in patients with Type 2 diabetes, and in the general population.

The investigators reported that medical interventions to reduce postprandial hyperglycemia decrease the risk of cardiovascular disorders linked to oxidative stress in etiology of cardiovascular disorders involving also postprandial hyperglycemia.

Acute hyperglycemia increases heart rate and arterial pressure, disturbs myocardial perfusion and contractility, and causes endothelial dysfunction, and atherosclerosis.

The authors recommended α-glucosidase inhibitors, glynides, ultrashort-acting insulin analogs, dipeptidylpeptidase-4 inhibitors, and/or exenatide (incretin mimetic) for patients with Type 2 diabetes and postprandial hyperglycemia (Shvarts. 2009).

A report in the journal *Diabetes Care* summarizes what is known about the increased risk of vascular disease linked to atherosclerosis in diabetic individuals compared to those free of the condition. The authors contend that diabetic large blood vessel disease also has a more severe course and a greater prevalence of multiple-vessel coronary artery disease with more diffuse and elongated atheromas in affected blood vessels.

They refer to epidemiological studies that suggest that the effect of hyperglycemia on cardiovascular risk is independent of other known risk factors, but aver that no data from primary interventional trials are available yet. They also pointed out that analysis of data sets from populations that included individuals with impaired glucose tolerance and impaired fasting glucose suggests that the damaging effect of hyperglycemia on the blood vessel wall already exists even in the early stages of glucose intolerance.

It seems to be the case that the effect of postprandial or post-challenge hyperglycemia is greater than the effect of fasting blood glucose abnormalities. The relationship of postprandial glycemia, fasting blood glucose, and cardiovascular risk in individuals with diagnosed (or overt) diabetes is less clear, although most reports indicate a greater pathogenic potential of postprandial hyperglycemia than fasting hyperglycemia.

It is concluded that the most appropriate targets in interventional trials are postprandial hyperglycemia or HbA1c (Milicevic, Raz, Beattie et al. 2008).

The *American Journal of Cardiology* reported a study to address "Absence of correlation between coronary arterial atherosclerosis and severity or duration of diabetes mellitus of adult onset" because the relation between the severity and duration of diabetes mellitus and the severity of ischemic heart disease is uncertain.

Clinical and autopsy findings were studied in patients with diabetes of adult onset who ranged in age from 37 to 91 years and had a clinical diagnosis of diabetes established in time spans ranging from a few days, to 50 years before death.

No statistically significant association was demonstrated between the clinically diagnosed severity or duration of diabetes, and either the overall coronary disease, the number of diseased vessels, or the number of myocardial infarctions.

However, comparison with age- and gender-matched control patients revealed that, on the average, diabetic patients have more overall coronary disease, more diffuseness of coronary disease, more coronary collateralization, more vessels involved in atherosclerosis, and more myocardial infarcts (Vigorita, Moore, and Hutchins. 1980).

3.4.1 SOME ANATOMICAL AND PATHOPHYSIOLOGICAL CHANGES IN THE HEART RELATED TO CHRONIC HYPERGLYCEMIA

The *International Journal of Cardiology* reported on aspects of the morphology of diabetic myocardium obtained by endomyocardial biopsy in diabetic patients. There were three sets of observations: The first consisted of patients with unexplained enlarged heart (cardiomegaly) and obscure congestive cardiac failure. The second group had no cardiac signs and symptoms, but exhibited abnormal systolic time intervals. The third group had no cardiac symptoms or signs and had normal systolic time intervals.

The vascular and extravascular changes observed were more pronounced in the symptomatic group, intermediate in the asymptomatic patients with abnormal intervals, and least in those without symptoms and normal intervals.

The investigators concluded that there is evidence of the existence of a specific primary myocardial disease in chronic hyperglycemia even with good structural function (Das, Das, and Chandrasekar. 1987). A similar conclusion was reported in the *Heart Journal*: the authors concluded that evidence has accumulated for the existence of a specific "diabetic" cardiomyopathy.

Abundant literature evidence supports the concept of myocardial dysfunction separate from epicardial coronary disease in diabetic individuals (Zarich, and Nesto. 1989).

The *American Journal of Medicine* reported that clinical and morphologic necropsy observations were made on patients with diabetes with onset of the disease after age 30, some patients without clinical evidence of coronary heart disease (DM – CHD), and some with both diabetes and clinical evidence of coronary heart disease (DM + CHD). These observations were compared to those in age- and sex-matched nondiabetic control participants who died from a fatal coronary event.

The average number of three major (right, left anterior descending, and left circumflex) coronary arteries per patient that narrowed more than 75% in cross-sectional area by atherosclerotic plaques was identical in the diabetic patients with diabetes only, and in those with both diabetes and coronary heart disease, as well as those in the control participants group (2.5/3.0). This similarity in the amount of coronary arterial narrowing was present irrespective of the age at onset (after 30 years) or duration of diabetes.

The DM + CHD patients were found to have more severe narrowing of the three major coronary arteries than did the DM – CHD patients. The amount of severe narrowing in the proximal halves of each of these three arteries was similar to that in the distal halves. The amount of severe narrowing—more than 75% in cross-sectional area—of the left main coronary artery was greater in the patients with diabetes than in the nondiabetic controls participants—13% versus 6%.

The type of treatment given the patients with diabetes, or their adherence to the therapeutic program as measured by the level of random fasting blood sugar, did not alter the amount of severe coronary narrowing observed at necropsy (Waller, Palumbo, Lie et al. 1980).

The *American Journal of Epidemiology* reported a study titled "Association of diabetes mellitus with coronary atherosclerosis and myocardial lesions. An autopsy study from the Honolulu Heart Program." It focused on the excess risk of clinical cardiovascular disease among persons with diabetes and noted that previous autopsy studies had failed to elucidate reasons for the excess, to assess potential selection bias, or to adjust for other cardiovascular risk factors.

Therefore, the study aimed to examine the relation between diabetes and autopsy evidence of coronary atherosclerosis, and myocardial lesions, in a population of Japanese–American men examined at baseline from 1965 to 1968 as part of the Honolulu Heart Program. A number of the participants were free of cardiovascular disease, and some of them died over a 17-year follow-up period.

Myocardial lesions (acute, healing, or fibrotic) occurred significantly more frequently among diabetes than among nondiabetes cohorts (77.7% vs. 63.4%), even after adjustment for other risk factors. It appears that the more adverse risk factor profile among diabetes sufferers accounts for some of the observed excess coronary atherosclerosis.

However, diabetes was independently associated with myocardial lesions, and these findings suggest a role for non-atherosclerotic mechanisms, such as clotting abnormalities or microvascular disease, in accounting for the excess clinical heart disease found in persons with diabetes (Burchfiel, Reed, Marcus et al. 1993).

There is a higher incidence of heart arrhythmias in persons diagnosed with Type 2 diabetes who also suffered myocardial infarction. A study published in the journal *Klinicheskaia Meditsina* revealed that arrhythmias, usually extrasystoles or atrial fibrillation, were more common in patients with Type 2 diabetes (42.1%) and 30.4% in those without that condition.

The frequency of these arrhythmias was directly correlated with coronary and myocardial dysfunction. In patients with diabetes, arrhythmias were also associated with the duration of the diabetes and with HbA1c level.

In severe metabolic decompensation (HbA1c greater than 8.5%) and in cases with a relatively low HbA1c level (less than 7%), arrhythmias were more frequent than in patients with an HbA1c level between 7.0% and 8.5%.

The authors concluded that cardiac arrhythmias, systolic dysfunction, and diabetes are "prognostically unfavorable factors" influencing the survival rate in patients with myocardial infarction and Type 2 diabetes (Panova, and Kruglova. 2008).

Further evidence of the hazard of chronic hyperglycemia to cardiovascular and heart function is reported in the journal *PLoS ONE*: A systematic review and meta-analysis of MEDLINE database prospective studies was undertaken to determine the association of HbA1c level with the risk of all-cause mortality and cardiovascular outcomes in patients with Type 2 diabetes. Twenty-six studies with a mean follow-up range of 2.2 to 16 years were included in this analysis.

It was found that the pooled relative risk associated with a 1% increase in HbA1c level among patients with Type 2 diabetes was 1.15 for all-cause mortality, 1.17 for cardiovascular disease, 1.15 for coronary heart disease, 1.11 for heart failure, 1.11 for stroke, and 1.29 for peripheral arterial disease. In addition, a positive dose–response trend existed between HbA1c level and cardiovascular outcomes.

The authors contend that there are biologically plausible mechanisms that explain why chronic hyperglycemia is associated with cardiovascular outcomes and all-cause mortality. For one thing, hyperglycemic periods play a major role in the activation of oxidative stress and overproduction of mitochondrial superoxide, which trigger various metabolic pathways of glucose-mediated vascular damage (Brownlee, and Hirsch. 2006; Monnier, Mas, Ginet et al. 2006). For another thing, glucose can react with proteins to form AGEs, which may contribute to long-term complications in diabetes, plaque formation, and atherosclerosis (Sheetz, and King. 2002) (see Chapter 7).

These effects are gradual and likely to be cumulative, occurring during decades of exposure to chronically elevated blood glucose levels, and it has been suggested that most previous studies, including clinical trials, may have had insufficient follow-up to detect a moderate increase in risk (Selvin, Marinopoulos, Berkenblit et al. 2004).

The authors concluded that *"chronic hyperglycemia is associated with an increased risk for cardiovascular outcomes and all-cause mortality among patients with Type 2 diabetes, likely independently from other conventional risk factors"* (Zhang, Hu, Yuan et al. 2012).

3.4.1.1 The Effect of Hyperglycemia on Heart Rate Variability

In normal circumstances, at rest, the rhythm of the heart follows the breathing cycle: pulse rate rises with inspiration and declines with expiration (Fried, and Grimaldi. 1993). Taken in toto, *this is the nature of heart rate variability* (HRV). Parenthetically, Hales noted in 1733 that blood pressure follows the same pattern (Dornhorst, Howard, and Leathhart. 1952).

HRV is considered a useful tool in determining the modulatory effects of the autonomic nervous system on the heart (Billman, Huikuri, Sacha et al. 2015). Historically, HRV was determined by the time distribution of pulse interbeat intervals and taken as a measure of the modulation of the Hering–Breuer reflex by sympathetic activation. Some years ago, this analysis was taken to task for failing to account for the sequential dependency of interbeat intervals, therefore defying any analysis then known, since these relied on sequential independence (Fried. 1972; Fried. 1993).

The interaction between the sympathetic and parasympathetic discharge to the heart is of course a major determinant of HRV and consequently cardiac autonomic modulations (Freeman, and Chapleau. 2013). Time and frequency domain analyses are commonly used to evaluate HRV and cardiac autonomic modulation. However, frequency domain is preferred if HRV measurements are derived from short-term (5-min) electrocardiograph (ECG) recording.

Natural logarithm of total power, very low frequency, low frequency and high frequency, low frequency/high frequency ratio, and normalized low frequency and high frequency are the main measurements used to express results of frequency domain HRV analysis (No authors listed. 1996; Lutfi. 2015). Of course, any repetitive observation has "frequency" but that does not mean that it is frequency-modulated because "modulated" here means *driven*; in other words, the "intelligence" in the signal is encoded in modulation. Both the electrocardiograph and the electroencephalograph are amplitude-modulated signals that have frequency as one aspect.

There is much more to this and some of it can be found in Lutfi, and Elhakeem (2016). But, more important, what is the effect of hyperglycemia on HRV, and what might be the consequence of such an effect?

This study on HRV as a function of blood glucose level, published in the journal *PLoS ONE*, demonstrates that an increase in blood glucose concentration, within physiological range, is associated with higher parasympathetic and lower sympathetic cardiac autonomic modulation. Combining results of previous reports and the present, the enhanced sympathetic discharge associated with hypoglycemia seems to extend to the lower range of normal fasting blood glucose, but decrease gradually and is replaced by enhanced parasympathetic modulations at a higher normal level of fasting blood glucose. Further research is needed to detect the glycemic threshold beyond which further increase in glucose level readjusts sympathovagal balance toward sympathetic predominance again (Lutfi, and Elhakeem. 2016).

The journal *Diabetic Medicine* reported a study that aimed to evaluate the relationships between dysglycemia, insulin resistance and metabolic variables, and heart rate, heart rate recovery, and HRV, part of the Epidemiological Study on the Insulin Resistance syndrome (DESIR) (9-year) study.

All participants reported that they were free of cardiac antecedents and were not taking drugs that alter heart rate. During five consecutive periods (rest, deep breathing, recovery, rest and lying, to standing), heart rate and HRV were measured and analyzed.

It was found that heart rate differed between glycemic groups, except during deep breathing. Between rest and deep-breathing periods, patients with diabetes had a lower increase in heart rate than others; between deep breathing and recovery, the heart rate of patients with diabetes continued to rise, and for others, heart rate declined. Heart rate correlated positively with capillary glucose and triglycerides during the five test periods.

HRV differed according to glycemic status, especially during the recovery period. After age, gender, and body mass index (BMI) adjustment, HRV was correlated with triglycerides at two test periods. Change in heart rate between recovery and deep breathing was inversely correlated with HRV at rest: lower resting HRV was associated with heart rate acceleration.

The investigators concluded that heart rate, but not HRV, was associated with glycemic status and capillary glucose. After deep breathing, heart rate recovery was altered in patients with known diabetes and was associated with reduced HRV (Valensi, Extramiana, Lange et al. 2011).

To what extent does hyperglycemia disrupt autonomic homeostasis? The journal *Diabetes Care* published a report titled "Diabetes, glucose, insulin, and heart rate variability: the Atherosclerosis Risk in Communities (ARIC) study." The aim of the study was to describe the progression of autonomic impairment among individuals with diabetes and prediabetic metabolic impairments. The study involved observation of changes in HRV over a 9-year period in a population-based cohort of individuals 45 to 64 years old at baseline, and cross-sectional associations among these individuals.

It was found that diabetic participants had a more rapid temporal decrease in HRV conditional on baseline HRV than nondiabetic participants. While the investigators found cross-sectional associations between decreased HRV and diabetic and nondiabetic hyperinsulinemia, and a weak inverse association with fasting glucose, neither impaired fasting glucose nor nondiabetic hyperinsulinemia was associated with a measurably more rapid decline in HRV than normal.

The investigators concluded that cardiac autonomic impairment appears to be present at early stages of diabetic metabolic impairment, and progressive worsening of autonomic cardiac function over 9 years was observed in diabetes participants (Schroeder, Chambless, Liao et al. 2005).

3.4.1.2   HRV and Blood Glucose Levels: Potential for Noninvasive Glucose Monitoring for Diabetes

There is a great need for a means of noninvasive glucose monitoring that is suitable for continuous monitoring. Such means do not presently exist, nor does it seem that they are in sight. There is presently a continuous monitoring unit on the market, but it is, albeit minimally, nevertheless invasive; it is expensive, and not readily available to the average consumer without a prescription from a physician.

Good glucose control cannot be established until antiglycemic means can be matched to blood levels of glucose patterns as these vary over the day.

The journal *Diabetes Technology and Therapeutics* reported that the dynamic physiological nature of HRV suggests a possible noninvasive measure of the autonomic nervous system as an alternative means of blood glucose monitoring.

The participants in this study were diabetes patients (average age, 40 years) and nondiabetes control participants (average age, 30 years).

Fasting preceded a 10-min, three-lead ECG, which was followed by a finger prick-blood glucose assessment. After this, a regular meal was consumed, and 30 min after ingestion, a second post-prandial 10-min ECG was obtained, and blood glucose assessment was conducted.

It was found that low-frequency power, high-frequency power, and total power of HRV were inversely associated with blood glucose level in participants with diabetes. Furthermore, the ratio of low-frequency power to high-frequency power was positively correlated with blood glucose level.

Duration of diabetes was also associated with multiple HRV parameters, with negative associations between both low-frequency power and high-frequency power parameters as well as total power.

The investigators concluded that the links between specific HRV factors, and blood glucose levels, could provide a unique and real-time method for monitoring blood glucose for continuous noninvasive prediction and/or management of diabetes (Rothberg, Lees, Clifton-Bligh et al. 2016).

3.5   DIABETES AND THYROID HORMONES

The pituitary gland controls the production of many hormones, including thyroid-stimulating hormone (TSH), which in turn determines how much T4 the thyroid gland will release. The TSH level in blood indicates how much T4 the pituitary gland is signaling the thyroid gland to make. Abnormally high TSH levels usually indicate underactive thyroid, that is, hypothyroidism. There are many explanations for hypothyroidism, but the most common cause of hypothyroidism in the United States is Hashimoto's thyroiditis, an autoimmune disorder. However, worldwide, insufficient iodine in the diet is the most common cause of hypothyroidism.

The thyroid gland also secretes the hormone triiodothyronine, known as T3, from T4. It is T3 that is actually the active hormone. If one is producing too little thyroid hormone, TSH rises, and if one makes too much of it, TSH declines.

What's normal can vary, depending on a number of factors, including the laboratory where the blood test is performed, but generally, the normal range for TSH in most laboratories is 0.4 milliunits per liter (mU/L) to 4.0 mU/L. Therefore, a TSH higher than 4.0 mU/L, on repeat tests, indicates the likelihood of hypothyroidism.

Most of the T4 in blood attaches to a protein, preventing it from entering body cells. Only "free" T4 can enter cells. There is a blood test that can measure the level of free T4 (FT4).

3.5.1   Hypothyroidism Raises the Risk of Diabetes

"The hypoglycemic side of hypothyroidism" is the title of a study published in the Indian *Journal of Endocrinology and Metabolism*. The authors contend that hypothyroidism is linked to various hormonal, biochemical, and nervous system abnormalities; among them, there is blunted hypothalamo-pituitary-adrenal response to hypoglycemia in hypothyroid persons (Kamilaris, DeBold, Pavlou et al. 1987).

The role of gluconeogenesis is reduced in hypothyroidism, both in skeletal muscle and in adipose tissue (McCulloch, Johnston, Baylis et al. 1983), as is also glycogenolysis. (McDaniel, Pittman, Oh et al. 1977). These biochemical defects lead to a delayed recovery from hypoglycemia.

Other abnormalities in hypothyroidism include a reduction in glucagon secretion (Clausen, Lins, Adamson et al. 1986), reduced effect of glucagon on hepatocytes in an animal model (Müller, and Seitz. 1987), and slowing of insulin clearance (Shah, Motto, Papagiannes et al. 1975). Contributory factors also include the effect of hypothyroidism on the gastrointestinal system: It slows gastric emptying and decreases intestinal absorption of glucose as well as portal venous flow (Holdsworth, and Besser. 1968).

There are also reports of the link between subclinical and overt hypothyroidism on one hand, and insulin resistance on the other (Singh, Goswami, and Mallika. 2010). This seeming paradox is explained by contrasting the insulin agonist actions of thyroid hormones, evident in peripheral tissues, with insulin antagonist activity in the liver (Brenta. 2011; see also Kalra, Unnikrishnan, and Sahay. 2014).

A recent study published in the journal *BMC Medicine* warned that low blood thyroid hormone—even low-normal—raises the risk of developing Type 2 diabetes, particularly in people with prediabetes. Adults in the lowest third of thyroid function levels had a 1.4 times higher risk of progressing from prediabetes to Type 2 diabetes than those in the highest third of thyroid function. Patients diagnosed with prediabetes, and hypothyroidism, have a 40% greater likelihood of developing diabetes.

In an interview, one of the authors of that study reported that, over a lifetime, 70% to 75% of people diagnosed with prediabetes will progress to diabetes (Chaker, Lighart, Korevaar. 2016). The data in that report were drawn from participants from the Rotterdam Study, a population-based study of adults, aged 45 or older, that reflects the general population in the Netherlands. The study had 58% women participants, aged 65, on average.

No patients had diabetes at baseline, and mean TSH and free thyroxine (FT4) were on par with that of the general population (1.91 mIU/L and 1.22 ng/dL, respectively). All participants were tested for blood sugar and thyroid function, and reexamined every 2 to 3 years to check for the development of Type 2 diabetes.

Patients with fasting glucose between 108 and 125 mg/dL (6 and 7 mmol/L) were considered to have prediabetes, and those with a fasting glucose of 125 mg/dL (7 mmol/L) or more were considered to have diabetes.

Over an average follow-up of nearly 8 years, higher TSH was linked to increased diabetes risk (hazard ratio = 1.13), even within the reference range of thyroid function. Risk for progression from prediabetes to diabetes was 1.4 times greater for participants in the lowest third of thyroid function levels compared with those in the highest third. Even people whose thyroid function was in the low-normal range had an increased risk of diabetes (Chaker, Ligthart, Korevaar et al. 2016).

Parenthetically, it was shown in a previously cited study that statins increased the risk of progression from prediabetes to diabetes (Chaker, Ligthart, Korevaar et al. 2016). The aim of a study published in the journal *Diabetes Care* was twofold: Phase one involved high-throughput in silico processing of biomedical data to identify risk factors for the development of statin-associated diabetes.

In phase two, the most prominent risk factor identified was confirmed in an observational cohort study at Clalit, the largest health care organization in Israel. Statin nonusers were matched by propensity score to highly compliant statin initiators in 2004 to 2005 and followed until the end of 2010.

It was found that hypothyroidism and subclinical hypothyroidism bore an increased risk for diabetes (RR, 1.53 and 1.75, respectively). Hypothyroidism increased diabetes risk irrespective of statin treatment (RR, 2.06 and 1.66 in statin users and nonusers, respectively). Subclinical hypothyroidism risk for diabetes was prominent only upon statin use (RR, 1.94 and 1.20 in statin users and nonusers, respectively).

It was concluded, first, that hypothyroidism is a risk factor for diabetes. Second, subclinical hypothyroidism-associated risk for diabetes was found to be prominent only with statin use. Third, identifying and treating hypothyroidism and subclinical hypothyroidism might reduce the risk of diabetes (Gronich, Deftereos, Lavi et al. 2015).

It has been reported that metformin, a first-line oral hypoglycemic agent, may tend to lower TSH. The aim of a study published in the *Canadian Medical Association Journal* was to determine whether the use of metformin monotherapy, when compared with sulfonylurea monotherapy, is associated with an increased risk of low TSH levels (less than 0.4 mIU/L) in patients with Type 2 diabetes.

Conventional statistical analysis indicated that the incidence of low TSH levels in diabetes patients (compared to euthyroid patients) with treated hypothyroidism observed during follow-up was 119.7/1000 person-years. Compared with sulfonylurea monotherapy, metformin monotherapy was associated with a 55% increased risk of low TSH levels in patients with treated hypothyroidism (incidence rate, 79.5/1000 person-years vs. 125.2/1000 person-years [adjusted hazard ratio = 1.55], with the highest risk 90 to 180 days after initiation [adjusted hazard ratio = 2.30]). No association was observed in euthyroid patients, whose data are not reported here.

It was concluded that metformin use was associated with an increased incidence of low TSH levels in patients with treated hypothyroidism (but not in euthyroid patients) (Fournier, Yin, Yu et al. 2014). "Euthyroid" describes abnormal findings on thyroid function tests that occur in the face of a nonthyroidal illness.

What is the effect of treating thyroid deficiency in Type 2 diabetes? The *World Journal of Diabetes* addressed exactly that question in a study titled "Effect of treatment of overt hypothyroidism on insulin resistance." The study aimed to determine the outcome of hypothyroidism and thyroxine therapy on insulin sensitivity in patients with overt hypothyroidism.

The study was conducted on overtly hypothyroid and on healthy euthyroid South Western Asian women. The two groups were matched for age and BMI. Physiological and pathological conditions as well as medications that may alter thyroid function, glucose homeostasis, or serum lipids were ruled out. Serum thyrotropin (TSH), free tetraiodothyronine (FT4), free triiodothyronine (FT3), fasting insulin, fasting plasma glucose, total cholesterol, and triglycerides were measured before and 6 months after initiating thyroxine therapy for hypothyroid patients, and once for the control group. Insulin resistance (IR) was estimated using homeostasis model assessment (HOMA-IR) and BMI was calculated.

It was shown that in both study groups, hypothyroid patients and euthyroid control participants, there was no significant difference in fasting plasma glucose, fasting insulin, insulin resistance, total cholesterol, and triglycerides between the hypothyroid patients and the euthyroid control group.

In the hypothyroid patients, triglycerides correlated positively with TSH and negatively with FT3. Similarly, total cholesterol correlated negatively with FT3. After thyroxine replacement and reaching an euthyroid state as confirmed by clinical and laboratory data, there was no significant change in fasting plasma glucose, insulin resistance, or triglyceride level, while total cholesterol significantly declined and fasting insulin significantly rose (Nada. 2013).

An interesting theoretical explanation of a flat glucose tolerance curve after oral glucose tolerance test is reported in a study published in the *Medical Journal, Armed Forces of India*. According to the authors, oral glucose load produces a flat glucose tolerance curve in patients with primary hypothyroidism. Delayed glucose absorption was proposed to explain the flat glucose tolerance curve, but the exact mechanism remains to be determined.

Therefore, they undertook to determine glucose and insulin response to oral glucose tolerance test and intravenous glucose tolerance test in newly diagnosed patients with hypothyroidism and healthy control participants matched for gender, age, BMI, and waist hip ratio. Other conventional controls such as family history, hypertension, and so on, were also applied.

Fasting plasma glucose levels were significantly lower in hypothyroid patients (78 ± 2.2 vs. 88 ± 4.4 mg/dL) than in the control participants.

The oral glucose tolerance curve was flat, with plasma glucose levels significantly lower at 30 min. The insulin levels during oral glucose tolerance test were found to be higher in the patients at all stages. There was loss of first-phase insulin response to the glucose load during the intravenous glucose tolerance test, which was blunted at all stages, and the difference was statistically significant at 0 and 3 min.

Loss of first-phase insulin response to intravenous glucose suggests that there is evidence of beta-cell dysfunction. Patients with hypothyroidism were more insulin sensitive than control participants and insulin secretion was comparable to that in controls.

The authors concluded that a flat glucose tolerance curve can be explained by the absence of an insulin priming effect leading to decreased glucose absorption, followed by increased glucose disposal, because of higher insulin levels after oral glucose test and increased glucose disposal caused by increased insulin sensitivity (Pakhetra, Garg, and Saini. 2001).

3.6 DIABETES, KIDNEY FUNCTION, AND KIDNEY STONE FORMATION

There is very little reason for the average person to think that there might be a link between diabetes and kidney stones, yet the link is quite well established.

There are two kidneys, bean-shaped organs each about the size of a fist, located just below the rib cage, one on each side of the spine. Every day, the two kidneys filter about 120 to 150 quarts of blood to produce about 1 to 2 quarts of urine, composed of wastes and extra fluid. The urine flows from the kidneys to the bladder through two thin muscle tubes (ureters), one on each side of the bladder. The bladder stores the urine.

The muscles of the bladder wall remain relaxed while the bladder fills with urine, but as the bladder fills to capacity, signals sent to the brain signal the urge to urinate. When the bladder empties, urine flows out of the body through the urethra, located at the bottom of the bladder (https://www .niddk.nih.gov/health-information/kidney-disease/kidneys-how-they-work).

3.6.1 TYPE 2 DIABETES IS LINKED TO KIDNEY DISEASE

The aim of a study published in the journal *BMC Nephrology* was to determine the prevalence of different types of renal disease in patients with Type 2 diabetes. The data were obtained by a cross-sectional study of a random sample of Type 2 diabetes patients in primary care. The variables considered were demographic and clinical characteristics, pharmacological treatments, and Type 2 diabetes complications such as diabetic foot ulcers, retinopathy, coronary heart disease, and stroke. Renal function variables were as follows:

1. Microalbuminuria: albumin excretion rate of 30 mg/g or 3.5 mg/mmol
2. Macroalbuminuria: albumin excretion rate of 300 mg/g or 35 mg/mmol
3. Kidney disease: glomerular filtration rate (GFR) according to modification of diet in renal disease less than 60 mL/min/1.73 m^2 and/or the presence of albuminuria
4. Renal impairment: GFR less than 60 mL/min/1.73 m^2
5. Nonalbuminuric renal impairment: GFR less than 60 mL/min/1.73 m^2 without albuminuria
6. Diabetic nephropathy: macroalbuminuria or microalbuminuria plus diabetic retinopathy

It was found that the prevalence of different types of renal disease in patients was as follows:

34.1% kidney disease
22.9% renal impairment
19.5% albuminuria
16.4% diabetic nephropathy

The prevalence of albuminuria without renal impairment was 13.5% and nonalbuminuric renal impairment was 14.7%. After adjusting for age, BMI, cholesterol, blood pressure, and macrovascular disease, renal impairment was found to be a significant factor in women (odds ratio [OR], 2.20), microvascular disease (OR, 2.14), and insulin treatment (OR, 1.82), and it was inversely related to HbA1c (OR, 0.85 for every 1% increase).

Albuminuria without renal impairment was inversely related to duration of diabetes (OR, 0.94) and directly related to HbA1c (OR, 1.19 for every 1% increase).

It was concluded that one-third of the population in this study suffered kidney disease. The presence or absence of albuminuria identified two subgroups with different characteristics related to gender, the duration of diabetes and the metabolic status of the patient (Coll-de-Tuero, Mata-Cases, Rodriguez-Poncelas et al. 2012).

The journal *Primary Care Diabetes* reported a study conducted in Finland to examine the prevalence of chronic kidney disease, and related cardiovascular morbidity, in a cross-sectional population in patients with type 2 diabetes treated in a primary care setting.

The patients ranged in age between 29 and 92 years, and the average age was 67 years; average BMI was 32.8 kg/m2; blood pressure ranged between 140 and 143/80–81 (average was 142/80 mmHg); the HbA1c range was 7.0% to 7.2% (53.8 mmol/mol, 53 to 55) with an average of 7.1%; the median duration of diabetes was 9.2 years, ranging from newly diagnosed to 43 years; 73.3% of the patients had a history of dyslipidemia, 27.8% had cardiovascular disease, and 82.7% had hypertension.

The primary endpoint, prevalence of chronic kidney disease of any grade (1 to 5) or albuminuria, was 68.6%; 16.2% of the patients had an estimated glomerular filtration rate (eGFR) less than 60 mL/min/1.72 m², and they were classified as having chronic kidney disease grade 3 to 5. Concerning renal damage, albuminuria was present in 24.3% of the patients, with microalbuminuria in 17.1% and macroalbuminuria in 7.2%.

Combining the patients with chronic kidney disease and/or the presence of albuminuria, 34.7% seemed to suffer from significant chronic kidney disease. The proportion of patients with albuminuria increased with a decrease in GFR. Historically, diabetic nephropathy had been diagnosed in 24.3% of the patients.

The authors reported that nearly 70% of patients with Type 2 diabetes in primary care, in Finland, have some sign of chronic kidney disease, and nearly half of all Type 2 diabetes patients have a significant chronic kidney disease. Parenthetically, only half of them were diagnosed and documented in their patient charts, thus highlighting the importance of performing routine screening of nephropathy by measuring both albuminuria and eGFR in patients with Type 2 diabetes (Metsärinne, Bröijersen, Kantola et al. 2015).

A study published in the *British Journal of General Practice*, conducted in two Dutch primary health care centers in the Netherlands, concerned the prevalence and severity of chronic kidney disease in primary care patients with diabetes or hypertension.

The patients were about 25 years old, on average, with Type 2 diabetes or hypertension. The initial screening uptake rates were assessed from the electronic patient records. The presence of albuminuria was determined, GFR was estimated, and clinical characteristics were extracted.

In initial screening, 93% were diagnosed with diabetes and 69% were diagnosed with hypertension. The prevalence of chronic kidney disease was 28% in those with diabetes only and 21% in those with hypertension only. The presence of diabetes was independently associated with albuminuria (OR, 4.23), but not with decreased eGFR (OR, 0.75). Age showed the strongest association with decreased eGFR (OR, 2.73).

The authors reported that in primary care, more than one-quarter of patients with diabetes and about one-fifth of patients with hypertension have chronic kidney disease (van der Meer, Wielders, Grootendorst et al. 2010).

3.6.1.1 A Note on eGFR

The eGFR is used to screen for and detect early kidney damage, to help diagnose chronic kidney disease, and to monitor kidney status. It is a calculation based on the results of a blood creatinine test along with other variables such as age, gender, and race (e.g., African-American, non–African-American), depending on the equation used.

Creatinine is a waste product produced by muscles from the breakdown of creatine. The more muscle mass a person has, the more creatinine will be produced.

Almost all creatinine is filtered from the blood by the kidneys and released into the urine, so blood levels are usually a good indicator of how well the kidneys are working. The creatinine blood test is frequently ordered along with a blood urea nitrogen (BUN) test or as part of a basic or comprehensive metabolic panel.

The National Kidney Disease Education Program, the American Society of Nephrology, and the National Kidney Foundation all recommend that an eGFR be calculated every time a creatinine blood test is done. The creatinine test is ordered frequently as part of a routine comprehensive metabolic panel (AKA basic metabolic panel) or along with a BUN test to evaluate the functional status of a person's kidneys.

Creatinine, along with eGFR, is often used to monitor people with known chronic kidney disease, and those with conditions such as diabetes and high blood pressure, that may lead to kidney damage.

Other tests that may be conducted at the same time to help detect kidney damage and/or evaluate kidney function include urine albumin (microalbumin) and albumin/creatinine ratio, used to screen people with chronic conditions, such as diabetes and hypertension, that put them at an increased risk of developing kidney disease; increased levels of albumin in the urine may indicate kidney damage; and urinalysis to help detect signs of kidney damage, such as the presence of blood or casts in the urine. A creatinine test and eGFR may be ordered to evaluate kidney function either as part of a health checkup, or if kidney disease is suspected.

Most men with normal kidney function have approximately 0.6 to 1.2 mg/dL of creatinine. Most women with normal kidney function have between 0.5 and 1.1 mg/dL of creatinine. Women usually have lower creatinine levels than men because women, on average, have less muscle mass than men. Other factors that may affect the level of creatinine in the blood include body size, activity level, and medications.

eGFR results are reported as mL/min/1.73m^2. Because some laboratories do not collect information on a patient's race when the sample is collected for testing, they may report calculated results for both African-Americans and non–African-Americans.

A normal eGFR for adults is greater than 90 mL/min/1.73m^2, according to the National Kidney Foundation.

An eGFR below 60 mL/min/1.73m^2 suggests that some kidney damage has occurred. Chronic kidney disease is diagnosed when a person has an eGFR less than 60 mL/min/1.73m^2 for more than 3 months.

3.6.1.2   GFR and Creatinine Normally Rise with Age

GFR and creatinine are major clinical indices of kidney function, and kidney function is adversely affected by Type 2 diabetes. According to the American Diabetes Association, the percentage of Americans who have diabetes and who are 65 years old and older remains high at 25.9%, or about 11.2 million seniors (http://www.diabetes.org/diabetes-basics/statistics/; accessed 6.25.17). The importance of these statistics is that it begs the need to determine whether clinical measures of kidney function take the natural changes in the aging population into account.

The last decade saw the introduction of a new paradigm where the true or measured GFR is estimated (eGFR) by formulas based on serum creatinine levels, and where these estimates are used in diagnosis of chronic kidney disease in the general population. These criteria for diagnosis of chronic kidney disease include an absolute threshold, unadjusted for the effects of age on the normal values for eGFR.

In consequence of these criteria, the frequency of chronic kidney disease in the general population is thought to be overestimated, and there may now be more "false positive" diagnoses of chronic kidney disease (Glassock, and Winearls. 2009).

However, a study published in *Transactions of the American Clinical and Climatological Association* holds that it has been well established since the 1930s that GFR declines predictably with normal aging, usually beginning after the age of 30 to 40. The rate of decline may accelerate after age 50 to 60 years. This decline appears to be a part of the normal physiologic process of cellular and organ senescence, and it is associated with structural changes in the kidneys.

In fact, there is a natural change in kidney function as we age that is imbedded in the clinical measures. According to *Molecular and Clinical Basics of Gerontology* (Kvell, Pongrácz, Székely et al. 2011), renal mass, renal blood flow, and the number of functioning nephrons in the kidneys decrease in the elderly, leading to both glomerular and tubular dysfunctions. The GFR also decreases progressively with age.

By the age of 80, GFR may decrease to 50%, resulting in the tendency for an elevation of BUN (azotemia) and serum creatinine levels, due to fall of kidney function (Kvell, Pongrácz, Székely et al. 2011; http://www.tankonyvtar.hu/en/tartalom/tamop425/0011_1A_Gerontologia_en_book/ch01s07.html).

The objective of a study reported in the journal *Cardiovascular Surgery* was to establish age-related reference intervals for serum creatinine, especially for those persons over 60 years of age, to assist in the clinical interpretation of creatinine levels in the years after a surgical procedure.

Serum creatinine concentration rose steadily with age; in women from the age of 40 years, and from 60 years for men. Reference intervals for men and women, ranging in age between 20 and 94 years, were established. It was found that advancing age affects serum creatinine levels, especially in the "vascular" age group of 60 to 80 years (Tiao, Semmens, Masarei et al. 2002).

According to the authors of a report, "Understanding and Estimating Glomerular Filtration Rate," on Medscape, the real problem clinicians face is to be able to determine who actually has chronic kidney disease, and who doesn't. For instance, normally, if serum creatinine is 1 mg/dL, GFR would be about 100 mL/min/1.73 m^2. Likewise, the journal *Nephrology, Dialysis and Transplantation* published a report titled "Serum creatinine is a poor marker of GFR in nephrotic syndrome" that illustrates the relationship between serum creatinine and GFR—the effects of age on renal function (Goldfarb, Fishbane, and Provenzano. 2017). The investigators point out that, at age 70 or older, the trend has shifted so that serum creatinine of 1 mg/dL now has a GFR that is about half of that in a younger person (hereabove labeled "normal"). The author, Goldfarb, presents the following analogy:

> This represents the relationship between creatinine production, levels of creatinine in the blood, and creatinine in the urine. I always like to analogize this to a reservoir; a reservoir's level will start to rise if outflow from the reservoir is impaired. However, if inflow and outflow are impaired equally, then the level doesn't rise, yet outflow is impaired. That's exactly what happens in elderly individuals; their production of creatinine falls dramatically because their muscle mass falls, even though their weight may not fall. Therefore, at any level of creatinine production, a serum creatinine that represents their outflow may be quite different from what it is in a normal individual. A youthful normal individual with serum creatinine of 2 mg/dL has a GFR that is half of normal, but an elderly individual may have a GFR that is half of normal when his or her serum creatinine is 1 mg/dL. Thus, we have a large number of patients with serum creatinines in the normal range, but in fact they have reduced GFRs; they have renal disease. [From Goldfarb, Fishbane, Provenzano et al. Patients with moderate chronic kidney disease: the emerging mandate. *Medscape CME & Education*. Published June 20, 2006 (expired CME activity). Available at: https://www.medscape.org/view article/533695. With permission.]

The *Journal of Pakistan Medical Association* reported a study aimed at determining the frequency of patients with underlying renal insufficiency scheduled for coronary angiography with normal serum creatinine less than 1.5 mg/dL. GFR was calculated for each patient using the Cockcroft–Gault equation and a GFR less than 80 ml/min was labeled as renal insufficiency. The mean age of men was 51.86 ± 10.19 years, and that of women was 51.52 ± 9.80 years.

Almost one-third of the patients had GFR less than 80 ml/min; 83.5% of patients had GFR less than 80 mL/min.

It is quite clear, looking at Table 3.2, that as men and women age from 40 to 70, the number of patients with GFR greater than 80 mL/min declines, and the number of them with GFR less than 80 mL/min rises.

TABLE 3.2
Age Bracket-Related Distribution of GFR in Men and Women

			GFR ml/min		
	No. of Subjects		<80	>80	p Value
Gender	Male	538	168(31.2%)	370(68.8%)	0.003
	Female	155	68(43.9%)	87(56.1%)	
Age groups	<40 years	67	7(10.4%)	60(89.6%)	0.001
	40–49 years	208	32(15.4%)	176(84.6%)	
	50–59 years	238	81(34.0%)	157(66.0%)	
	60–69 years	142	83(58.5%)	59(41.5%)	
	≥ 70 years	38	33(86.8%)	5(13.2%)	

Source: Mujtaba, Ashraf, Mahmood et al. 2010. *Journal of Pakistan Medical Association*, Nov; 60(11): 915–917. With permission.

The investigators concluded that, in this study conducted in Pakistan, most of the patients with normal serum creatinine have abnormal GFR. Serum creatinine, which is considered to be an important screening test in patients with renal impairment, might remain in the normal range despite the renal function being significantly impaired. Therefore, GFR should be considered as an estimate of renal insufficiency, regardless of serum creatinine levels being in normal range.

It should be noted that an increase in the mean value of serum creatinine was observed particularly in aging women. This emphasizes the importance of validating an age-specific reference range for serum creatinine in any population (Mujtaba, Ashraf, Mahmood et al. 2010).

A study reported in the *Indian Journal of Clinical Biochemistry* aimed to determine calculated reference interval for serum creatinine levels of healthy normal individuals in different gender and age groups, compared with the established interval in a sample from a population in India. The calculated reference intervals for serum creatinine level were as follows:

- For age groups 21–40 years, 0.4 to 1.3 mg/dL
- For age groups 41–60 years, 0.6 to 1.3 mg/dL

The difference between the mean serum creatinine values in men and women, in the age range 21 to 60 years, was statistically significant. When men and women participants were analyzed by age group, the data showed a significant difference between mean serum creatinine values in the three age groups 21 to 30, 31 to 40, and 41 to 50 years. In the older age group 51 to 60 years, the difference was nonsignificant (Verma, Khadapkar, Sahu et al. 2006).

It stands to reason that there may be slight differences in clinical kidney function test measures obtained from people in widely different world geographical regions but, bottom-line, regardless of the region, these measures can be expected to follow the pattern of age-related changes.

3.6.2 DIABETES AND KIDNEY STONES

Urine contains many dissolved minerals and salts that, when concentrated, can form "stones." Kidney stones usually start small but they can grow larger in size, even filling the inner hollow structures of the kidney. Some stones stay in the kidney and do not cause any problems. But sometimes, the kidney stone can travel down the ureter, reach the bladder, and pass out of the body in urine. If the stone becomes lodged in the ureter, it blocks the urine flow from that kidney, causing intense pain.

Kidney stones come in many different types and colors. How they are treated, how they can be stopped, and how to prevent new stones from forming depends on the type of stone:

Calcium stones, the most common type of kidney stone (about 80%), come in two types: calcium oxalate and calcium phosphate. Calcium oxalate is by far the most common type of calcium stone. Some people have too much calcium in their urine, raising their risk of calcium stones. Even with normal amounts of calcium in the urine, calcium stones may form for other reasons.

Uric acid stones (5% to 10% of stones) come from chemical changes in the body. Uric acid crystals do not dissolve well in acidic urine and instead will form a uric acid stone. Having acidic urine may come from

- Being overweight
- Chronic diarrhea
- Type 2 diabetes (hyperglycemia)
- Gout
- A diet that is high in animal protein and low in fruits and vegetables

There are other less common forms of stones, for example, struvite/infection stones (about 10% of stones) and cystine stones (less than 1% of stones).

It is generally held that kidney stone formation is promoted by dietary constituents, such as oxalate, that promote stones, inadequate hydration that leads to crystal concentration in the bladder, and urinary pH: alkaline pH favors the crystallization of calcium- and phosphate-containing stones, whereas an acidic urine pH promotes uric acid or cystine stones (Wagner, and Mohebbi. 2010).

Insulin resistance plays a key role in Type 2 diabetes, and it has been linked to uric acid stone formation. A study published in the journal *Advanced Biomedical Research* focused on patients presenting with renal stones for surgical management. BMI was calculated by noting the weight and height of the patient. The extracted stone/stone fragments were analyzed to determine the chemical composition. Urinary pH was similarly noted in all.

It was found that the mean BMI among the nondiabetic patients was 23.41 ± 2.85, ranging from 17.71 to 31.62. The mean BMI of the diabetic patients was 26.35 ± 5.20, ranging from 17.75 to 35.60. The difference was statistically significant.

The incidence of uric acid calculi in the diabetic patients was significantly elevated compared to the nondiabetic patients. The mean urinary pH of the diabetic patients was 5.61 ± 0.36, and that of the nondiabetics was significantly higher—6.87 ± 0.32.

The investigators contend that there is a strong association between Type 2 diabetes and uric acid stone formation. There is also a strong association between diabetes, elevated BMI, and low urinary pH, the latter a known causal factor in stone formation (Nerli, Jali, Guntaka et al. 2015).

In this study also, published in the journal *European Urology*, the investigators sought to determine the link between the severity of Type 2 diabetes, glycemic control, insulin resistance, and kidney stone disease. Their data were based on adult participants in the 2007 to 2010 National Health and Nutrition Examination Survey. A history of kidney stone disease was obtained by self-report.

Type 2 diabetes was defined by self-reported history, related medication usage, and reported diabetic comorbidity. Insulin resistance was estimated using fasting plasma insulin levels and the homeostasis model assessment of insulin resistance (HOMA-IR). Glycemic control was classified by HbA1c and fasting plasma glucose levels.

When adjusting for patient factors, a history of Type 2 diabetes, the use of insulin, fasting plasma insulin, and HgbA1c remained significantly associated with kidney stone disease. Furthermore, the more severe the diseases, the greater the risk of developing kidney stones (Weinberg, Patel, Chertow et al. 2014).

It seems that full-blown diabetes may not be required to form kidney stones. The investigators of a study published in the *Diabetes and Metabolism Journal* aimed to determine whether impaired fasting glucose and kidney stone disease are linked because up to that point in time, no studies examining the relationship between impaired glucose tolerance and kidney stone disease were reported.

They examined a population that underwent health checkups between January 2000 and August 2009 at the Health Evaluation Center of National Cheng Kung University Hospital, Taiwan. Glycemic status was based on the 2009 American Diabetes Association criteria: normal glucose tolerance, isolated impaired glucose tolerance, isolated impaired fasting glucose, combined impaired fasting glucose/impaired glucose tolerance, and diabetes.

The existence of kidney stone disease was evaluated using renal ultrasonography, and the presence of any *hyperechoic* structures causing acoustic shadowing was considered to be indicative of kidney stone disease. It was found that the prevalence of kidney stone disease was as follows:

- 7.4% in participants with normal fasting glucose tolerance
- 9.3% in participants with isolated impaired glucose tolerance
- 10.8% in participants with isolated impaired fasting glucose
- 12.0% in participants with combined impaired fasting glucose/impaired glucose tolerance
- 11.3% in participants with diabetes

Isolated impaired fasting glucose, combined with impaired fasting glucose/impaired glucose tolerance, and diabetes were associated with kidney stone disease after adjusting for other clinical variables, but isolated impaired glucose tolerance was not. Age, gender, hypertension, and hyperuricemia were also independently associated with kidney stone disease.

The investigators concluded that isolated impaired fasting glucose, combined impaired fasting glucose/impaired glucose tolerance, and diabetes, but not isolated impaired glucose tolerance, were associated with a higher risk of kidney stone disease (Lien, Wu, Yang et al. 2016).

3.7 DIABETES-RELATED IMPAIRED WOUND HEALING

Chronic wounds that resist healing are rarely seen in persons who are otherwise healthy. In fact, chronic wound patients frequently suffer from "highly branded" diseases such as diabetes and obesity. Eight million Americans annually suffer from a chronic wound, and 15% of people with diabetes will have a non-healing wound sometime during their lifetime. Without proper treatment, these non-healing, open ulcers, can be so severe that they may lead to amputation. Wounds are most commonly found on the feet, ankles, heels, and calves. For those who cannot walk, wounds are commonly found on hips, thighs, and buttocks.

Typically, a wound that does not respond to normal medical care within 30 days is considered a "chronic wound." These may include a diabetic food ulcer, a venous-related ulceration, a non-healing surgical wound, a pressure ulcer, or a wound that repeatedly breaks down.

According to Dr. VR Driver, professor of orthopedic surgery, Brown University, Providence, Rhode Island, "…an estimated prevalence rate for chronic, non-healing wounds in the United States is 2 percent of the general population. The staggering cost of managing these patients' wounds exceeds $50 billion per year. This is 10 times more than the annual budget of the World Health Organization. The prevalence of chronic wounds is thought to be comparable to heart failure. However, unlike heart failure, little is known about the value of the treatments administered, or the outcome of these patients" (http://www.futureofhealthcarenews.com/patient-safety/the-little-known-silent-epidemic-of-non-healing-wounds; accessed 6.30.17).

The Journal of Clinical Investigation reported in 2007 that approximately 15% of all diabetic patients experience foot ulcers at some point in their lives (Brem, and Tomic-Canic. 2007). Venous ulcers are the most common type of leg ulcers, accounting for approximately 70% of cases, while arterial disease accounts for another 5% to 10% of leg ulcers (Brem, and Tomic-Canic. 2007); most of the others are due to either diabetes or a combination of those diseases (Casey. 2004; Sarkar, and Ballantyne. 2000; Moloney, and Grace. 2004; see also Agale. 2013).

Diabetic neuropathy, defined by damage to the sensory nerves of the foot, contributes to foot deformities and/or ulcers that increase the chance of lower-extremity amputations unless treated timely. It is estimated that up to 25% of all persons with diabetes will develop a diabetic foot ulcer (Singh, Armstrong, and Lipsky. 2005) and that about 71,000 nontraumatic lower-limb amputations were performed in people with diabetes, in 2004 (No authors listed. 2008).

3.7.1 VENOUS ULCERS

In the United States, it has been estimated that venous ulcers cause the loss of 2 million working days per year (Fishman. 2007). They account for 70% to 90% of ulcers found on the lower leg (Fife, Walker, Thomson et al. 2007). In individuals 65 years and older in the United States, venous leg ulcers affect approximately 1.69% of the population. Up to one-third of treated patients experience four or more episodes of recurrence (Fishman. 2007).

Similar findings were found in other geographical regions, including Europe. In a Spanish study appearing in *Wounds—A Compendium of Clinical Research and Practice,* it was reported that 81% of all of the leg ulcers occurred in patients aged over 65 (Soldevilla, Torra, Verdu et al. 2006). In Ireland, as reported in the *Journal of Wound Care,* the prevalence of leg ulcers in the general population is estimated at 0.12%, rising to 1.2% in the population over 70 years of age (Clarke-Moloney, Keane, and Kavanagh. 2006).

3.7.2 THE ROLE OF ENDOTHELIUM IN WOUND HEALING

A report in the journal *Clinics in Podiatric Medicine and Surgery* proposes that wound healing is defective principally because of impairment of the microcirculation; that is, the dysfunction of the endothelium has emerged now as the prominent abnormality related to vascular disease in diabetes (Veves. 1998; see also Sen, Gordillo, Roy et al. 2009). In a report in the *International Journal of Vascular Medicine,* wound healing defect in patients with Type 2 diabetes is attributed to endothelial dysfunction as these patients frequently suffer ischemic vascular disease. The complications of diabetes, that is, atherosclerosis, endothelial cell dysfunction, glycosylation of extracellular matrix proteins, and vascular denervation, interfere with neovascularization and diabetic wound healing (Kolluru, Bir, and Kevil. 2012).

The method by which neovascularization is impaired in diabetes is proposed in a report in the journal *Cell Metabolism*: Endothelial cell migration is required to repair damage to blood vessels, or to recover from injuries that require angiogenesis, and endothelial cells are dysfunctional in individuals with diabetes (Wong. 2014). A report in that journal implicates transcriptional coactivator PGC-1α, a powerful regulator of metabolism: Endothelial PGC-1α expression is high in diabetic rodents and humans, and it blocks endothelial migration in cell culture and vasculogenesis, *in vivo.*

PGC-1α renders endothelial cells unresponsive to established angiogenic factors, and, predictably, removing endothelial PGC-1α rescues impaired wound healing and promotes recovery from hind-limb ischemia seen in Type 1 and Type 2 diabetes.

Endothelial PGC-1α thus potently inhibits endothelial function and angiogenesis, and induction of endothelial PGC-1α contributes to multiple aspects of vascular dysfunction in diabetes (Sawada, Jiang, Takizawa et al. 2014).

Another theory of the possible mechanisms involved in impaired wound healing in Type 2 diabetes concerns microRNAs (miRNA/miR) stably present in body fluids and increasingly explored as disease biomarkers. The authors of a study published in the journal *Arteriosclerosis, Thrombosis and Vascular Biology* aimed to determine the influence of impaired wound healing on the plasma miRNA signature and their functional importance in patients with Type 2 diabetes: miRNA array profiling identified 41 miRNAs significantly deregulated in diabetic controls, when compared with patients with diabetes-associated peripheral arterial disease and chronic wounds.

Quantitative real-time polymerase chain reaction validation confirmed decrease in circulating miR-191 and miR-200b levels in Type 2 diabetes versus healthy controls. This was reversed in diabetic participants with associated peripheral arterial disease and chronic wounds, who also exhibited higher circulating C-reactive protein and proinflammatory cytokine levels compared with diabetic controls. miR-191 and miR-200b were significantly correlated with C-reactive protein or cytokine levels in patients with diabetes.

Proinflammatory stress was found to increase endothelial- or platelet-derived secretion of miR-191 or miR-200b. In addition, dermal cells took up endothelial-derived miR-191 leading to downregulation of the miR-191 target zonula occludens-1. Altered miR-191 expression influenced angiogenesis and migratory capacity of diabetic dermal endothelial cells, or fibroblasts, respectively, partly via its target zonula occludens-1.

The investigators concluded that inflammation underlying non-healing wounds in patients with Type 2 diabetes influences plasma miRNA concentrations and that miR-191 modulates cellular migration, and angiogenesis, via paracrine regulation of zonula occludens-1, to delay the tissue repair process (Dangwal, Stratmann, Bang et al. 2015).

3.8 DIABETES IMPAIRS SEXUAL FUNCTION BOTH IN MEN AND IN WOMEN BY JEOPARDIZING ENDOTHELIUM HEALTH

There are three major components of normal sexual response in men and in women. The first is sexual desire, that is, libido. Libido, in a sense, motivates or instigates sexual behavior. The second is the sequence of sexual arousal, and what can at best be described as sexual "performance." Arousal depends on the stimulation and consequent activity of hormones, and responses depend on the capacity of the cardiovascular system to support physical response by a process that depends on the healthy endothelium to support increased blood flow to the sex organs. This results from forming adequate amounts of blood vessel–dilating NO when needed in arousal (Fried. 2014).

Blood vessel dilation results mostly in engorgement of the labia and clitoris in women, supported by the hormone estradiol that contributes to vaginal changes and lubrication. In men, blood vessel dilation leads to relaxation of the cavernosae chambers of the penis, and increased blood inflow, that is, erection of the penis.

The mechanism that leads to increased blood inflow into the penis is largely the same NO-dependent process that results in engorgement of the clitoris and labia (Etgen, and Pfaff. 2009).

The third factor is the social component of sexual behavior, which is largely dictated by social/cultural conventions.

Sex hormones supply the principal basis for sexual drive in both men and women and their activity varies with age. Men and women produce both estrogens and testosterone in different amounts, and at different times and stages in the life span, but it is testosterone that drives sexual desire both in men and in women.

Parenthetically, the *Journal of the American Medical Association*, reported a meta-analysis of sex differences of endogenous sex hormones and risk of Type 2 diabetes that concluded that "…sex hormones may differentially modulate glycemic status and risk of Type 2 diabetes in men and women. High testosterone levels are associated with higher risk of Type 2 diabetes in women but with lower risk in men; the inverse association of sex hormone-binding globulin (SHBG) with risk was stronger in women than in men" (Ding, Song, Malik et al. 2006).

In men, the steroid hormone testosterone peaks in the middle years, and as it declines, it is supplemented by the formation of dihydrotestosterone (DHT) that both maintains desire and can cause benign prostate enlargement and male pattern hair loss. In women, testosterone levels decline as estradiol, an estrogen and the primary female sex hormone, declines in menopause.

Clearly, the physiological basis of sexual desire over the life span affects different aspects of sexual function in men and in women: age-related testosterone decline in men is not as precipitous as it is in women where, compounded by loss of estrogens, sexual intercourse can become problematic as well.

It is against this complex background that the effects of diabetes must be evaluated.

A report in the journal *Diabetes, Metabolic Syndrome and Obesity: Targets and Therapy* summarizes a study titled "Diabetes and sexual dysfunction: current perspectives." According to this study, diabetes puts men at a threefold risk of erectile dysfunction in comparison to nondiabetic men. Although the association between diabetes and sexual dysfunction in women is less clear-cut, there is a higher prevalence of female sexual dysfunction (FSD) in diabetic women than in nondiabetic women.

Hyperglycemia, which is a main determinant of vascular and microvascular diabetic complications, is thought to contribute to the pathogenetic mechanisms of sexual dysfunction in diabetes. Furthermore, people with diabetes may present additional clinical conditions including hypertension, overweight and obesity, metabolic syndrome, cigarette smoking, and atherogenic dyslipidemia, all of which are themselves risk factors for sexual dysfunction, both in men and in women.

The authors hold that the adoption of a "healthy lifestyle" may reduce endothelial dysfunction and oxidative stress—associated with sexual dysfunction in both men and women—which are desirable achievements in diabetic patients (Maiorino, Bellastella, and Esposito. 2014).

3.8.1 DIABETES IMPAIRS SEXUAL FUNCTION IN WOMEN

The *Journal of Sexual Medicine* reported a meta-analysis to determine the frequency of FSD in diabetic women, and clinical and metabolic correlates. The analysis encompassed MEDLINE, EMBASE, Cochrane Library, and reference lists of articles and systematic reviews for clinical studies published as full articles reporting on FSD in women with and women without diabetes.

Measures obtained were frequency of FSD and the score of Female Sexual Function Index (FSFI), as a function of patient details (age, BMI, duration of diabetes, metabolic control [HbA1c], chronic complications, and Beck Depression Inventory [BDI] score).

The analysis revealed that the frequency of FSD was higher in women with Type 1 diabetes (OR, 2.27) and Type 2 diabetes (OR, 2.49) than in those women who did not have diabetes. The FSFI score was lower (worse) in women with Type 1 diabetes, or in those with Type 2 diabetes, than in the diabetes free-control participants.

Depression was significantly more frequent in the women with diabetes than in those who did not have diabetes, and low FSFI score is associated with high BMI. The authors concluded that FSD is more frequent in women with diabetes than in those women without it (Pontiroli, Cortelazzi, and Morabito. 2013).

What is different about sexual arousal in diabetic women compared to women who don't have that condition? The journal *Archives of Sexual Behavior* reported that past research is based on self-report measures and may, therefore, be a flawed methodology due to response bias. Nevertheless, the investigators undertook to determine whether women with diabetes differed from a matched non-diabetic control group both in their physiological and in their subjective response to erotic stimuli.

Vaginal photoplethysmographic measures of capillary engorgement were taken while participants individually viewed counterbalanced erotic, and non-erotic, videotape presentations. A plethysmograph reflects changes in volume. A photoplethysmogram is an optically obtained plethysmograph, often obtained by using a pulse oximeter that illuminates the skin and measures changes in light absorption reflecting blood vessel volume and changes in volume as blood pressure varies in the vessel.

The analysis indicated that women with diabetes showed significantly less physiological arousal to erotic stimuli than nondiabetic women even though their subjective responses were comparable (Wincze, Albert, and Bansal. 1993).

The study points to impaired blood vessel relaxation and impaired blood inflow increase in the arousal sequence—NO/cGMP pathway—jeopardizing vaginal and clitoral engorgement. This arousal response is analogous to that in men as shown by the elucidation of "The neurovascular mechanism of clitoral erection: Nitric oxide and cGMP-stimulated activation of BKCa channels," reported in the *FASEB Journal* (Federation of American Societies for Experimental Biology) (Gragasin, Michelakis, Hogan et al. 2004).

The need for viability of the endothelium underscores also what is understood to be the analogous clitoral erection, dependent as is the penis—and as are all arterial blood vessels in the body, in fact—on NO relaxation of smooth muscle to promote increased blood flow. The results of the study by Gragasin, Michelakis, Hogan et al. (2004), described below, are based on an animal model.

The investigators proposed that rat clitoris relaxes by a mechanism similar to that in the penis. Rat clitoris expresses components of the proposed pathway: neuronal and endothelial NO synthases (NOSs), soluble guanylyl cyclase (sGC), type 5 phosphodiesterase (5-PDE), and BKCa channels. The NO donor diethylamine NONOate (DEANO), the PKG activator 8-pCPT-cGMP, and the PDE-5 inhibitor sildenafil cause dose-dependent clitoral relaxation that is inhibited by antagonists of PKG (Rp-8-Br-cGMPS) or BKCa channels (iberiotoxin).

The results of their study are illustrated in their Figure 2. Relaxation of the clitoris induced by the NO donor DEANO and the cGMP analog 8-pCPT-cGMPS. It appeared in Gragasin, Michelakis, Hogan et al. (2004). The neurovascular mechanism of clitoral erection: NO and cGMP-stimulated activation of BKCa channels. *FASEB Journal*, Sep; 18(12): https://doi.org/10.1096/fj.04-1978com. This illustration can be accessed at http://www.fasebj.org/doi/10.1096/fj.04-1978com.

Electrical field stimulation (EFS) induced tetrodotoxin-sensitive NO release and vessel relaxation that was inhibited by the Na+ channel blocker, tetrodotoxin, or the sGC inhibitor 1H-(1,2,4) oxadiozolo(4,3-a)quinoxalin-1-one.

Human BKCa channels, transferred to Chinese hamster ovary cells via an adenoviral vector, and endogenous rat clitoral smooth muscle K+ current were activated by this PKG-dependent mechanism. Laser confocal microscopy revealed protein expression of BKCa channels on clitoral smooth muscle cells; these cells exhibited BKCa channel activity that is activated by both DEANO and sildenafil.

The investigators concluded that neurovascular-derived NO resulted in clitoral relaxation via a PKG-dependent activation of BKCa channels just as it occurs in the penis. Parenthetically, EFS is similar to a TENS unit used to stimulate nerves to induce relaxation or abate pain.

L-NAME is Nω-nitro-L-arginine methyl ester that competes with and inhibits NOS, thus reducing NO formation.

The Na+ channel blocker tetrodotoxin physically blocks the flow of sodium ions through the channel, thereby preventing action potential generation and propagation.

Both of these agents were used in the study to either impair NO formation or interfere with its smooth blood vessel relaxation action. Both of these agents effectively inhibited the action of EFS in triggering NO synthesis.

The investigators concluded that engorgement and erection in the clitoris, as well as in the penis, are endothelium NO-dependent.

Furthermore, as described in the book *Human Sexuality—Basics of Functional Biology with Behavioral and Clinical Considerations*, contrary to common understanding, there is no known glandular vaginal lubrication. Glandular lubricant is available at the entrance to the vagina (Bartholin's glands) and usually introduced into the vagina by insertion of the penis in intercourse or by other means. Vaginal lubrication proper is actually achieved when blood pressure in the vaginal wall rises as a result of arousal increased blood inflow, and higher blood pressure, thus exuding serum from the vaginal wall arterial vasculature into the vagina proper (Fried. 2010).

Because of the analogous blood flow–dependent characteristics of vaginal engorgement and penile erection, it has been proposed that sildenafil citrate (Viagra® Pfizer, New York, New York), indicated for the treatment of erectile dysfunction in men, may be effective in treatment of estrogen-deficient women with sexual dysfunction that included female sexual arousal disorder (Basson, McInnes, Smith et al. 2004).

In a study published in the journal *Acta Diabetologica*, the investigators aimed to determine clinical, metabolic, psychological, cardiovascular, and neurophysiologic correlates of sexual dysfunction in diabetic premenopausal women. The collected data used the FSFI, BDI, Michigan Diabetic Neuropathy Index (DNI), and the symptoms of diabetic neuropathy (SDN) questionnaires, metabolic variables, endothelial vascular function (flow-mediated dilation, FMD), echocardiography, and electromyography.

The participants ranged in age between 18 and 50 years: One subgroup had Type 1 diabetes and the other group had Type 2 diabetes. These two groups were compared to a third group of healthy women.

In addition, the participants were evaluated for physical activity, smoking habits, parity, BMI, waist circumference, HOMA-IR index, fibrinogen, cholesterol (total, HDL, LDL), triglycerides, HbA1c, high-sensitivity C-reactive protein, total testosterone, and estradiol, as well as echocardiography, assessment of IMT, FMD, ECG (heart rate and Qtc, indexes of sympathetic activity), and electromyography. It was found, first, that

- The FSFI total score and score for arousal, lubrication, and orgasm domains were lower in diabetes sufferers than in the healthy control group.

Second, women with diabetes had

- Higher BDI scores
- Doppler A wave peak velocity, an index of diastolic dysfunction that can eventually lead to heart failure
- Higher DNI scores
- SDN

Doppler E wave peak velocity, a marker of the function of the left ventricle of the heart, is an index of diastolic dysfunction, and it can eventually lead to the symptoms of heart failure.

Peroneal, posterior tibial and sural nerve conduction velocity and amplitude are an index of nerve damage. They were found to be lower (worse) in women with diabetes than in the healthy control group.

The FSFI score was positively correlated with physical activity.

The Doppler E wave peak velocity and peroneal nerve amplitude were inversely related to the BDI score, parity, IMT, SDN, and HbA1c. These cardiac and neural markers point to some basic concerns about diabetes and cardiovascular and heart risk. Of note is that negative score on SDN score and Doppler E wave peak velocity reliably predicted FSFI score.

The investigators concluded that cardiovascular and neurological impairments are associated with FSD in women with diabetes (Cortelazzi, Marconi, Guazzi et al. 2013).

How does Type 2 diabetes affect women's sexual function as they age? This question was addressed in a study titled "Diabetes mellitus and sexual function in middle-aged and older women," published in the journal *Obstetrics and Gynecology*.

The investigators examined the relationship between diabetes and sexual function in middle-aged and older women (average age, 55 ± 9.2 years) in a cross-sectional cohort of ethnically diverse women ranging in age between 40 and 80 years.

Self-administered questionnaires were given to the participants with the intent of comparing self-reported level of sexual desire, frequency of sexual activity, overall sexual satisfaction, and specific sexual problems such as poor lubrication, low arousal, orgasm, or pain, among insulin-treated diabetic, non-insulin-treated diabetic, and nondiabetic women. The investigators also assessed relationships between diabetic end-organ complications such as heart disease, stroke, renal dysfunction, peripheral neuropathy, and sexual function.

It was reported that in non-Latina white women, 21.4% had diabetes, and 6.1% were taking insulin. In comparisons, 19.3% of nondiabetic women, 34.9% of insulin-treated diabetic women, and 26.0% of non-insulin-treated diabetic women (adjusted OR, 1.42) reported low overall sexual satisfaction.

Among sexually active women, insulin-treated diabetic women were more likely to report problems with lubrication (OR, 2.37) and orgasm (OR, 1.80) than nondiabetic women. Among all diabetic women, end-organ complications such as heart disease, stroke, renal dysfunction, and peripheral neuropathy were associated with decreased sexual function in at least one domain.

The investigators concluded that, compared to nondiabetic women, diabetic women are more likely to report low overall sexual satisfaction. Insulin-treated diabetic women also appear at higher risk for problems such as difficulty with lubrication and orgasm. Furthermore, prevention of end-organ complications may be important in preserving sexual activity and function in diabetic women (Copeland, Brown, Creasman et al. 2012).

3.8.1.1   Is Sexual Dysfunction More Prevalent in Type 1 or Type 2 Diabetes?

This question was addressed in a study published in the journal *Diabetes, Metabolic Syndrome and Obesity*. A group of women with Type 1 diabetes and another group with Type 2 diabetes were selected, as well as an additional group of nondiabetic women. Each participant was asked to complete the nine-item FSFI questionnaire. The metabolic profile was evaluated by BMI and glycosylated hemoglobin assay (HbA1c).

It was found that the prevalence of sexual dysfunction (total FSFI score greater than or equal to 30) was significantly higher in the Type 1 and Type 2 diabetes groups than in the healthy control group.

The mean total score was significantly lower in the Type 1 diabetes group than in the control group, but there was no significant difference between the Type 2 diabetes group and the control group.

Concerning specific questionnaire items, the mean values for *arousal, lubrication, dyspareunia, and orgasm* were significantly lower in the Type 1 diabetes group than in the control group. The mean values for *desire* were lower than those of the control group in Type 1 and Type 2 diabetes.

The investigators concluded that Type 1 diabetes is associated with sexual dysfunction due, perhaps, to classic neurovascular complications or to the negative impact of the disease on psychological and social factors (Mazzilli, Imbrogno, Elia et al. 2015).

The conclusion of these investigators is particularly noteworthy insofar as these conclusions set conventional psychosomatic theory on its head: Historically, psychosomatic theory (see the next study) proposed that psychological (now also psychosocial) stressors, conscious or otherwise, translate into disease entities. In the abovementioned study, we see the opposite posited: disease entities translate into psychological stress.

The preponderance of the evidence in clinical reports is that diabetes affects sexual function in women because of the adverse impact of hyperglycemia on physical function. While there is some degree of focus on the subjective aspects of sexual dysfunction—perhaps more so than is found in clinical reports about men's sexual dysfunction—the focus is typically on physical symptoms that point to cardiovascular and blood vessel impairment.

On the other hand, not everyone is onboard, and that may be due, in part, to the vagueness of the linkage between endothelial failure as clearly seen in male sexual dysfunction and in the female counterpart. It is pretty clear when and why the penis fails to erect, but the comparable female anatomy is not quite so distinct. In fact, most studies of comparable pathophysiology are largely performed on animal models.

A study reported in the *Journal of Sexual Medicine* aimed to establish the "mediators" of sexual functions in women with diabetes. Women aged 18 to 55 years old with both form of diabetes were enrolled in a questionnaire-based, cross-sectional study. Sexual function was compared between women with Type 1 and those with Type 2 diabetes.

It was found that sexual dysfunction was identified in 32.65% of women with diabetes. Those with Type 2 diabetes scored significantly lower in all FSFI domains except pain, compared to Type 1 respondents.

Neither the presence of comorbidities, the duration of diabetes, the presence of diabetes complications, nor glycemic control was shown to be a moderator of FSD. The strongest significant predictors of FSD were the presence of depressive symptoms, the importance of sex to the respondent, and satisfaction with the partner as a lover.

The authors concluded that diabetes-related factors have little impact on sexual functions in women and that depression symptoms, partner-related factors, and individual perception of sexuality should be evaluated when counseling such women (Nowosielski, and Skrzypulec-Plinta. 2011).

3.8.2 Diabetes Impairs Sexual Function in Men

The physiology of dysfunctional penile erection in sexual arousal and sexual "performance" in men provides a good window into the devastation of cardiovascular and blood vessel function caused by any form of diabetes. Many studies connect erectile dysfunction to cardiovascular and heart disease, and the common link is invariably endothelium impairment and consequent NO unavailability.

In an article in the *Journal of Endocrinological Investigation*, the authors address the "Pathophysiology of diabetic sexual dysfunction" with several proposals: Sexual dysfunction, common in patients with diabetes, invariably involves vascular, neurological, and hormonal alterations. Many studies showed altered endothelium-dependent and neurogenic relaxations in the *corpus cavernosum* from diabetic patients with erectile dysfunction. These alterations induced by diabetes are commonly associated with reduced NO production and a significant increase in the number of binding sites for NO that are present in the enzyme NOS, which means that this particular enzyme is being underutilized.

AGEs contribute to diabetic vascular complications by quenching NO activity and by increasing the expression of mediators of vascular damage such as VEGF, having neoangiogenic effects, and endothelin-1 (ET-1), with vasoconstricting and mitogenic action. Mitogens trigger signal transduction pathways where mitogen-activated protein kinase leads to mitosis, or cell division.

Moreover, the differential gene expression for various growth factors in penile tissues may be involved in the pathophysiology of erectile dysfunction associated with diabetes.

Neuropathy is an important aspect of diabetic erectile dysfunction: morphological alterations of autonomic nerve fibers in cavernosal tissue of patients with diabetic erectile dysfunction have been demonstrated. Also, androgens enhance NOS gene expression in the penile *corpus cavernosum* of rats, suggesting that they play a role in maintaining NOS activity (Morano. 2003).

The reduced ability to convert L-arginine to L-citrulline via NOS in diabetes is another approach to understanding reduced NO availability. This was proposed in a study published in the journal *Biochemical and Biophysical Research Communications*.

The major cause of erectile dysfunction in diabetic patients is reduced NO synthesis in the penis *corpora cavernosa*. The enzyme arginase shares a common substrate with NOS, thereby downregulating NO production because it competes with NOS for the substrate L-arginine.

The aim of a study was to compare arginase gene expression, protein levels, and enzyme activity in diabetic human cavernosal tissue. It was determined that diabetic *corpus cavernosum* from erectile dysfunction sufferers had higher levels of arginase II protein, gene expression, and enzyme activity than normal cavernosal tissue. In contrast, gene expression and protein levels of arginase I were not significantly different in diabetic cavernosal tissue when compared to control tissue.

The reduced ability of diabetic tissue to convert L-arginine to L-citrulline via NOS was reversed by the selective inhibition of arginase by 2(S)-amino-6-boronohexanoic acid.

These data suggested to the investigators that the increased expression of arginase II in diabetic cavernosal tissue may contribute to the erectile dysfunction associated with this common disease process and may play a role in other manifestations of diabetic disease in which NO production is decreased (Bivalacqua, Hellstrom, Kadowitz et al. 2001).

3.8.2.1 The ACh/NO/cGMP Pathway

In the early 1900s, the Austrian pharmacologist Otto Loewi discovered a substance made by cells in the nervous system that he termed *"vagus material."* Some years later, Sir Henry Dale, with whom Loewi later collaborated at the University of London, and with whom he shared the 1936 Nobel Prize in Medicine, named it "acetylcholine" (ACh). ACh was found to relax arterial smooth muscles, and this seemed a promising road to lower blood pressure to treat hypertension. However, it did so unreliably and unpredictably. No one knew why.

In 1980, Dr. RF Furchgott, professor of pharmacology at Downstate Medical Center in Brooklyn, New York, published his findings in the journal NATURE that ACh relaxation of arterial smooth muscle depended on the simultaneous presence of a mysterious substance made by the *endothelium*. It was termed *"endothelium derived relaxing factor"* (EDRF), and ACh relaxed the vessels only when EDRF was also present (Furchgott, and Zawadzki. 1980). The identity of EDRF was a mystery.

In 1993, Dr. S Moncada at Wellcome Research Labs, UK, who had previously first identified EDRF as a gas, NO, detailed its role in health and disease in the *New England Journal of Medicine* (Moncada, and Higgs. 1993). Then, in 1998, Dr. Furchgott and two colleagues were awarded the Nobel Prize in Medicine for the discovery of the biological role of NO in blood vessel, cardiovascular and heart function, and the nervous system and brain. One of the three recipients, Dr. LJ Ignarro, detailed how ACh in sexual arousal caused increased and sustained production of NO, synthesized from the amino acid L-arginine by the endothelium lining the spongy chambers of the penis *cavernosa(e)*. This causes them to relax (dilate), allowing increased blood inflow.

3.8.2.2 NO from L-Arginine

Three isofroms of NOSs form the free radical NO: endothelial NOS (eNOS), neuronal NOS (nNOS), and inducible NOS (iNOS). Each has a different function. The neuronal enzyme (NOS-1) and the endothelial isoform (NOS-3) are calcium-dependent and produce low levels of this gas as a cell signaling molecule. The inducible isoform (NOS-2) is calcium-independent and produces large amounts of gas that can be cytotoxic.

NOS oxidizes the guanidine group of L-arginine in a process that results in the formation of NO with the formation also of L-citrulline. The process involves the oxidation of NADPH and the reduction of molecular oxygen. The transformation occurs at a catalytic site adjacent to a specific binding site of L-arginine (Ignarro. 1990).

3.8.2.3 The Role of Citrulline in NO Formation

L-citrulline is a naturally occurring nonessential amino acid present in all living organisms. The body produces it, and it can also be found naturally in certain foods such as watermelons, cucumbers, pumpkins, muskmelons, bitter melons, squashes, and gourds. About 80% of citrulline is converted to arginine in the kidney, recycling arginine to citrulline and NO, thus serving as a potent arginine precursor.

Citrulline has been shown to be an effective substitute to restore NO production in situations of limited arginine availability, and supplementation holds promise as a therapeutic adjunct in clinical conditions associated with arginine-derived NO deficiency and/or endothelial dysfunction (Kaore, and Kaore. 2014; Habib, and Ali. 2011).

3.8.3 THE PATHWAY TO PENILE ERECTION

In sexual arousal, the brain sends signals via the nervous system and bloodstream to the spongy expandable *cavernosae* of the penis:

1. Components of the central nervous system release the chemical messenger acetylcholine that signals the cells of the endothelium to form NO from L-arginine by the enzyme NOS (eNOS), facilitated by a co-factor, tetrahydrobiopterin.

2. In the vascular smooth muscle of the penis *cavernosae*, NO signals the release of another enzyme, GC (*guanylate cyclase*), that helps form cGMP (*cyclic guanosine monophosphate*) from GTP (*guanosine-5′-triphosphate*).
3. cGMP is the vasodilator that actually relaxes the *cavernosae* smooth muscle, increasing blood inflow via relaxation that follows sequestration of myoplasmic Ca2+ (Murphy, and Walker. 1998).
4. As blood inflow rises in the *cavernosae*, increased inflow and pressure cause shear stress on the endothelium that results in additional release of eNOS, and further maintenance of NO formation.
5. As blood fills the *cavernosae*, they expand, exerting pressure on the veins that lie between the *albuginea* and the *tunica*. This pressure constricts the veins, thus limiting blood outflow.
6. However, at the same time, there is also the formation and buildup of phosphodiesterase type-5 (PDE5) that breaks down cGMP to end the erection cycle.

PDE5 rapidly breaks down cGMP, causing reabsorption of the constituents and thereby ending erection.

The *cavernosae* can be thought of as variants of arterial blood vessels, and their endothelium reacts in the same way. Thus, sexual arousal and penile erection are a particular case of systemic autonomic arousal and cardiovascular response patterns. Therefore, before considering the impact of chronic hyperglycemia—as in Type 2 diabetes—on erectile function, it is instructive to look at the impact of cardiovascular and heart disease on erectile function since it has already been established that diabetes is a risk factor for dysfunction.

3.8.3.1 "The Canary in the Coal Mine"

The journal *Atherosclerosis* reported a study that found that men with erectile dysfunction of unknown cause (idiopathic) present evidence of endothelial dysfunction in forearm resistance vessels observed by FMD, increased pulse pressure, and impaired HRV. They concluded that erectile dysfunction is a predictor of cardiovascular dysfunction and a precursor of clinical cardiovascular disease (Stuckey, Walsh, Ching et al. 2006).

In fact, a report in the *American Journal of Medicine* refers to Type 2 diabetes as a coronary heart disease "risk equivalent." The study aimed to determine whether in an older adult population, where both glucose disorders and preexisting atherosclerosis are common, cardiovascular and all-cause mortality rates would be similar in participants with prevalent coronary heart disease, versus those with diabetes.

The investigators concluded that among older adults, diabetes alone confers a similar risk for cardiovascular mortality as established clinical coronary heart disease (Carnethon, Biggs, Barzilay et al. 2010).

Writing in the *Journal of the American College of Cardiology*, investigators concluded that in men under the age of 60, and in men with diabetes, or hypertension, erectile dysfunction can be a critical warning sign for existing or impending cardiovascular disease, and risk of death. Their article is titled "The link between erectile and cardiovascular health: the canary in the coal mine" (Meldrum, Gambone, Morris et al. 2011).

Again, the *Journal of the American College of Cardiology* reported a study where a cohort of men between the ages of 55 and 88 years, with Type 2 diabetes, were enrolled in ADVANCE (Action in Diabetes and Vascular Disease: Preterax and Diamicron Modified-Release Controlled Evaluation). Baseline medical examination included inquiries about erectile dysfunction.

Over 5 years of follow-up during which participants attended repeat clinical examinations, the occurrence of fatal and nonfatal cardiovascular episodes, cognitive decline, and dementia were ascertained. After adjusting for a range of cofactors such as existing illness, psychological health, and classic cardiovascular risk factors relative to those who were free of the condition, baseline erectile dysfunction was associated with an elevated risk of all cardiovascular events, coronary heart disease, stroke, and dementia.

Men who experienced erectile dysfunction at baseline, and at 2-year follow-up, were at the highest risk for these events (Batty, Li, Czernichow et al. 2010). See also Roth, Kalter-Leibovici, Kerbis et al. (2003) in the journal *Clinical Cardiology:* "Erectile dysfunction is common among patients at high risk for cardiovascular disease because of diabetes and/or [hypertension]. Diabetic men are affected earlier than those with [hypertension]...."

3.8.4 How Does Diabetes Lead to Erectile Dysfunction?

According to a report in the *American Journal of Physiology—Heart and Circulatory Physiology*, the endothelial cell dysfunction caused by hyperglycemia is mediated by free radicals. The authors propose treatment with antioxidants to protect against impaired endothelium-dependent relaxations caused by elevated glucose (Tesfamariam, and Cohen. 1992). A report titled "Reactive oxygen-derived free radicals are key to the endothelial dysfunction of diabetes" appeared in the *Journal of Diabetes.*

Elevated levels of oxygen-derived free radicals are the initial source of endothelial dysfunction in diabetes. Oxygen-derived free radicals not only reduce NO bioavailability but also facilitate the production and/or action of the antagonist—endothelial derived contracting factors—causing the endothelial balance to tip toward vasoconstrictor responses over the course of diabetes (Shi, and Vanhoutte. 2009).

According to the *International Journal of Vascular Medicine*, Type 2 diabetes accelerates atherosclerosis and endothelial cell dysfunction (Kolluru, Bir, and Kevil. 2012). In fact, a report in the *International Journal of Impotence Research* addressed the erectile dysfunction link between erectile dysfunction at the level of the endothelium.

The aim of the study was to assess systemic vascular function in patients with erectile dysfunction: Patients were diagnosed by Doppler Ultrasound and the International Index of Erectile Function 5-item questionnaire, and asymptomatic men were the control group enrolled in the study. They all underwent the tests including serum glucose and lipid levels. Echocardiography and exercise stress test was performed routinely.

It was found that baseline factors such as BMI, heart rate and blood pressures, and fasting glucose and lipid levels were not significantly different between patients and asymptomatic participants.

Endothelial-dependent brachial artery flow-mediated vasodilation and brachial artery response to 0.4 mg nitroglycerine were measured: Participants were negative on the exercise stress test, and echocardiographic parameters including ejection fraction were similar.

However, endothelial-dependent brachial artery percent diameter change with flow-mediated dilation (6.01 ± 2.9 vs. 12.3 ± 3.5) and brachial artery response to nitroglycerine (12.8 ± 4.2 vs. 17.8 ± 5.2) were significantly different between groups.

The authors concluded that endothelial function was impaired in patients with no apparent cardiovascular disease or diabetes, and they hypothesized that the impaired function might be explained by the abnormality in the systemic NO–cyclic guanosine monophosphate vasodilator system and suggest that erectile dysfunction and vascular disease may be linked at the level of the endothelium (Kaya, Uslu, and Karaman. 2006).

However, an article in the *British Journal of Pharmacology* that reviewed studies on the dysfunction of endothelium-dependent vasodilation in diabetes highlighted the disparity in the clinical and experimental findings and cautions that the susceptibility of tissues to the damaging effects of elevated serum glucose may vary.

The article further cautions that the process of endothelium-dependent vasodilation may be quite different in blood vessels of different size and in different anatomical locations. Thus, it may be hazardous to extrapolate conclusions drawn from one vessel type, or diabetes model, to another. It is said to be important to select clinically relevant models for future studies on endothelial dysfunction (De Vriese, Verbeuren, Van de Voorde et al. 2000).

It should be noted that the concern of the authors of the study cited above, namely, that it is hazardous to extrapolate conclusions about NO-dependent vasodilation drawn from one vessel type, is not supported by the evidence gathered in studies of peripheral artery disease and evidence of comparable endothelial blood vessel damage in other arterial vessels. However, this excludes coronary arteries where it has been shown that it is quite possible to have advanced atheromas, absent that condition elsewhere in the body (Fried. 2014).

Most authorities agree that Type 2 diabetes is characterized by oxidative stress, which in turn causes endothelial dysfunction. The *Journal of Diabetes Complications* reports that antioxidant treatment with glicazide, an antidiabetic drug with antioxidant properties, improves both antioxidant status, and NO-mediated vasodilation in diabetic patients (De Mattia, Laurenti, and Fava. 2003).

A review appearing in the journal *Cardiovascular Research* holds that damaged endothelium may be the key factor in diabetic impairments of endothelium- and NO-dependent microvascular function. This may contribute to several other clinical aspects of diabetes such as hypertension, abnormal amounts of blood lipids, and insulin resistance.

There are now several reports describing elevations in specific oxidant stress markers in both insulin resistance syndrome and diabetes, together with determinations of reduced total antioxidant defense and depletions in individual antioxidants.

The pro-oxidant environment in diabetes may disrupt endothelial function through the inactivation of NO, resulting in the reduction of basic anti-atherogenic functions and an increase above normal glucose concentrations. One clinical study showed that the supplementation of insulin-resistant or diabetic states, with antioxidants such as vitamin E, reduces oxidant stress and improves both endothelium-dependent vasodilation and insulin sensitivity (Laight, Carrier, and Anggard. 2000).

Endocrinological Reviews published a very comprehensive review titled *"Diabetes and Endothelial Dysfunction: A Clinical Perspective"* (Calles-Escandon, and Cipolla. 2001). Only highlights are reported below and in abbreviated form:

The effects of aging, elevated serum lipids, hypertension, and other factors add to the complexity of the role of endothelial dysfunction in Type 2 diabetes, making it more complicated than Type 1. For one thing, markers of endothelial dysfunction are often elevated years before any evidence of damage to small blood vessels becomes evident.

A major element of Type 2 diabetes is insulin resistance. As a result, a great research effort has been focused on defining the possible contribution of insulin resistance to endothelial dysfunction. In patients with Type 2 diabetes, endothelial dysfunction occurs with insulin resistance and precedes elevated serum glucose. It follows that the metabolic abnormalities of insulin resistance may lead to endothelial dysfunction.

Endothelial cells are easily damaged by oxidative stress, a characteristic of the diabetic state where there is often an increased tendency for oxidative stress and high levels of oxidized lipoproteins, especially the so-called small, dense LDL-C. High levels of fatty acids and elevated serum glucose have both been shown to induce an increased level of oxidation of phospholipids (a class of lipids that are a major component of all cell membranes) as well as proteins. This has been proposed to be one of the causal factors in inducing endothelial dysfunction in Type 2 diabetes.

Type 2 diabetes is associated also with increased blood platelet aggregation (clumping) and a prothrombotic (blood coagulation and clot formation) tendency that may be related to diminished NO formation.

The report also addresses L-arginine supplementation and antioxidants—one may reasonably assume that L-arginine supplementation would activate eNOS and produce more NO with greater vasodilation since L-arginine is a substrate for eNOS. In fact, this idea has been implemented in different cases including reversal of endothelial dysfunction associated with chronic heart failure and diabetes.

However, it is not clear how elevated L-arginine plasma levels could produce more eNOS activation: In the normal state, L-arginine is present at concentrations that would support maximum enzymatic turnover of arginine to citrulline and NO. It is possible that in the cases where L-arginine supplementation restored normal endothelial function, arginine levels were low to begin with. However, it is difficult to know what intracellular L-arginine levels actually are, and there is some evidence that arginine transporters can concentrate arginine against a concentration gradient (see the "arginine paradox"). Therefore, even measuring arginine levels would not necessarily result in accurate conclusions about intracellular arginine levels.

3.9   A NOTE ON OBSTRUCTIVE SLEEP APNEA AND HEART ARRHYTHMIAS IN TYPE 2 DIABETES

Apnea is a transient suspension of breathing lasting more than 10 seconds. Obstructive sleep apnea (OSA) is a common type of sleep apnea typically lasting 20 to 40 s. Sufferers are often unaware of this condition, even on awakening.

Sleep apnea is preceded by a period of hypocapnia (low alveolar PCO_2) typically induced by open mouth breathing, with more CO_2 being "blown off" than usual, followed by temporary suspension of breathing, which is then often but not invariably followed by sudden awakening. This excess loss of CO_2 causes the body to lose acidity (i.e., to shift toward alkalinity), which in this case is termed respiratory alkalosis. The respiratory alkalosis causes hemoglobin to lose some of its affinity for oxygen, causing a leftward shift of the oxygen dissociation curve. With less oxygen being delivered to the tissues, there is a period of hypoxia of undetermined length and, therefore, hypoxemia preceding the apnea and, to some extent, afterward.

A number of theories have been advanced to explain OSA: Some theories look to sleep-induced dysregulation of brain breathing-regulation centers—central sleep apnea—disturbing upper chest and respiratory muscle function. More popular theories look to nasal and throat congestion and blockage, attributed to various causes including the collapse of the soft tissues in the back of the throat called the "pharyngeal tissue" and the supine sleep position.

Treatment typically centers on preventing hypoxia and often involves methods such as the continuous positive airway pressure, a form of ventilator, which applies mild air pressure on a continuous basis during sleep. Parenthetically, the body is relatively insensitive to low arterial blood O_2, but is sensitive to low arterial blood CO_2 level (Fried. 1993), and the sleeper awakens in response to the low $PaCO_2$ (not to low PaO_2).

There are many adverse metabolic sequelae of hypocapnia, not the least of which is that it affects heart function: Depression of cardiac aerobic metabolism is dangerous because the heart is the driving force for its own perfusion and oxygen supply.

In an estimated 30% to 50% of sufferers, OSA can cause numerous disturbances, including cardiac arrhythmias (including but not limited to ventricular extrasystoles), heart failure, and stroke (https://www.diabetesself management.com/blog/sleep-apnea-increases-type-2-diabetes-risk/; accessed 2.9.18; see also Sleep Apnea and Heart Disease, Stroke, American Heart Association (AHA), http://www.heart.org/HEARTORG/Conditions/More/MyHeartandStrokeNews/Sleep-Apnea-and-Heart-Disease-Stroke_UCM_441857_Article.jsp#.Wn8wLORy7cs; accessed 2.9.18)

A comprehensive review published in the *World Journal of Diabetes* reports that OSA is frequently associated with obesity, metabolic syndrome, and also Type 2 diabetes. Because both Type 2 diabetes and metabolic syndrome are often found in the same individuals, these conditions may have a common pathophysiological basis in the development of insulin resistance:

The authors report that there is extensive published literature exploring the cause–effect relationship between OSA and Type 2 diabetes, and in their review, they provide an in-depth analysis of the complex pathophysiological mechanisms linking OSA to Type 2 diabetes. It focuses on the effect of OSA on the microvascular complications of Type 2 diabetes (Nannapaneni, Ramar, and Surani. 2013; see also Pamidi, and Tasali. 2012).

The journal *Chest* published a report titled "Obstructive sleep apnea and type 2 diabetes: interacting epidemics." According to the authors, the majority of patients with Type 2 diabetes also have OSA. They assert that OSA is a significant risk factor for cardiovascular disease and mortality.

Epidemiological and clinical studies suggest that OSA is also independently associated with alterations in glucose metabolism, and it is an increased risk factor for development of Type 2 diabetes. Intermittent hypoxia and sleep fragmentation have adverse effects on glucose metabolism.

The authors propose that clinicians need to address the risk of OSA in patients with Type 2 diabetes and evaluate the presence of Type 2 diabetes in patients with OSA. They concluded that there is need for a better understanding of the relationship between OSA and Type 2 diabetes (Tasali, Mokhlesi, and Van Cauter. 2008).

Furthermore, a report in the *American Journal of Respiratory and Critical Care Medicine* demonstrated a link between the severity of OSA and the risk of developing Type 2 diabetes. Investigators from the University of Toronto, Canada, examined adults with suspected OSA who underwent a sleep study between 1994 and 2010. The severity of sleep apnea was evaluated using an Apnea–Hypopnea Index (AHI), which indicates the number of times a person stops breathing or breathes irregularly each hour.

Based on the results, the participants were assigned to one of four OSA categories—none, mild, moderate, or severe—and they were then followed through May 2011 to determine whether they developed diabetes. It was found that 11.7% of the participants developed Type 2 diabetes.

After adjusting for risk factors known to increase the chances of developing diabetes, including age, gender, BMI, neck circumference, smoking, and income status, participants with severe OSA were found to have a 30% higher risk of developing Type 2 diabetes than those without OSA.

Furthermore, participants with mild or moderate OSA were found to have a 23% increased risk of developing Type 2 diabetes compared to those without OSA. Additional risk factors for diabetes included experiencing breathing difficulties during the rapid eye movement stage of sleep, low oxygen levels in the blood, sleep deprivation, and activation of the sympathetic nervous system as indicated by increased heart rate.

The investigators concluded that after adjusting for other potential causes, there is a significant link between OSA severity and the risk of developing diabetes (Kendzerska, Gershon, Hawker et al. 2014).

The aim of a study using polysomnography, published in the *American Journal of Respiratory Care and Medicine*, was to determine the impact of OSA on HbA1c, the major clinical indicator of glycemic control in patients with Type 2 diabetes. It was found that 77% of patients with diabetes had OSA with an AHI greater than 5. Increasing OSA severity was associated with poorer glucose control, after controlling for age, gender, race, BMI, number of diabetes medications, level of exercise, years of diabetes, and total sleep time.

Compared to patients without OSA, the adjusted mean HbA1c was higher by 1.49% in patients with mild OSA; it was higher by 1.93% in patients with moderate OSA, and higher by 3.69% in patients with severe OSA. These differences were statistically significant.

Measures of OSA severity, including total AHI, rapid eye movement AHI, and the oxygen desaturation index during total and rapid eye movement sleep were positively correlated with higher HbA1c levels.

It was concluded that in patients with Type 2 diabetes, increasing severity of OSA is associated with poorer glucose control, independent of adiposity and other confounders (Aronsohn, Whitmore, Van Cauter et al. 2010).

Most publications consider OSA to be a consequence of Type 2 diabetes. However, a review in *Chest* concludes that the relationship between OSA and Type 2 diabetes may actually be bidirectional, given that diabetic neuropathy of the autonomic system (as opposed to peripheral neuropathy) can affect central control of respiration and upper airway neural reflexes, thereby promoting sleep-disordered breathing (Reutrakul, and Mokhlesi. 2017).

REFERENCES

Agale SV. 2013. Review article. Chronic leg ulcers: Epidemiology, aetiopathogenesis, and management. *Ulcers*, (2013), Article ID 413604, 9 pages. http://dx.doi.org/10.1155/2013/413604.

Arcidiacono MV, Traveset A, Rubinat E, Ortega E, Betriu A, Hernández M, Fernández E, and D Mauricio. 2013. Microangiopathy of large artery wall: a neglected complication of diabetes mellitus. *Atherosclerosis*, May; 228(1): 142–147. DOI: 10.1016/j.atherosclerosis.2013.02.011.

Aronsohn RS, Whitmore H, Van Cauter E, and E Tasali1. 2010. Impact of untreated obstructive sleep apnea on glucose control in Type 2 diabetes. *American Journal of Respiratory Care and Medicine*. Mar; 181(5): 507–513. DOI: 10.1164/rccm.200909-1423)C.

Basson R, McInnes R, Smith MD, Hodgson G, and N Koppiker. 2004. Efficacy and safety of Sildenafil citrate in women with sexual dysfunction associated with female sexual arousal disorder. *Journal of Women's Health & Gender-Based Medicine*. Jul; 11(4): 367–377. https://doi.org/10.1089/152460902317586001.

Batty GD, Li Q, Czernichow S, Neal B, Zoungas S, Huxley R, Patel A, de Galan BE, Woodward M, Hamet P, Harrap SB, Poulter N, and J Chalmers. 2010. Erectile dysfunction and later cardiovascular disease in men with type 2 diabetes: prospective cohort study based on the ADVANCE (Action in Diabetes and Vascular Disease: Preterax and Diamicron Modified-Release Controlled Evaluation) trial. *Journal of the American College of Cardiology*. Nov; 56(23): 1908–1913. DOI: 10.1016/j.jacc. 2010.04.067.

Billman GE, Huikuri HV, Sacha J, and K Trimmel. 2015. An introduction to heart rate variability: methodological considerations and clinical applications. *Frontiers in Physiology*. Feb; 6: 55 DOI: 10.3389/fphys.2015.00055.

Bivalacqua TJ, Hellstrom WJ, Kadowitz PJ, and HC Champion. 2001. Increased expression of arginase II in human diabetic corpus cavernosum: in diabetic-associated erectile dysfunction. *Biochemical and Biophysical Research Communications*, May; 83(4): 923–927. DOI: 10.1006/bbrc.2001.4874.

Brem H, and M Tomic-Canic. 2007. Cellular and molecular basis of wound healing in diabetes. *The Journal of Clinical Investigation*, May; 117(5): 1219–1222. DOI: 10. 1172/JCI32169.

Brenta G. 2011. Why can insulin resistance be a natural consequence of thyroid dysfunction? *Journal of Thyroid Research*, 2011:152850. DOI: 10.4061/2011/152850. Epub 2011 Sep 19. PMCID: PMC3175696.

Brownlee M, and IB Hirsch. 2006. Glycemic variability: a hemoglobin A1c-independent risk factor for diabetic complications. *Journal of the American Medical Association*, Apr; 295(14): 1707–1708. DOI: 10 .1001/jama.295.14.1707.

Burchfiel CM, Reed DM, Marcus EB, Strong JP, and T Hayashi. 1993. Association of diabetes mellitus with coronary atherosclerosis and myocardial lesions. An autopsy study from the Honolulu Heart Program. *American Journal of Epidemiology*, Jun 15; 137(12): 1328–1340. PMID: 8333414.

Calles-Escandon J, and M Cipolla. 2001. Diabetes and endothelial dysfunction: a clinical perspective. *Endocrine Reviews*, Feb; 22(1): 36–52.

Carnethon MR, Biggs ML, Barzilay J, Kuller LH, Mozaffarian D, Mukamal K, Smith NL, and D Siscovick. 2010. Diabetes and coronary heart disease as risk factors for mortality in older adults. *American Journal of Medicine*, Jun; 123(6): 556.e1–559.el. DOI: 10.1016/j.amjmed.2009.11.023. DOI: 10.1016/j.amjmed.2009.11.023.

Casey G. 2004. Causes and management of leg and foot ulcers. Nursing Standard, Jul; 18(4): 57–58.

Chaker L, Ligthart S, Korevaar TIM, Hofman A, Franco OH, Peeters RP, and A Dehghan. 2016. Thyroid function and type 2 diabetes risk: a population-based prospective cohort study. *BMC Medicine*, 201614:150. DOI: 10.1186/s12916-016-0693-4.

Chawla A, Chawla R, and S Jaggi. 2016. Microvasular and macrovascular complications in diabetes mellitus: distinct or continuum? *Indian Journal of Endocrinology and Metabolism*, Jul–Aug; 20(4): 546–551. DOI: 10.4103/2230-8210.183480.

Chen G, McAlister FA, Walker RL, Hemmelgarn BR, and NR Campbell. 2010. Cardiovascular outcomes in framingham [sic] participants with diabetes: the importance of blood pressure. *Hypertension*, May; 57(5): 891–897. DOI: 10.1161/HYPERTENSION AHA.110.162446.

Cheung BMY, and C Li. 2012. Diabetes and hypertension: is there a common metabolic pathway? *Current Atherosclerosis Reports*, Apr; 14(2): 160–166. DOI: 10.1007/s11883-012-0227-2.

Chilelli NC, Burlina S, and A Lapolla. 2013. AGEs, rather than hyperglycemia, are responsible for microvascular complications in diabetes: a "glycoxidation-centric" point of view. *Nutrition, Metabolism and Cardiovascular Diseases*, Oct; 23(10): 913–919. DOI: 10.1016/j.numecd.2013.04.004.

Clarke-Moloney M, Keane N, and E Kavanagh. 2006. An exploration of current leg ulcer management practices in an Irish community setting. *Journal of Wound Care,* Oct; 15(9): 407–410. PMID: 17044358. DOI: 10.12968/jowc.2006.15.9.26963.

Clausen N, Lins PE, Adamson U, Hamberger B, and S Efendić. 1986. Counterregulation of insulin-induced hypoglycaemia in primary hypothyroidism. *Acta Endocrinologica* (Copenh), Apr; 111(4): 516–521. PMID: 3518323.

Colette C, and L Monnier. 2007. Acute glucose fluctuations and chronic sustained hyperglycemia as risk factors for cardiovascular diseases in patients with type 2 diabetes. *Hormones and Metabolic Research,* Sep; 39(9): 683–686. DOI: 10.1055/s-2007-985157.

Coll-de-Tuero G, Mata-Cases M, Rodriguez-Poncelas A, Pepió JM, Roura P, Benito B, Franch-Nadal J, and M Saez. 2012. Chronic kidney disease in the type 2 diabetic patients: prevalence and associated variables in a random sample of 2642 patients of a Mediterranean area. *BMC Nephrology,* Aug 20; 13: 87. DOI: 10.1186/1471-2369-13-87.

Copeland KL, Brown JS, Creasman JM, Van Den Eeden SK, Subak LL, Thom DH, Ferrara A, and AJK Huang. 2012. Diabetes mellitus and sexual function in middle-aged and older women. *Obstetrics and Gynecology,* Aug; 120(2 Pt 1): 331–340. DOI: 10.1097/AOG.0b013e31825ec5fa.

Cortelazzi D, Marconi A, Guazzi M, Cristina M, Zecchini B, Veronelli A, Cattalini C, Innocenti A, Bosco G, and AE Pontiroli. 2013. Sexual dysfunction in pre-menopausal diabetic women: clinical, metabolic, psychological, cardiovascular, and neurophysiologic correlates. *Acta Diabetologica,* Dec; 50(6): 91191–91197. DOI: 10. 1007/s00592-013-0482-x.

Cosentino F, and TF Lüscher. 2001. Effects of blood pressure and glucose on endothelial function. *Current Hypertension Reports,* 3(1): 79–88. DOI:10.1007/s11906-001-0085-8.

Dangwal S, Stratmann B, Bang C, Lorenzen JM, Kumarswamy R, Fiedler J, Falk CS, Scholz CJ, Thum T, and D Tschoepe. 2015. Impairment of wound healing in patients with Type 2 diabetes mellitus influences circulating microRNA patterns via inflammatory cytokines. *Arteriosclerosis, Thrombosis, and Vascular Biology,* Jun; 35(6): 1480–1488. DOI: 10.1161/ATVBAHA.114.305048.

Das AK, Das JP, and S Chandrasekar. 1987. Specific heart muscle disease in diabetes mellitus—a functional structural correlation. *International Journal of Cardiology,* Dec; 17(3): 299–302. PMID: 3679609.

De Mattia G, Laurenti O, and D Fava. 2003. Diabetic endothelial dysfunction: effect of free radical scavenging in Type 2 diabetic patients. *Journal of Diabetes and Its Complications,* Mar–Apr; 17(2 Suppl): 30–35. PMID: 12623166.

De Vriese AS, Verbeuren TJ, Van de Voorde J, Lameire NH, and PM Vanhoutte. 2000. Endothelial dysfunction in diabetes. *British Journal of Pharmacology,* Jul; 130(5): 963–974. DOI: 10.1038/sj.bjp .0703393.

Ding EL, Song Y, Malik VS, and S Liu. 2006. Sex differences of endogenous sex hormones and risk of type 2 diabetes: a systematic review and meta-analysis. *Journal of the American Medical Association* (JAMA), Mar 15; 295(11): 1288–1299. DOI: 10.1001/jama.295.11.1288.

Dornhorst AC, Howard P, and GL Leathhart. 1952. Respiratory variations in blood pressure. *Circulation,* 6: 553–558. DOI: 10.1161/01.CIR.6.4.553.

Endemann DH, and EL Schiffrin. 2004. Endothelial dysfunction. *Journal of the American Society of Nephrology,* Aug: 15(8): 1983–1992. DOI: 10.1097/01.ASN. 0000132474.50966.DA JASN.

Epstein M, and JR Sowers. 1992. Brief review. Diabetes mellitus and hypertension. *Hypertension,* 19: 403–418. DOI: 10.1161/01.HYP.19.5.403.

Etgen AM, and DW Pfaff. 2009. Clinical aspects of CNS arousal mechanisms. In: *Molecular Mechanisms of Hormone Actions on Behavior.* New York: Academic Press. pp. 87–88.

Fife C, Walker D, Thomson B, and M Carter. 2007. Limitations of daily living activities in patients with venous stasis ulcers undergoing compression bandaging: Problems with the concept of self-bandaging. *Wounds,* Oct; 19(10): 255–257. PMID: 25942507.

Fishman T. 2007. How to manage venous stasis ulcers. *Podiatry Today,* May; 20: 66–72.

Fournier J-P, Yin H, Yu OHY, and L Azoulay. 2014. Metformin and low levels of thyroid-stimulating hormone in patients with type 2 diabetes mellitus. *Canadian Medical Association Journal,* Oct 21; 186(15): 1138–1145. DOI: 10.1503/cmaj. 140688.

Fox CS. 2010. Cardiovascular disease risk factors, type 2 diabetes mellitus, and the Framingham Heart Study. *Trends in Cardiovascular Medicine,* Apr; 20(3): 90–95. DOI: 10.1016/j.tcm.2010.08.001.

Freeman R, and MW Chapleau. 2013. Testing the autonomic nervous system. *Handbook of Clinical Neurology,* 115: 115–136. DOI: 10.1016/B978-0-444-52902-2.00007-2.

Fried R, and J Grimaldi. 1993. *The Psychology and Physiology of Breathing in Behavioral Medicine, Clinical Psychology and Psychiatry.* New York: Springer Publishing.

Fried R. 1972. Cardiac arrhythmia computer. US Patent No. 3,698,386.

Fried R. 1993. *The Psychology and Physiology of Breathing in Behavioral Medicine, Clinical Psychology and Psychiatry.* New York: Springer/Plenum Press.

Fried R. 2010. *Human Sexuality—Basics of Functional Biology with Behavioral and Clinical Considerations.* New York: Whittier Publishing.

Fried R. 2014. *Erectile Dysfunction as a Cardiovascular Impairment.* Amsterdam: Academic Press/Elsevier.

Furchgott RF, and J V Zawadzki. 1980. The obligatory role of endothelial cells in the relaxation of arterial smooth muscle by acetylcholine. *Nature,* Nov; 288: 373–376. DOI: 10.1038/288373a0.

Glassock RFJ, and C Winearls. 2009. Ageing and the glomerular filtration rate: Truths and consequences. *Transactions of the American Clinical and Climatological Association,* 120: 419–428. PMCID: PMC2744545.

Goldfarb S, Fishbane S, and R Provenzano. 2017. Patients with moderate chronic kidney disease (CKD): the emerging mandate. Recognition and staging of CKD presented by Stanley Goldfarb, MD. Medscape, http://www.medscape.org/view article/533695; accessed 6.26.17.

Gragasin FS, Michelakis ED, Hogan A, Moudgil R, Hashimoto K, Wu X, Bonnet S, Haromy A, and SL Archer. 2004. The neurovascular mechanism of clitoral erection: nitric oxide and cGMP-stimulated activation of BKCa channels. *FASEB J* (Federation of American Societies for Experimental Biology). Sept; 18(12): 1382–1391. DOI: 10.1096/fj.04-1978com.

Gronich N, Deftereos SN, Lavi I, Persidis AS, Abernethy DA, and G Rennert. 2015. Hypothyroidism is a risk factor for new-onset diabetes mellitus: a cohort study. *Diabetes Care,* Jun; dc142515. https://doi.org/10.2337/dc14-2515.

Habib S, and A Ali. 2011. Biochemistry of nitric oxide. *Indian Journal of Clinical Biochemistry,* Jan; 26(1): 3–17. DOI: 10.1007/s12291-011-0108-4.

Holdsworth CD, and GM Besser. 1968. Influence of gastric emptying-rate and of insulin response on oral glucose tolerance in thyroid disease. *Lancet,* Sep 28; 2(7570): 700–702. PMID: 4175086.

Hu G, Jousilahti P, and J Tuomilehto. 2007. Joint effects of history of hypertension at baseline and type 2 diabetes at baseline and during follow-up on the risk of coronary heart disease. *European Heart Journal,* Dec; 28(24):3059–3066. DOI: 10.1093/eurheartj/ehm501.

Ignarro LJ. 1990. Nitric oxide. A novel signal transduction mechanism for transcellular communication. *Hypertension,* Nov; 16(5):477–483. PMID: 1977698.

Järvilehto M, and P Tuohimaa. 2009. Vasa vasorum hypoxia: initiation of atherosclerosis. *Medical Hypotheses,* Jul; 73(1): 40–41. DOI: 10.1016/j.mehy. 2008.11.046.

Joshi SR, Saboo B, Vadivale M, Dani SI, Mithal A, Kaul U, Badgandi M, Iyengar SS, Viswanathan V, Sivakadaksham N, Chattopadhyaya PS, Arup Das Biswas AD, Jindal S, Khan IA, Sethi BK, Rao VD, and JJ Dalal, on behalf of the SITE Investigators. 2012. Prevalence of diagnosed and undiagnosed diabetes and hypertension in India—Results from the Screening India's Twin Epidemic (SITE) Study. *Diabetes Technology and Therapeutics.* 14(1): DOI: 10.1089/dia.2011.0243.

Kalra S, Unnikrishnan AG, and R Sahay. 2014. The hypoglycemic side of hypothyroidism. *Indian Journal of Endocrinology and Metabolism,* Jan–Feb; 18(1): 1–3. DOI: 10.4103/2230-8210.12 6517.

Kamilaris TC, DeBold CR, Pavlou SN, Island DP, Hoursanidis A, and DN Orth. 1987. Effect of altered thyroid hormone levels on hypothalamic-pituitary-adrenal function. *The Journal of Clinical Endocrinology and Metabolism,* Nov; 65(5): 994–999. DOI: 10.1210/jcem-65-5-994.

Kaore SN, and NM Kaore. 2014. Citrulline: pharmacological perspectives and role as a biomarker in diseases and toxicities. In RC Gupta (Ed.), *Biomarkers in Toxicology.* Amsterdam: Academic Press/Elsevier, pp. 883–905. https://doi.org/10.1016/B978-0-12-404630-6.00053-1.

Katte J-C, Dzudie A, Sobngwi E, Mbong EN, Fetse GT, Kouam CK, and A-P Kengne. 2014. Coincidence of diabetes mellitus and hypertension in a semi-urban Cameroonian population: a cross-sectional study. *BMC BioMed Central Public Health,* 14:696. DOI: 10.1186/1471-2458-14-696.

Kaya C, Uslu Z, and I Karaman. 2006. Is endothelial function impaired in erectile dysfunction patients? *International Journal of Impotence Research,* Jan–Feb; 18(1): 55–60. DOI: 10.1038/sj.ijir.3901371.

Kendzerska T, Gershon AS, Hawker G, Tomlinson G, and RS. Leung. 2014. Obstructive sleep apnea and incident diabetes: a historical cohort study. *American Journal of Respiratory and Critical Care Medicine,* Jul; 180(2): Published online https://doi.org/10.1164/rccm.201312-2209OC; DOI: 10.1164/rccm.201312-2209OC.

Kolluru GK, Bir SC, and CG Kevil. 2012. Endothelial dysfunction and diabetes: effects on angiogenesis, vascular remodeling, and wound healing. *International Journal of Vascular Medicine,* 2012: 918267. 30 pages. DOI: 10.1155/2012/918267.

Kvell K, Pongrácz J, Székely M, Balaskó M, Pétervári E, and G Bakó. 2011. *Molecular and Clinical Basics of Gerontology.* Copyright © 2011 Dr. Krisztián Kvell, University of Pécs, Hungary.

Laight DW, Carrier MJ, and EE Anggard. 2000. Antioxidants, diabetes and endothelial dysfunction. *Cardiovascular Research,* Aug; 47(3): 457–464. PMID: 10963719.

Lastra G, Syed S, Kurukulasuriya R, Manrique C, and JR Sowers. 2014. Type 2 diabetes mellitus and hypertension: an update. *Endocrinology and Metabolism Clinics of North America,* Mar; 43(1): 103–122. DOI: 10.1016/j.ecl.2013.09.005.

Lien T-H, Wu J-S, Yang Y-C, Sun Z-J, and C-J Chang. 2016. The effect of glycemic status on kidney stone disease in patients with prediabetes. *Diabetes and Metabolism Journal,* 2016 Apr; 40(2): 161–166. DOI: 10.4093/dmj.2016.40.2.161.

Lutfi MF, and RF Elhakeem. 2016. Effect of fasting blood glucose level on heart rate variability of healthy young adults. *PLoS ONE,* 11(7): e0159820. DOI: 10.1371/journal.pone.0159820.

Lutfi MF. 2015. Patterns of heart rate variability and cardiac autonomic modulations in controlled and uncontrolled asthmatic patients. *BMC Pulmonary Medicine.* Oct; 15: 119. DOI: 10.1186/s12890-015-0118-8.

Maiorino MI, Bellastella J, and K Esposito. 2014. Diabetes and sexual dysfunction: current perspectives. *Diabetes, Metabolic Syndrome and Obesity: Targets and Therapy,* 7: 95–105. Published online 2014 Mar 6. DOI: 10.2147/DMSO.S36455.

Mazzilli R, Imbrogno N, Elia J, Delfino M, Bitterman O, Napoli A, and F Mazzilli. 2015. Sexual dysfunction in diabetic women: prevalence and differences in type 1 and type 2 diabetes mellitus. *Diabetes, Metabolic Syndrome and Obesity,* Feb; 8: 97–101. DOI: 10.2147/DMSO.S71376.

McAlpine CS, Bowes AJ, and GH Werstuck. 2010. Diabetes, hyperglycemia and accelerated atherosclerosis: evidence supporting a role for endoplasmic reticulum (ER) stress signaling. *Cardiovascular and Hematological Disorders Drug Targets,* 2010 Jun; 10(2): 151–157. PMID: 20350283.

McCulloch AJ, Johnston DG, Baylis PH, Kendall-Taylor P, Clark F, Young ET, and KG Alberti. 1983. Evidence that thyroid hormones regulate gluconeogenesis from glycerol in man. *Clinical Endocrinology* (Oxf), Jul; 19(1): 67–76. PMID: 6688558.

McDaniel HG, Pittman CS, Oh SJ, and S DiMauro. 1977. Carbohydrate metabolism in hypothyroid myopathy. *Metabolism,* Aug; 26(8): 867–873. PMID: 875732.

Meldrum DR, Gambone JC, Morris MA, Meldrum DA, Esposito K, and LJ Ignarro. 2011. The link between erectile and cardiovascular health: the canary in the coal mine. *American Journal of Cardiology,* Aug; 108(4):599–606.

Metsärinne K, Bröijersen A, Kantola I, Niskanen L, Rissanen A, Appelroth T, Pöntynen N, Poussa T, Koivisto V, Virkamäki A; STages of NEphropathy in Type 2 Diabetes Study Investigators. 2015. High prevalence of chronic kidney disease in Finnish patients with type 2 diabetes treated in primary care. *Primary Care Diabetes,* Feb; 9(1): 31–38. DOI: 10.1016/j.pcd.2014.06.001.

Milicevic Z, Raz I, Beattie SD, Campaigne BN, Sarwat S, Gromniak E, Kowalska I, Galic E, Tan M, and M Hanefeld. 2008. Natural history of cardiovascular disease in patients with diabetes: role of hyperglycemia. *Diabetes Care,* Feb; 31 Suppl 2: S155–160. DOI: 10.2337/dc08-s240.

Moloney MC, and P Grace. 2004. Understanding the underlying causes of chronic leg ulceration. *Journal of Wound Care,* 13(5): 215–218.

Moncada S, and A Higgs. 1993. The L-Arginine–nitric oxide pathway. *The New England Journal of Medicine* (NEJM), Dec; 329: 2002–2012. DOI: 10.1056/NEJM199312303292706.

Monnier L, Mas E, Ginet C, Michel F, Villon L, Crisrol JP, and CC Colette. 2006. Activation of oxidative stress by acute glucose fluctuations compared with sustained chronic hyperglycemia in patients with type 2 diabetes. *Journal of the American Medical Association,* Apr; 295(14): 1681–1687. DOI: 10.1001/jama.295.14.1681.

Morano S. 2003. Pathophysiology of diabetic sexual dysfunction. *Journal of Endocrinological Investigation,* 26(3 Suppl): 65–69. PMID: 12834025.

Mujtaba SH, Ashraf T, Mahmood SN, and Q Anjum. 2010. Assessment of renal insufficiency in patients with normal serum creatinine levels undergoing angiography. *Journal of Pakistan Medical Association,* Nov; 60(11): 915–917. PMID: 21375194.

Muller MD, Reed AB, Leuenberger UA, and LI Sinowa. 2013. Physiology in medicine: Peripheral arterial disease. Journal of Applied Physiology (1985), Nov 1; 115(9): 1219–1226. Published online 2013 Aug 22. DOI: 10.1152/japplphysiol.00885.2013.

Müller MJ, and HJ Seitz. 1987. Interrelation between thyroid state and the effect of glucagon on gluconeogenesis in perfused rat livers. *Biochemical Pharmacology,* May 15; 36(10): 1623–1627. PMID: 2439088.

Murphy RA, and JS Walker. 1998. Inhibitory mechanisms for cross-bridge cycling: the nitric oxide-cGMP signal transduction pathway in smooth muscle relaxation. *Acta Physiologica Scandinavica,* Dec; 164(4): 373–380. DOI: 10.1046/j.1365-201X.1998.00434.x.

Nada AM. 2013. Effect of treatment of overt hypothyroidism on insulin resistance. *World Journal of Diabetes,* Aug 15; 4(4): 157–161. Published online 2013 Aug 15. DOI: 10.4239/wjd.v4.i4.157 PMCID: PMC3746089.

Nannapaneni S, Ramar K, and S Surani. 2013. Effect of obstructive sleep apnea on type 2 diabetes mellitus: a comprehensive literature review. *World Journal of Diabetes,* Dec; 4(6): 238–244. DOI: 10.4239/wjd.v4.i6.238.

Nerli R, Jali M, Guntaka AK, Patne P, Patil S, and MB Hiremath. 2015. Type 2 diabetes mellitus and renal stones. *Advanced Biomedical Research,* 4: 180. Published online 2015 Aug 31. DOI: 10.4103/2277-9175.164012.

Newman AB. 2000. Peripheral arterial disease: insights from population studies of older adults. *Journal of the American Geriatrics Society,* Sep; 48(9): 1157–1162. PMID: 10983919.

No authors listed. 1996. Task Force of the European Society of Cardiology and the North American Society of Pacing and Electrophysiology. Heart rate variability standards of measurement, physiological interpretation and clinical use. *Circulation,* Mar; 93(5): 65-1043. PMID: 8598068.

No authors listed. 2008. Center for Disease Control and Prevention. National diabetes fact sheet: general information and national estimates on diabetes in the United States, 2007. U.S. Department of Health and Human Services, Centers for Disease Control and Prevention; Atlanta, GA.

Nowosielski K, and V Skrzypulec-Plinta. 2011. Mediators of sexual functions in women with diabetes. *Journal of Sexual Medicine,* Sep; 8(9): 2532–2545. DOI: 10. 1111/j.1743-6109.2011.02336.x.

Nuutila P, Mäki M, Laine H, Knuuti MJ, Ruotsalainen U, Luotolahti M, Haaparanta M, Solin O, Jula A, and VA Koivisto. 1995. Insulin action on heart and skeletal muscle glucose uptake in essential hypertension. *The Journal of Clinical Investigation,* Aug; 96(2): 1003–1009. DOI: 10.1172/JCI118085.

Pakhetra R, Garg MK, and JS Saini. 2001. Is beta cell dysfunction responsible for flat glucose tolerance curve in primary hypothyroidism? (A hypothesis). *Medical Journal, Armed Forces of India,* 2001 Apr; 57(2):120–125. DOI: 10.1016/S0377-1237(01)80129-5.

Pamidi S, and E Tasali. 2012. Obstructive sleep apnea and type 2 diabetes: Is there a link? *Frontiers in Neurology,* Aug; 3: 126. DOI: 10.3389/fneur.2012.00126.

Panova E, and NE Kruglova. 2008. Factors associated with cardiac arrhythmias in patients with type 2 diabetes mellitus and myocardial infarction (Article in Russian). *Klinicheskaia Meditsina* (Mosk), 86(1): 23–26. PMID: 18326278.

Pontiroli AE, Cortelazzi D, and A Morabito. 2013. Female sexual dysfunction and diabetes: a systematic review and meta-analysis. *Journal of Sexual Medicine,* Apr; 10(4): 1044–1051. DOI: 10.1111/jsm.12065. PMID: 23347454.

Ramasamy R, Yan SF, and AM Schmidt. 2006. Glycation and RAGE: Common links in the pathogenesis of microvascular and macrovascular complications of diabetes. *Canadian Journal of Diabetes,* 30(4): 422–429 DOI: http://dx.doi.org/10.1016/S1499-2671(06)04007-X.

Reutrakul S, and B Mokhlesi. 2017. Obstructive sleep apnea and diabetes. A state of the art review. *Chest,* 152(5): 1070–1086. http://journal.chestnet.org/article/S0012-3692(17)30930-3/pdf.

Roth A, Kalter-Leibovici O, Kerbis Y, Tenenbaum-Koren E, Chen J, Sobol T, and I Raz. 2003. Prevalence and risk factors for erectile dysfunction in men with diabetes, hypertension, or both diseases: a community survey among 1,412 Israeli men. *Clinical Cardiology,* Jan; 26(1): 25–30. PMID: 12539809.

Rothberg LJ, Lees T, Clifton-Bligh R, and S Lal. 2016. Association between heart rate variability measures and blood glucose levels: implications for noninvasive glucose monitoring for diabetes. *Diabetes Technology and Therapeutics,* Jun; 18(6): 366–376. DOI: 10.1089/dia.2016.0010.

Ruilope LM, and R García-Robles.1997. How far should blood pressure be reduced in diabetic hypertensive patients? *Journal of Hypertension Supplement,* Mar; 15(2): S63–65. PMID: 9218201.

Sarkar PK, and S Ballantyne. 2000. Management of leg ulcers. *Postgraduate Medical Journal,* 76(901): 674–682.

Sarwar N, Gao P, Seshasai SR, Gobin R, Kaptoge S, Di Angelantonio E, Ingelsson E, Lawlor DA, Selvin E, Stampfer M, Stehouwer CD, Lewington S, Pennells L, Thompson A, Sattar N, White IR, Ray KK, and J Danesh. 2010. Diabetes mellitus, fasting blood glucose concentration, and risk of vascular disease: a collaborative meta-analysis of 102 prospective studies. *Lancet,* Jun 26; 375(9733): 2215–2222. DOI: 10.1016/S0140-6736(10)60484-9. PMCID: PMC2904878.

Sawada N, Jiang A, Takizawa F, Safdar A, Manika A, Tesmenitsky Y, Kang KT, Bischoff J, Kalwa H, Sartoretto JL, Kamei Y, Benjamin LE, Watada H, Ogawa Y, Higashikuni Y, Kessinger CW, Jaffer FA, Michel T, Sata M, Croce K, Tanaka R, and Z Arany. 2014. Endothelial PGC-1α mediates vascular dysfunction in diabetes. *Cell Metabolism,* Feb 4; 19(2): 2462–2458. DOI: 10.1016/j.cmet.2013.12.014.

Schutta MH. 2007. Diabetes and hypertension: epidemiology of the relationship and pathophysiology of factors associated with these comorbid conditions. *Journal of the Cardiometabolic Syndrome,* Spring; 2(2): 124–130. PMID: 17684469.

Schroeder EB, Chambless LE, Liao D, Prineas RJ, Evans GW, Rosamond WD, G Heiss. and the Atherosclerosis Risk in Communities (ARIC) study. 2005. Diabetes, glucose, insulin, and heart rate variability: the Atherosclerosis Risk in Communities (ARIC) study. *Diabetes Care,* Mar; 28(3): 668–674. PMID: 15735206.

Scotland R, Vallance P, and A Ahluwalia. 1999. On the regulation of tone in vasa vasorum. *Cardiovascular Research,* Jan; 41(1): 237–245. DOI: https://doi.org/10. 1016/S0008-6363(98)00223-5.

Selvin E, Marinopoulos S, Berkenblit G, Rami T, Brancati FL, Rami T, Brancati FL, Powe NR, and SH Golden. 2004. Meta-analysis: glycosylated hemoglobin and cardiovascular disease in diabetes mellitus. *Annals of Internal Medicine,* Sept; 141(6): 421–431. PMID: 15381515.

Sen CK, Gordillo GM, Roy S, Kirsner R, Lambert L, Hunt TK, Gottrup F, Gurtner GC, and MT Longaker. 2009. Human skin wounds: a major and snowballing threat to public health and the economy. *Wound Repair and Regeneration,* Nov–Dec; 17(6): 763–771. DOI: 10.1111/j.1524-475X.2009.00543.x.

Shah JH, Motto GS, Papagiannes E, and GA Williams. 1975. Insulin metabolism in hypothyroidism. Diabetes, Oct; 24(10): 922–925. PMID: 1175861.

Sheetz MJ, and GL King. 2002. Molecular understanding of hyperglycemia's adverse effects for diabetic complications. *Journal of the American Medical Association,* Nov; 288(20): 2579–2588. PMID: 12444865.

Shi Y, and PM Vanhoutte. 2009. Reactive oxygen-derived free radicals are key to the endothelial dysfunction of diabetes. *Journal of Diabetes,* Jun; 1(3): 151–162. DOI: 10.1111/j.1753-0407.2009.00030.x.

Shvarts V. 2009. The role of postprandial hyperglycemia in the development of cardiovascular diseases in type 2 diabetes mellitus [article in Russian]. *Klinicheskaia meditsina (Mosk),* 87(11): 17–24. PMID: 20143560.

Singh BM, Goswami B, and V Mallika. 2010. Association between insulin resistance and hypothyroidism in females attending a tertiary care hospital. *Indian Journal of Clinical Biochemistry,* Apr; 25(2): 141–145. DOI: 10.1007/s12291-010-0026-x. Epub 2010 May 27.

Singh N, Armstrong DG, and BA Lipsky. 2005. Preventing foot ulcers in patients with diabetes. *Journal of the American Medical Association,* Jan; 293(2): 217–228. DOI: 10.1001/jama.293.2.217.

Soldevilla J, Torra JE, Verdu J, Rueda J, Martinez F, and E Roche. 2006. Epidemiology of chronic wounds in Spain: Results of the First National Studies on Pressure and Leg Ulcer Prevalence. *Wounds—A Compendium of Clinical Research and Practice.* 18: 213–226.

Sowers JR, Khoury S, Standley P, Zemel P, and M Zemel. 1991. Mechanisms of hypertension in diabetes. *American Journal of Hypertension,* Feb; 4(2 Pt 1): 177–182. PMID: 2021449.

Sowers JR. 1990. Insulin resistance and hypertension. *Molecular and Cell Endocrinology,* Dec 3; 74(2): C87–C89. PMID: 2090512.

Sowers JR. 2013. Diabetes mellitus and vascular disease. *Hypertension,* May; 61(5): 943–947. DOI: 10.1161 /HYPERTENSIONAHA.111.00612.

Stamler J, Vaccaro O, Neaton JD, and D Wentworth. 1993. Diabetes, other risk factors, and 12-yr cardiovascular mortality for men screened in the Multiple Risk Factor Intervention Trial. *Diabetes Care,* Feb; 16(2): 434–444. PMID: 8432214.

Statsenko ME, and MV Derevianchenko. 2015. Possibilities of correction of endothelial dysfunction at the background of combined antihypertensive therapy in patients with arterial hypertension and Type 2 diabetes (Article in Russian). Kardiologiia, 55(3): 17–20. PMID: 26320285.

Stuckey BG, Walsh JP, Ching HL, Stuckey AW, Palmer NR, Thompson PL, and GF Watts. 2007. Erectile dysfunction predicts generalised cardiovascular disease: evidence from a case–control study. *Atherosclerosis,* Oct; 194(2), 458–464. DOI: 10.1016/j.atherosclerosis.2006.08.043.

Tasali E, Mokhlesi B, and E Van Cauter. 2008. Obstructive sleep apnea and type 2 diabetes: interacting epidemics. Chest, Feb; 133(2): 496–506. DOI: 10.1378/chest. 07-0828.

Tesfamariam B, and RA Cohen. 1992. Free radicals mediate endothelial cell dysfunction caused by elevated glucose. *American Journal of Physiology* – Heart, Aug; 263 (2 Pt 2): H321–H326. PMID: 1510128.

Tiao JY, Semmens JB, Masarei JR, and MM Lawrence-Brown. 2002. The effect of age on serum creatinine levels in an aging population: relevance to vascular surgery. Cardiovascular Surgery (London, England), Oct; 10(5): 445–451. PMID: 12379401.

Uribarri J, Woodruff S, Goodman S, Cai W, Chen X, Pyzik R, Yong A, Striker GE, and H Vlassara. 2010. Advanced glycation end products in foods and a practical guide to their reduction in the diet. *Journal of the American Dietetic Association,* Jun; 110(6): 911–916.e12. DOI: 10.1016/j.jada.2010.03.018.

Valensi P, Extramiana F, Lange C, Cailleau M, Haggui A, Maison Blanche P, Tichet J, and B Balkau. 2011. And, the DESIR Study Group collaborators: Balkau P, Ducimetière E, Eschwège E, Alhenc-Gelas F, Gallois Y, Girault A, Fumeron F, Marre M, Bonnet F, Froguel P, Cogneau J, Born C, Caces E, Cailleau M,

Lantieri O, Moreau JG, Rakotozafy F, Tichet J, and S Vol. Influence of blood glucose on heart rate and cardiac autonomic function. The DESIR study. *Diabetic Medicine,* Apr; 28(4): 440–449. DOI: 10.1111/j.1464-5491.2010.03222.x.

van der Meer V, Wielders HPM, Grootendorst DC, de Kanter JS, Sijpkens YWJ, Assendelft WJJ, Gussekloo J, Dekker FW, and Y Groeneveld, 2010. Chronic kidney disease in patients with diabetes mellitus type 2 or hypertension in general practice. British *Journal of General Practice,* Dec; 60(581): 884–890. DOI: 10.3399/bjgp 10X544041.

Veerman KJ, Venegas-Pino DE, Shi Y, Khan MI, Gerstein HC, and GH Werstuck. 2013. Hyperglycaemia is associated with impaired vasa vasorum neovascularization and accelerated atherosclerosis in apolipoprotein-E deficient mice. *Atherosclerosis,* Apr; 227(2): 250258. DOI: 10.1016/j.atherosclerosis.2013.01.018.

Verma M, Khadapkar R, Sahu PS and BR Das. 2006. Comparing age-wise reference intervals for serum creatinine. *Indian Journal of Clinical Biochemistry,* Sept; 21(2): 90–94. DOI: 10.1007/BF02912919.

Veves A. 1998. The role of endothelial function on the foot. Microcirculation and wound healing in patients with diabetes. *Clinics in Podiatric Medicine and Surgery,* Jan; 15(1): 85–93. PMID: 9463769.

Vigorita VJ, Moore GW, and GM Hutchins. 1980. Absence of correlation between coronary arterial atherosclerosis and severity or duration of diabetes mellitus of adult onset. *American Journal of Cardiology,* Oct; 46(4): 535–542. PMID: 7416013.

Wagner CA, and N Mohebbi. 2010. Urinary pH and stone formation. *Journal of Nephrology,* Nov-Dec; 23 Suppl 16: S165–169. PMID: 21170875.

Waller BF, Palumbo PJ, Lie JT, and WC Roberts. 1980. Status of the coronary arteries at necropsy in diabetes mellitus with onset after age 30 years. Analysis of 229 diabetic patients with and without clinical evidence of coronary heart disease and comparison to 183 control subjects. *The American Journal of Medicine,* Oct; 69(4): 498–506.

Weinberg AE, Patel CJ, Chertow GM, and JT. Leppert. 2014. Diabetic severity and risk of kidney stone disease. *European Urology,* Jan: 65(1): 242–247. DOI: 10. 1016/j.eururo.2013.03. 026.

Wincze JP, Albert A, and S Bansal. 1993. Sexual arousal in diabetic females: physiological and self-report measures. *Archives of Sexual Behavior,* Dec; 22(6): 587–601. PMID: 8285846.

Wong W. 2014. Why wounds won't heal for diabetics. *Science Signaling,* Feb; 7(314). DOI: 10.1126/scisignal .2005210.

Zarich SW, and RW Nesto. 1989. Diabetic cardiomyopathy. *American Heart Journal,* Nov; 118(5 Pt 1): 1000–1012. PMID: 2683698.

Zhang Y, Hu G, Yuan Z, and L Chen. 2012. Glycosylated hemoglobin in relationship to cardiovascular outcomes and death in patients with Type 2 diabetes: A systematic review and meta-analysis. *PLoS ONE,* August 9; https://doi.org/10.1371/journal.pone.0042551.

4 Hyperglycemia Impairs the Functions of Blood

And so I conclude that blood lives and is nourished of itself and in no way depends on any other part of the body as being prior to it or more excellent... So that from this we may perceive the causes not only of life in general... but also of longer or shorter life, of sleeping and waking, of skill, of strength and so forth.

William Harvey (1651)

4.1 BLOOD—SOME BASICS

Healthy functioning requires the unimpeded circulation of blood throughout the body. Anything that changes the character of blood so that it becomes sluggish will become a major threat to health, even to life.

In a test tube of blood standing for half an hour, the blood separates into three layers, as the denser constituents sink to the bottom of the tube, and fluid remains at the top. The light fluid top layer is the plasma, which constitutes about 60% of blood. The middle layer is composed of white blood cells (WBCs) and platelets, and the bottom red layer consists mostly of red blood cells (RBCs). These bottom two layers of cells constitute about 40% of the blood.

Plasma is mainly water, much like seawater, but it also contains many important substances such as proteins, albumin, clotting factors, antibodies, enzymes, hormones, sugars (glucose), and fat particles.

All of the cells found in the blood come ultimately from the bone marrow: They begin as stem cells, and they mature into three main types of cells: RBCs (erythrocytes), WBCs, and platelets.

There are three types of WBCs: lymphocytes, monocytes, and granulocytes, and there are three main types of granulocytes: neutrophils, eosinophils, and basophils.

RBCs are the most common type of cell in the blood, circulating in the body for up to 120 days, at which point the old or damaged RBCs are removed from the circulation by macrophages and are disposed of in the spleen and liver.

Mature RBCs lack a nucleus. This conveniently allows for more room to store hemoglobin, the oxygen-binding protein, enabling the RBCs to transport more oxygen.

The RBCs have a biconcave shape, which increases their surface area and thereby allows for greater diffusion of oxygen. Contrary to common understanding, they are, on average, larger than the diameter of the smallest capillaries through which they must course. They therefore do so under pressure, allowing the maximum cell-wall to vessel-wall contact with the capillary.

WBCs make up part of the immune system. They come in many different shapes and sizes. Some have nuclei with multiple lobes, whereas others contain one large, round nucleus. Some contain packets of granules in their cytoplasm and so are known as granulocytes.

Despite differences in appearance, all of the various types of WBCs play a role in the immune response: They circulate in blood and become activated when they receive a signal, including interleukin 1 (IL-1), a molecule secreted by macrophages that contributes to fever in infections, and histamine, which is released by circulating basophils and tissue mast cells, and contributes to the symptoms of allergic reactions. In response to these signals, WBCs pass through "pores" in the blood vessel wall and migrate to the source of the signal to begin the healing process.

Neutrophils digest bacteria. They belong to a group of WBCs known as granulocytes because their cytoplasm is dotted with granules that contain enzymes that help them digest pathogens.

Monocytes, young WBCs, circulate in the blood, maturing into macrophages after they have left the blood and migrated into tissue. There they provide an immediate defense because they can engulf (phagocytose) and digest pathogens before other types of WBCs reach the area.

In the liver, tissue macrophages (Kupffer cells) remove harmful agents from blood that has left the gut. In the lungs, alveolar macrophages remove harmful agents that may have been inhaled. Macrophages in the spleen remove old or damaged RBCs and platelets from the circulation. Macrophages activated in host defense do so by triggering the release of nitric oxide (NO) with which they destroy pathogens.

Macrophages are also "antigen-presenting cells," presenting foreign protein antigens to other immune cells, thus triggering an immune response.

Lymphocytes are round cells containing a single large nucleus. There are two main classes of lymphocytes: the B-cells, which mature in the bone marrow, and the T-cells, which mature in the thymus gland. When "activated," the B-cells and T-cells trigger different types of immune responses: The activated B-cells (plasma cells) produce highly specific antibodies that bind to the agent that triggered the immune response. The T-cells (helper T cells) secrete chemicals that recruit other immune cells and help coordinate their attack. Another group, called cytotoxic T-cells, attacks cells invaded by viruses.

Platelets help to clot blood. Platelets are irregularly shaped fragments of cells that circulate in the blood until they are either activated to form a blood clot, or are removed by the spleen. Platelets also originate from stem cells in the bone marrow. They circulate for about 9 days. When they encounter damage to a blood vessel wall, they adhere to the damaged area and become activated to form a blood clot (Dean. 2005).

In short, in order for the body to thrive, the blood must flow unimpeded, and the formed parts (those with a form), the cells, and so on, must perform their individual function(s) without interference. Hyperglycemia actually interferes with both fluid flow and cell function.

There are conditions—chronic systemic inflammation, for one, as in atherosclerosis—that cause blood platelets to clump together (aggregate) (Gawaz, Langer, and May. 2005). Blood platelets can be damaged by reactive oxygen species (ROS) generated by inflammation, causing them to release substances, including serotonin, that promote aggregation. To ameliorate that condition, patients are prescribed blood "thinners."

When the free radical/antioxidant balance is tipped in favor of free radicals in Type 2 diabetes, the RBCs are now also compromised, causing a tendency to aggregate. Red cell aggregation is one of the factors that cause changes in how blood flows in the circulation, leading to increased cardiovascular risks.

4.2 HYPERGLYCEMIA AND BLOOD VISCOSITY

The viscosity of blood changes as a function of shear rate related to velocity. When blood moves quickly as in peak systole, it is actually thinner, whereas when it moves slowly during end diastole, it is thicker and stickier. This is due to red cell aggregation. The phenomenon is known as the "shear-thinning, non-Newtonian behavior of whole blood" (Cokelet, and Meiselman. 2007).

During each cardiac cycle, blood viscosity varies dynamically from high shear to low shear: At systole (high shear rate), blood is thinner, while at diastole (low shear rate), blood is two to five times thicker. The Edinburgh Artery Study published in the *British Journal of Haematology* in the late 1990s followed a random population of about 1600 middle-aged adults for an average of 5 years. It showed that blood viscosity, after adjustment for age and gender, was significantly higher in patients experiencing heart attacks and strokes than in those who did not. The 20% of individuals with the highest viscosity had 55% of the heart attacks and strokes during the 5-year period. In contrast, only 4% of those in the lowest-viscosity group had any significant cardiovascular or heart events.

It should be noted that these findings were *based solely* on measuring systolic blood viscosity (i.e., high shear rate viscosity), where the variation range is very narrow. The association between systolic viscosity, and cardiovascular events, was stronger for instance than that between smoking and cardiovascular events (Lowe, Lee, Rumley et al. 1997).

In a study of obese people (body mass index [BMI] greater than 28 kg/m^2) compared to non-obese healthy controls, published in the *International Journal of Obesity*, it was found that diastolic blood viscosity was 15% higher in the obese than in the nonobese patients.

In this study, whole blood, plasma, and erythrocyte viscosity values were determined with a Contraves LS30 viscometer. Plasma and whole blood viscosity were significantly increased in the obese participants. The increased low shear erythrocyte viscosity suggested diminished erythrocyte deformability in obesity. The rheological (flow) abnormalities were present even in the absence of impaired glucose tolerance, diabetes, hypertension, or hyperlipidemia. In the obese group, during an oral glucose tolerance test, the rheological parameters showed significant correlations with BMI, insulin, or C-peptide during an oral glucose tolerance test and plasma lipids. The investigators concluded that obesity *per se* may be associated with abnormal blood viscosity properties (Rillaerts, van Gaal, Xiang et al. 1989).

Other studies have also shown that persons with Type 2 diabetes have higher systolic and diastolic viscosity than healthy nondiabetic people. Patients with metabolic syndrome have higher viscosity than those without that condition, and viscosity scores can predict diabetes, and predict a tendency to develop diabetes in initially nondiabetic adults (Holsworth, and Cho. 2012). A study published in the journal *Diabetes Care* was conducted to determine parameters of blood viscosity in relation to blood glucose in individuals with normal glucose or prediabetes because little is known about that population.

Participants were assigned to one of three groups according to fasting blood glucose: group A, blood glucose less than 90 mg/dL; group B, blood glucose ranging from 90 to 99 mg/dL; and group C, blood glucose ranging from 100 to 125 mg/dL. Blood viscosity was measured at 37°C with a cone-plate viscometer at shear rates ranging from 225 to 22.5 s^{-1}. Shear rate is the rate of change of velocity at which one layer of fluid passes over an adjacent layer.

It was found that blood pressure, blood lipids, fibrinogen, and plasma viscosity were similar in the three groups. BMI and waist circumference were significantly increased in group C. Hematocrit and blood viscosity were significantly higher in groups B and C, compared to group A.

Blood glucose was significantly inversely correlated with high-density lipoprotein (HDL) cholesterol and directly with BMI, waist, hematocrit, and blood viscosity (from 225 to 22.5 s^{-1}). Blood viscosity at shear rate 225 s^{-1} was independently associated with blood glucose.

The investigators concluded that there is a direct relationship between blood viscosity and blood glucose level in nondiabetic participants. It is so much the case that even within glucose values considered completely normal, individuals with higher blood glucose levels have higher blood viscosity, comparable to that observed in participants with prediabetes (Irace, Carallo, Scavelli et al. 2014).

A report in the *American Journal of Epidemiology* proposes that elevated blood viscosity may predispose to insulin resistance and Type 2 diabetes by limiting delivery of glucose, insulin, and oxygen, to metabolically active tissues. To test this hypothesis, the investigators analyzed longitudinal data on about 13,000 initially nondiabetic adults 45 to 64 years old, who were participants in the Atherosclerosis Risk in Communities Study between 1987 and 1998.

Whole blood viscosity was estimated by using a validated formula based on hematocrit and total plasma proteins at baseline: At baseline, estimated blood viscosity was independently associated with several features of the metabolic syndrome. In models adjusted simultaneously for known predictors of diabetes, estimated whole blood viscosity and hematocrit predicted the tendency to develop Type 2 diabetes in a graded fashion.

Compared with their counterparts in the lowest quartiles, adults in the highest quartile of blood viscosity (hazard ratio = 1.68) and hematocrit (hazard ratio = 1.63) were more than 60% more likely to develop diabetes. Therefore, elevated blood viscosity and hematocrit deserve attention as emerging risk factors for insulin resistance and Type 2 diabetes (Tamariz, Young, Pankow et al. 2008). The hematocrit is the percentage of blood, by volume, that is composed of RBCs.

4.3 HYPERGLYCEMIA IMPEDES BLOOD FLOW BY INCREASING VISCOSITY

The term "hemorheology" is the combination of archaic Greek words that mean blood, flow, and study—in other words, the study of blood flow. One measure of blood flow is viscosity, the inherent resistance of blood to flow through a vessel. Blood viscosity is the degree of "thickness" and "stickiness of blood." Normal adult blood viscosity is 40/100, which is read as "forty over one hundred" and reported in units of *millipoise*. A *poise* is a unit of dynamic viscosity equal to one dyne-second, per square centimeter. A dyne is a unit of force that, acting on a mass of 1 g, increases its velocity by 1 cm/s, every second.

Increased blood viscosity is the only biological parameter that has been linked to all of the other major cardiovascular risk factors: In an article titled "A unifying theory of atherogenesis" published in the journal *Medical Hypotheses*, the author proposes that all major risk factors, including atherosclerosis, high blood pressure, elevated low-density lipoprotein (LDL) cholesterol, low HDL, Type 2 diabetes, metabolic syndrome, obesity, smoking, age, and male gender, cause the interaction of atherogenic elements with the endothelium by increasing viscosity, thereby creating larger areas of decreased blood flow (Sloop. 1996).

In fact, the *American Heart Journal* reported a study titled "Hematocrit and the risk of cardiovascular disease—the Framingham study: a 34-year follow-up" in the early 1990s. This study concluded that:

> … there was an increased risk of all-cause death as well as morbidity and mortality due to CVD in subjects with HCT values in the highest quintile. There was no evidence of a decrease risk of CVD in men with lower than median HCT values, and women actually showed increased risk of CVD events with lower HCT values, indicating a J- or U-shaped relationship between HCT and CVD events.
>
> The impact of HCT on CVD events appears to differ for different age groups and by sex [gender]. HCT is significantly related to the incidence of CVD, including CHD, MI, angina pectoris, stroke, and IC in younger men. In younger women, HCT is related to the incidence of CVD, CHD, MI and mortality from CVD and CHD. A negative association with CHF incidence and stroke death is noted in elderly women. These results support the hypothesis that HCT is an important risk factor for some CVD events, an association that merits further investigation. (From Gagnon, Zhang, Brand et al. 1994. *American Heart Journal*, Mar; 127(3): 674–682. With permission.)

(HCT is hematocrit; CVD is cardiovascular disease; and CHD is coronary heart disease.)

This is, of course, about viscosity, and it should raise the question, Why do people residing at sea level have the hematocrit of people adapted to living at high altitude?

Since red cell formation is driven by oxygen needs, perhaps, from a physiological perspective, their tissues were in fact somewhat oxygen deprived. LDL causes increased viscosity by fostering erythrocyte aggregation. HDL protects against atherosclerosis by antagonizing erythrocyte aggregation, thereby decreasing viscosity (Sloop. 1996).

4.3.1 HYPERGLYCEMIA IMPEDES CORONARY BLOOD FLOW

A clinical study published in the journal *Experimental and Clinical Cardiology* compared the coronary blood flow in diabetic, prediabetic, and nondiabetic patients all with angiographically normal coronary arteries. The participants in this study underwent coronary angiography between January 2010 and July 2011. The angiograms of eligible patients were reviewed again for thrombolysis in myocardial infarction (TIMI) frame counts. Thrombolysis is a treatment to dissolve dangerous clots in blood vessels, improve blood flow, and prevent damage to tissues and organs.

Patients were subsequently grouped according to their diabetes status: group 1, nondiabetic; group 2, prediabetic; and group 3, diabetes.

TIMI frame counts for each of three coronary arteries were found to be significantly different. TIMI frame counts for left anterior descending artery and TIMI frame counts for left circumflex and right coronary arteries, respectively, in the three groups, are as follows: group 1: 20.2 ± 6.8, 18.8 ± 5.4, and 19.9 ± 8.7; group 2: 22.2 ± 8.0, 20.8 ± 7.9, and 22.2 ± 8.8; group 3: 22.3 ± 9.2, 21.6 ± 10.2, and 22.3 ± 10.6, for each coronary artery.

When the groups were compared with one another using post hoc tests, group 2 and group 3 had similar TIMI frame counts for all three coronary arteries, but both of these groups had significantly higher TIMI frame counts than group 1.

The investigators were able to show for the first time that coronary blood flow measured by TIMI frame count is slower, that is to say, more sluggish, in prediabetic patients than in nondiabetic patients, and it is similar to coronary flow in diabetic patients. This result led the investigators to conclude that endothelial dysfunction develops in the prediabetic phase, before overt diabetes is manifest (Arslan, Balc, and Kocaoglu. 2012).

4.3.2   Elevated WBC Count in Type 2 Diabetes—Chronic Inflammation

The *International Journal of Environmental Research and Public Health* reported a large-scale study of the relationship between WBC count and glucose metabolism in a Chinese population. The participants were classified into groups including those with normal glucose tolerance, those with isolated impaired fasting glucose, and those with impaired glucose tolerance and Type 2 diabetes.

It was found that WBC count rose as glucose metabolism disorders worsened. WBC count was positively correlated with waist–hip ratio, BMI, smoking, triglycerides, glycosylated hemoglobin A1c (HbA1c), and 2-h postprandial glucose.

The investigators concluded that elevated WBC count is independently associated with worsening glucose metabolism in the middle-aged and elderly (Jiang, Yan, Li et al. 2014). An elevated WBC count signals that there is a tendency to inflammation in one or more tissues. So what this study reveals is that disordered glucose metabolism is linked to systemic inflammation that varies with the severity of the metabolic disorder.

4.3.3   Hyperglycemia Can Cause Red Cell Membrane Lipid Peroxidation and Fragility

The aim of this study published in the *Journal of Biological Chemistry* was to determine the effect of elevated glucose levels on membrane lipid peroxidation and osmotic fragility in human RBC. Defibrinated whole blood, or RBCs, were incubated with varying concentrations of glucose at 37°C for 24 h.

RBCs incubated with elevated levels of glucose showed a significantly increased membrane lipid peroxidation, when compared to control RBCs. A significant positive correlation was observed between the extent of glucose-induced membrane lipid peroxidation and the osmotic fragility of treated RBCs.

Glucose-induced membrane lipid peroxidation and osmotic fragility were blocked when RBCs were pretreated with fluoride, an inhibitor of glucose metabolism; with vitamin E, an antioxidant; with para-chloromercurobenzoate and metyrapone, inhibitors of the cytochrome P-450 system; or with dimethylfurane, diphenylamine, and thiourea, scavengers of oxygen radicals.

RBCs exposed to elevated glucose concentrations also showed an increase in NADPH levels. Exogenous addition of NADPH to normal RBC lysate induced membrane lipid peroxidation similar to that observed in the glucose-treated RBCs. These data suggest that elevated glucose levels can cause the adverse peroxidation of membrane lipids in human RBCs (Jain. 1989).

4.3.4   Increased Red Cell Aggregation in Diabetes Raises Cardiovascular Risk Factors

Red cell aggregation has been shown to be higher in diabetic patients, and it may predispose to cardiovascular disease. In a study published in the journal *Diabetic Medicine*, red cell aggregation was measured by a simple photometric method in diabetic patients, and matched control participants, to determine its relationship to cardiovascular risk factors.

Red cell aggregation was significantly increased in both Type 1 (4.3 ± 1.3 vs. 3.4 ± 1.2) and Type 2 diabetic patients (5.5 ± 1.5 vs. 3.2 ± 1.3). In all diabetic patients, aggregation varied directly with the levels of triglycerides and very-low-density lipoprotein (VLDL) and inversely with levels of HDL; in Type 2 diabetic patients, aggregation varied directly with BMI and hypertension and with the duration of diabetes. Triglycerides and BMI showed an independent association with red cell aggregation, and in Type 2 diabetic patients, smoking was also associated with increased red cell aggregation.

It was concluded that increased red cell aggregation may be one mechanism by which some cardiovascular risk factors could promote cardiovascular disease in diabetes (MacRury, Lennie, McColl et al. 1993).

The *New England Journal of Medicine* published a clinical study that concluded that patients with Type 2 diabetes, who have not had a myocardial infarction, have a risk of infarction similar to that in nondiabetic patients who have had a prior myocardial infarction.

This observation, combined with the results of previous studies showing the efficacy of lipid-lowering therapy in diabetic patients with coronary heart disease (Pyorala, Pedersen, Kjekshus et al. 1997; Sacks, Pfeffer, Moye et al. 1996) and the high mortality (including prehospital mortality) after myocardial infarction (Abbott, Donahue, Kannel et al. 1988; Herliz, Karlson, Edvardsson et al. 1992), suggests that all persons with diabetes could be treated as if they had prior coronary heart disease (Haffner, Lehto, Rönnemaa et al. 1998).

4.3.4.1   Glycemic Control Reduces Red Cell Aggregation

A study published in the journal *Diabetic Medicine* was designed to test the hypothesis that intensified management of Type 2 diabetes with diet, exercise, and insulin would reduce RBC aggregation. Blood samples were obtained from participants before and after 14 ± 3 weeks of intensified management. RBC aggregation was measured *in vitro* for cells in plasma, or in an aggregating 70-kD dextran solution. Plasma viscosity and whole blood viscosity were also measured.

It was found that during treatment, fasting glucose declined by 27%, HbA1c declined by 21%, and serum triglycerides and total cholesterol declined by 28% and 12%, respectively.

The extent and strength of RBC aggregation in plasma declined by 10% and 13%, respectively. Similar decreases in RBC aggregation were seen for cells suspended in dextran. Plasma viscosity decreased by 3% and high shear blood viscosity decreased by 6% to 7%.

Changes in RBC aggregation in plasma and in dextran were significantly correlated, supporting a cellular rather than a plasma origin for these changes. However, there were no significant correlations between RBC aggregation changes and changes of fasting glucose, HbA1c, serum triglycerides, serum cholesterol, or plasma fibrinogen.

The investigators concluded that intensified metabolic control results in a reduction of RBC aggregation that appears to be intrinsic to RBCs (Chong-Martinez, Buchanan, Wenby et al. 2003).

4.3.5   Hyperglycemia Alters Fibrin Clotting Properties

Fibrin is a protein involved in the clotting of blood. It is formed by the action of thrombin on fibrinogen, which causes it to polymerize. The polymerized fibrin together with platelets forms a clot over a wound site.

When the lining of a blood vessel is ruptured, platelets are attracted, forming a platelet plug. These platelets have thrombin receptors on their surfaces that bind serum thrombin molecules, which, in turn, convert soluble fibrinogen in the serum into fibrin at the wound site. Fibrin forms long strands of tough insoluble protein that are bound to the platelets. The cross-linking of fibrin hardens and contracts, forming a mesh over the platelet plug that completes the clot.

Excessive generation of fibrin due to activation of the coagulation cascade leads to thrombosis, the blockage of a vessel by an agglutination of RBCs, platelets, polymerized fibrin, and other components.

The journal *Diabetologia* published a study titled "The influence of type 2 diabetes on fibrin structure and function." The aim of the study was to determine the role of fibrin clot structure, in Type 2 diabetic patients, in order to assess the potential mechanism whereby diabetes influences CVD risk.

In this study, fibrin clots were formed from fibrinogen purified from participants with Type 2 diabetes and varying degrees of glycemic control (assessed by HbA1c) and from matched control participants. Clot structure was assessed by turbidity, permeation, and confocal microscopy. The specific effect of glucose itself was assessed by analyzing the structure of clots formed from purified fibrinogen in the presence of increasing concentrations of the sugar.

It was found that clots formed by fibrinogen purified from Type 2 diabetic participants had a denser, less porous, structure than those from control participants. The structural changes that were found were related to the individual's glycemic control.

HbA1c correlated inversely with permeation coefficient (K) values (indicates clot pore size) and positively with maximum absorbance (indicator of fiber size), branch point number, and fiber density. The ambient glucose level influenced clot structure: hypoglycemia (less than 5 mmol/L) and hyperglycemia (greater than or equal to 10 mmol/L) were both associated with a reduction in K values and maximum absorbance, and with increased fiber density and branch point number within clots.

The investigators concluded that the structural differences found in Type 2 diabetes, and in association with hypo- and hyperglycemia, may confer increased resistance to fibrinolysis, and in consequence contribute to the increase in CVD risk in diabetic patients (Dunn, Ariëns, and Grant. 2005). The term *fibrinolysis* refers to the enzymatic breakup of clots, which is an important mechanism to keep clots in check. So when high or low levels of glucose cause increased *resistance* to fibrinolysis, that means the patient is more likely to have clots, and that the clots are more likely to increase in size, increasing the risk of arterial blockage (e.g., myocardial infarction and/or strokes).

A study published in the journal *Thrombosis and Haemostasis* showed that glycemic control could reduce the risk of clots: Persons with diabetes have demonstrably altered fibrin network structures thought to result from high blood glucose. Therefore, the aim of this study was to determine whether glycemic control could modify the altered fibrin network structures due to decreased fibrinogen glycation.

Patients with uncontrolled Type 2 diabetes were treated with insulin to achieve glycemic control. Age- and BMI-matched nondiabetic participants were included as a reference group. Purified fibrinogen, isolated from plasma samples, was used for analysis.

There was a significant decrease in fibrinogen glycation (6.81 to 5.02 mol glucose/mol fibrinogen) with a corresponding decrease in rate of lateral aggregation (5.86 to 4.62), increased permeability (2.45 to 2.85 × 10⁻⁸ cm²), and lysis rate (3.08 to 3.27 µm/min) in the diabetic patients following glycemic control. These variables correlated positively with markers of glycemic control.

On the other hand, fibrin clots of nondiabetic participants had a significantly higher ratio of inelastic to elastic deformation than those of the diabetic patients.

Although there was no difference in median fiber diameter between diabetic patients and nondiabetic participants, there was a small increase in the proportion of thicker fibers in the diabetic samples after glycemic control.

Results from SDS-PAGE (a common method for separating proteins by electrophoresis) indicated no detectable difference in factor XIIIa cross-linking of fibrin clots between uncontrolled and controlled diabetic samples. Diabetic patients may have altered fibrin network formation kinetics, which contributes to decreased pore size and lysis rate of fibrin clots. Achievement of glycemic control, and decreased fibrinogen glycation level, improves permeability and lysis rates in a purified fibrinogen model (Pieters, Covic, van der Westhuizen et al. 2008).

4.3.6 TYPE 2 DIABETES MAY FEATURE LOW HEMOGLOBIN CONCENTRATION AND ANEMIA

Reduced hemoglobin concentrations—even anemia—are common findings in diabetic patients (Thomas, MacIsaac, Tsalamandris et al. 2003) and low hemoglobin levels have been linked to cardiovascular disease in these patients (McFarlane, Salifu, Makaryus et al. 2006; Vlagopoulos, Tighiouart, Weiner et al. 2005).

It has been reported that hemoglobin levels were lower in diabetic patients than in nondiabetic individuals (Ishimura, Nishizawa, Okuno et al. 1998) and that red cell survival decreased by about 13% in hyperglycemic states (Redondo-Bermejo, Pascual-Figal, Hurtado-Martínez et al. 2007). It has also been reported in an article published in the *Journal of the Association of Physicians of India* that patients with diabetes durations of more than 5 years have about a 1.5-fold higher risk of developing anemia than those with diabetes durations of less than 5 years (Ranil, Raman, Rachepalli et al. 2010). In fact, a number of studies have suggested that it is this resulting anemia that may exacerbate the severity of microangiopathy in diabetic patients and impair treatment outcomes. Lower hemoglobin concentrations not only might be a consequence of diabetes (Deray, Heurtier, Grimaldi et al. 2004) but also may accelerate microvascular damage.

The *Korean Journal of Internal Medicine* published a study that aimed to determine whether there is an association between hemoglobin concentrations and various clinical parameters, including metabolic factors, plasma C-peptide response after a meal tolerance test, and microvascular complications with Type 2 diabetes.

Male patients with Type 2 diabetes were recruited, given a meal tolerance test, and underwent assessment of hemoglobin levels, fasting and postprandial β-cell responsiveness, and microvascular complications.

Patients with lower hemoglobin concentrations were shown to have a longer duration of diabetes, a lower BMI, and lower concentrations of total cholesterol, triglycerides, and LDL cholesterol. They also had lower levels of postprandial C-peptide, Δ C-peptide, and postprandial β-cell responsiveness. They also had a higher prevalence of retinopathy and nephropathy. It was found that there was a significant association between nephropathy and hemoglobin concentration. Also, hemoglobin concentrations were independently associated with Δ C-peptide levels, and postprandial β-cell responsiveness (Kwon, and Ahn. 2012).

C-peptide is generally found in amounts equal to insulin in the blood because insulin and C-peptide are linked when first made by the pancreas. Therefore, it can show how much insulin is being made by the pancreas. C-peptide does not affect the blood sugar level in the body. A C-peptide test measures the level of this peptide in the blood.

4.3.6.1 Hypothesis: Hypoxemia Promotes β-Cell Failure in Type 2 Diabetes Mellitus

Reduced oxygen delivery and therefore hypoxia of pancreatic islets have been proposed to be possible etiologic factors in β-cell failure in Type 2 diabetes (Tal. 2009; Dynyak, Dynyak, and Popova. 2010). Pancreatic islets comprise only approximately 2% of the pancreas mass, but they consume about 20% of the oxygen in the arterial blood supply; consequently, they may be highly susceptible to hypoxia.

Erythrocytes of diabetic individuals were also reported to show impaired deformability and increased hemoglobin-oxygen affinity, which impairs oxygen delivery to tissues (McMillan, Utterback, and La Puma. 1978; Ditzel. 1979). Thus, a subtle reduction in oxygen delivery to the islets may impair β-cell function under conditions of pancreatic microvascular changes due to chronic hyperglycemia.

4.3.7 Hemoglobin Glycation and Oxihemoglobin Dissociation

The oxygen saturation of hemoglobin is largely pH dependent; likewise, the dissociation of oxygen from hemoglobin in body tissue (it is also body core temperature related). Ordinarily, the body tolerates some degree of pH deviation from normal (pH = 7.4) in alkalosis, but not so in acidosis. One deviation from normal pH is diabetic ketoacidosis.

Acidosis alters oxihemoglobin saturation/dissociation: At lower pH, hemoglobin binds less oxygen (Bohr effect), but there are also other conditions that affect how hemoglobin transports and delivers oxygen. One of these is glycation.

Hemoglobin glycation (attachment of glucose) of RBCs is an irreversible stable product, formed at rates that increase with increasing plasma glucose and fructose concentrations in blood. Glycated hemoglobin is less saturated with oxygen, and in extreme cases, there is no oxygen at all. Therefore, the tissue and organs of people with high levels of glycated hemoglobin may be oxygen deficient (hypoxic).

In a study titled "Oxygen transport impairment in diabetes," published in the journal *Diabetes*, oxyhemoglobin dissociation curves (ODCs) from zero to full saturation were developed from tests performed on whole blood from various groups of diabetic and nondiabetic healthy participants.

The underlying hypothesis was developed in an earlier study that suggested that elevated levels of 2,3-diphosphoglycerate (2,3-DPG), found to be a feature in diabetic patients, led to tissue hypoxia because 2,3-DPG competes with oxygen for binding with hemoglobin (Ditzel, and Standl. 1975).

2,3-DPG is an intermediate product of glycolysis in RBCs, and it is rapidly consumed under conditions of normal oxygen tension. However, in hypoxia in peripheral tissues, the concentration of 2,3-DPG can accumulate to significant levels within hours. At these higher concentrations, 2,3-DPG can bind to hemoglobin and reduce its affinity for oxygen, resulting in a right shift of the ODC.

The P50 at *in vivo* pH was slightly but significantly lower than normal in ambulatory non-acidotic, uncomplicated juvenile diabetics (26.0 vs. 27.3 mmHg) despite increased red cell 2,3-DPG concentrations in diabetic erythrocytes (15.0 vs. 13.7 μmol/g Hb). This combination of changes is in keeping with the presence of increased proportions of HbA1c in insulin-treated diabetics. The "P50" is the oxygen tension (pressure) at which hemoglobin is 50% saturated. The normal P50 is 26.7 mmHg.

The position of the oxygen dissociation curve was positively correlated with the 2,3-DPG concentration, which varied in response to fluctuations in plasma concentration of inorganic phosphate (Pi).

2,3-DPG acts as a heteroallosteric effector (affecting the binding affinity) of hemoglobin, lowering the affinity of hemoglobin for oxygen by binding preferentially to deoxyhemoglobin. An increased concentration of 2,3-DPG in RBCs favors formation of the low-affinity state of hemoglobin, and so the oxygen-binding curve will shift to the right. Optimal metabolic control may lead to a normalization of the oxygen dissociation curve in association with increased concentrations of red cell 2,3-DPG.

When the diabetes was uncontrolled, the oxygen dissociation curve was usually unchanged during the acidotic phase because the lowered pH balanced the effect of diminished 2,3-DPG concentration on the oxygen dissociation curve. After correction of acidosis, the disproportion between erythrocyte 2,3-DPG and pH became quite prominent, accompanied by a corresponding fall in P50 (21.0 vs. 26.1 mmHg).

Following ketoacidosis, with a persistently lowered Pi, it may take up to 1 week for 2,3-DPG to return to an approximately normal level, and the P50 will be impaired for the same period. A diphosphonate (EHDP) known to enhance tubular phosphate reabsorption in man was given to non-acidotic insulin-treated diabetic and healthy volunteers for 28 days. It caused a statistically significant and beneficial increase in mean Pi and in oxygen saturation (P50) in both healthy and diabetic patients.

When a dietary supplement of dibasic calcium phosphate was given to diabetic patients for 28 days, a significant increase in P50 also occurred (25.2 vs. 27.2 mmHg).

The investigators recommended that the diabetes diet be supplemented by dibasic calcium phosphate to prevent the inhibitory effect of a low concentration of Pi on red cell oxygen delivery (Ditzel. 1976).

Parenthetically, elevated levels of hemoglobin 2,3-DPG have been reported in a number of other pathophysiological conditions involving hypoxia, including respiratory alkalosis in hyperventilation syndrome (Fried. 1993).

4.3.7.1 Elevated HbA1c Can Lead to False Pulse-Oximetry Readings

Nonenzymatic glycation alters the structure and function of hemoglobin in the direction of increasing hemoglobin–oxygen affinity, which results in lower oxygen delivery to the tissues.

The aim of a study published in the journal *Cardiovascular Diabetology* was to determine whether elevated blood concentration of glycosylated hemoglobin (HbA1c) could induce falsely high pulse-oximeter oxygen saturation (SpO_2) in Type 2 diabetic patients. Arterial oxygen saturation (SaO_2) and partial pressure of oxygen (PO_2) were determined with simultaneous monitoring of SpO_2 in Type 2 diabetic patients during ventilation or oxygen inhalation.

It was found that blood concentration of glycosylated hemoglobin was greater than 7% in 114 patients, and less than or equal to 7% in 147 patients. Both SaO_2 (96.2% ± 2.9% vs. 95.1% ± 2.8%) and $SpO2$ (98.0% ± 2.6% vs. 95.3% ± 2.8%) were significantly higher in patients with HbA1c greater than 7% than in those with less than or equal to 7%. However, PO_2 did not differ significantly between the two groups. Bland–Altman analysis demonstrated a significant bias between SpO_2 and SaO_2 and limits of agreement in patients with HbA1c greater than 7%. The differences between SpO_2 and SaO_2 correlated closely with blood HbA1c levels.

The investigators concluded that elevated blood HbA1c levels lead to an overestimation of SaO_2 by SpO_2, suggesting that arterial blood gas analysis may be needed for Type 2 diabetic patients with poor glycemic control during the treatment of hypoxemia (Pu, Shen, Lu et al. 2012).

4.3.8 THE EFFECT OF HYPERGLYCEMIA ON BLOOD PLATELETS

Blood platelets (thrombocytes) are the "corks" of the blood vessels. Their function is to plug leaks in injured vessels and so stem blood loss. According to a report in the journal *Current Pharmaceutical Design*, in Type 2 diabetes, hypersensitivity of platelets to agonists are a prominent feature, including altered adhesion and aggregation. Disturbed carbohydrate and lipid metabolism lead to changes in cell membrane dynamics and consequently result in the problem of increased exposure of surface membrane receptors (Watala. 2005).

According to a report in the journal *Diabetes Care*, intact healthy vascular endothelium is central to the normal functioning of smooth muscle contractility, as well as its normal interaction with platelets. What is not clear is the role of hyperglycemia in the functional and organic microvascular deficiencies and platelet hyperactivity in individuals with diabetes.

The entire coagulation cascade is dysfunctional in diabetes: Increased levels of fibrinogen and plasminogen activator inhibitor 1 favor both thrombosis and defective dissolution of clots once formed. Platelets in Type 2 diabetic individuals adhere to vascular endothelium, and they aggregate more readily than those in healthy people. Loss of sensitivity to the normal restraints exercised by prostacyclin [PGI(2)] and NO, generated by the vascular endothelium, presents as the major defect in platelet function.

Insulin is a natural antagonist of platelet hyperactivity. It sensitizes the platelet to PGI(2) and enhances endothelial generation of PGI(2), and NO. Thus, the defects in insulin action in diabetes create a milieu of disordered platelet activity conducive to macrovascular and microvascular events (Vinik, Erbas, Park et al. 2001).

People with diabetes, particularly those with Type 2 diabetes, show increased platelet reactivity. Hyperglycemia contributes to greater platelet reactivity by promoting glycation of platelet proteins. Hypertriglyceridemia is another factor that increases platelet reactivity. Both insulin resistance and insulin deficiency increase platelet reactivity: Insulin antagonizes activation of platelets.

The aim of a study, published in the *Journal of Laboratory Physicians*, was to determine the mean platelet volume in diabetic and nondiabetic patients, to determine whether there is a difference in mean platelet volume between diabetic patients with and without vascular complications, and to determine the correlation of mean platelet volume with fasting blood glucose, glycosylated hemoglobin (HbA1c), BMI, and duration of diabetes in the diabetic patients.

Following conventional laboratory procedures, the mean platelet counts and mean platelet volume were found to be higher in diabetic patients than those in the nondiabetic patients (277.46 ± 81 × 10^9/L vs. 269.79 ± 78 × 10^9/L; 8.29 ± 0.74 fl vs. 7.47 ± 0.73 fl, respectively). Mean platelet volume showed a strong positive correlation with fasting blood glucose, postprandial glucose, and HbA1C levels.

The investigators concluded that the significantly higher mean platelet volume in diabetic patients, than in the nondiabetic patients, indicates that elevated mean platelet volume could be a cause of vascular complications (Kodiatte, Manikyam, Rao et al. 2012).

Diabetes is associated with oxidative stress and inflammation. Consequent endothelial dysfunction promotes activation of platelets by decreasing production of NO that would otherwise attenuate platelet reactivity. Oxidative stress accentuates this effect by attenuating activity of NO and thereby promoting platelet activation.

Inflammation and platelet activation are reciprocally related: Inflammation promotes platelet activation that, in turn, promotes inflammation. Accordingly, improved metabolic control achieved with regimens that improve insulin sensitivity and preserve pancreatic β-cell function is likely to decrease platelet reactivity and enhance effects of antiplatelet agents (Schneider. 2009).

Hyperglycemia can increase platelet reactivity by inducing nonenzymatic glycation of proteins on the surface of the platelet. Such glycation decreases membrane fluidity and increases the propensity of platelets to activate (Winocour, Watala, and Kinglough-Rathbone. 1992). The osmotic effect of glucose is a second mechanism whereby hyperglycemia can increase platelet reactivity (Keating, Sobel, and Schneider. 2003). It was also found that brief exposure of platelets *in vitro* to hyperglycemia or a similar concentration of mannitol increased their reactivity (Schneider. 2009).

Activation of protein kinase C is a third mechanism whereby hyperglycemia can increase platelet reactivity (Assert, Scherk, Bumbure et al. 2001). Protein kinase C is an essential mediator of platelet activation. People with diabetes exhibit increased expression of the surface glycoproteins Ib and IIb/IIIa (Tschoepe, Roesen, Kaufmann et al. 1990). These glycoproteins mediate platelet adhesion and adherence.

Although hyperglycemia is the *sine qua non* of diabetes, abnormalities of lipid metabolism are uniformly observed as well. People with diabetes typically manifest hypertriglyceridemia. VLDL that is rich in triglycerides increases platelet reactivity (Pedreño, Hurt-Camejo, Wiklund et al. 2000). This effect appears to be mediated, in part, by apolipoprotein E. Thus, both hyperglycemia and hypertriglyceridemia increase platelet reactivity in persons with diabetes.

4.3.8.1 Insulin Resistance, Insulin Deficiency, and Platelet Function

It is now generally accepted that most people who develop Type 2 diabetes show insulin resistance and consequent hyperinsulinemia for one to two decades before manifesting diabetes. During this interval, hyperinsulinemia compensates for insulin resistance and fasting hyperglycemia is not evident. Obesity can induce and exacerbate insulin resistance.

Apoptosis of pancreatic β-cells leads to a relative, and ultimately absolute, deficiency of insulin. Progressive insulin deficiency is seen after Type 2 diabetes becomes manifest. Both insulin resistance and insulin deficiency can alter platelet reactivity (Schneider. 2009).

Insulin antagonizes the effect of platelet agonists such as collagen, ADP, epinephrine, and platelet-activating factor (Westerbacka, Yki-Järvinen, Turpeinen et al. 2002). This antagonism is mediated by activation of an inhibitory G protein by insulin receptor substrate (IRS)-1 (Ferreira, Eybrechts, Mocking et al. 2004).

Insulin resistance reflects impaired insulin signaling predominantly mediated by IRS-1. Thus, resistance by the platelet to the effects of insulin (relative insulin deficiency) or absolute deficiency of insulin attenuates insulin-mediated antagonism of platelet activation and thereby increases platelet reactivity.

Obese persons who are insulin resistant exhibit increased activation of platelets. Platelet activation identified by the measurement of a thromboxane metabolite in urine, and the concentration of CD40 ligand in blood, was higher in obese compared to lean women. Decreased insulin resistance achieved by weight loss, or treatment with pioglitazone (without weight loss), reduced the concentrations of these markers (Basili, Pacini, Guagnano et al. 2006).

A study published in the journal *Thrombosis Research* quantified the concentration of platelet-derived microparticles in blood, which are released during the activation of platelets. They were increased in obese persons. Similar to results in the previous study, the concentration of micropartices was decreased after weight reduction (Murakami, Horigome, Tanaka et al. 2007). Thus, insulin resistance appears to increase the activation of platelets, consistent with increased platelet reactivity.

Persons with Type 2 diabetes exhibit progressive deficiency of insulin due to pancreatic β-cell apoptosis. A consequence of pancreatic β-cell apoptosis is absolute deficiency of insulin. Accordingly, the relative deficiency of insulin imparted by insulin resistance is magnified by the superimposition of insulin deficiency. Platelet reactivity that is increased in obese persons manifesting insulin resistance will be greater when Type 2 diabetes is also manifest and accompanied by absolute deficiency of insulin.

A recent study published in the journal *Cell Metabolism* suggested that resistance to the effects of insulin is apparent in pathways independent of IRS in addition to those dependent on IRS (Hoehn, Hohnen-Behrens, Cederberg et al. 2008). Consistent with this observation, platelets from participants with insulin resistance show diminished sensitivity to the actions of NO and prostacyclin (Betteridge, El Tahir, Reckless et al. 1982; Anfossi, Mularoni, Burzacca et al. 1988).

NO and prostacyclin are produced by the intact endothelium and retard platelet activation by increasing intraplatelet concentrations of the cyclic nucleotides cyclic guanosine monophosphate and cyclic adenosine monophosphate. Thus, resistance of the platelet to the effects of these agents promotes increased platelet reactivity. Accordingly, insulin resistance attenuates tonic antagonism of platelet activation and thereby increases platelet reactivity (Schneider. 2009).

4.3.8.2   Diabetes, Inflammation, and Platelet Function

A report in the *Journal of Clinical Investigation* concluded that diabetes is associated with systemic inflammation and oxidative stress that may contribute to increased platelet reactivity. Superoxide has been shown to increase platelet reactivity (Handin, Karabin, and Boxer. 1977).

Superoxide may increase platelet reactivity by enhancing intraplatelet release of calcium after activation (Schaeffer, Wascher, Kostner et al. 1999). In addition, it limits the biologic activity of NO (Freedman. 2008). Reducing the effect of NO would likely increase platelet reactivity.

Impaired endothelial function also decreases the production of prostacyclin (Schäfer, and Bauersachs. 2008). Accordingly, oxidative stress that accompanies diabetes promotes greater platelet reactivity through direct effects on platelets and by inducing endothelial dysfunction. Endothelial dysfunction increases platelet reactivity because of decreased production of NO, along with decreased production of prostacyclin.

An additional mechanism by which inflammation can increase platelet reactivity is by increasing expression of proteins that participate in the activation of platelets. For example, people with diabetes exhibit increased expression of Fcγ receptor type IIa (FcγRIIa) and associated increased platelet activation in response to collagen (Calverley, Hacker, Loda et al. 2003). According to a report in the journal *Arthritis and Rheumatism*, inflammation appears to increase expression of FcγRIIa and reduced inflammation decreases expression of FcγRIIa (Belostocki, Pricop, Redecha et al. 2008).

Human platelets express FcγRIIa, the low-affinity receptor for the constant fragment (Fc) of immunoglobulin G that is also found on neutrophils, monocytes, and macrophages. Engagement of this receptor on platelets by immune complexes triggers intracellular signaling events that lead to platelet activation and aggregation. Importantly, these events occur *in vivo*, particularly in response to pathological immune complexes, and engagement of this receptor on platelets has been causally linked to pathology (Qiao, Al-Tamimi, Baker et al. 2015).

Thus, the inflammation that accompanies diabetes contributes to increased platelet reactivity that, in turn, contributes to greater inflammation (Schneider. 2009).

4.4   HYPERGLYCEMIA IMPEDES RED CELL FORM AND FUNCTION

A report in the *Journal of Diabetes Science and Technology* concluded that in Type 2 diabetes, the erythrocyte deformability is reduced, while at the same time, its aggregation increases, both of which make whole blood more viscous, compared to that of healthy individuals. The increased blood viscosity adversely affects the microcirculation, leading to microangiopathy (Cho, Michael, Mooney et al. 2008).

An analysis of this phenomenon was detailed in a study published in the journal *Cardiovascular Diabetology*. The authors reported that RBCs are ordinarily highly deformable and possess a robust membrane that can withstand shear force. However, previous research showed that in diabetic patients, there is a changed RBC ultrastructure, where these cells are elongated and twist around spontaneously formed fibrin fibers. These changes may affect their function.

The investigators examined the membrane roughness and ultrastructural changes in RBCs of Type 2 diabetes patients. Atomic force microscopy (AFM) was used to study membrane roughness, and it was compared to scanning electron microscopy (SEM) of RBCs of healthy individuals. The combined AFM and SEM analyses of RBCs gave valuable information about the disease status of patients with diabetes.

Figure 4.1 shows an RBC from a healthy individual and Figure 4.2a and b show RBCs from a diabetic patient. These results are comparable to previously published results (Lipinski, and Pretorius. 2012).

In the healthy group, RBCs show the typical concave shape. However, in diabetes, the RBCs are elongated and their membranes form extended projections and twist spontaneously around fibrin fibers as shown in Figure 4.2a and b.

Atomic force measurement indicated that erythrocytes from patients suffering from diabetes are smaller, with a reduced concave depth. Measurement of the surface roughness, of three orders of spatial domains, contributes to the topography of the erythrocyte membrane (as shown in the authors' Table 2. Go to: https://doi.org/10.1186/1475-2840-12-25). A decrease of roughness by about half was noted in the erythrocytes of diabetic patients.

In the current analysis, a difference in diameter, height, and concave depth between cells from the healthy and diabetic individuals was seen (Table 1, ibid). This correlates with the SEM visual analysis, where the RBCs from diabetic patients differ in shape and size from RBCs from healthy individuals, as shown in Figures 4.1 and 4.2a and b.

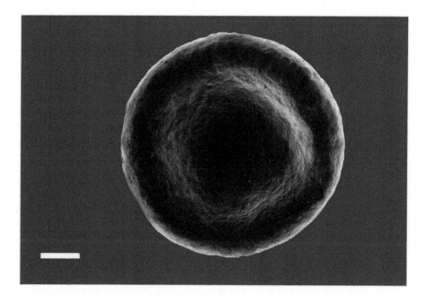

FIGURE 4.1   SEM micrograph of an RBC from a healthy individual showing the typical concave morphology. Scalebar = 1 μm. (From Buys, Van Rooy, Soma et al. 2013. *Cardiovascular Diabetology*, Jan; 12:25. With permission.)

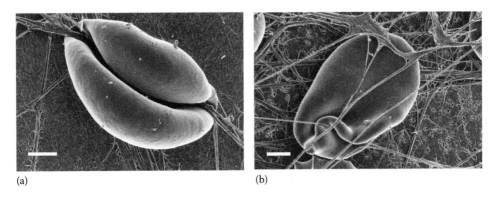

(a)   (b)

FIGURE 4.2   SEM micrograph of an RBC from a diabetic individual. (a) RBC with very smooth membrane twisted around spontaneously formed fibrin fibers. (b) RBC showing lengthened ultrastructure. Scalebar = 1 μm. (From Buys, Van Rooy, Soma et al. 2013. *Cardiovascular Diabetology*, Jan; 12:25. With permission.)

It has been shown that the topographical nanostructure of the erythrocyte membrane and the roughness of these structures can be classified as independent morphological parameters of the membrane, describing both the primary and the altered structure and functional status of the membrane (Kozlova, Chernysh, Moroz et al. 2013; Girasole, Dinarelli, and Boumis. 2012; Girasole, Pompeo, Cricenti et al. 2007; Girasole, Pompeo, Cricenti et al. 2010).

AFM is an ideal method to analyze the structure of the erythrocyte membrane, its main advantage being that qualitative images are accompanied by the corresponding quantitative height data, which allows for further measurements and analysis, for example, *Fourier Transform*. The selection of the size of the spectral domains is guided by the structural properties of the erythrocyte membrane (Moroz, Chernysh, Kozlova et al. 2010).

The first-order surface of the erythrocyte membrane represents the accepted undulate nature of the erythrocyte membrane relating to the macroparameters of the cell. The second-order surface correlates with the underlying spectrin–actin cytoskeletal complex, and the third-order surface represents the uppermost protein, protein cluster, and other membrane macromolecular topography.

Measurement of surface roughness indicated alterations in the first-order surface of the cell, relating to the cell's macro parameters, as is also seen in the macro parameter measurements; the roughness of the second-order surface is also decreased in diabetic patients, indicating alterations in the cytoskeletal matrix, and the connections between band 3 and 4 proteins and the matrix.

A decrease in roughness measurements in the third-order surface indicates superficial protein structure rearrangement. This corresponds with the SEM visual analysis where the diabetes RBCs visibly appear smoother than that of the healthy RBCs (Figures 4.1 and 4.2).

It has been found that the cytoskeletal proteins of RBCs from diabetic patients are heavily glycosylated and that spectrin is oxidatively damaged (Garnier, Attali, Valensi et al. 1990); also, several lipids (free cholesterol, sphingomeyelin, and phosphatidylcholine) on the outer surface of the phospholipid bilayer are significantly decreased (Garnier, Attali, Valensi et al. 1990; Labrouche, Freyburger, Gin et al. 1996). This directly correlates with the ultrastructural roughness results seen by the AFM of the second and third order, respectively.

The investigators concluded by suggesting that the combined AFM and SEM analyses of RBCs might give valuable information about the disease status of patients with diabetes. However, the ultrastructural changes seen in this study are not visible using a traditional light microscope. They believe that ultrastructural analysis of RBCs in inflammatory diseases can no longer be ignored and should form a fundamental research tool in clinical studies. Efficacy of treatment regimes on the integrity, cell shape, and roughness and health status of RBCs may be tracked, as this cell health status is crucial to the overall wellness of the diabetic patient (Buys, Van Rooy, Soma et al. 2013).

Red cell exposure to high glucose concentrations *in vitro* is often employed as a model for understanding erythrocyte modifications in diabetes. The journal *Redox Biology* reported a study that aimed to compare alterations in various red cell parameters, in this type of experiment, to differentiate between those affected by glycoxidation and those affected by energy imbalance.

Erythrocytes were incubated with 100 mM glucose for up to 72 hours.

It was found that high glucose concentrations intensified lipid peroxidation and loss of activity of the erythrocyte enzymes glutathione *S*-transferase and glutathione reductase.

However, hemolysis, eryptosis, calcium accumulation, loss of glutathione, and increase in the ratio of GSSG/GSH (oxidized to reduced glutathione) were attenuated by high glucose, apparently due to maintenance of energy supply to the cells. Loss of plasma membrane Ca^{2+}-ATPase activity and decrease in superoxide production were not affected by glucose concentration, being seemingly determined by processes independent of both glycoxidation and energy depletion.

These results point to the necessity of careful interpretation of data obtained in experiments, where erythrocytes are subject to treatment with high glucose concentrations *in vitro* (Viskupicova, Blaskovic, Galiniak et al. 2015).

4.4.1 As Hyperglycemia Impairs Red Cell Form and Function, It Impairs Longevity

According to a report in the journal *Clinical Biochemistry*, alterations of RBC plasma membrane appear both in diabetes and during the physiological aging process. It decreases RBC life span and, therefore, it may change the plasma membrane by acting through its effect on the aging process.

RBCs from normal people and from insulin-dependent diabetic patients were fractionated in five subpopulations of different mean age from fraction 1, early young RBC, to fraction 5, mature RBCs.

Thereafter, plasma membranes were prepared and enzymatic activity, membrane fluidity, and lipid peroxidation were evaluated.

It was found that Na^+, $K(+)$-ATPase activity decreased during aging, and it was higher in all RBC subpopulations from normal participants, in comparison to diabetic patients.

Next, it was also found that lipid peroxidation and fluidity increased during aging in both the study groups; in this case, however, in all subpopulations, except for that from fraction 1, RBCs from diabetic patients showed higher membrane fluidity and lipid peroxidation in comparison to those from healthy participants.

These findings suggest that diabetes affects the plasma membrane independently of lipid peroxidation and fluidity, or dependent on Na^+, $K(+)$-ATPase. In the case of lipid peroxidation and fluidity, diabetes seems to affect the membrane, thus decreasing RBC life span, whereas in the case of Na^+, $K(+)$-ATPase, it seems to alter this enzymatic activity, which, in turn, might affect RBC aging.

Acetylcholinesterase activity decreased during aging in RBCs from healthy participants, but it increased in RBCs from diabetic patients. RBC subpopulations from fraction 1, on the other hand, showed similar values in normal participants and diabetic patients. In this case, the effect of diabetes appears only during aging (Mazzanti, Faloia, Rabini et al. 1992).

4.4.1.1 Blood Cell Telomeres Mirror Incipient and Developing Diabetes

Life, as we understand it, results from the aggregate of body cell functions. Human health and disease—indeed life span—are intimately tied to ordinary cellular recycling as body cells age and are replaced. Cell recycling can be accelerated by consistent unopposed exposure to free radicals, and that acceleration can be observed in the rate at which DNA telomeres shorten with each cell cycle.

Type 2 diabetes has all the ingredients necessary for more rapidly abbreviating telomeres, thus shortening life span: chronic inflammation and the accompanying unopposed free radical load said to contribute to cardiovascular and heart disease are more than up to the task. This process is nowhere more evident than in our blood cells.

In a review and meta-analysis (PubMed, Web of Science, and EMBASE) reported in the journal *PLoS ONE*, the investigators aimed to assess the association of telomere length with incident Type 2 diabetes in prospective cohort studies.

Leukocyte relative telomere length (RTL) was measured using quantitative polymerase chain reaction in participants of the prospective population-based Bruneck Study, with repeat leukocyte RTL measurements performed in year 2005 and year 2010.

Hazard ratios for Type 2 diabetes were calculated across quartiles of baseline RTL adjusted for age, gender, BMI, smoking, socioeconomic status, physical activity, alcohol consumption, HDL cholesterol, log high-sensitivity C-reactive protein, and waist–hip ratio.

Over 15 years of follow-up, 44 out of 606 participants, free of diabetes at baseline, developed incident Type 2 diabetes. The adjusted hazard ratio for Type 2 diabetes comparing the bottom versus the top quartile of baseline RTL (i.e., shortest vs. longest) was 2.00 and 2.31, comparing the bottom quartile versus the remainder (1.21 to 4.41). The corresponding hazard ratios corrected for within-person RTL variability were 3.22 (1.27 to 8.14) and 2.86 (1.45 to 5.65).

In a random-effects meta-analysis of three prospective cohort studies involving 6991 participants and 2011 incident Type 2 diabetes events, the pooled relative risk was 1.31 (1.07 to 1.60).

The authors concluded that low leukocyte telomere relative length is independently associated with the risk of incident Type 2 diabetes (Willeit, Raschenberger, Heydon et al. 2014).

A study published in the journal *Experimental Biology and Medicine* (Maywood) compared leukocyte telomere length and fasting, or post-load glucose levels, in persons who do not receive glucose-lowering treatment. Randomly selected rural Ukrainian residents aged 45 or older, not previously diagnosed with Type 2 diabetes, were administered the WHO oral glucose tolerance test, and anthropometric measurements were collected.

Leukocyte telomere length was measured by the standardized method of quantitative monochrome multiplex polymerase chain reaction in real time.

The 2-h post-load plasma glucose levels demonstrated an inverse correlation with leukocyte telomere length, whereas no association between fasting plasma glucose and leukocyte telomere length was found. Waist circumference and systolic blood pressure were inversely related to leukocyte telomere length in men. Oral glucose tolerance test result-based glycemic categories did not show differences between mean leukocyte telomere length in categories of normal fasting plasma glucose and 2-h post-load plasma glucose, diabetes, and impaired fasting glucose/tolerance levels.

The association between leukocyte telomere length and fasting plasma glucose was confirmed in diabetes group only, and increased 2-h post-load plasma glucose—but not fasting plasma glucose—level improved the chances of finding short telomeres (OR, 1.52).

After the adjustment for age, gender, waist circumference, systolic blood pressure, and fasting plasma glucose, the investigators concluded that 2-h post-load plasma glucose, but not fasting plasma glucose, is inversely related to leukocyte telomere length (Khalangot, Krasnienkov, Vaiserman et al. 2017).

There is ample evidence that prematurely short telomeres reflect unopposed free radical damage to cell structures, but the role of free radicals in etiology of disease remains to be detailed. This is also clear in the following study published in the *International Journal of Cardiology*, titled "Telomere length, antioxidant status and incidence of ischaemic heart disease in type 2 diabetes."

In their *introduction*, the investigators state that Type 2 diabetes is associated with an increased risk of ischemic heart disease. An accelerated process of vascular aging induced by an increased oxidative stress exposure is suggested as the pathway accounting for this association. However, no studies have explored the relationship between markers of vascular aging, measures of oxidative stress, and risk of ischemic heart disease in Type 2 diabetes.

They therefore undertook to determine the association between plasma antioxidant status, marker of cellular aging, that is, leukocyte telomere length, and 10 years risk of ischemic heart disease in patients with Type 2 diabetes.

In patients with Type 2 diabetes, plasma total antioxidant status and leukocyte telomere length were measured by photometric microassay and RT-PCR (a technique commonly used in molecular biology to detect RNA expression), respectively. The incidence of ischemic heart disease over 10 years was determined through linkage with the national clinical audit of acute coronary syndrome in UK.

It was found that at baseline, total antioxidant status was associated with leukocyte telomere length. After 10 years, 61 patients developed ischemic heart disease. Lower total antioxidant status and shorter leukocyte telomere length at baseline predicted an increased ischemic heart disease risk at follow-up. These associations were independent of age, gender, cardiovascular risk factors, circulating levels of C-reactive protein, and medication differences.

The investigators concluded that reduced total antioxidant status and short leukocyte telomere length are interrelated pathways that predict risk of ischemic heart disease in patients with Type 2 diabetes. These findings suggest that antioxidant defenses are important to maintain telomere integrity, potentially reducing the progression of vascular aging in patients with Type 2 diabetes (Masi, D'Aiuto, Cooper et al. 2016).

In an article published in the journal *Geriatrics and Gerontology International*, the authors report that in patients with Type 2 diabetes, or impaired glucose tolerance, oxidative stress shortens telomeres. They suggest that telomere length is a good surrogate marker for mortality and diabetic complications in diabetes patients.

They found that telomere length in pancreatic β-cells is also shortened in Type 2 diabetes, potentially leading to impaired capacity for proliferation and insulin secretion, and accelerated cell death.

Taken together, the available data suggest that hyperglycemia, oxidative stress, and telomere attrition in pancreatic β-cells and adipocytes create a vicious cycle that underlies the pathophysiology of Type 2 diabetes. They conclude that prevention of telomere attrition in various organs, including pancreatic β-cells, could be a new approach for preventing the progression of diabetes and its complications (Tamura, Takubo, Aida et al. 2016).

Glycemic control *can* attenuate telomere shortening: A study published in the journal *Experimental Gerontology* aimed to assess the effect of glycemic control on telomeres in arterial blood vessel cells of patients undergoing coronary artery bypass and in mononuclear blood cells of other (Type 1 and Type 2) diabetic patients—comparing well-controlled to uncontrolled patients. All were compared to the age-dependent curve of healthy controls.

It was found that telomeres were significantly shorter in the arteries of diabetic patients as compared to nondiabetic patients and in mononuclear cells of both Type 1 and Type 2 diabetes patients. However, in all groups in the study, good glycemic control attenuated shortening of the telomeres.

In arterial cells, good glycemic control attenuated but did not abolish the telomere shortening. In Type 2 diabetes, the mononuclear telomere abbreviation was completely prevented by adequate glycemic control.

Telomere shortening in mononuclear cells of Type 1 diabetic patients was attenuated but not prevented by good glycemic control.

The investigators concluded that diabetes is associated with premature cellular senescence, but it can be prevented by good glycemic control in Type 2 diabetes and reduced in Type 1 (Uziel, Singer, Danicek et al. 2007).

It was reported earlier that low hemoglobin concentration and even anemia have been found to be a common feature of Type 2 diabetes. A clue to why this may be the case may be found in a study on telomere length in blood cells titled "Association between telomere length and complete blood count in US adults" published in the journal *Archives of Medical Science*.

The investigators aimed to determine the relationship between telomere length and complete blood count in a sample of healthy US adults. The participants in this study were drawn from the National Health and Nutrition Examination Survey (NHANES) recruited between 1999 and 2002 with essential data on total complete blood count and telomere length.

A significant inverse relationship was found between telomere length and monocyte count, mean cell hemoglobin, and red cell distribution.

The authors concluded that telomere attrition may be a marker of reduced proliferative reserve in hematopoietic progenitor cells (Mazidi, Penson, and Banach. 2017). Hematopoietic stem cells, or hemocytoblasts, are the stem cells that give rise to all the other blood cells through the process of hematopoiesis. They are located in the red bone marrow that is contained in the core of most bones.

"Reduced proliferative reserve in hematopoietic progenitor cells" is one theory, but in the case of diabetes, where the undercurrent is free radical damage to cells, another theory is destruction of red cells by ROS, a known occurrence: Free radicals have been found responsible for shortened red cell life span in a large series of hemolytic disorders including diabetes (Bracci. 1999).

Were that the case, one ready solution to the problem can be found in a report titled "Nutritional programming of coenzyme Q: potential for prevention and intervention?" published in *The Journal of the Federation of American Societies of Experimental Biology*. The aim of the study was to determine whether aortic and WBC CoQ10 could prevent programmed accelerated aging.

It was found that recuperated male rats had reduced aortic CoQ10, accelerated aortic telomere shortening, increased DNA damage, increased oxidative stress, and decreased mitochondrial complex II–III activity.

WBC CoQ10 levels correlated with aortic telomere length, suggesting its potential as a diagnostic marker of vascular aging (Tarry-Adkins, Fernandez-Twinn, Chen et al. 2014).

This study suggests that CoQ10 (ubiquinol) might be a valuable adjunct in integrative treatment of Type 2 diabetes.

4.5   CHRONIC HYPERGLYCEMIA AND MANAGEMENT OF RBC IRON

Iron is an important constituent in many body processes, but especially so in blood. How does diabetes affect iron metabolism and storage in the blood? This question was addressed in a study published in the journal *Biochimica Biophysica Acta*. It was reported that iron is a strong pro-oxidant, and high body iron levels are associated with increased level of oxidative stress that may elevate the risk of Type 2 diabetes.

Several epidemiological studies have reported a positive association between high body iron stores as measured by circulating ferritin level, and the risk of Type 2 diabetes, and of other insulin-resistant states such as the metabolic syndrome.

Increased dietary intake of iron, especially heme iron (from ingesting animal products), is associated with risk of Type 2 diabetes in apparently healthy populations.

Several clinical trials have suggested that phlebotomy-induced reduction in body iron levels may improve insulin sensitivity in humans; however, no interventional studies have yet directly evaluated the effect of reducing iron intake, or body iron levels, on the risk of developing Type 2 diabetes. Such studies are required to prove the causal relationship between moderate iron overload and diabetes risk (Rajpathak, Crandall, Wylie-Rosett et al. 2009).

It is difficult to reconcile such reports, and there are others, with reports of anemia in Type 2 diabetes.

Most of the iron stored in the body is bound to ferritin, a protein in the body. Ferritin is found in the liver, the spleen, skeletal muscles, and bone marrow. Only a small amount of ferritin is found in the blood, but the amount of ferritin in the blood indicates how much iron is stored in the body.

A study published in the *Journal of the Pakistan Medical Association* aimed to determine the levels of high-sensitivity C-reactive protein and ferritin in blood and to assess their association with inflammation in people with Type 2 diabetes.

Fasting blood samples from randomly selected patients and healthy control participants were analyzed for blood glucose, insulin, high-sensitivity C-reactive protein, and iron status. The study population was 38.6 ± 1.56 years old, on average, and their mean fasting blood sugar was 110.78 ± 3.795 mg/dL, on average. Group 1 consisted of healthy controls, while Group 2 was composed of diabetic patients.

Mean elevated serum ferritin levels (233.11 ± 43.84 ng/mL), insulin (29.94 ± 2.19), homeostasis model of insulin resistance (10.23 ± 0.89), and high-sensitivity C-reactive protein (5.29 ± 0.80 mg/L) with low serum iron levels (1.07 ± 0.115 μg/dL) were found in Group 2, the diabetic patients.

There was positive correlation between the homeostasis model of insulin resistance and fasting blood sugar, serum ferritin, insulin, and total iron-binding capacity. There was negative correlation with serum iron and transferrin saturation.

The investigators concluded that elevated ferritin levels, without evident iron overload, may affect glucose homeostasis, leading to insulin resistance in conjunction with inflammatory changes, as seen by elevated C-reactive protein levels (Alam, Fatima, Orakzai et al. 2014).

A review in the journal *Cell Metabolism* reports that Type 2 diabetes is marked by chronic inflammation (Hotamisligil. 2006). It is known that ferritin levels increase with inflammation. The question therefore arose whether high iron, the best biomarker being high ferritin, *causes* diabetes, or whether diabetes *causes* high ferritin.

In the study of metabolic syndrome quoted (Hotamisligil. 2006), independent markers of inflammatory stress such as C-reactive protein did not account for the association of ferritin with diabetes (Jehn, Clark, and Guallar. 2004).

Other studies have also concluded that the diabetes risk associated with high iron is not accounted for by inflammation, but rather it is related to dietary iron overload (Fleming, Jacques, Tucker et al. 2001).

Two recent studies of gestational diabetes have reported that the increased risk is associated in particular with dietary heme iron, which is more efficiently absorbed than nonheme iron (Bowers, Yeung, Williams et al. 2011; Qiu, Zhang, Gelaye et al. 2011). However, the best evidence for the causal role of iron comes from studies where reversal of diabetes occurs with iron reduction.

Increased iron stores are also associated with the development of typical Type 2 diabetes (Fernández-Real, López-Bermejo, and Ricart. 2002). For example, in approximately 9500 adults in the United States studied as part of the NHANES, the odds ratios for newly diagnosed diabetes in those with elevated serum ferritin levels are 4.94 for men and 3.61 for women (Ford, and Cogswell. 1999). This iron-associated risk approaches the relative risk of obesity (Kriska, Saremi, Hanson et al. 2003).

The NHANES population data also confirm that high ferritin approximately doubles the risk for metabolic syndrome after accounting for age, race, alcohol, smoking, and inflammatory state as assessed by C-reactive protein levels (Jehn, Clark, and Guallar. 2004). High ferritin is also positively correlated with central adiposity (Gillum. 2001; Iwasaki, Nakajima, Yoneda et al. 2005; Dongiovanni, Fracanzani, Fargion et al. 2011) and cardiovascular disease.

Epidemiologic studies established a clear association between tissue iron stores and diabetes risk. Some of these studies suggest that it is causal; that is, high iron is sufficient to cause diabetes. However, iron has a multiplicity of effects in many tissues that can be either pro- or antidiabetic at the ends of a spectrum that runs from iron deficiency to iron excess.

In the β-cell, for example, excess iron is toxic, but there is clearly also a minimum level required for full "metallation" of the proteins needed for glucose oxidation and glucose sensing. Likewise, although iron overload is associated with diabetes risk, iron deficiency is associated with another major risk factor for diabetes, obesity.

The phenotypes of iron excess and obesity are certainly not mutually exclusive, however, and it might be in fact that the combination of obesity and iron overload is particularly prone to causing diabetes through its resulting combination of insulin deficiency and insulin resistance (Simcox, and McClain. 2013).

REFERENCES

Abbott RD, Donahue RP, Kannel WB, and PW Wilson. 1988. The impact of diabetes on survival following myocardial infarction in men vs. women: the Framingham Study. *Journal of the American Medical Association*, Dec; 260(23): 3456–3460. PMID: 2974889.

Alam F, Fatima F, Orakzai S, Iqbal N, and SS Fatima. 2014. Elevated levels of ferritin and hs-CRP in type 2 diabetes. *The Journal of the Pakistan Medical Association*, Dec; 64(12): 13891391. PMID: 25842584.

Anfossi G, Mularoni EM, Burzacca S, Ponziani MC, Massucco P, Mattiello L, Cavalot F, and M Trovati. 1988. Platelet resistance to nitrates in obesity and obese NIDDM, and normal platelet sensitivity to both insulin and nitrates in lean NIDDM. *Diabetes Care*, Jan; 21(1): 121–126. PMID: 9538982.

Arslan U, Balc MM, and İ Kocaoglu. 2012. Coronary blood flow is slower in prediabetic and diabetic patients with normal coronary arteries compared with nondiabetic patients. *Experimental and Clinical Cardiology*, Winter; 17(4): 187–190. PMCID: PMC3627272.

Assert R, Scherk G, Bumbure A, Pirags V, Schatz H, and AF Pfeiffer. 2001. Regulation of protein kinase C by short term hyperglycaemia in human platelets in vivo and in vitro. *Diabetologia*, Feb; 44(2): 188–195. DOI: 10.1007/s001250051598.

Basili S, Pacini G, Guagnano MT, Manigrasso MR, Santilli F, Pettinella C, Ciabattoni G, Patrono C, and G Davì. 2006. Insulin resistance as a determinant of platelet activation in obese women. *Journal of the American College of Cardiology*, Dec; 48(12): 2531–2538. DOI: 10.1016/j.jacc.2006.08.040.

Belostocki K, Pricop L, Redecha PB, Aydin A, Leff L, Harrison MJ, and JE Salmon. 2008. Infliximab treatment shifts the balance between stimulatory and inhibitory Fcgamma receptor type II isoforms on neutrophils in patients with rheumatoid arthritis. *Arthritis and Rheumatism*, Feb; 58(2): 384–388. DOI: 10.1002/art.23200.

Betteridge D, El Tahir K, Reckless J, and K Williams. 1982. Platelets from diabetic subjects show diminished sensitivity to prostacyclin. *European Journal of Clinical Investigation*, Oct, 12(5): 395–398. PMID: 6816610.

Bowers K, Yeung E, Williams MA, Qi L, Tobias DK, Hu FB, and C Zhang. 2011. A prospective study of prepregnancy dietary iron intake and risk for gestational diabetes mellitus. *Diabetes Care*, Jul; 34(7): 1557–1563. DOI: 10.2337/dc11-0134.

Bracci R. 1999. Normal and abnormal effects of free radicals in blood cells. *Paediatric Research*, 45: 771–771. DOI: 10.1203/00006450-1999050100-00203.

Buys AV, Van Rooy M-J, Soma P, Van Papendorp D, Lipinski B, and E Pretorius. 2013. Changes in red blood cell membrane structure in type 2 diabetes: a scanning electron and atomic force microscopy study. *Cardiovascular Diabetology*, Jan; 12:25; https://doi.org/10.1186/1475-2840-12-25.

Calverley DC, Hacker MR, Loda KA, Brass E, Buchanan TA, Tsao-Wei DD, and S Groshen 2003. Increased platelet Fc receptor expression as a potential contributing cause of platelet hypersensitivity to collagen in diabetes mellitus. *British Journal of Haematology*, Apr; 121(1): 139–142. PMID: 12670344.

Cho YI, Mooney MP, and DJ Cho. 2008. Hemorheological disorders in diabetes mellitus. *Journal of Diabetes Science and Technology*, Nov; 2(6): 1130–1138. DOI: 10.1177/193229680800200622.

Chong-Martinez B, Buchanan TA, Wenby RB, and HJ Meiselman. 2003. Decreased red blood cell aggregation subsequent to improved glycaemic control in Type 2 diabetes mellitus. *Diabetic Medicine*, Apr; 20(4): 301–306. PMID: 12675644.

Cokelet GR, and HJ Meiselman. 2007. Macro- and microrheological properties of blood. In: *Handbook of Hemorheology and Hemodynamics*. Baskurt OK, Hardeman MR, Rampling MW, and HJ Meiselman (Eds.). Amsterdam, Berlin, Oxford, Tokyo, Washington, DC: IOS Press, pp. 45–71.

Dean L. 2005. *Blood Groups and Red Cell Antigens*. Bethesda, MD: National Center for Biotechnology Information (US); https://www.ncbi.nlm.nih.gov/books/NBK 2263/; accessed 8.30.17.

Deray G, Heurtier A, Grimaldi A, Launay Vacher V, and C Isnard Bagnis. 2004. Anemia and diabetes. *American Journal of Nephrology*, Sep–Oct; 24(5): 522–526. DOI: 10. 1159/000081058.

Ditzel J and E Standl. 1975. The problem of tissue oxygenation in diabetes mellitus. *Acta Medica Scandinavica Supplementum*, 578: 59–68. PMID: 239528.

Ditzel J. 1976. Oxygen transport impairment in diabetes. *Diabetes*, 25(2 Suppl): 832–838. PMID: 9322.

Ditzel J. 1979. Changes in red cell oxygen release capacity in diabetes mellitus. *Federation Proceedings*, Oct; 38(11): 2484–2488. PMID: 39792.

Dongiovanni P, Fracanzani AL, Fargion S, and L Valenti. 2011. Iron in fatty liver and in the metabolic syndrome: a promising therapeutic target. *Journal of Hepatology*, Oct; 55(4): 920–932. DOI: 10.1016/j.jhep.2011.05.008.

Dunn EJ, Ariëns RA, and PJ Grant. 2005. The influence of type 2 diabetes on fibrin structure and function. *Diabetologia*, Jun; 48(6): 1198–1206. DOI: 10.1007/s00125-005-1742-2.

Dynyak AK, Dynyak AA, and FV Popova. 2010. Diabetes mellitus: hypoxia of the islets of Langerhans resulting from the systematic rest prone on the back after a meal? *Medical Hypotheses*, Jun; 74(6): 1002–1005. DOI: 10.1016/j.mehy.2010.01.016.

Fernández-Real JM, López-Bermejo A, and W Ricart. 2002. Cross-talk between iron metabolism and diabetes. *Diabetes*, Aug; 51(8): 2348–2354. https://doi.org/10.2337/diabetes.51.8.2348.

Ferreira IA, Eybrechts KL, Mocking AI, Kroner C, and JW Akkerman. 2004. IRS-1 mediates inhibition of Ca^{2+} mobilization by insulin via the inhibitory G-protein Gi. *The Journal of Biological Chemistry*, Jan 30; 279(5): 3254–3264. DOI: 10.1074/jbc. M305474200.

Fleming DJ, Jacques PF, Tucker KL, Massaro JM, D'Agostino RB Sr, Wilson PW, and RJ Wood. 2001. Iron status of the free-living, elderly Framingham Heart Study cohort: an iron-replete population with a high prevalence of elevated iron stores. *American Journal of Clinical Nutrition*, Mar; 73(3): 638–646. PMID: 11237943.

Ford ES, and ME Cogswell. 1999. Diabetes and serum ferritin concentration among U.S. adults. *Diabetes Care*, Dec; 22(12): 1978–1983. PMID: 10587829.

Freedman JE. 2008. Oxidative stress and platelets. *Arteriscleriosis, Thrombosis and Vascular Biology*, Mar; 28(3): s11–s16. DOI: 10.1161/ATVBAHA.107.159178.

Fried. R. 1993. *The Psychology and Physiology of Breathing in Behavioral Medicine, Clinical Psychology, and Psychiatry*. New York: Plenum Press.

Gagnon DR, Zhang TJ, Brand FN, and WB Kannel. 1994. Hematocrit and the risk of cardiovascular disease—the Framingham study: a 34-year follow-up. *American Heart Journal*, Mar; 127(3): 674–682. PMID: 8122618.

Garnier M, Attali JR, Valensi P, Delatour-Hanss E, Gaudey F, and D Koutsouris. 1990. Erythrocyte deformability in diabetes and erythrocyte membrane lipid composition. *Metabolism*, Aug; 39(8): 794–798. PMID: 2377077.

Gawaz M, Langer H, and AE May. 2005. Platelets in inflammation and atherogenesis. *Journal of Clinical Investigation*, Dec; 115(12): 3378–3384. DOI: 10.1172/JCI27196.

Gillum RF. 2001. Association of serum ferritin and indices of body fat distribution and obesity in Mexican American men—the Third National Health and Nutrition Examination Survey. *International Journal of Obesity and Related Metabolic Disorders*, May; 25(5): 639–645. DOI: 10.1038/sj.ijo.0801561.

Girasole M, Dinarelli S, and G Boumis. 2012. Structure and function in native and pathological erythrocytes: a quantitative view from the nanoscale. *Micron (Oxford, England)*, Dec; 43(12): 1273–1286. DOI: 10.1016/j.micron.2012.03.019.

Girasole M, Pompeo G, Cricenti A, Congiu-Castellano A, Andreola F, Serafino A, Frazer BH, Boumis G, and G Amiconi. 2007. Roughness of the plasma membrane as an independent morphological parameter to study RBCs: a quantitative atomic force microscopy investigation. *Biochimica Biophysica Acta*, May; 1768(5): 1268–1276. DOI: 10.1016/j.bbamem.2007.01.014.

Girasole M, Pompeo G, Cricenti A, Longo G, Boumis G, Bellelli A, and S Amiconi. 2010. The how, when, and why of the aging signals appearing on the human erythrocyte membrane: an atomic force microscopy study of surface roughness. *Nanomedicine*, Dec; 6(6): 760–768. DOI: 10.1016/j.nano.2010.06.004.

Haffner SM, Lehto S, Rönnemaa T, Pyörälä K, and M Laakso. 1998. Mortality from coronary heart disease in subjects with Type 2 diabetes and in nondiabetic subjects with and without prior myocardial infarction. *New England Journal of Medicine*, Jul; 339: 229–234. DOI: 10.1056/NEJM199807233390404.

Handin R, Karabin R, and GJ Boxer. 1977. Enhancement of platelet function by superoxide anion. *Journal of Clinical Investigation*, May; 59(5): 959–965. DOI: 10. 1172/JCI108718.

Herliz J, Karlson BW, Edvardsson N, Emanuelsson H, and A Hjalmarson. 1992. Prognosis in diabetics with chest pain or other symptoms suggestive of acute myocardial infarction. *Cardiology*, 1992; 80(3–4): 237–245. PMID: 1511471.

Hoehn KL, Hohnen-Behrens C, Cederberg A, Wu LE, Turner N, Yuasa T, Ebina Y, and DE James. 2008. IRS1-independent defects define major nodes of insulin resistance. *Cell Metabolism*, May; 7(5): 421–433. DOI: 10.1016/j.cmet.2008.04.005.

Holsworth RE, and YI Cho. 2012. Hyperviscosity syndrome: a nutritionally-modifiable cardiovascular risk factor. In: *Advancing Medicine with Food and Nutrients*, Second Edition. I Kohlstadt (Ed.). Boca Raton: CRC Press.

Hotamisligil GS. 2006. Inflammation and metabolic disorders. *Nature*, Dec; 444(7121): 860–867. DOI: 10.1038/nature05485.

Irace C, Carallo C, Scavelli F, De Franceschi MS, Esposito T, and A Gnasso. 2014. Blood viscosity in subjects with normoglycemia and prediabetes. *Diabetes Care*, Feb; 37(2): 488–492. DOI: 10.2337/dc13-1374.

Ishimura E, Nishizawa Y, Okuno S, Matsumoto N, Emoto M, Inaba M, Kawagishi T, Kim CW, and H Morii. 1998. Diabetes mellitus increases the severity of anemia in non-dialyzed patients with renal failure. *Journal of Nephrology*, Mar–Apr; 11(2): 83–86. PMID: 9589379.

Iwasaki T, Nakajima A, Yoneda M, Yamada Y, Mukasa K, Fujita K, Fujisawa N, Wada K, and Y Terauchi. 2005. Serum ferritin is associated with visceral fat area and subcutaneous fat area. *Diabetes Care*, Oct; 28(10): 2486–2491. PMID: 16186284.

Jain SK. 1989. Hyperglycemia can cause membrane lipid peroxidation and osmotic fragility in human red blood cells. *Journal of Biological Chemistry*, Dec; 264(35): 21340–21345. PMID: 2592379.

Jehn M, Clark JM, and E Guallar. 2004. Serum ferritin and risk of the metabolic syndrome in U.S. adults. *Diabetes Care*, Oct; 27(10): 2422–2428. PMID: 15451911.

Jiang H, Yan W-H, Li C-J, Wang A-P, Dou J-T, and Y-M. Mu 2014. Elevated white blood cell count is associated with higher risk of glucose metabolism disorders in middle-aged and elderly Chinese people. *International Journal of Environmental Research and Public Health*, May; 11(5): 5497–5509. DOI: 10.3390/ijerph110505497.

Keating FK, Sobel BE, and DJ Schneider. 2003. Effects of increased concentrations of glucose on platelet reactivity in healthy subjects and in patients with and without diabetes mellitus. *American Journal of Cardiology*, Dec 1; 92(11): 1362–1365. PMID: 14636925.

Khalangot M, Krasnienkov D, Vaiserman A, Avilov I, Kovtun V, Okhrimenko N, Koliada A, and Kravchenko V. 2017. Leukocyte telomere length is inversely associated with post-load but not with fasting plasma glucose levels. *Experimental Biology and Medicine* (Maywood), Apr; 242(7): 700–708. DOI: 10.1177/1535370217694096.

Kodiatte TA, Manikyam UK, Rao SB, Jagadish TM, Reddy M, Lingaiah HKM, and V Lakshmaiah. 2012. Mean platelet volume in Type 2 diabetes mellitus. *Journal of Laboratory Physicians*, Jan–Jun; 4(1): 5–9. DOI: 10.4103/0974-2727.98662.

Kozlova EK, Chernysh AM, Moroz VV, and AN Kuzovlev. 2013. Analysis of nanostructure of red blood cells membranes by space Fourier transform of AFM images. *Micron (Oxford, England)*, Jan; 44: 218–227. DOI: 10.1016/j.micron. 2012.06.012.

Kriska AM, Saremi A, Hanson RL, Bennett PH, Kobes S, Williams DE, and WC Knowler. 2003. Physical activity, obesity, and the incidence of type 2 diabetes in a high-risk population. *American Journal of Epidemiology*, Oct; 158(7): 669–675. PMID: 14507603.

Kwon E, and C Ahn. 2012. Low hemoglobin concentration is associated with several diabetic profiles. *Korean Journal of Internal Medicine*, Sep; 27(3): 273–274. DOI: 10.3904/kjim.2012.27.3.273.

Labrouche S, Freyburger G, Gin H, Boisseau MR, and C Cassagne. 1996. Changes in phospholipid composition of blood cell membranes (erythrocyte, platelet, and polymorphonuclear) in different types of diabetes—clinical and biological correlations. *Metabolism*, Jan; 45(1): 57–71. PMID: 8544778.

Lipinski B, and E Pretorius. 2012. Novel pathway of iron-induced blood coagulation: implications for diabetes mellitus and its complications. *Polskie Archiwum Medycyny Wewnetrznej*, 122(3): 115–122. PMID: 22460041.

Lowe GD, Lee AJ, Rumley A, Price JF, and FG Fowkes. 1997. Blood viscosity and risk of cardiovascular events: the Edinburgh Artery Study. *British Journal of Haematology*, Jan; 96(1): 168–173. PMID: 9012704.

MacRury SM, Lennie SE, McColl P, Balendra R, MacCuish AC, and GD Lowe. 1993. Increased red cell aggregation in diabetes mellitus: association with cardiovascular risk factors. *Diabetic Medicine*, Jan–Feb; 10(1): 21–26. PMID: 8435983.

Masi S, D'Aiuto F, Cooper J, Salpea K, Stephens JW, Hurel SJ, Deanfield JE, and SE Humphries. 2016. Telomere length, antioxidant status and incidence of ischaemic heart disease in type 2 diabetes. *International Journal of Cardiology*, Aug; 216: 159164. DOI: 10.1016/j.ijcard.2016.04.130.

Mazidi M, Penson P, and M Banach. 2017. Association between telomere length and complete blood count in US adults. *Archives of Medical Science*, Apr; 13(3): 601–605. DOI: 10.5114/aoms.2017.67281.

Mazzanti L, Faloia E, Rabini RA, Staffolani R, Kantar A, Fiorini R, Swoboda B, De Pirro R, and E Bertoli. 1992. Diabetes mellitus induces red blood cell plasma membrane alterations possibly affecting the aging process. *Clinical Biochemistry*, Feb; 25(1): 41–46. PMID: 1312917.

McFarlane SI, Salifu MO, Makaryus J, and JR Sowers. 2006. Anemia and cardiovascular disease in diabetic nephropathy. *Current Diabetes Reports*, Jun; 6(3): 213–218. PMID: 16898574.

McMillan DE, Utterback NG, and J La Puma. 1978. Reduced erythrocyte deformability in diabetes. *Diabetes*, Sept; 27(9): 895–901. PMID: 689301.

Moroz VV, Chernysh AM, Kozlova EK, Borshegovskaya PY, Bliznjuk UA, Rysaeva RM, and OY Gudkova. 2010. Comparison of red blood cell membrane microstructure after different physicochemical influences: atomic force microscope research. *Journal of Critical Care*, Sept; 25 (3): 539.e1–539.e12. DOI: http://dx.doi.org/10.1016/j.jcrc.2010. 02.007.

Murakami T, Horigome H, Tanaka K, Nakata Y, Ohkawara K, Katayama Y, and A Matsui. 2007. Impact of weight reduction on production of platelet-derived microparticles and fibrinolytic parameters in obesity. *Thrombosis Research*, 119(1):45–53. DOI: 10.1016/j.thromres.2005.12.013.

Pedreño J, Hurt-Camejo E, Wiklund O, Badimón L, and L Masana. 2000. Platelet function in patients with familial hypertriglyceridemia: evidence that platelet reactivity is modulated by apolipoprotein E content of very-low-density lipoprotein particles. *Metabolism*, Jul; 49(7): 942–949. PMID: 10910008.

Pieters M, Covic N, van der Westhuizen FH, Nagaswami C, Baras Y, Loots DT, Jerling JC, Elgar D, Edmondson KS, van Zyl DG, Rheeder P, and JW Weisel. 2008. Glycaemic control improves fibrin network characteristics in type 2 diabetes—a purified fibrinogen model. *Thrombosis and Haemostasis*, Apr; 99(4): 691–700. DOI: 10.1160/TH07-11-0699.

Pu LJ, Shen Y, Lu L, Zhang RY, Zhang Q, and WF Shen. 2012. Increased blood glycohemoglobin A1c levels lead to overestimation of arterial oxygen saturation by pulse oximetry in patients with type 2 diabetes. *Cardiovascular Diabetology*, Sept; 11: 110. DOI: 10.1186/1475-2840-11-110.

Pyorala K, Pedersen TR, Kjekshus J, Faergeman O, Olsson AG, and G Thorgeirsson. 1997. Cholesterol lowering with simvastatin improves prognosis of diabetic patients with coronary heart disease: A subgroup analysis of the Scandinavian Simvastatin Survival Study (4S). *Diabetes Care*, Apr; 20(4): 614–620. PMID: 9096989 [Erratum, *Diabetes Care* 1997; 20: 1048].

Qiao J, Al-Tamimi M, Baker RI, Andrews RK, and EE Gardiner. 2015. The platelet Fc receptor, FcγRIIa. *Immunological Reviews*, Nov; 268(1): 241–252. DOI: 10.1111/imr.12370.

Qiu C, Zhang C, Gelaye B, Enquobahrie DA, Frederick IO, and MA Williams. 2011. Gestational diabetes mellitus in relation to maternal dietary heme iron and nonheme iron intake. *Diabetes Care*, Jul; 34(7): 1564–1569. DOI: 10.2337/dc11-0135.

Rajpathak SN, Crandall JP, Wylie-Rosett J, Kabat GC, Rohan TE, and FB Hu. 2009. The role of iron in type 2 diabetes in humans. *Biochimica Biophysica Acta*, Jul; 1790(7): 671–681. DOI: 10.1016/j.bbagen .2008.04.005.

Ranil PK, Raman R, Rachepalli SR, Pal SS, Kulothungan V, Lakshmipathy P, Satagopan U, Kumaramanickavel G, and T Sharma. 2010. Anemia and diabetic retinopathy in type 2 diabetes mellitus. *The Journal of the Association of Physicians of India*, Feb; 58: 91–94. PMID: 20653149.

Redondo-Bermejo B, Pascual-Figal DA, Hurtado-Martínez JA, Montserrat-Coll J, Peñafiel-Verdú P, Pastor-Pérez F, Giner-Caro JA, and M Valdés-Chávarri. 2007. Clinical determinants and prognostic value of hemoglobin in hospitalized patients with systolic heart failure [Article in Spanish]. *Revista Espanola de Cardiologia*, Jun; 60(6): 597–606. PMID: 17580048.

Rillaerts E, van Gaal L, Xiang DZ, Vansant G, and I De Leeuw. 1989. Blood viscosity in human obesity: relation to glucose tolerance and insulin status. *International Journal of Obesity*, 13(6): 739–745. PMID: 2695480.

Sacks FM, Pfeffer MA, Moye LA, Rouleau JL, Rutherford JD, Cole TG, Brown L, Warnica JW, Arnold JM, Wun CC, Davis BR, and E Braunwald. 1996. The effect of pravastatin on coronary events after myocardial infarction in patients with average cholesterol levels. *New England Journal of Medicine*, Oct; 335(14): 1001–1009. DOI: 10.1056/NEJM199610033351401.

Schaeffer G, Wascher TC, Kostner GM, and WF Graier. 1999. Alterations in platelet Ca^{2+} signalling in diabetic patients is due to increased formation of superoxide anions and reduced nitric oxide production. *Diabetologia*, Feb; 42(2): 167–176. DOI: 10.1007/s001250051135.

Schäfer A, and J Bauersachs. 2008. Endothelial dysfunction, impaired endogenous platelet inhibition and platelet activation in diabetes and atherosclerosis. *Current Vascular Pharmacology*, Jan; 6(1): 52–60. PMID: 18220940.

Schneider DJ. 2009. Factors contributing to increased platelet reactivity in people with diabetes. *Diabetes Care*, Apr; 32(4): 525–527. DOI: 10.2337/dc08-1865.

Simcox JA, and DA McClain. 2013. Iron and diabetes risk. *Cell Metabolism*, Mar; 17(3): 329–341. DOI: 10.1016 /j.cmet.2013.02.007.

Sloop GD. 1996. A unifying theory of atherogenesis. *Medical Hypotheses*, Oct; 47(4): 321–325. https://doi .org/10.1016/S0306-9877(96)90073-0.

Tal MG. 2009. Type 2 diabetes: microvascular ischemia of pancreatic islets? *Medical Hypotheses*, Sept; 73(3):357–358. DOI: 10.1016/j.mehy.2009.03.034.

Tamariz LJ, Young H, Pankow JS, Yeh H-C, Schmidt MI, Astor B, and FL Brancati. 2008. Blood viscosity and hematocrit as risk factors for Type 2 diabetes mellitus. The Atherosclerosis Risk in Communities (ARIC) Study. *American Journal of Epidemiology*, Nov; 168(10): 1153–1160. DOI: 10.1093/aje /kwn243.

Tamura Y, Takubo K, Aida J, Araki A, and H Ito. 2016. Telomere attrition and diabetes mellitus. *Geriatrics and Gerontology International*, Mar; 16 Suppl 1: 66–74. DOI: 10.1111/ggi.12738.

Tarry-Adkins JL, Fernandez-Twinn DS, Chen J-H, Hargreaves IP, Malgorzata S. Martin-Gronert MS, McConnell JM, and SE Ozanne. 2014. Nutritional programming of coenzyme Q: potential for prevention and intervention? *The Journal of the Federation of American Societies of Experimental Biology*, Dec; 28(12): 5398–5405. DOI: 10.1096/fj.14-259473.

Thomas MC, MacIsaac RJ, Tsalamandris C, Power D, and G Jerums. 2003. Unrecognized anemia in patients with diabetes: a cross-sectional survey. *Diabetes Care*, Apr; 26(4): 1164–1169. PMID: 12663591.

Tschoepe D, Roesen P, Kaufmann L, Schauseil S, Kehrel B, Ostermann H, and FA Gries. 1990. Evidence for abnormal platelet glycoprotein expression in diabetes mellitus. *European Journal of Clinical Investigation*, Apr; 20(2): 166–170. PMID: 2112481.

Uziel O, Singer JA, Danicek V, Sahar G, Berkov E, Luchansky M, Fraser A, Ram R, and M Lahav. 2007. Telomere dynamics in arteries and mononuclear cells of diabetic patients: effect of diabetes and of glycemic control. *Experimental Gerontology*, Oct; 42(10): 971–978. DOI: 10.1016/j.exger.2007.07.005.

Vinik AI, Erbas T, Park TS, Nolan R, and GL Pittenger. 2001. Platelet dysfunction in type 2 diabetes. *Diabetes Care*, Aug; 24(8): 1476–1485. PMID: 11473089.

Viskupicova J, Blaskovic D, Galiniak S, Soszyński M, Bartosz G, Horakova L, and I Sadowska-Bartosz. 2015. Effect of high glucose concentrations on human erythrocytes in vitro. *Redox Biology*, Aug; 5: 381–387. DOI: 10.1016/j.redox.2015.06.011.

Vlagopoulos PT, Tighiouart H, Weiner DE, Griffith J, Pettitt D, Salem DN, Levey AS, and MJ Sarnak. 2005. Anemia as a risk factor for cardiovascular disease and all-cause mortality in diabetes: the impact of chronic kidney disease. *Journal of the American Society of Nephrology*, Nov; 16(11): 3403–3410. DOI: 10.1681/ASN.2005030226.

Watala C. 2005. Blood platelet reactivity and its pharmacological modulation in (people with) diabetes mellitus. *Current Pharmaceutical Design*, 11(18): 2331–2365. PMID: 16022671.

Westerbacka J, Yki-Järvinen H, Turpeinen A, Rissanen A, Vehkavaara S, Syrjälä M, and R Lassila. 2002. Inhibition of platelet-collagen interaction: an in vivo action of insulin abolished by insulin resistance in obesity. *Arteriosclerosis, Thrombosis, and Vascular Biology*, Jan; 22(1): 167–172. PMID: 11788478.

Willeit P, Raschenberger J, Heydon EE, Sotirios Tsimikas S, Haun M, Mayr A, Weger S, Witztum JL, Butterworth AS, Willeit J, Kronenberg F, and S Kiechl. 2014. Leucocyte telomere length and risk of Type 2 diabetes mellitus: new prospective cohort study and literature-based meta-analysis. *PLoS ONE*, Nov. 12. https://doi.org/10.1371/journal.pone.0112483.

Winocour PD, Watala C, and RL Kinglough-Rathbone. 1992. Membrane fluidity is related to the extent of glycation of proteins, but not to alterations in the cholesterol to phospholipid molar ratio in isolated platelet membranes from diabetic and control subjects. *Thrombosis and Haemostasis*, May 4; 67(5): 567–571. PMID: 1519216.

5 Chronic Hyperglycemia Impairs Vision, Hearing, and Sensory Function

The best and most beautiful things in the world cannot be seen or even touched – they must be felt with the heart.

Hellen Keller

5.1 DIABETES CAUSES RETINAL VASCULAR DYSFUNCTION, RETINAL DETACHMENT, AGE-RELATED MACULAR DEGENERATION, AND CATARACT FORMATION

Some retinal changes occur over time in almost all people with diabetes, even if they are on insulin therapy, and those who also have high blood pressure are at much higher risk of developing diabetic retinopathy because both conditions tend to damage the retina.

Repeated exposure to high levels of glucose in the blood makes small blood vessel walls, including those in the retina, weaker and, therefore, more prone to damage. Damaged retinal blood vessels leak blood and fluid into the retina. Unlike Type 1 diabetes, diagnosis of Type 2 diabetes may not occur for years, so retinopathy may be present—even advanced—by the time some people are diagnosed with Type 2 diabetes.

Diabetes mellitus can cause two types of changes in the eye: Nonproliferative diabetic retinopathy occurs first. Proliferative diabetic retinopathy occurs after nonproliferative diabetic retinopathy, and it is more severe. In nonproliferative diabetic retinopathy, small blood vessels in the retina leak fluid or blood and may develop small bulges. Areas of the retina affected by leakage may swell, causing damage to parts of the field of vision. At first, the effects on vision may be minimal, but gradually vision may become impaired. Blind spots may appear, although these may not be noticed at first, and they are usually discovered only during testing.

If there is leakage near the macula, central vision may be blurry. The macula is the central area of the retina that affords the greatest acuity in vision. Swelling of the macula (macular edema) due to leakage of fluid from blood vessels can eventually cause significant loss of vision.

In proliferative diabetic retinopathy, retinal damage stimulates abnormal growth of new blood vessels, sometimes leading to bleeding, scarring, or even detachment of the retina. Proliferative diabetic retinopathy results in greater loss of vision than does nonproliferative diabetic retinopathy, and it can result in total or near-total blindness due to a large hemorrhage into the substance that fills the back of the eyeball (the vitreous humor) or to a type of retinal detachment called traction retinal detachment (see below).

Symptoms of proliferative diabetic retinopathy may include blurred vision, floaters (black spots), or flashing lights in the field of vision, and sudden, severe, painless vision loss. The damage done by hyperglycemia to the retina is better known than that done to the lens. This may be due in part to the fact that the damage done to the retina is basically (micro-)vascular damage, unlike that done to the lens, and vascular impairment in other parts of the body is pretty well detailed now.

A report in the *Journal of Ophthalmic and Vision Research* titled "Diabetes and retinal vascular dysfunction" details the impairments that diabetes imposes on vision (Shin, Sorenson, and

Sheibani. 2014). According to this report, one could conclude that vision impairment results primarily from oxidative stress caused by inflammatory mediators and reactive oxygen species (ROS) due to hyperglycemia.

Diabetes mainly affects the microvascular circulation of the retina, resulting in a range of structural changes that ultimately lead to altered permeability, hyperproliferation of endothelial cells, edema, and abnormal vascularization.

5.1.1 THE RETINA

The retina is composed of endothelial cells, pericytes, and astrocytes. In addition, there are cells that mediate vision. Photoreceptors, scotopic "rods," and photopic "cone" cells convert light information into signals and send those to an intermediate layer that, in turn, relays them to the 20 or so distinct types of retinal ganglion cells.

Diabetes affects the integrity of the blood–retinal barrier by altering the structure of the retina (Figure 5.1).

The blood–retinal barrier is composed of both an inner and an outer barrier. The outer blood–retinal barrier refers to the barrier formed at the retinal pigment epithelial cell layer, and it functions, in part, to regulate the movement of solutes and nutrients from the choroid to the subretinal space. In contrast, the inner blood–retinal barrier, similar to the blood–brain barrier, is located in the inner retinal microvasculature and comprises the microvascular endothelium that lines these vessels.

The tight junctions located between these cells mediate highly selective diffusion of molecules from the blood to the retina, and the barrier is essential in maintaining retinal homeostasis (Campbell, and Humphries. 2012).

In the diabetic retina, there are increases in the level of vascular endothelial growth factor (VEGF), a signal protein from cells that stimulates angiogenesis, contributing to vascular leakage (Kim, Kim, Roh et al. 2012). VEGF activates factors that contribute to increased vascular permeability (Murakami, Frey, Lin et al. 2012). Alterations in vascular structure under diabetic conditions result in the breakdown of the blood–retinal barrier and, thus, diabetic edema (Bandello, Lattanzio, Zucchiatti et al. 2013).

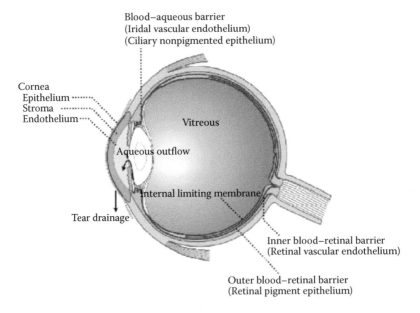

FIGURE 5.1 Diagram of the structure of the eye showing the location of the retinal–blood barriers. (From Araki, Tanaka, and Ebihara. 2013. *International Journal of Nanomedicine*, Feb: 8: 495–504. With permission.)

Pericytes maintain vascular stability, and their early depletion leads to formation of *pericyte ghosts* and the increased proliferation of endothelial cells, contributing to microaneurysm formation in retinal vessels. The density of pericytes inversely correlates with vascular abnormalities of the retina, and their reduction leads to diabetic retinopathy (Enge, Bjarnegard, Gerhardt et al. 2002). Loss and degeneration of pericytes damage the integrity and maintenance of the blood–retinal barrier, and it induces proliferative neovascularization, leading to retinal detachment and impairment of vision. Consequently, pericyte dysfunction leads to capillary dilation, microaneurysms, and increased vascular permeability, resulting in vascular leakage and macular edema (Bandello, Lattanzio, Zucchiatti et al. 2013).

Retinal endothelial cells are the main components in the inner blood–retinal barrier forming the physical barriers between the vascular lumen and the retina (Armulik, Genové, Mäe et al. 2010). Transport of metabolites and nutrients between blood and the retina is selectively regulated by this physical barrier (Al Ahmad, Gassmann, and Ogunshola. 2009).

5.1.2 HYPERGLYCEMIA DAMAGES RETINAL BLOOD VESSEL ENDOTHELIAL CELL MITOCHONDRIA

Hyperglycemia exposes the mitochondria of retinal blood vessel endothelial cells to high concentrations of glucose (Joussen, Smyth, and Niessen. 2007). High concentrations of glucose increase membrane potential and ROS in bovine retinal endothelial cell mitochondria, which correlates with the rate of apoptosis (Cui, Xu, Bi et al. 2006).

High glucose in rat retinas was also shown to increase mitochondrial fragmentation and increase cytochrome c release leading to apoptosis (Trudeau, Molina, Guo et al. 2010). Paradoxically, the majority of *in vitro* studies do not report apoptosis in retinal microvascular endothelial cells exposed to high glucose, especially those from the retina (Huang, and Sheibani. 2008). However, this may not be the case *in vivo* where the loss of endothelial cells may result from loss of pericytes leading to vascular dysfunction and formation of acellular capillaries.

Retinal endothelial cell adhesive and migratory activities are critical for angiogenesis. Increased migration under high glucose conditions contributes to increased angiogenic activity and is consistent with downregulation of thrombospondin-1 (TSP-1) in microvascular endothelial cells, as well as with enhanced migration of TSP-1–deficient retinal endothelial cells (Sheibani, Sorenson, Cornelius et al. 2000; Huang, and Sheibani. 2008; Su, Sorenson, and Sheibani. 2003). TSP-1 is an adhesive glycoprotein that mediates cell-to-cell and cell-to-matrix interactions (see also Shin, Sorenson, and Sheibani. 2014).

5.1.3 DIABETIC RETINOPATHY, HYPOXIA, AND OXIDATIVE STRESS

According to a report in the journal *Current Diabetes Reviews*, retinal hypoxia precedes oxidative stress: The vascular cells first affected in small animal models of diabetic retinopathy are found throughout the inner retina and not specifically associated with small blood vessels until later in the development of retinopathy. On the other hand, the small retinal blood vessels are selectively affected in human disease.

The earliest retinal pathology and the earliest biochemical changes appear to begin within 1 week of the time when experimental animals become diabetic and are provoked by hyperglycemia. These changes include alterations to the appearance of microglia, the formation of advanced glycation end products (AGEs), the overproduction of VEGF and its mRNA, and consequent leakage of capillary endothelial cells. Microglia are a type of macrophage cells that act as the main form of active immune defense mostly in the central nervous system.

These early pro-inflammatory changes can directly cause hypoxia in the retina and not necessarily via ROS. Experiments on isolated cells indicate that retinal capillaries are less susceptible to hyperglycemia than other retinal cells, but *in vivo* are selectively damaged, possibly via paracrine changes. This suggests a new concept: Although the changes in blood vessels may be a consequence of gradual and cumulative development of oxidative stress, the preceding paracrine and other changes that cause the development of oxidative stress are highly significant to the understanding and treatment of diabetic retinopathy.

The clinical importance of these findings is that about the time that oxidative stress becomes easily demonstrable, the progress of diabetic retinopathy is already irreversible. A number of methods of treatment of diabetic retinopathy depend on the relief of retinal hypoxia (Arden, and Sivaprasad. 2011).

5.1.4 VASCULAR LESIONS IN DIABETIC RETINOPATHY

The Romanian journal, *Oftalmologia*, reported a study comparing normal eye to ocular globes from patients with diabetic retinopathy preserved in different stages of evolution, fixed and stained by classic histological techniques. The investigators focused on the histopathological examinations of arterial and venous morphology in different retinal areas (central and peripheral).

Vascular lesions of all types were observed in capillaries, arterioles, and venules, and they corresponded to the stage of the disease. They were manifest principally in thickening of the basal membrane, the degeneration of pericytes, the proliferation of the endothelial cells, microaneurysms, neovessels, and vascular hyalinization. Diabetes increased the rate of death of capillary cells and retinal neurons (Craitoiu, Mocanu, Olaru et al. 2005).

5.1.5 HYPERGLYCEMIA AND RETINAL DETACHMENT

In retinal detachment, the retina separates from the choroid, the underneath layer to which it normally adheres. This may present to the patient as flashes of light and disruption of the periphery of the visual field. It is most common in people who are in their 60s or 70s, and men are more often affected than women. In about 7% of the cases, both eyes are affected. Without treatment, permanent loss of vision may occur (Mitry, Charteris, Fleck et al. 2010).

Generally, there is a tear in the retina and that allows the fluid in the eye to seep behind the retina. There are medical interventions intended to prevent it becoming a detachment, and these include using a laser device.

There are three types of retinal detachment: The rhegmatogenous retinal detachment, the most common type, is caused by retinal tears. A retinal tear allows vitreous fluid from the middle of the eye to pass through the breach and settle under the retina. As the fluid builds up under the retina, it pushes the retina away from the layer beneath it. The most frequent cause of retinal tears is posterior vitreous detachment (PVD), a normal, usually harmless part of aging.

Retinal tears that occur with new symptoms, such as floaters, flashes of light, or other visual disturbances, are much more likely to progress to detachments.

Traction retinal detachment occurs when scar tissue or other abnormal tissue grows on the surface of the retina, pulling the retina away from the layer beneath it. This does not cause a specific tear or break in the retina. The leading cause of traction retinal detachment is proliferative retinopathy, a condition most frequently caused by diabetes.

Exudative retinal detachment occurs when blood or fluid from the middle layer of tissue that forms the eyeball flows into the space under the retina and separates the retina from the layer beneath it. The detachment does not involve tears in the retina or traction from the vitreous. Exudative retinal detachment is most often a complication of other diseases or conditions such as severe macular degeneration, eye tumors, inflammation in the choroid or the retina, or severe high blood pressure.

It is not common knowledge among laypeople that retinal detachment can be caused by diabetes. However, this information is readily available on many popular medical information websites. For instance, the Mayo Clinic website lists "Advanced diabetes" as a cause (http://www.mayoclinic.org /diseases-conditions/retinal-detachment/symptoms-causes/dxc-20197292).

Massive periretinal proliferation is a serious complication of retinal detachment caused by proliferation and fibrous change of cells to a form not normally present in that tissue (metaplasia), mostly deriving from retinal pigment epithelium and retinal glial cells. The late signs such as starfolds, irregular retinal folds, circumferential folds, and funnel-shaped detachments are well documented (Machemer. 1978).

A study conducted in Japan, and published in the journal *Ophthalmologica*, addressed the relationship between the diabetic state and massive periretinal proliferation in idiopathic retinal detachment. It was found that in 3.5% of their cases of idiopathic retinal detachment, massive periretinal proliferation occurred before or after retinal detachment surgery. In a number of those cases, a diabetic or suspected diabetic state was found. Half of those cases were receiving treatment for diabetes and never developed massive periretinal proliferation, while one-third of the patients who were not being treated had massive periretinal proliferation.

This suggested that massive periretinal proliferation in retinal detachment may easily be induced by the diabetic state and could be prevented by treatment for diabetes (Amemiya, Yoshida, Harayama1 et al. 1979; see also Jalali. 2003).

As said above, the second most common type of retinal detachment is a tractional retinal detachment. "Tractional" means that there is pulling on the retinal surface and the pulling is strong enough to separate the light-sensing retina from the back of the eye. The traction comes from extensive growth of abnormal blood vessels in proliferative diabetic retinopathy. The abnormal blood vessels grow from the damaged vasculature of the retina into the jelly of the eye called the *vitreous.*

As these blood vessels grow into the jelly, they become denser and mature into membranes of fibrous scar tissue. Eventually, the scar tissue contracts and detaches the retina. Sometimes, the stress on the retina is so great that tears or holes are formed.

A report in the journal *Klinische Monatsblatter fur Augenheilkunde (Clinical Ophthalmology Monthly)* paints a bleak picture of the prognosis of diabetic tractional retinal detachment. The author reports that although tractional detachment can remain stable for a long time, so long as the center of the macula is not threatened, it can cause edema and reduced vision.

Retinal breaks, or tears due to tractional membranes, can cause a traction-rhegmatogenous retinal detachment, which is usually rapidly progressive and requires early surgery. In cases of tractional detachment of the macula, there is no alternative to surgery. Where there is long-standing and complete tractional detachment with severe retinal ischemia, the prognosis even after successful surgery is poor (Helbig. 2002).

5.1.6 HYPERGLYCEMIA AND MACULAR PUCKER (EPIRETINAL MEMBRANE)

A macular pucker is scar tissue that formed on the macula, the light-sensitive tissue in the center of the retina. A macular pucker can cause blurred and distorted central vision.

The cause of epiretinal membrane (ERM) is a defect in the surface layer of the retina where glial cells can migrate and grow into a membranous sheet on the retinal surface. This membrane can appear like cellophane and over time may contract and cause traction (or pulling) and puckering of the retina, leading to decreased vision and visual distortion.

The most common cause of macular pucker is an age-related condition called PVD where the vitreous gel that fills the back half of the eye separates from the retina, causing micro-tears and symptoms of floaters and flashes. If there is no specific cause such as a PVD, the ERM is called idiopathic (of unknown origin).

The *Canadian Journal of Ophthalmology* recently reported a study that aimed to determine the prevalence of ERM in patients with Type 2 diabetes and to assess the associated risk factors.

Patients with Type 2 diabetes seen for annual follow-up between 2009 and 2010 were evaluated by digital nonmydriatic retinal photography for the detection of diabetic retinopathy. Retinal photographs were assessed by a retina specialist. Nonmydriatic fundus photography allows for imaging of the retina and optic nerve without pharmacologic pupil dilation because it uses infrared light, which does not trigger a pupillary response.

ERM was present in 6.5% of patients with Type 2 diabetes. The prevalence of ERM was significantly associated with age: 1.2% for those below 49 years, 4% for those 50 to 59 years old, 8.2% for those 60 to 69 years old, and 9.6% for those older than 70 years; with cataract surgery, diabetic nephropathy, and chronic renal failure. In any case, according to a report published in the journal *Clinical and Experimental Optometry*, the likelihood of developing an ERM increases following cataract surgery (Kopsachilis, Carifi, and Cunningham. 2014). Prevalence was similar for both genders.

The investigators concluded that the prevalence of ERM in patients with Type 2 diabetes was not significantly different from that in the general population, except that it was significantly associated with age, diabetic nephropathy, and cataract surgery (Knyazer, Schachter, Plakht et al. 2016).

However, an earlier study published in the journal *PLoS ONE*, based on a Chinese population, arrived at a different conclusion.

The latter study was intended to determine the prevalence of idiopathic epiretinal membrane (iERM) and possible demographic, systemic, and ocular factors associated with it. Each participant underwent a standardized interview and comprehensive ophthalmic examination. iERM was identified and graded from retinal photographs, and then those participants with iERM were compared to those without it to further determine the associations between iERM and blood biochemical test results (including fasting plasma glucose, serum creatinine, total cholesterol, and triglyceride), ocular biological parameters (including the axial length, corneal curvature, refractive diopter, intraocular pressure, and anterior chamber depth), and the data of optical coherence tomography.

The prevalence of iERM was found to be 1.02%, and it was significantly associated with diabetes (odds ratio [OR], 2.457).

Blood biochemical test results and ocular biological parameters showed no significant differences between the iERM group and control groups, whereas the incidence of PVD in the iERM group was higher, albeit not significantly so, than in the control group (26.5% vs. 8.8%). Moreover, iERM significantly adversely affected visual acuity.

The investigators concluded that in their Shanghai population, iERM was relatively rare, but that it was strongly linked to diabetes (Zhu, Peng, Zou et al. 2012).

5.1.7 HYPERGLYCEMIA AND THE CORNEA

The cornea is the transparent front part of the eye—the dome—that covers the iris, pupil, and anterior chamber. Together with the anterior chamber and the lens, the cornea refracts light, accounting for approximately two-thirds of the total optical power of the eye.

According to a report in the journal *Nutrition and Diabetes*, different parts of the cornea such as the epithelium, the nerves, immune cells, and the endothelium entail specific complications of diabetes: corneal nerve changes reflect peripheral and autonomic neuropathy, and alterations of immune cells in the cornea indicate an inflammatory component in diabetic complications. Furthermore, impaired corneal epithelial wound healing may also imply more widespread disease.

Hyperglycemia and formation of AGEs affect different parts of the cornea, resulting in three principal types of tissue dysfunction with physiological effects that can be measured:

- Defective wound healing in the corneal epithelium
- Abnormalities of subbasal nerves
- Loss of corneal endothelial pump function

The investigators reported an extensive review of publications on the damaging effect of diabetes on the cornea in the journal *Nutrition and Diabetes* (Shih, Lam, and Tong. 2017). Certain elements of their extensive findings stand out. For instance, the eyes of diabetes sufferers are at increased risk of dry eye, superficial punctate keratitis, recurrent corneal erosion syndrome, and persistent epithelial defects (Ye, and Lu. 2015; Achtsidis, Eleftheriadou, Kozanidou et al. 2014).

The corneal epithelium is the first layer of the eye, so it is constantly subjected to wear and tear and it needs to be constantly regenerated. Any process such as diabetes that affects wound healing or the speed of epithelial regeneration will have physiological impact and will increase morbidity including ocular pain and redness (Xu, Li, Ljubimov, and Yu. 2009; Funari, Winkler, Brown et al. 2013).

Recently, a study reported in the journal *The Ocular Surface* showed for the first time that tear levels of Type 1 and Type 2 diabetic individuals had significantly higher insulin-like growth factor binding protein (IGFBP3) compared with age-matched normal adults. IGFBP3 is a protein that is known to play a negative regulatory role in IGF signaling by binding and sequestrating it, competing with its cellular receptor IGFR-1. IGFs are proteins with high similarity to insulin. IGFs are part of a complex system that cells use to communicate with their physiologic environment.

IGFBP3 increases insulin resistance and induces apoptosis and oxidative damage. The processes regulating the secretion of IGFBP3 from corneal epithelial tissue is not known, but in experiments with human corneal epithelial cells, it was found that high levels of glucose in the culture medium can induce the production of IGFBP3, suggesting that the hyperglycemia in patients may be the cause of the IGFBP3 upregulation (Wu, Buckner, Zhu et al. 2012).

Investigators reported in the journal *Graefe's Archive for Clinical and Experimental Ophthalmology* that one of the molecular changes observed in animal eyes is the measurement of levels of AGEs. AGEs are considered to be the mediator for all chronic diabetes complications including macrovascular and microvascular complications such as diabetic retinopathy in the eye. The accumulation of AGEs in the cornea epithelium-basement membrane shifts local cell signaling toward pro-apoptotic and proliferative pathways and increases oxidative stress and inflammation (Kim, Kim, Sohn et al. 2011).

5.1.7.1 Corneal Neuropathy

Corneal nerves are branches of the ophthalmic nerve, which in turn is a branch of the trigeminal cranial nerve. They perforate the corneal stroma at the medial and lateral positions and branch into neurites that eventually sprout nerve endings anteriorly into the corneal epithelium (Bikbova, Oshitari, Tawada et al. 2012). The cornea is the most densely innervated structure in humans, with nerve fibers playing an important neurotrophic role in the development of a healthy corneal surface.

Loss of neurotrophic function may result in a nonhealing or persistent cornea epithelial defect, or neurotrophic ulcer. Neurotrophins are proteins that promote the survival, development, and function of neurons. They belong to a class of growth factors, which are secreted proteins that are capable of signaling particular cells to survive, differentiate, or grow.

In both Type 1 and Type 2 diabetes, corneal nerve density is reduced and corneal nerve abnormalities are increased (Shih, Lam, and Tong. 2017). Reduction in corneal nerve fiber density is a characteristic manifestation of diabetic corneal neuropathy, with progression demonstrated over time.

5.1.7.2 Mechanisms of Corneal Neuropathy

It is generally understood that AGEs initiate damage to the pericytes and to the endothelium of capillaries, thus reducing microvascular supply to Schwann cells and neurons. This adversely affects neuronal function. Microvascular abnormalities are observed in the cornea: Reduction of cornea nerve fiber density, or length, has been shown to predict the development of diabetic retinopathy as well as other sight-threatening retinopathies (Messmer, Schmid-Tannwald, Zapp et al. 2010; Bitirgen, Ozkagnici, Malik et al. 2014).

Changes in corneal nerve structure lead to functional alteration. Corneal esthesiometry is used to evaluate corneal sensitivity, which is a functional outcome of nerve innervation. An association has been found between corneal nerve parameters and corneal sensitivity (Efron. 2011; Bitirgen, Ozkagnici, Malik et al. 2014; Pritchard, Edwards, Vagenas et al. 2012).

Loss of corneal sensation also reduces lacrimal tear production, since the corneal sensory receptors are the afferent limb of the lacrimal reflex arc. The reduction of corneal innervation has been linked to abnormal tear function as well as more frequent and severe symptoms of dry eye in diabetes patients.

5.1.7.3 Corneal Hysteresis

The Reichert Ocular Response Analyzer facilitates the determination of the relationship between ocular hysteresis, corneal resistance factor, and central corneal thickness in normal eyes (Shaha, Laiquzzamana, Cunliffea et al. 2006). Hysteresis is the force required to indent the cornea as well as the recovery from the indentation. Resistance force is the hysteresis normalized to the cornea shape. A higher hysteresis suggests a more rigid and less deformable cornea.

The *substantia propria* is the fibrous, tough, unyielding, and perfectly transparent, stroma of the cornea. At its center, human cornea stroma is composed of about 200 flattened layers of collagen fibrils superimposed one on another. They are each about 1.5 to 2.5 μm in thickness.

A study reported in the *Journal of Cataract and Refractive Surgery* compared diabetic patients and healthy participants. It was found that the mean corneal hysteresis was 9.3 ± 1.4 (SD) mmHg in the control group and 10.7 ± 1.6 mmHg in the patients, and the mean corneal resistance factor was 9.6 ± 1.6 mmHg in the control group and 10.9 ± 1.7 mmHg in the diabetic group. Diabetic corneas were significantly thicker; the mean central corneal thickness was 530.3 ± 35.9 μm in the control group and 548.7 ± 33.0 μm in the diabetic group.

The investigators concluded that diabetes affects biomechanical parameters of the human cornea, including increased corneal hysteresis, corneal resistance factor, and central corneal thickness (Goldich, Barkana, Gerber et al. 2009).

A number of clinic-based studies including those in Western Europe, Brazil, the United States, Israel, and Iran have reported that individuals with Type 1 or Type 2 diabetes have higher hysteresis. These reports may be found in Shih, Lam, and Tong (2017). This includes one study conducted in Turkey that found them to have a lower hysteresis, compared with age-matched controls.

The reason why diabetes may be causally linked to greater corneal hysteresis or thicknesses is thought to be due to the accumulation of AGEs in the corneal stroma. This was shown in diabetic monkeys in a study reported in the journal *Cornea* (Zou, Wang, Huang et al. 2012). This finding is consistent with evidence of AGE-induced cross-linking of the extracellular matrix (ECM) in diabetes, resulting in increased arterial stiffness, as reported in the journal *Circulation* (Goldin, Beckman, Schmidt et al. 2006).

5.1.7.4 Corneal Endothelial Disease

The corneal endothelial cells in the innermost layer of the cornea help to keep the stroma relatively dehydrated by the pumping action of fluid from the cornea out to the anterior chamber. A study published in the *European Journal of Ophthalmology* aimed to elucidate the status of the corneal endothelium in diabetes and identify risk factors contributing to compromised corneal endothelium.

Diabetic and nondiabetic patients were given detailed slit lamp and fundus tests and evaluated with the Nidek Confoscan 2. Cell density, percentage polymegathism, and pleomorphism were calculated. Polymegathism is the variation in cell size within the endothelial monolayer, and pleomorphism is the variation in the size and shape of cells of their nuclei. Controls were instituted for possible confounding factors such as hypertension, hyperlipidemia, age, gender, type, duration, glycemic control, and grades of diabetic retinopathy in both diabetic and nondiabetic participants.

It was found that the mean corneal density in diabetic patients was 175 cells/mm fewer than in healthy controls. The number of corneal endothelial cells with polymegathism, and with pleomorphism of the nuclei, was significantly greater in the diabetic patients than in the controls.

The authors concluded that the corneal endothelium in diabetic patients seems to be compromised and that evaluation of the corneal endothelium should be part of the protocol for eye care of diabetic patients (Shenoy, Khandekar, Bialasiewicz et al. 2009).

The aims of a study titled "Manifestations of type 2 diabetes in corneal endothelial cell density, corneal thickness and intraocular pressure" published in *The Journal of Biomedical Research* were to evaluate central corneal thickness, corneal endothelial cell density, and intraocular pressure in patients with Type 2 diabetes and to determine the potential differences due to diabetes duration and treatment modality in a prospective, randomized study.

Endothelial cell density, central corneal thickness, and intraocular pressure were measured in patients with Type 2 diabetes 57 years old, on average, and compared to age-matched, nondiabetic, control participants. Observations were analyzed for association with diabetes duration and glucose control modalities (insulin injection or oral medication) while controlling for age.

In the diabetic group, the mean endothelial cell density (2511 ± 252 cells/mm^2), mean central corneal thickness (539.7 ± 33.6 μm), and mean intraocular pressure (18.3 ± 2.5 mmHg) differed significantly from those in the control group (endothelial cell density: 2713 ± 132 cells/mm^2, central corneal thickness: 525.0 ± 45.3 μm, and intraocular pressure: 16.7 ± 1.8 mmHg). Endothelial cell density was significantly reduced by about 32 cells/mm^2 for diabetes patients with more than 10 years disease duration, when compared to those with duration of less than 10 years. Central corneal thickness was thicker and intraocular pressure was higher in diabetic patients with duration of more than 10 years than in those with disease duration of less than 10 years.

It was concluded that patients with Type 2 diabetes have significant changes in endothelial cell density, intraocular pressure, and central corneal thickness, which, however, are not correlated with disease duration or with whether the patients are on insulin injection or on oral medications (Briggs, Osuagwu, and Al Harthi. 2016).

The reference to intraocular pressure in the study cited above will be revisited in a later section on glaucoma. The following study addresses again the destructive role of AGEs, this time in the cornea.

The journal *Investigative Ophthalmology and Visual Science* featured a report titled "Advanced glycation end products in diabetic corneas." The aim of this study was to determine the role of AGEs in the pathogenesis of diabetic keratopathy because, as the authors pointed out, corneas in diabetic patients are exposed to increased glucose concentration despite their relatively avascular property, and this condition may contribute to the accumulation of AGEs. Keratopathy is any corneal disease, damage, dysfunction, or abnormality. There are several varieties.

Here is the procedure the investigators employed: An anti-AGE monoclonal antibody (6D12), which recognizes an N(epsilon)-carboxymethyl lysine (CML)–protein adduct as an epitope, was prepared. Immunohistochemical localization of CML was examined in human age-matched diabetic and nondiabetic corneas (8 of each). *In vitro*, type I collagen-, type IV collagen-, or laminin-coated 96-well plates were glycated by glucose-phosphate. In some experiments, aminoguanidine was present in the incubation mixture.

The amounts of CML–protein adducts in the ECM were determined by enzyme-linked immunosorbent assay using 6D12. SV40-immortalized human corneal epithelial cells (from diabetic as well as nondiabetic patients) were seeded onto modified or unmodified ECM in 96-well plates and allowed to attach for 3 h. Attached cells were fixed, and the areas of attached cells in each condition were measured. Attached cells without fixation were removed, and cell number was counted.

Here is what they found: In all of the diabetic corneas, CML immunoreactivity was observed in the epithelial basement membrane, whereas CML immunoreactivity was not found in the corresponding area in seven of eight nondiabetic corneas. *In vitro*, nonenzymatic glycation of laminin on the culture dish attenuated adhesion and spreading of corneal epithelial cells. The presence of aminoguanidine in the incubation mixture during glycation inhibited CML formation and promoted the adhesion and spreading of corneal epithelial cells in a dose-dependent manner.

It was concluded that the accumulation of AGEs on the basement membrane, particularly on laminin, may play a causative role in the corneal epithelial disorders of diabetic patients (Kaji, Usui, Oshika et al. 2000).

In a study published in the journal *Experimental and Therapeutic Medicine*, the investigators aimed to determine the effect of diabetes on cornea optical density, central corneal thickness, and corneal endothelial cell count. Diabetic patients were enrolled in the study during the period from March 2012 to March 2013. The patients were divided into three age groups: younger than 5, 5 to 10, and older than 10 years. During the same period, nondiabetic participants were selected and labeled as the normal control group.

The Pentacam (OCULUS Pentacam) was used to measure the corneal optical density and central corneal thickness. Specular microscopy was used to examine the corneal endothelial cell density.

The corneal optical density in the diabetes group was greater than that in the normal control group. The medial and intimal corneal optical density and central corneal thickness were positively correlated with the course of the disease. However, the corneal endothelial cell density was not associated with the course of diabetes. There was a positive association between the medial and intimal corneal optical density and central corneal thickness of the diabetic patients.

The study shows that medial and intimal corneal optical density and central corneal thickness are sensitive indicators of early diabetic keratopathy (Gao, Lin, and Pan. 2016).

5.1.8 HYPERGLYCEMIA AND GLAUCOMA

When most people consider glaucoma, it is usually high blood pressure that comes to mind but that is often because of the confusion between systemic blood pressure and intraocular pressure. While, as it will be shown, there is a relationship between systemic diastolic blood pressure and intraocular fluid pressure—at least in some people—the relationship is hardly as strong as one might think.

Normal (intraocular) eye pressure ranges from 12 to 22 mmHg, and eye pressure of greater than 22 mmHg, absent other evidence of glaucoma, is considered ocular hypertension. However, some people can have glaucoma at pressures between 12 and 22 mmHg. Eye pressure is unique to each person.

Glaucoma is characterized by optic nerve damage caused by consistently elevated intraocular pressure and, in far too many cases, it causes blindness. In fact, in the United States, it is the leading cause of blindness in people over 60 years old, even though it can often be prevented with early treatment. How does glaucoma come about?

The clear fluid inside the eye in front of the lens, known as the aqueous humor, is produced by the ciliary body, a small, circular structure behind the iris (the pigmented portion of the eye). The aqueous humor flows behind the iris and through the pupil, the opening in the middle of the iris. It then fills the anterior chamber, the space between the back of the clear cornea, and the front of the lens.

The aqueous humor exits the eye through the drainage angle, which is the angle formed inside the anterior chamber between the iris and the peripheral cornea. The aqueous humor filters through this angle and through the sclera, the white part of the eye, and then joins with the network of veins outside the eye. Any disruption of this outflow of aqueous humor can result in an increase in intraocular pressure.

The eye drainage angle can be structurally either "open" or "closed" (narrow). The narrower the angle, the more difficult it is for the aqueous humor to flow through it.

There are two major types of glaucoma: Primary open-angle glaucoma is the most common type. It occurs gradually when the eye does not drain fluid as it should: eye pressure builds and starts to damage the optic nerve. This type of glaucoma is painless and causes no vision changes at first.

The second type is angle-closure glaucoma or "narrow-angle glaucoma." This happens when the iris is very close to the drainage angle in the eye and blocks the drainage angle. Angle-closure glaucoma can cause blindness if not treated right away.

Since it has been previously shown that there is a greater likelihood of elevated blood pressure in persons with diabetes, these two factors, blood pressure and diabetes, need to be considered in determining the role of diabetes in glaucoma. To that end, investigators reported a longitudinal study on intraocular pressure and systemic blood pressure in the *British Journal of Ophthalmology*.

The aim of the study was to determine the relation between change in systemic blood pressures and change in intraocular pressure.

This was a population-based study of people 43 to 86 years old living in Beaver Dam, Wisconsin. Measurements of systemic blood pressures, intraocular pressures, and history of use of blood pressure medications were obtained at baseline (1988 to 1990) and then 5 years later.

It was reported that intraocular pressures were positively correlated with systolic and diastolic blood pressures at both baseline and follow-up. Changes in systemic blood pressures varied directly with changes in intraocular pressure with a 0.21-mmHg increase in intraocular pressure for a 10-mmHg increase in systolic blood pressure, and a 0.43-mmHg increase in intraocular pressure for a 10-mmHg increase in diastolic blood pressure.

Decreased systolic or diastolic blood pressures of more than 10 mmHg over 5 years were significantly associated with decreased intraocular pressure, and so the authors concluded that lower systemic blood pressure is associated with lower intraocular pressure (Klein, Klein, and Knudtson. 2005).

There is one dissenting opinion: Patrick Quaid, MD, head of the Guelph Vision Therapy Center in Canada, conducted research that showed a critical balance between blood pressure and eye pressure: hypertensive patients should be encouraged to keep blood pressures from falling too low because that, he claims, can cause eye problems. Dr. Quaid suggests that the perfusion pressure should remain above 50 to 55 mmHg (https://amsurgcontent.com/news/item/low-blood-pressure-linked-to-glaucoma-01262015; accessed 7.7.17).

What are the risk factors for glaucoma? A study published in the *American Journal of Preventive Medicine* reported that patients with well-documented glaucomatous visual field loss were matched by age, race, and gender to control participants and then both groups completed a detailed interview about past and current ocular and systemic diseases, plus a history of medication, alcohol, and cigarette use. Blood pressure measurements were taken at the time of the interview.

Diabetes showed the closest association with glaucoma (OR, 2.80). A history of hypertension and/or medication use was not associated with glaucoma, but elevated diastolic blood pressure showed some association (OR, 2.40). Separate analyses for white and black participants showed diabetes to be a risk factor for both groups (Katz, and Sommer. 1988).

5.1.9 Hyperglycemia and Cataracts

A comprehensive review in the *Journal of Ophthalmology* provides an overview of the pathogenesis of diabetic cataract, clinical studies investigating the association between diabetes and cataract development, and current treatment of cataract in diabetics (Pollreisz, and Schmidt-Erfurth. 2010). Evidently, cataract development occurs more frequently, and at an earlier age, in diabetic compared to nondiabetic patients (Klein, Klein, and Moss. 1985; Nielsen, and Vinding. 1984).

The Framingham (and other eye studies) reported a three- to fourfold increased prevalence of cataract in patients with diabetes under the age of 65 and up to a twofold excess prevalence in patients above 65 (Klein, Klein, and Moss. 1985; Ederer, Hiller, and Taylor. 1981). The greater the duration of diabetes, and the poorer the control of blood glucose, the greater the risk of cataracts.

The most frequently seen type of cataract in diabetics is the age-related or senile variety, which tends to occur earlier and progresses more rapidly in diabetics than in nondiabetics. However, in young Type 1 diabetic individuals, cataracts may be reversible with improvement in metabolic control (Jin, Huang, Zou et al. 2012).

The Wisconsin Epidemiologic Study of Diabetic Retinopathy investigated the incidence of cataract extraction in people with diabetes. Predictors of increased risk of needing cataract surgery included age and use of insulin in Type 2 diabetics, and the 10-year cumulative incidence of cataract surgery was 24.9% (Klein, Klein, and Moss. 1985). Data for the Beaver Dam Eye Study cohort and a follow-up are reported in Klein, Klein, and Lee (1998) and in Klein, Klein, Wang et al. (1995).

A population-based cross-sectional investigation, the Blue Mountains Eye Study reported the relationship between nuclear, cortical, and posterior subcapsular cataract in participants between the years 1992 and 1994 (Rowe, Mitchell, Cumming et al. 2000). The study supported the previous findings of the harmful effects of diabetes on the lens. Posterior subcapsular cataract was shown to be significantly associated with diabetes.

Many other studies conducted in other regions of the world arrived at similar conclusions. For instance: The Visual Impairment Project showed that diabetes was an independent risk factor for posterior subcapsular cataract when present for more than 5 years (Mukesh, Le, Dimitrov et al. 2006). The Barbados Eye study reported an 18% prevalence of lens changes when there is a history of diabetes, especially at younger ages (Leske, Wu, Hennis et al. 1999).

5.1.9.1   Cataracts, Blood Glucose, and the Polyol Pathway: The Osmotic Hypothesis

The enzyme aldose reductase reduces glucose to sorbitol through the polyol pathway, a process linked to the development of diabetic cataract. The intracellular accumulation of sorbitol leads to changes resulting in lens fibers that swell and take up fluid (hydropic), and degenerate, forming sugar cataracts (Kinoshita, Fukushi, Kador et al. 1979).

In the lens, sorbitol is produced faster than it can be converted to fructose by the enzyme sorbitol dehydrogenase, and the polar nature of sorbitol prevents its intracellular removal through diffusion. The increased accumulation of sorbitol creates a hyperosmotic effect that results in an infusion of fluid to countervail the osmotic gradient.

Animal studies have shown that the intracellular accumulation of polyols leads to a collapse and liquefaction of lens fibers that ultimately results in the formation of lens opacities (Kinoshita. 1965, 1974).

These findings have led to the "Osmotic Hypothesis" of sugar cataract formation that the intracellular increase of fluid in response to aldose reductase–mediated accumulation of polyols results in lens swelling and other changes that lead to cataract formation (Kador, and Kinoshita. 1984; Suzen, and Buyukbingol. 2003). The osmotic stress in the lens induces apoptosis in lens epithelial cells leading to the development of cataract (Li, Kuszak, Dunn et al. 1995). Impairments in the osmoregulation may render the lens susceptible to even small increases of aldose reductase–mediated osmotic stress, potentially leading to progressive cataract formation.

The polyol pathway is the primary mediator of diabetes-induced oxidative stress in the lens (Chung, Ho, Lam et al. 2003). In the cells of the lens, osmotic stress caused by the accumulation of sorbitol induces stress in the endoplasmic reticulum, the principal site of protein synthesis, ultimately leading to the generation of free radicals. Endoplasmic reticulum stress may also result from fluctuations of glucose levels initiating an unfolded protein response that generates ROS and causes oxidative stress damage to lens fibers (Mulhern, Madson, Danford et al. 2006).

While it is clear that free radicals and ROS play a role in cataract formation, there is no evidence that they initiate the process, but rather that they may accelerate and aggravate cataract development. Hydrogen peroxide (H_2O_2), elevated in the aqueous humor of diabetics, may induce hydroxyl radicals (OH^-) after entering the lens through processes described as "Fenton reactions" (Bron, Sparrow, Brown et al. 1993).

Increased glucose levels in the aqueous humor may induce glycation of lens proteins resulting in the generation of superoxide radicals ($O2^-$) and in the formation of AGEs—the *Maillard Reaction* (Stitt. 2005). The interaction of AGE with cell surface receptors such as receptor for advanced glycation end-products (rAGE) in the epithelium of the lens increases $O2^-$ and H_2O_2 formation (Hong, Lee, Handa et al. 2000).

The lenses of diabetic individuals have impaired antioxidant capacity, increasing their susceptibility to oxidative stress. This is exacerbated by inactivation of lens antioxidant enzymes like copper-zinc superoxide dismutase 1 (SOD1), the most dominant superoxide dismutase enzyme in the lens (Ookawara, Kawamura, Kitagawa et al. 1992; Behndig, Karlsson, Johansson et al. 2001). The enzyme SOD1 degrades superoxide radicals ($O2^-$) into hydrogen peroxide (H_2O_2) and oxygen. The importance of SOD1 in protection against cataract development in the presence of diabetes is the reason for its being featured in a later chapter.

In addition, investigators reported in the *Journal of Enzyme Inhibition and Medicinal Chemistry* that extracts and organic fractions of lychee nut (*Litchi chinensis*) yielded a methanol (MeOH) extract and an ethyl acetate (EtOAc) fraction found to be potent inhibitors of rat lens aldose reductase (RLAR) in vitro—their IC_{50} values being 3.6 and 0.3 µg/mL, respectively. From the active ethyl acetate fraction, four minor compounds were isolated and identified. Among these, delphinidin 3-O-β-galactopyranoside-39-O-β-glucopyranoside was found to be the most potent RLAR inhibitor (IC_{50} = 0.23 µg/mL) and may be useful in the prevention and/or treatment of diabetic complications (Lee, Park, and Moon. 2009).

5.1.10 Hyperglycemia and Age-Related Macular Degeneration

Macular degeneration causes loss in the center of the field of vision. In dry macular degeneration, the center of the macula deteriorates. With wet macular degeneration, leaky blood vessels grow under the retina. The National Eye Institute of the National Institutes of Health has a website titled "What you should know about age-related macular degeneration." It features "What is AMD?"

> AMD is a common eye condition and a leading cause of vision loss among people age 50 and older. It causes damage to the macula, a small spot near the center of the retina and the part of the eye needed for sharp, central vision, which lets us see objects that are straight ahead.
>
> In some people, AMD advances so slowly that vision loss does not occur for a long time. In others, the disease progresses faster and may lead to a loss of vision in one or both eyes. As AMD progresses, a blurred area near the center of vision is a common symptom. Over time, the blurred area may grow larger or you may develop blank spots in your central vision. Objects also may not appear to be as bright as they used to be. AMD by itself does not lead to complete blindness, with no ability to see. However, the loss of central vision in AMD can interfere with simple everyday activities, such as the ability to see faces, drive, read, write, or do close work, such as cooking or fixing things around the house.

And,

Who is at risk?

> Age is a major risk factor for AMD. The disease is most likely to occur after age 60, but it can occur earlier. Other risk factors for AMD include:
>
> - Smoking. Research shows that smoking doubles the risk of AMD.
> - Race. AMD is more common among Caucasians than among African-Americans or Hispanics/Latinos.
> - Family history and Genetics. People with a family history of AMD are at higher risk....

(https://nei.nih.gov/health/maculardegen/armd_facts; accessed 7.4.17)

No mention is made of diabetes, although diabetes is consistently cited in research reports as a significant factor in this visual disorder.

It is not surprising that many persons with early age-related macular degeneration (AMD) are not aware of the diabetes connection. Yet, diabetic retinopathy and AMD are two of the most common eye diseases in the United States. The aim of a study published in the *American Journal of Preventive Medicine* was to examine the frequency and predictors of unawareness of diabetic retinopathy and AMD. To that end, the study examined data from the 2005 to 2008 National Health and Nutrition Examination Survey consisting of collected digital retinal images of survey participants aged 40 years or older that were graded for diabetic retinopathy and AMD using standard protocols.

A sample of individuals with diabetic retinopathy was created, as was a separate sample of individuals with AMD. Individuals were categorized as "unaware of their condition" if they did not report that they had the condition.

An estimated 73% of individuals with diabetic retinopathy and 84% of individuals with AMD were unaware of their condition. The odds of unawareness of diabetic retinopathy were higher for individuals with less-severe diabetic retinopathy, shorter diabetes duration, smaller families, or who had not had a recent eye examination. The odds of unawareness of AMD were higher for individuals with "early" AMD or who were younger, less educated, or not primarily English speaking.

It was concluded that the very high frequency of unawareness of diabetic retinopathy and AMD suggests that unawareness of these conditions should be a major public health concern and that efforts are needed to increase the frequency of eye exams among those at risk for these conditions (Gibson. 2012).

The journal *PLoS ONE* reported a meta-analysis based on MEDLINE, EMBASE, and the Cochrane Library to evaluate data of diabetes as an independent factor for AMD. Reports of relative risks, hazard ratios, ORs, or evaluation data of diabetes as an independent factor for AMD were included.

In seven cohort studies, diabetes was shown to be a risk factor for AMD. Results of nine cross-sectional studies revealed consistent association of diabetes with AMD (OR, 1.21), especially for late AMD (OR, 1.48). Similar association was also detected for AMD (OR, 1.29) and late AMD (OR, 1.16) in 11 case–control studies.

The pooled ORs for risk of neovascular AMD (nAMD) were 1.10, 1.48, and 1.15 from cohort, cross-sectional, and case–control studies, respectively. No obvious divergence existed among different ethnic groups.

The authors concluded that diabetes is a risk factor for AMD, stronger for late AMD than earlier stages (Chen, Rong, Xu et al. 2014). AMD is also an independent risk factor for cardiovascular mortality in Type 2 diabetic patients: A study published in the journal *Diabetes Care* aimed to determine the evolution of visual acuity, AMD, and its relation to 10-year cardiovascular mortality and risk factors, in patients with newly diagnosed Type 2 diabetes, compared to control participants.

It was found that by the 10-year follow-up, visual acuity had declined more markedly in the diabetic patients than in the control participants. Although the frequency of AMD was nearly the same in both groups, it decreased visual acuity earlier in the diabetic patients than in the control participants. AMD at baseline predicted 10-year cardiovascular mortality independently of adjustment for other risk factors in the diabetic patients (OR, 4.7).

It was concluded that visual acuity deteriorated earlier in newly diagnosed Type 2 diabetic patients than in the control group, although the cross-sectional frequency of AMD was nearly the same in both groups. It is noteworthy that AMD was an independent risk factor for cardiovascular mortality in Type 2 diabetic patients. It is not known why that is so (Voutilainen-Kaunisto, Teräsvirta, Uusitupa et al. 2000).

The journal *Retina* reported a 10-year-long study aimed at determining the incidence of dry and wet AMD in Medicare beneficiaries either free of diabetes, diabetes without retinopathy sufferers, nonproliferative diabetic retinopathy sufferers, and proliferative diabetic retinopathy sufferers. The data were based on Medicare claimants older than 69.

It was found that newly diagnosed nonproliferative diabetic retinopathy was associated with significantly increased risk of incident diagnosis of dry AMD (hazard ratio, 1.24) and wet AMD (hazard ratio, 1.68).

Newly diagnosed proliferative diabetic retinopathy was associated with significantly increased risk of wet AMD only (hazard ratio, 2.15). Diabetes without retinopathy did not affect risk of dry or wet AMD. There was no difference in risk of wet AMD in proliferative diabetic retinopathy compared to nonproliferative diabetic retinopathy.

It was concluded that elderly persons with nonproliferative or proliferative diabetic retinopathy may be at higher risk of AMD compared to those without diabetes or diabetic retinopathy (Hahn, Acquah, Cousins et al. 2013).

5.2 CHRONIC HYPERGLYCEMIA IMPAIRS HEARING

Hearing loss is a major public health issue that is the third most common physical condition after arthritis and heart disease. About 20% of Americans, about 48 million, report some degree of hearing loss, and by the age of 65, one out of three people has some hearing loss. Sixty percent of the people with hearing loss are either in the workforce or in educational settings (http://www.hearing loss.org/content/basic-facts-about-hearing-loss; accessed 7.7.17). Gradual hearing loss can affect people of all ages—varying between mild and profound. Depending on the cause, it can be mild or severe, temporary or permanent.

The pathologic changes that accompany diabetes could plausibly cause injury to the vasculature or the neural system of the inner ear, resulting in sensorineural hearing impairment. Evidence of such pathology, including sclerosis of the internal auditory artery, thickened capillaries of the *stria vascularis*, atrophy of the spiral ganglion, and demyelination of the eighth cranial nerve, have variously been observed in autopsied patients with diabetes (Makishima, and Tanaka. 1971; Jorgensen. 1961).

There has for some time been sporadic evidence of a possible link between diabetes and hearing impairment, but it was limited to several small studies of the duration of the diabetes and the level of hearing loss: for instance, between hearing and diabetic neuropathy, in *Archives of Internal Medicine*, in 1978; hearing in diabetics, in *Acta Otolaryngologica Supplementum*, in 1978; and hearing threshold in patients with diabetes in *The Journal of Laryngology and Otology*, in 1989. *Diabetes Care* also published epidemiological evidence from one population-based cohort study in 1998 that suggested a modest association (Dalton, Cruickshank, Klein et al. 1998).

In 2008, the journal *Annals of Internal Medicine* reported a survey aimed to determine whether hearing impairment is more prevalent among US adults with diabetes than among those without diabetes. The premise underlying this survey was that there is reason to believe, based on previous reports, that the vasculature and neural systems of the inner ear may be affected by diabetes. The investigators therefore undertook a cross-sectional analysis of nationally representative data from the National Health and Nutrition Examination Survey, 1999 to 2004. Data were collected from adult participants aged 20 to 69 years old, who underwent audiometric testing.

Hearing impairment was assessed from the pure tone average of thresholds over low/mid frequencies (500, 1000, and 2000 Hz) and high frequencies (3000, 4000, 6000, and 8000 Hz), and defined for mild or greater severity (pure tone average greater than 25 decibels hearing level (dB HL) and moderate or greater severity (pure tone average greater than 40 dB HL).

It was found that for low/mid-frequency hearing impairment of mild or greater severity assessed in the worse ear, age-adjusted prevalence estimates were 21.3% among the participants with diabetes and 9.4% among the participants without diabetes.

For high-frequency hearing impairment of mild or greater severity, assessed in the worse ear, age-adjusted prevalence estimates were 54.1% among those with diabetes and 32.0% among those without it.

Adjusted ORs of 1.82 and 2.16 for the low/mid-frequency and high-frequency impairments, respectively, indicated that differences in sociodemographic characteristics, noise exposure, ototoxic medication use, and smoking did not account for the association between diabetes and hearing impairment.

Diagnosed diabetes was based on self-report and did not distinguish between Type 1 and Type 2 diabetes. Noise exposure assessments were based on participant recall. The investigators concluded that persons with diabetes have a higher occurrence of hearing impairment than those without diabetes (Bainbridge, Hoffman, and Cowie, 2008).

The journal *Laryngoscope* reported a meta-analysis of multiple databases pooled data using Cochrane's Review Manager. Hearing loss was defined by all studies as pure tone average greater than 25 dB in the worse ear.

The incidence of hearing loss ranged between 44% and 69.7% for Type 2 diabetes sufferers—significantly more frequent than in normal hearing controls (OR, 1.91). The mean pure tone audiometry thresholds were greater in the diabetes sufferers than in controls for all frequencies.

Auditory brainstem response (ABR) wave V latencies were also significantly longer in diabetics when compared to control groups (OR, 3.09). (For wave V, see below.)

The authors concluded that there is a significantly higher incidence for at least a mild degree of hearing loss in Type 2 diabetic patients, when compared to controls. Mean pure tone audiometry thresholds were greater in diabetic patients for all frequencies, but they were more clinically relevant at 6000 and 8000 Hz. Prolonged ABR wave V latencies in the diabetes group suggest retrocochlear involvement.

Age and duration of diabetes play important roles in the occurrence of diabetes-related hearing loss (Akinpelu, Mujica-Mota, and Daniel. 2014). Based on data from the Blue Mountains Hearing Study cited earlier in connection with vision, as reported in the journal *Diabetic Medicine*, it was shown that age-related hearing loss was present in 50% of diabetic participants, compared to 38.2% in nondiabetic participants (OR, 1.55) after adjusting for multiple risk factors. A relationship between diabetes duration and hearing loss was also demonstrated.

After 5 years, progression of existing hearing loss (greater than 5 dB) was significantly greater in participants with newly diagnosed diabetes (69.6%), than in those without diabetes (47.8%) over this period (adjusted OR, 2.71).

The authors concluded that Type 2 diabetes was associated with *prevalent*, but not *incident* hearing loss in an older population. Accelerated hearing loss progression over 5 years was more than doubled in persons newly diagnosed with diabetes. These data support a link between Type 2 diabetes and age-related hearing loss (Mitchell, Gopinath, McMahon et al. 2009).

A study reported in the journal *Laryngoscope* was conducted on veterans to investigate the relationship between diabetes severity and hearing in participants with and without Type 2 diabetes, who had no more than a moderate hearing loss. It was found that diabetes is associated with an increased risk of hearing loss, and this difference is manifest particularly in adults below the age of 50 (Austin, Konrad-Martin, Griest et al. 2009).

Another study was reported in the journal *Ear and Hearing* conducted on a cohort of veterans with Type 2 diabetes and relatively good hearing. Significant effects of disease severity were found for hearing thresholds at a subset of frequencies, and for one of the three Quality of Life Scale (QOL) subscales. The QOLs were adapted for use in chronic illness groups (Burckhardt, and Anderson. 2003).

Significant differences were found among those veterans with poorly controlled diabetes based on their current HbA1c. Results suggested that the observed hearing dysfunction in Type 2 diabetes might be prevented, or delayed, by tight metabolic control (Konrad-Martin, Reavis, Austin et al. 2015).

A number of reports have now confirmed the link between diabetes and hearing impairment (hypoacusia) (Vesperini, Di Giacobbe, Passatore et al. 2011; Cowie, Rust, Byrd-Holt et al. 2006). Some studies have shown that the magnitude of hearing loss in patients with diabetes is related to the duration of the disease and age, and affects principally the auditory threshold to high frequencies. (See below.)

For instance, a study in the journal *Hearing Research* reports that age-related hearing loss (presbycusis) is the number one communication disorder and a significant chronic medical condition of the aged. Up to now, however, little was known about the link between presbycusis and Type 2 diabetes, another prevalent age-related medical condition, and so the study aimed to determine the characteristics of hearing impairment in aged Type 2 diabetes sufferers. Hearing tests measuring both peripheral (cochlear) and central (brainstem and cortex) auditory processing were administered. The majority of differences between the hearing ability of the aged diabetes sufferers, and their age-matched control participants, were found in measures of inner ear function.

For all frequencies tested, diabetes participants had higher tone thresholds than nondiabetes participants, but the differences were greater at low frequencies, and they were greater for the right ear compared to the left. For example, large differences were found in pure tone audiograms, wideband noise and speech reception thresholds, and otoacoustic emissions (OAEs). An OAE is a low-level sound emitted by the cochlea either spontaneously, or evoked by an auditory stimulus.

The greatest deficits tended to be at low frequencies.

In addition, there was a strong tendency for diabetes to affect the right ear more than the left. One possible interpretation is that as one develops presbycusis, the right ear advantage is lost, and this decline is accelerated by diabetes. In contrast, auditory processing tests that measure both peripheral and central processing showed less decline between the elderly diabetes sufferers and the control group (Frisina, Mapes, Kim et al. 2006).

In another study published in *Clinical Otolaryngology and Allied Sciences*, it was also found that there is a link between the duration of diabetes and hearing loss (Tay, Ray, Ohri et al. 1995). The auditory system requires glucose and high-energy utilization for its complex signal processing. This suggests that the cochlea may be yet another target organ for the ill effects of hyperglycemias: Increased glucose exposure, even for short periods, initiates a metabolic cascade that could disrupt the cochlea both anatomically and physiologically (Jorgensen. 1961).

Hearing depends on small blood vessels and nerves of the inner ear that are affected by the high blood sugar level in diabetic patients. Outer hair cells modulate auditory reception in the inner ear: Consequently, OAE screening is commonly considered a useful index of cochlear function (Martin, Probst, and Lonsbury-Martin. 1990).

Consistent with the complications of diabetes in other organs, such as retinopathy, nephropathy, and peripheral neuropathy resulting from pathogenic changes to the microvasculature and sensory nerves, in a similar manner, diabetes leads to commonplace problems of the organs of hearing, producing symptoms such as tinnitus, dizziness, and typically bilateral and progressive hearing impairment (Lisowska, Namysłowski, Morawski et al. 2002).

5.2.1 ABR Wave V Latencies

Auditory evoked potentials are used to determine the integrity of hearing and to make inferences about how well it works. The ABR is an auditory *evoked potential* observed in ongoing electrical activity in the brain and recorded by means of electrodes placed on the scalp. The measured recording is a series of six to seven vertex positive waves, of which I through V are evaluated. These waves, labeled with Roman numerals (V is 5), occur in the first 10 ms after onset of an auditory stimulus. The ABR is considered an exogenous response because it depends on external factors (Hall. 2007; Eggermont, Burkard, and Manuel. 2007).

The auditory structures that generate the ABR are believed to be waves I through III—generated by the auditory branch of cranial nerve VIII and lower—and waves IV and V—generated by the upper brainstem (Moore. 1983; Hall. 2007; DeBonis, and Donohue. 2007). The ABR technology is used to identify the response to auditory stimulation by bypassing hearing organs and observing brain orienting response to sound stimulation.

The *Journal of Neurology and Psychiatry* reported that diabetic patients have longer latencies in the brainstem auditory evoked response than do age-matched control participants. They hold that the delay is not related to clinical hearing loss or even to blood glucose level at the time of testing, but because it occurs between waves II and V, it reflects altered transmission time in auditory brainstem and midbrain structures. This suggested to the authors the presence of a central neuropathy in patients with diabetes (Donald, Bird, Lawson et al. 1981). In a sense, they conclude that hearing loss in diabetes is a neuropathy equivalent, that is, two sides of the same coin. (Neuropathy is detailed in a following section of this chapter.)

The idea that hearing loss in diabetes is a neuropathy equivalent may be supported by the following study, and it raises the question what other impairments due to diabetes are more nearly "central"—in the sense of neuropathy—than previously thought.

The *Indian Journal of Endocrinology and Metabolism* reported a study of "Type-2 diabetes and auditory brainstem response." The objective of the study was to find evidence of central neuropathy in diabetes patients by analyzing brainstem audiometry electric response, obtained by auditory evoked potentials, to quantify the characteristic of auditory brain response in long standing diabetes.

The participants were men and women older than 30 years, with Type 2 diabetes duration greater than 5 years. The brainstem evoked response audiometry (BERA) was performed by universal smart box manual version 2.0 at 70, 80, and 90 dB. The wave latency pattern and interpeak latencies were estimated. The data were compared to those of healthy men and women control participants.

It was found that 52% of Type 2 diabetes sufferers had diabetic neuropathy, of which 92% showed abnormal BERA. In non-neuropathic participants, only 50% showed abnormal BERA.

The authors concluded that delay in absolute latencies and interpeak latencies, by BERA, demonstrates defect at the level of the brainstem and midbrain in long-standing Type 2 diabetes participants, which is more pronounced in those with neuropathy (Siddiqi, Gupta, Mohd et al. 2013).

The Greek *Hippokratia Medical Journal* featured a study that aimed to determine the impact of the duration of diabetes, and the control of hyperglycemia on the auditory function of patients with Type 2 diabetes. Using the same hearing methodology, they determined that the hearing threshold in Type 2 diabetes patients was significantly higher than normal for 1000, 2000, 4000, and 8000 Hz. In other words, their hearing was significantly poorer in that range.

Absolute latencies of brainstem auditory evoked potentials revealed significant differences between average absolute latencies for waves I, III, and V, as well as interwave latencies I to V and I to III. A significant difference was noted in the presence of transient evoked OAEs (TEOAE).

The cochlear apparatus in the ear normally does not simply receive sound but, as noted above, it also produces low-intensity sounds called "otoacoustic emissions" (OAEs). These sounds are produced specifically by the cochlea and, most probably, by the cochlear outer hair cells as they expand and contract.

There are four known OAEs. The one of concern in the study cited here is the spontaneous OAEs—sounds emitted without a sound stimulus. However, the transient OAEs, or TEOAEs, are sounds emitted in response to an acoustic stimulus of very short duration—like a click.

In the patients with poor glycemic control, where the glycated hemoglobin (HbA1c) was above 7%, the hearing threshold levels were significantly higher in both ears at 8000 Hz and at 2000 Hz in the right ear and the absolute latency of wave V was prolonged in the right ear. However, there was no evidence that the duration of diabetes significantly affected the auditory threshold absolute and interwave brainstem auditory evoked potentials latencies.

The investigators concluded that the patients displayed an increased hearing threshold, qualitative changes in brainstem auditory evoked potentials, and the absence of transitory OAEs. The duration of poorly controlled glycemia had a greater effect on auditory function in the patients than the duration of their diabetes (Zivkovic-Marinkov, Milisavljevic, Stankovic et al. 2016).

5.2.2 Hyperglycemia and Tinnitus

Tinnitus is a sound sensation that appears to be in one or both ears, occurring absent acoustic impulses from the environment. It is often referred to as "ringing in the ears," but it can also be perceived in many different ways as hissing, clicking, or whistling. It is said to be more prevalent in elderly persons. The *Brazilian Jornal da Sociedade Brasileira de Fonoaudiologia* (...of the Brazilian Society of Speech Therapy), which is dedicated to contributing to the scientific and technical knowledge in communication sciences and disorders, and associated areas, published a report titled "Prevalence of tinnitus complaints and probable association with hearing loss, diabetes mellitus and hypertension in elderly."

Tinnitus may be linked to hypertension as well as to diabetes in the elderly: The Brazilian study examined participants of both genders, older than 60 (median age = 69 years), who underwent audiological evaluation (pure tone audiometry and history) and answered a comorbidity questionnaire.

It was found that the prevalence of tinnitus was 42.77%; bilateral tinnitus, 58.68%; and unilateral tinnitus, 41.31%. There was a difference between tinnitus and hearing loss, but there was no difference between tinnitus and hypertension and between tinnitus and diabetes alone.

The authors concluded that the prevalence of tinnitus is considerable in the elderly. Furthermore, there are differences between tinnitus and hearing loss, with association between the side affected by tinnitus and the side of hearing loss. Also, only the association of diabetes and hypertension was found to be an independent risk factor for tinnitus (Gibrin, Melo, and Marchiori. 2013).

The link between tinnitus and HbA1c was detailed in the Hungarian medical journal *Orvosi Hetilap* that reported a study aimed to determine the prevalence of hearing impairment and tinnitus in Type 2 diabetes patients and to examine the possible associations between hearing impairment and/or tinnitus and increased HbA1c levels.

Patients with Type 2 diabetes, ranging in age between 33 and 88 years, were evaluated in this study at the Second Department of Medicine, Semmelweis University. The results were compared to those obtained from another sample of Type 2 diabetic men and women, ranging in age between 26 and 97 years, and nondiabetic patients ranging in age between 26 and 98 years, who participated in a comprehensive health screening program in Hungary. Hearing impairment was determined using the Interacoustics model AS608 Screening Audiometer in all patient groups. Tinnitus was evaluated with responses to a questionnaire.

It was found that hearing impairment and/or tinnitus occurred in 80% of diabetic patients, a very high proportion of Type 2 diabetic patients evaluated at the Second Department of Medicine, Semmelweis University, in comparison to 14% of nondiabetic patients enrolled in the national health screening program. There was no significant correlation between higher HbA1c levels, and hearing impairment, or tinnitus, in Type 2 diabetic patients. The investigators concluded that the prevalence of hearing impairment and tinnitus is higher, and it develops at an earlier age in patients with Type 2 diabetes (Somogyi, Rosta, and Vaszi. 2013).

Type 2 diabetes and hypertension were also shown to be closely linked. It is not surprising therefore that hypertension is also linked to tinnitus. A study published in the journal *Frontiers in Neurology* aimed to evaluate the link between arterial hypertension in tinnitus and non-tinnitus patients and to analyze differences between tinnitus impact and psychoacoustic measurements in hypertensive and normotensive patients. In addition, it aimed to evaluate the association between the presence of tinnitus and diverse antihypertensive drugs treatment.

The investigators compared two groups of participants for demographic, audiometric, and psychoacoustics characteristics—one group was tinnitus sufferers and another was a control participant group free of tinnitus. They reported that the prevalence of hypertension in tinnitus sufferers was 44.4%, as compared to 31.4% in the control participants. There was a significant positive correlation between tinnitus and hypertension, and with hypertension treatment with angiotensin-converting enzyme (ACE) inhibitors, thiazide diuretics, potassium-sparing diuretics, and calcium channel blockers.

It was concluded that a link exists between tinnitus and arterial hypertension and that it is particularly strong in older patients. The investigators also pointed out that, given that the treatment of hypertension with diuretics, ACE inhibitors, and calcium channel blockers is more prevalent in tinnitus patients, this suggests a possible ototoxicity of these drugs that needs to be investigated (Figueiredo, Azevedo, and Penido. 2016).

5.3 DIABETIC NEUROPATHY

Consistent hyperglycemia can cause nerve injury throughout the body, but it is typically observed earlier in the legs and feet. Symptoms of diabetic neuropathy can range from pain and numbness in the extremities to problems with the digestive system, urinary tract, blood vessels, and the heart. For some people, these symptoms are mild, whereas for others, they can be painful, disabling, and even fatal.

There are four main types of diabetic neuropathy that usually develop gradually and may not be noticed until there is some tissue damage:

1. Peripheral neuropathy: This is the most common form. The feet and legs are often affected first, followed by the hands and arms. Signs and symptoms of peripheral neuropathy are often worse at night, and may include the following:
   - Numbness or reduced ability to feel pain or temperature changes
   - A tingling or burning sensation
   - Sharp pains or cramps
   - Increased sensitivity to touch—for some people, even the weight of a bed sheet can be agonizing
   - Muscle weakness; loss of reflexes, especially in the ankle; loss of balance and coordination
   - Serious foot problems, such as ulcers, infections, deformities, and bone and joint pain

2. Autonomic neuropathy: The autonomic nervous system affects the heart, bladder, lungs, stomach, intestines, sex organs, and eyes. Diabetes can affect functions, possibly causing a lack of awareness of low blood sugar levels (hypoglycemia):
   - Bladder problems, including urinary tract infections or urinary retention or incontinence
   - Constipation, uncontrolled diarrhea, or a combination of these
   - Slow stomach emptying (gastroparesis), leading to nausea, vomiting, bloating, and loss of appetite; difficulty swallowing; erectile dysfunction in men; vaginal dryness and other sexual difficulties in women
   - Increased or decreased sweating; inability of the body to adjust blood pressure and heart rate, leading to sharp drops in blood pressure after sitting or standing that may cause fainting or feeling lightheaded
   - Problems regulating body temperature changes in the way the eyes adjust from light to dark; and increased heart rate when at rest

3. Radiculoplexus neuropathy (diabetic amyotrophy): This affects nerves in the thighs, hips, buttocks, or legs. Also called femoral neuropathy or proximal neuropathy, this condition is more common in people with Type 2 diabetes and older adults. Symptoms are usually on one side of the body, though in some cases, symptoms may spread to the other side.

   Most people improve at least partially over time, though symptoms may worsen before they get better. This condition is often marked by
   - Sudden, severe pain in the hip and thigh or buttock
   - Gradually developing weakness and atrophy of the thigh muscles
   - Difficulty rising from a sitting position
   - Abdominal swelling, if the abdomen is affected; and weight loss

4. Mononeuropathy: Also called focal neuropathy, it involves damage to a specific nerve, perhaps in the face, torso, or leg. It is most common in older adults and it often comes on suddenly. Although mononeuropathy can cause severe pain, it usually doesn't cause long-term problems. Symptoms usually diminish and disappear on their own over a few weeks or months. Signs and symptoms of mononeuropathy depend on the nerve involved and may include the following:
   - Difficulty focusing the eyes, double vision, or aching behind one eye
   - Paralysis on one side of the face (Bell's palsy)
   - Pain in the shin or foot
   - Pain in the lower back or pelvis
   - Pain in the front of the thigh
   - Pain in the chest or abdomen

Sometimes, mononeuropathy occurs when a nerve is compressed, as in carpal tunnel syndrome, a common type of compression neuropathy in people with diabetes. Signs and symptoms of carpal tunnel syndrome include numbness or tingling in the fingers or hand, especially in the thumb, index finger, middle finger, and ring finger; a sense of weakness in the hand; and a tendency to drop things.

5.3.1 DIABETIC PERIPHERAL NEUROPATHY

The journal *F1000 Research* recently published a report titled "Updates in diabetic peripheral neuropathy" (Juster-Switlyka and Smith. 2016). It states that diabetes causes a wide variety of acute, chronic, focal, and diffuse neuropathy syndromes, but the most common, accounting for 75% of diabetic neuropathies, is peripheral neuropathy. The other patterns of nerve injury include diabetic autonomic neuropathy, cranial neuropathy, mononeuritis multiplex, mononeuropathy, radiculo-plexus neuropathies, diabetic neuropathic cachexia, and treatment-induced neuropathy in diabetes (Tracy, and Dyck. 2008).

Preceding the joint meeting of the 19th annual Diabetic Neuropathy Study Group of the European Association for the Study of Diabetes and the 8th International Symposium on Diabetic Neuropathy in Toronto, Canada, 13 to 18 October 2009, expert panels were convened to provide updates on classification, definitions, diagnostic criteria, and treatments of diabetic peripheral neuropathies, autonomic neuropathy, painful diabetic peripheral neuropathies, and structural alterations in diabetic peripheral neuropathy.

Diabetic peripheral neuropathy was defined by the *Toronto Consensus Panel on Diabetic Neuropathy* as a "symmetrical, length-dependent sensorimotor polyneuropathy attributable to metabolic and microvessel alterations as a result of chronic hyperglycemia exposure and cardiovascular risk covariates" (Tesfaye, Boulton, Dyck et al. 2010).

Subsequently, the journal *Diabetes/Metabolism Research and Reviews* reported that diabetic peripheral neuropathy affects up to 50% of patients with diabetes. Its clinical manifestations were said to include painful neuropathic symptoms and insensitivity, which increases the risk for burns, injuries, and foot ulceration. Several recent studies had implicated poor glycemic control, duration of diabetes, hyperlipidemia (particularly hypertryglyceridemia), elevated albumin excretion rates, and obesity as risk factors for the development of diabetic peripheral neuropathy.

Although there is now strong evidence for the importance of nerve microvascular disease in the pathogenesis of diabetic peripheral neuropathy, the risk factors for painful diabetic peripheral neuropathy are not known. However, emerging evidence regarding the central correlates of painful diabetic peripheral neuropathy is now afforded by brain imaging. The diagnosis of diabetic peripheral neuropathy begins with a careful history of sensory and motor symptoms.

The quality and severity of neuropathic pain, if present, should be assessed using a suitable scale. Clinical examination should include inspection of the feet and evaluation of reflexes and sensory responses to vibration, light touch, pinprick, and the 10-g monofilament.

The authors further state that glycemic control and addressing cardiovascular risk is now considered important in the overall management of the neuropathic patient (Tesfaye, and Selvarajah. 2012). They describe the following pattern of symptom progression:

Sensory symptoms start in the toes and over time affect the upper limbs in a distribution classically described as a "stocking and glove" pattern. Motor involvement is not typically seen in the early stages of diabetic peripheral neuropathy but patients describe a range of sensory symptoms that may include loss of pain sensation or insensitivity, tingling, "pins and needles" sensation, burning, "electric shocks," painful sensations to an inoffensive stimulus, and increased sensitivity to painful stimuli.

Symptoms are typically not predictable indicators of the severity of axonal loss. Often those with the most severe painful symptoms have minimal or no sensory deficit on exam or electrodiagnostic studies (Tesfaye, and Selvarajah. 2012). However, neuropathic pain affects up to 20% to 30% of patients with diabetic peripheral neuropathy and is one of the main reasons this group seeks medical care (Tesfaye, Vileikyte, Rayman et al. 2011; Quattrini, and Tesfaye. 2003; Callaghan, Cheng, Stables et al. 2012).

5.3.2 Paradoxical Treatment-Induced Neuropathy in Diabetes—"Insulin Neuritis"

In a seemingly paradoxical relationship, both poor glucose control and rapid treatment of hyperglycemia can be associated with an increased risk of neuropathy. A clinically distinct form of neuropathy that deserves mention is treatment-induced neuropathy in diabetes (Juster-Switlyka, and Smith. 2016). This underdiagnosed iatrogenic small-fiber neuropathy is defined as the "acute onset of neuropathic pain and/or autonomic dysfunction within eight weeks of a large improvement in glycemic control specified as a decrease in glycosylated HbA1c of more than two percent points over three months."

A study published in the journal *Annals of Neurology* aimed to report the natural history, clinical, neurophysiological, and histological features and treatment outcomes in diabetes patients presenting with acute painful neuropathy, associated with glycemic control, also referred to as "insulin neuritis."

Patients with acute painful neuropathy had neurological and retinal examinations, standard laboratory studies, autonomic testing, and pain assessments over 18 months. A subsample of patients had skin biopsies for evaluation of intraepidermal nerve fiber density.

It was found that all patients developed severe pain within 8 weeks of intensive glucose control including a high prevalence of autonomic cardiovascular, gastrointestinal, genitourinary, and sudomotor symptoms (relating to sweat glands) in all patients. Orthostatic hypotension and parasympathetic dysfunction were seen in 69% of patients. Orthostatic, or postural, hypotension can manifest as weakness, dizziness, and fainting. Retinopathy worsened in all subjects.

Reduced intraepidermal nerve fiber density was seen in all tested patients. Intraepidermal nerve fibers (small fibers) innervate the skin and are involved in temperature perception, nociception (pain), and autonomic regulation. Symptoms of small fiber neuropathy correlate with a decrease in the number, density, and length of small nerve fibers in the epidermis of skin biopsy specimens.

After 18 months of glycemic control, there were substantial improvements in pain, autonomic symptoms, autonomic test results, and intraepidermal nerve fiber density. After 18 months also, greater improvements were seen in cardiovascular, gastrointestinal, genitourinary, autonomic sympathetic, and parasympathetic function tests in Type 1 than in Type 2 diabetes patients.

The authors concluded that treatment-induced neuropathy is characterized by acute, severe pain, peripheral nerve degeneration, and autonomic dysfunction after intensive glycemic control. The neuropathy occurred in parallel with worsening diabetic retinopathy, suggesting a common underlying pathophysiological mechanism. Clinical features and objective measures of small myelinated and unmyelinated nerve fibers can improve in these diabetic patients, despite a prolonged history of poor glucose control, with greater improvement seen in patients with Type 1 diabetes (Gibbons, and Freeman. 2010).

Treatment-induced neuropathy in diabetes was recognized soon after the introduction of insulin and named "insulin neuritis" (Ellenberg. 1974). It is most common in Type 1 diabetes treated with insulin, although rapid glucose correction can occur in both types of diabetes as a result of either insulin or, less frequently, oral agents.

5.3.3 Pathogenesis of Diabetic Polyneuropathy

Treating hyperglycemia in Type 1 diabetes can significantly reduce the incidence of neuropathy by up to 60% to 70%. In fact, according to the results of a study in the *New England Journal of Medicine*, intensive therapy even effectively delays the onset and slows the progression of diabetic retinopathy, nephropathy, and neuropathy (Nathan, Genuth, Lachin et al. 1993). However, glucose control in Type 2 diabetes produces only a marginal 5% to 7% reduction in the development of neuropathy. Likewise, investigators reporting in the *Lancet* found that intensive therapy did not significantly reduce the risk of advanced measures of microvascular outcomes, but delayed the onset of albuminuria and some measures of eye complications and neuropathy (Ismail-Beigi, Craven, Banerji et al. 2010).

A study conducted at the University of Michigan (Ann Arbor, Michigan), reported that over 40% of patients with diabetes develop neuropathy despite good glucose control, suggesting that other factors are driving nerve injury (Callaghan. 2015).

Type 2 diabetes is linked to obesity. About 90% of the risk of diabetes is attributable to excess weight. Thus, the notion that diabetic peripheral neuropathy results only after longstanding hyperglycemia needs reexamination because even those with good glycemic control (HbA1c of less than 5.4%) are at risk.

To that end, the EURODIAB IDDM Complications Study of the "Prevalence of diabetic peripheral neuropathy and its relation to glycaemic control and potential risk factors...." was reported in the journal *Diabetologia*. The study examined insulin-dependent patients with diabetes in treatment in European countries, assessing neurological function including neuropathic symptoms and physical signs, vibration perception threshold, autonomic function, and the prevalence of impotence. Adjustments were made for age, duration of diabetes, and HbA1c.

It was found that the prevalence of diabetic neuropathy was 28% across Europe, with no significant geographical differences.

Significant linkage was found between diabetic peripheral neuropathy by age, by duration of diabetes, by quality of metabolic control, and by height; by the presence of background or proliferative diabetic retinopathy, cigarette smoking, and high-density lipoprotein cholesterol; and by the presence of cardiovascular disease. This confirmed previously known associations.

The authors also reported finding new associations with diabetes: elevated diastolic blood pressure, severe ketoacidosis, increased levels of fasting triglycerides, and microalbuminuria (Tesfaye, Stevens, Stephenson et al. 1996). Other studies have reported oxidative stress, mitochondrial dysfunction, activation of the polyol pathway, accumulation of AGEs, and elevation of inflammatory markers (Singh, Kishore, and Kaur. 2014; Juster-Switlyka, and Smith. 2016).

REFERENCES

Achtsidis V, Eleftheriadou I, Kozanidou E, Voumvourakis KI, Stamboulis E, Theodosiadis PG, and N Tentolouris. 2014. Dry eye syndrome in subjects with diabetes and association with neuropathy. *Diabetes Care*, Oct; 37(10): e210–e211. DOI: 10.2337/dc14-0860.

Akinpelu OV, Mujica-Mota M, and SJ Daniel. 2014. Is type 2 diabetes mellitus associated with alterations in hearing? A systematic review and meta-analysis. *Laryngoscope*, Mar; 124(3): 767–776. DOI: 10.1002/lary.24354.

Al Ahmad A, Gassmann M, and OO Ogunshola. 2009. Maintaining blood–brain barrier integrity: pericytes perform better than astrocytes during prolonged oxygen deprivation. *Journal of Cellular Physiology*, Mar; 218(3): 612–622. DOI: 10.1002/jcp.21638.

Amemiya T, Yoshida H, Harayama K, and N Yokoo. 1979. Massive periretinal proliferation in retinal detachment in relation to diabetes mellitus. *Ophthalmologica*. 179(3): 148–152. DOI: 10.1159/000308883.

Araki Y, Tanaka M, and N Ebihara. 2013. Liposomes and nanotechnology in drug development: focus on ocular targets. *International Journal of Nanomedicine*, Feb: 8: 495–504. DOI: 10.2147/IJN.S30725. https://www.researchgate.net/publication/235729464_Liposomes_and_nanotechnology_in_drug_development_Focus_on_ocular_targets.

Arden GB, and S Sivaprasad. 2011. Hypoxia and oxidative stress in the causation of diabetic retinopathy. *Current Diabetes Reviews*, Sep; 7(5): 291–304. PMID: 21916837.

Armulik A, Genové G, Mäe M, Nisancioglu MH, Wallgard E, Niaudet C, He L, Norlin J, Lindblom P, Strittmatter K, Johansson BR, and C Betsholtz. 2010. Pericytes regulate the blood–brain barrier. *Nature*, Nov; 468(7323): 557–561. DOI: 10.1038/nature09522.

Austin DF, Konrad-Martin D, Griest S, McMillan GP, McDermott D, and S Fausti. 2009. Diabetes-related changes in hearing. *Laryngoscope*, Sep; 119(9): 1788–1796. DOI: 10.1002/lary.20570.

Bainbridge KE, Hoffman HJ, and CC Cowie, 2008. Diabetes and hearing impairment in the United States: audiometric evidence from the National Health and Nutrition Examination Surveys, 1999–2004. *Annals of Internal Medicine*, Jul; 149(1): 1–10. Published online 2008 Jun 16. PMCID: PMC2803029.

Bandello F, Lattanzio R, Zucchiatti I, and C Del Turco. 2013. Pathophysiology and treatment of diabetic retinopathy. *Acta Diabetologica*, Feb; 50(1): 1–20. DOI: 10.1007/s00592-012-0449-3.

Behndig A, Karlsson K, Johansson BO, Brännström T, and SL Marklund. 2001. Superoxide dismutase isoenzymes in the normal and diseased human cornea. *Investigative Ophthalmology and Visual Science*,
Sep; 42(10): 2293–2296. PMID: 11527942.

Bikbova G, Oshitari T, Tawada A, and S Yamamoto. 2012. Corneal changes in diabetes mellitus. *Current
Diabetes Reviews*, Jul 1; 8(4): 294–302. PMID: 22587515.

Bitirgen G, Ozkagnici A, Malik RA, and H Kerimoglu. 2014. Corneal nerve fibre damage precedes diabetic
retinopathy in patients with type 2 diabetes mellitus. *Diabetic Medicine*, Apr; 31(4): 431–438. DOI:
10.1111/dme.12324.

Briggs S, Osuagwu UL, and EM AlHarthi. 2016. Manifestations of type 2 diabetes in corneal endothelial cell
density, corneal thickness and intraocular pressure. *The Journal of Biomedical Research*, Jan; 30(1):
46–51. Published online 2015 Jul 8. DOI: 10.7555/JBR.30.20140075.

Bron AJ, Sparrow J, Brown NA, Harding JJ, and R Blakytny. 1993. The lens in diabetes. *Eye* (Lond). 7 (Pt 2):
260–275. DOI: 10.1038/eye.1993.60.

Burckhardt CS, and KL Anderson. 2003. The Quality of Life Scale (QOLS): reliability, validity, and utilization. *Health and Quality of Life Outcomes*, 1:60. DOI: 10.1186/1477-7525-1-60.

Callaghan BC, Cheng HT, Stables CL, Smith AL, and EL Feldman. 2012. Diabetic neuropathy: clinical manifestations and current treatments. *The Lancet. Neurology*, Jun; 11(6): 521–534. DOI: 10.1016/S1474
-4422(12)70065-0.

Callaghan BC. 2015. The impact of the metabolic syndrome on neuropathy. http://grantome.com/grant/NIH
/K23-NS079417-02; accessed 7.12.17.

Campbell M, and P Humphries. 2012. The blood–retina barrier: tight junctions and barrier modulation.
Advances in Experimental Medicine and Biology, 763: 70–84. PMID: 23397619.

Casey G. 2004. Causes and management of leg and foot ulcers. *Nursing Standard*, Jul; 18(4): 57–58.

Chen X, Rong SS, Xu Q, Tang FY, Liu Y, Gu H, Tam POS, Chen LJ, Brelén ME, Pang CP, and C Zhao. 2014.
DmMeta-analysis. *PLoS ONE,* Sep. 19. https://doi.org/10.1371/journal.pone.0108196.

Chung SS, Ho EC, Lam KS, and SK Chung. 2003. Contribution of polyol pathway to diabetes-induced oxidative stress. *Journal of the American Society of Nephrology*, Aug; 14(8 Suppl 3): S233–S236. PMID:
12874437.

Cowie CC, Rust KF, Byrd-Holt DD, Eberhardt MS, Flegal KM, Engelgau MM, Saydah SH, Williams DE,
Geiss LS, and EW Gregg. 2006. Prevalence of diabetes and impaired fasting glucose in adults in the
U.S. population: National Health and Nutrition Examination Survey 1999–2002. *Diabetes Care*, Jun;
29(6): 1263–1268. DOI: 10.2337/dc06-0062.

Craitoiu S, Mocanu C, Olaru C, and M Rodica. 2005. Retinal vascular lesions in diabetic retinopathy [article
in Romanian]. *Oftalmologia*, 49(1): 82–87. PMID: 15934345.

Cui Y, Xu X, Bi H, Zhu Q, Wu J, Xia X, Qiushi R, and PCP Ho. 2006. Expression modification of uncoupling
proteins and MnSOD in retinal endothelial cells and pericytes induced by high glucose: the role of
reactive oxygen species in diabetic retinopathy. *Experimental Eye Research*, Oct; 83(4): 807–816. DOI:
10.1016/j.exer.2006.03.024.

Dalton DS, Cruickshanks KJ, Klein R, Klein BE, and TL Wiley. 1998. Association of NIDDM and hearing
loss. *Diabetes Care*, Sep; 21(9): 1540154-4. PMID: 9727906.

DeBonis DA, and CL Donohue. 2007. *Survey of Audiology: Fundamentals for Audiologists and Health
Professionals* (2nd Ed.). Boston, MA: Allyn and Bacon.

Donald, MW, Bird CE, Lawson JS, Letemendia FJJ, Monga, TN, Surridge DHC, Varête-Cerre P, Williams,
DL, Williams DML, and DL Wilson. 1981. Delayed auditory brainstem response in diabetes mellitus.
Journal of Neurology and Psychiatry. 44: 641–644.

Ederer F, Hiller R, and HR Taylor. 1981. Senile lens changes and diabetes in two population studies. *American
Journal of Ophthalmology*, Mar; 91(3): 381–395. PMID: 7211996.

Efron N. 2011. The Glenn A. Fry award lecture 2010: ophthalmic markers of diabetic neuropathy. *Optometry
and Vision Science*, 88: 661–683.

Eggermont JJ, Burkard RF, and D Manuel. 2007. *Auditory Evoked Potentials: Basic Principles and Clinical
Application*. Hagerstwon, MD: Lippincott Williams & Wilkins.

Ellenberg M. 1974. Diabetic neuropathic cachexia. *Diabetes*, May; 23(5): 418–423. PMID: 4364389.

Enge M, Bjarnegård M, Gerhardt H, Gustafsson E, Kalén M, Asker N, Hammes HP, Shani M, Fässler R, and
C Betsholtz. 2002. Endothelium-specific platelet-derived growth factor-B ablation mimics diabetic retinopathy. *The EMBO Journal*, Aug; 21(16): 4307–4316. PMCID: PMC126162.

Figueiredo RR, Azevedo AA, and ND-O Penido. 2016. Positive association between tinnitus and arterial
hypertension. *Frontiers in Neurology*, 7: 171. DOI: 10.3389/fneur.2016.00171.

Frisina ST, Mapes F, Kim S, Frisina DR, and RD Frisina. 2006. Characterization of hearing loss in aged type II diabetics. *Hearing Research*, Jan; 211(1–2): 103–113. Epub 2005 Nov 23. DOI: 10.1016/j.heares .2005.09.002.

Funari VA, Winkler M, Brown J, Dimitrijevich SD, Ljubimov AV, and M Saghizadeh. 2013. Differentially expressed wound healing-related microRNAs in the human diabetic cornea. *PLoS ONE*, Dec 20; 8(12): e84425. DOI: 10.1371/journal.pone.0084425.eCollection 2013.

Gao F, Lin T, and Y Pan. 2016. Effects of diabetic keratopathy on corneal optical density, central corneal thickness, and corneal endothelial cell counts. *Experimental and Therapeutic Medicine*, Sep; 12(3): 1705–1710. DOI: 10.3892/etm.2016.3511.

Gibbons CH, and R Freeman. 2010. Treatment-induced diabetic neuropathy: a reversible painful autonomic neuropathy. *Annals of Neurology*, Apr; 67(4): 534–541. DOI: 10.1002/ana.21952.

Gibrin PC, Melo JJ, and LL Marchiori. 2013. Prevalence of tinnitus complaints and probable association with hearing loss, diabetes mellitus and hypertension in elderly. *CoDAS*, 25(2): 176–180. PMID: 24408248.

Gibson DM. 2012. Diabetic retinopathy and age-related macular degeneration in the U.S. *American Journal of Preventive Medicine*, Jul; 43(1): 48–54. DOI: 10.1016/j.amepre.2012.02.028.

Goldich Y, Barkana Y, Gerber Y, Rasko A, Morad Y, Harstein M, Avni I, and D Zadok. 2009. Effect of diabetes mellitus on biomechanical parameters of the cornea. *Journal of Cataract and Refractive Surgery*, Apr; 35(4): 715–719. DOI: 10.1016/j.jcrs.2008.12.013.

Goldin A, Beckman JA, Schmidt AM, and MA Creager. 2006. Advanced glycation end products: sparking the development of diabetic vascular injury. *Circulation*, Aug 8; 114(6): 597–605. DOI: 10.1161 /CIRCULATIONAHA.106.621854.

Gössl M, Malyar NM, Rosol M, Beighley PE, and EL Ritman. 2003. Impact of coronary vasa vasorum functional structure on coronary vessel wall perfusion distribution. *American Journal of Physiology - Heart and Circulatory Physiology*, Nov; 285(5): H2019–H2026. DOI: 10.1152/ajpheart.00399.2003.

Hahn P, Acquah K, Cousins SW, Lee PP, and FA Sloan. 2013. Ten-year incidence of age-related macular degeneration according to diabetic retinopathy classification among Medicare beneficiaries. *Retina*, May; 33(5): 911–919. DOI: 10.1097/IAE.0b013e3182831248.

Hall JW. 2007. *New Handbook of Auditory Evoked Responses*. Boston: Pearson.

Helbig H. 2002. Diabetic tractional retinal detachment [article in German]. *Klinische Monatsblatter fur Augenheilkunde* (Clinical Ophthalmology Monthly) Apr; 219(4): 186–190. DOI: 10.1055/s-2002-30664.

Hong SB, Lee KW, Handa JT, and CK Joo. 2000. Effect of advanced glycation end products on lens epithelial cells in vitro. *Biochemical and Biophysical Research Communications*, Aug; 275(1):53–59. PMID: 10944440 DOI: 10.1006/bbrc.2000.3245.

Huang Q, and N Sheibani. 2008. High glucose promotes retinal endothelial cell migration through activation of Src, PI3K/Akt1/eNOS, and ERKs. *American Journal of Physiology. Cell Physiology*, Dec; 295(6): C1647–1457. DOI: 10.1152/ajpcell.00322.2008.

Ismail-Beigi F, Craven T, Banerji MA, Basile J, Calles J, Cohen RM, Cuddihy R, Cushman WC, Genuth S, Grimm RH Jr, Hamilton BP, Hoogwerf B, Karl D, Katz L, Krikorian A, O'Connor P, Pop-Busui R, Schubart U, Simmons D, Taylor H, Thomas A, Weiss D, Hramiak I, and the ACCORD trial group. 2010. Effect of intensive treatment of hyperglycaemia on microvascular outcomes in type 2 diabetes: an analysis of the ACCORD randomised trial. *Lancet*. Aug 7; 376(9739): 419–430. DOI: 10.1016/S0140-6736(10)60576-4.

Jalali S. 2003. Retinal detachment. *Community Eye Health Journal*, 16(46): 25–26. PMCID: PMC1705859.

Jin YY, Huang K, Zou CC, Liang L, Wang XM, and J Jin. 2012. Reversible cataract as the presenting sign of diabetes mellitus: report of two cases and literature review. *Iranian Journal of Pediatrics*, Mar; 22(1): 125–128. PMCID: PMC3448229.

Jorgensen MB. 1961. The inner ear in diabetes mellitus. Histological studies. *Archives of Otolaryngology*, Oct; 74:373–381. PMID: 14452477.

Joussen AM, Smyth N, and C Niessen. 2007. Pathophysiology of diabetic macular edema. *Development in Ophthalmology*, 39: 1–12. DOI: 10.1159/000098495.

Juster-Switlyka K, and AG Smith. 2016. Updates in diabetic peripheral neuropathy. *Version 1. F1000Research*, 5: F1000 Faculty Rev-738. Published online 2016 Apr 25. DOI: 10.12688/f1000research.7898.1. https:// www.ncbi.nlm.nih.gov/pmc/articles/PMC4847561/

Kaji Y, Usui T, Oshika T, Matsubara M, Yamashita H, Araie M, Murata T, Ishibashi T, Nagai R, Horiuchi S, and S Amano. 2000. Advanced glycation end products in diabetic corneas. *Investigative Ophthalmology and Visual Science*, Feb; 41(2): 362–368. PMID: 10670463.

Katz J, and A Sommer. 1988. Risk factors for primary open angle glaucoma. *American Journal of Preventive Medicine*, Mar; 4(2): 110–114. PMID: 3395491.

Kim J, Kim CS, Sohn E, Jeong IH, Kim H, and JS Kim. 2011. Involvement of advanced glycation end products, oxidative stress and nuclear factor-kappaB in the development of diabetic keratopathy. *Graefe's Archive for Clinical and Experimental Ophthalmology*, 249: 529–536.

Kim YH, Kim YS, Roh GS, Choi WS, and GJ Cho. 2012. Resveratrol blocks diabetes-induced early vascular lesions and vascular endothelial growth factor induction in mouse retinas. *Acta Ophthalmologica*, Feb;90(1):e31–37. DOI: 10.1111/j.1755-3768.2011.02243.x.

Kinoshita JH, Fukushi S, Kador P, and LO Merola. 1979. Aldose reductase in diabetic complications of the eye. *Metabolism*, Apr; 28(4 Suppl 1): 462–469. PMID: 45423.

Kinoshita JH. 1965. Cataracts in galactosemia. The Jonas S. Friedenwald Memorial Lecture. *Investigative Ophthalmology*, Oct; 4(5): 786–799. PMID: 5831988.

Kinoshita JH. 1974. Mechanisms initiating cataract formation. Proctor lecture. *Investigative Ophthalmology*, Oct; 13(10): 713–724. PMID: 4278188.

Klein BE, Klein R, and KE Lee. 1998. Diabetes, cardiovascular disease, selected cardiovascular disease risk factors, and the 5-year incidence of age-related cataract and progression of lens opacities: the Beaver Dam Eye Study. *American Journal of Ophthalmology*, Dec; 126(6): 782–790. PMID: 9860001.

Klein BE, Klein R, and SE Moss. 1985. Prevalence of cataracts in a population-based study of persons with diabetes mellitus. *Ophthalmology*, Sep; 92(9): 1191–1196. PMID: 4058882.

Klein BE, Klein R, Wang Q, and SE Moss. 1995. Older-onset diabetes and lens opacities. The Beaver Dam Eye Study. *Ophthalmic Epidemiology*, Mar; 2(1):49–55. PMID: 7585233.

Klein BEK, Klein R, and MD Knudtson. 2005. Intraocular pressure and systemic blood pressure: longitudinal perspective: the Beaver Dam Eye Study. *British Journal of Ophthalmology*, Mar; 89(3): 284–287. DOI: 10.1136/bjo.2004.048710.

Knyazer B, Schachter O, Plakht Y, Serlin Y, Smolar J, Belfair N, Lifshitz T, and J Levy. 2016. Epiretinal membrane in diabetes mellitus patients screened by nonmydriatic fundus camera. *Canadian Journal of Ophthalmology*, Feb; 51(1): 41–46. DOI: 10.1016/j.jcjo.2015.09.016.

Konrad-Martin D, Reavis KM, Austin D, Reed N, Gordon J, McDermott D, and MF Dille. 2015. Hearing impairment in relation to severity of diabetes in a veteran cohort. *Ear and Hearing*, Jul–Aug; 36(4): 381–394. DOI: 10.1097/AUD.0000000000000137.

Kopsachilis N, Carifi G, and C Cunningham. 2014. Rapid exaggeration of a pre-existing epiretinal membrane following uneventful cataract surgery. *Clinical and Experimental Optometry*, Oct; 98(1): 94–96. DOI:10.1111/cxo.12222.

Kvell K, Pongrácz J, Székely M, Balaskó M, Pétervári E, and G Bakó. 2011. *Molecular and Clinical Basics of Gerontology*. Copyright © 2011 Dr. Krisztián Kvell, University of Pécs, Hungary.

Lee S-J, Park W-H, and H-I Moon. 2009. Aldose reductase inhibitors from *Litchi chinensis* Sonn. *Journal of Enzyme Inhibition and Medicinal Chemistry*, Apr; 24(4): 957–959. http://dx.doi.org/10.1080/14756360802560867.

Leske MC, Wu SY, Hennis A, Connell AM, Hyman L, and A Schachat. 1999. Diabetes, hypertension, and central obesity as cataract risk factors in a black population. The Barbados Eye Study. *Ophthalmology*, Jan; 106(1): 35–41. PMID: 9917778.

Li WC, Kuszak JR, Dunn K, Wang RR, Ma W, Wang GM, Spector A, Leib M, Cotliar AM, Weiss M, Espy J, Howard G, Farris RL, Auran J, Donn A, Hofeldt A, Mackay C, Merriam J, Mittl R, and TR Smith. 1995. Lens epithelial cell apoptosis appears to be a common cellular basis for non-congenital cataract development in humans and animals. *The Journal of Cell Biology*, Jul; 130(1): 169–181. PMCID: PMC2120521.

Lisowska G, Namysłowski G, Morawski K, and K Strojek. 2002. Otoacoustic emissions and auditory brain stem responses in insulin dependent diabetic patients [article in Polish]. *Otolaryngologia Polska*, 56(2): 217–225. PMID: 12094649.

Machemer R. 1978. Pathogenesis and classification of massive periretinal proliferation. *British Journal of Ophthalmology*, 62(11): 737–747. http://dx.doi.org/10.1136/bjo.62.11.737.

Makishima K, and K Tanaka. 1971. Pathological changes of the inner ear and central auditory pathway in diabetics. *The Annals of Otology, Rhinology, and Laryngology*, Apr; 80(2): 218–228. PMID: 5550775 DOI: 10.1177/000348947108000208.

Martin GK, Probst R, and BL Lonsbury-Martin. 1990. Otoacoustic emissions in human ears: normative findings. *Ear and Hearing*, Apr; 11(2): 106–120. PMID: 2187724.

Messmer EM, Schmid-Tannwald C, Zapp D, and A Kampik. 2010. In vivo confocal microscopy of corneal small fiber damage in diabetes mellitus. *Graefes Archive for Clinical and Experimental Ophthalmology*, 248: 1307–1312.

Mitchell P, Gopinath B, McMahon CM, Rochtchina E, Wang JJ, Boyages SC, and SR Leeder. 2009. Relationship of Type 2 diabetes to the prevalence, incidence and progression of age-related hearing loss. *Diabetic Medicine*, May; 26(5): 483–488. DOI: 10.1111/j.1464-5491.2009.02710.x.

Mitry D, Charteris DG, Fleck BW, Campbell H, and J Singh. 2010. The epidemiology of rhegmatogenous retinal detachment: geographical variation and clinical associations. *British Journal of Ophthalmology*, Jun; 94(6): 678–684. DOI: 10.1136/bjo.2009.157727.

Moore, EJ. 1983. *Bases of Auditory Brain Stem Evoked Responses*. New York: Grune and Stratton.

Mukesh BN, Le A, Dimitrov PN, Ahmed S, Taylor HR, and CA McCarty. 2006. Development of cataract and associated risk factors: the Visual Impairment Project. *Archives of Ophthalmology*, Jan; 124(1): 79–85. DOI: 10.1001/archopht.124.1.79.

Mulhern ML, Madson CJ, Danford A, Ikesugi K, Kador PF, and T Shinohara. 2006. The unfolded protein response in lens epithelial cells from galactosemic rat lenses. *Investigative Ophthalmology and Visual Science*, Sep; 47(9):3951–3959. DOI: 10.1167/iovs.06-0193.

Murakami T, Frey T, Lin C, and DA Antonetti. 2012. Protein kinase cβ phosphorylates occludin regulating tight junction trafficking in vascular endothelial growth factor-induced permeability in vivo. *Diabetes*, Jun; 61(6): 1573–1583. DOI: 10.2337/db11-1367.

Nathan DM, Genuth S, Lachin J, Cleary P, Crofford O, Davis M, Rand L, and C Siebert (Diabetes Control and Complications Trial Research Group). 1993. The effect of intensive treatment of diabetes on the development and progression of long-term complications in insulin-dependent diabetes mellitus. *New England Journal of Medicine*, Sep; 329(14): 977–986. DOI: 10.1056/NEJM199309303291401.

Nielsen NV, and T Vinding. 1984. The prevalence of cataract in insulin-dependent and non-insulin-dependent-diabetes mellitus. *Acta Ophthalmologica* (Copenh), Aug; 62(4): 595–602. PMID: 6385608.

Ookawara T, Kawamura N, Kitagawa Y, and N Taniguchi. 1992. Site-specific and random fragmentation of Cu, Zn-superoxide dismutase by glycation reaction. Implication of reactive oxygen species. *The Journal of Biological Chemistry*, Sep; 267(26):18505–18510. PMID: 1326527.

Pollreisz A, and U Schmidt-Erfurth. 2010. Diabetic cataract—pathogenesis, epidemiology and treatment. *Journal of Ophthalmology*, 2010: 608751. Published online 2010 Jun 17. DOI: 10.1155/2010/608751. PMCID: PMC2903955.

Pritchard N, Edwards K, Vagenas D, Russell AW, Malik RA, and N Efron. 2012. Corneal sensitivity is related to established measures of diabetic peripheral neuropathy. *Clinical and Experimental Optometry*, Apr; 95, pp. 355–361. DOI: 10.1111/j.1444-0938.2012.00729.x.

Quattrini C, and S Tesfaye. 2003. Understanding the impact of painful diabetic neuropathy. *Diabetes/Metabolism Research and Reviews*, Jan–Feb; 19 Suppl 1: S2–8. DOI: 10.1002/dmrr.360.

Rowe NG, Mitchell PG, Cumming RG, and JJ Wans. 2000. Diabetes, fasting blood glucose and age-related cataract: the Blue Mountains Eye Study. *Ophthalmic Epidemiology*, Jun; 7(2): 103–114. PMID: 10934461.

Shaha S, Laiquzzamana M, Cunliffea I, S Mantrya. 2006. The use of the Reichert ocular response analyser to establish the relationship between ocular hysteresis, corneal resistance factor and central corneal thickness in normal eyes. *Contact Lens and Anterior Eye*, Dec; 29(5): 257–262. https://doi.org/10.1016/j.clae.2006.09.006.

Sheibani N, Sorenson CM, Cornelius LA, and WA Frazier. 2000. Thrombospondin-1, a natural inhibitor of angiogenesis, is present in vitreous and aqueous humor and is modulated by hyperglycemia. *Biochemical and Biophysical Research Communications*, Jan; 267(1): 257–2561. DOI: 10.1006/bbrc.1999.1903.

Shenoy R, Khandekar R, Bialasiewicz A, and A Al Muniri. 2009. Corneal endothelium in patients with diabetes mellitus: a historical cohort study. *European Journal of Ophthalmology*, May; 19(3): 369–375. PMID:19396780.

Shih KC, Lam KS-L, and L Tong. 2017. A systematic review on the impact of diabetes mellitus on the ocular surface. *Nutrition and Diabetes*, 7, e251; DOI:10.1038/nutd.2017.4.

Shin ES, Sorenson CM, and N Sheibani. 2014. Diabetes and retinal vascular dysfunction. *Journal of Ophthalmic and Vision Research*, Jul-Sep; 9(3): 362–373. DOI: 10.4103/2008-322X.143378.

Siddiqi SS, Gupta R, Mohd Aslam M, Hasan SA, and SA Khan. 2013. Type-2 diabetes mellitus and auditory brainstem response. *Indian Journal of Endocrinology and Metabolism*, Nov–Dec; 17(6): 1073–1077. DOI: 10.4103/2230-8210.122629.

Singh R, Kishore L, and N Kaur. 2014. Diabetic peripheral neuropathy: current perspective and future directions. *Pharmacological Research*, Feb; 80: 21–35. DOI: 10.1016/j.phrs.2013.12.005.

Somogyi A, Rosta K, and T Vaszi. 2013. Hearing impairment and tinnitus in patients with type 2 diabetes [article in Hungarian]. *Orvosi Hetilap*, Mar; 154(10): 363–368. DOI: 10.1556/OH.2013.29562.

Stamler J, Vaccaro O, Neaton JD, and D Wentworth. 1993. Diabetes, other risk factors, and 12-yr cardiovascular mortality for men screened in the Multiple Risk Factor Intervention Trial. *Diabetes Care*, Feb; 16(2): 434–444. PMID: 8432214.

Stitt AW. 2005. The maillard reaction in eye diseases. *Annals of the NY Academy of Sciences*, Jun; 1043: 582–597. PMID: 16037281. DOI: 10.1196/annals.1338.066.

Su X, Sorenson CM, and N Sheibani. 2003. Isolation and characterization of murine retinal endothelial cells. *Molecular Vision*, May; 9: 171–178. PMID: 12740568.

Suzen S, and E Buyukbingol. 2003. Recent studies of aldose reductase enzyme inhibition for diabetic complications. *Current Medicinal Chemistry*, Aug; 10(15): 1329–1352. PMID: 12871133.

Tay HL, Ray N, Ohri R, and NJ Frootko. 1995. Diabetes mellitus and hearing loss. *Clinical Otolaryngology and Allied Sciences*, Apr; 20(2): 130–134. PMID: 7634518.

Tesfaye S, and D Selvarajah. 2012. Advances in the epidemiology, pathogenesis and management of diabetic peripheral neuropathy. *Diabetes/Metabolism Research and Reviews*, Feb; 28 Suppl 1:8–14. DOI: 10.1002/dmrr.2239.

Tesfaye S, Boulton AJM, Dyck PJ, Freeman R, Horowitz M, Kempler P, Lauria G, Malik RA, Spallone V, Vinik A, Bernardi L, P Valensi, and on behalf of the Toronto Diabetic Neuropathy Expert Group. 2010. Diabetic neuropathies: update on definitions, diagnostic criteria, estimation of severity, and treatments. *Diabetes Care*, Oct; 33(10): 2285–2293. DOI: 10.2337/dc10-1303.

Tesfaye S, Stevens LK, Stephenson JM, Fuller JH, Plater M, Ionescu-Tirgoviste C, Nuber A, Pozza G, and JD Ward. 1996. Prevalence of diabetic peripheral neuropathy and its relation to glycaemic control and potential risk factors: the EURODIAB IDDM Complications Study. *Diabetologia*, Nov; 39(11): 1377–1384. PMID: 8933008.

Tesfaye S, Vileikyte L, Rayman G, Sindrup SH, Perkins BA, Baconja M, Vinik AI, and AJ Boulton AJ; Toronto Expert Panel on Diabetic Neuropathy. 2011. Painful diabetic peripheral neuropathy: consensus recommendations on diagnosis, assessment and management. *Diabetes/Metabolism Research and Reviews*, Oct; 27(7): 629–638. DOI: 10.1002/dmrr.1225.

Tracy JA, and PJ Dyck. 2008. The spectrum of diabetic neuropathies. *Physical Medicine and Rehabilitation Clinics of North America*, Feb; 19(1): 1–26, v. DOI: 10.1016/j. pmr.2007.10.010.

Trudeau K, Molina AJ, Guo W, and S Roy. 2010. High glucose disrupts mitochondrial morphology in retinal endothelial cells: implications for diabetic retinopathy. *The American Journal of Pathology*, Jul; 177(1): 447–455. DOI: 10.2353/ajpath.2010.091029.

Vesperini E, Di Giacobbe F, Passatore M, Vesperini G, Sorgi C, and G Vespasiani. 2011. Audiological screening in people with diabetes. First results. *Audiology Research*, May 10; 1(1): e8. DOI: 10.4081/audiores .2011.e8.

Vigorita VJ, Moore GW, and GM Hutchins. 1980. Absence of correlation between coronary arterial atherosclerosis and severity or duration of diabetes mellitus of adult onset. *American Journal of Cardiology*, Oct; 46(4): 535–542. PMID: 7416013.

Voutilainen-Kaunisto RM, Teräsvirta ME, Uusitupa MI, and LK Niskanen. 2000. Age-related macular degeneration in newly diagnosed type 2 diabetic patients and control subjects: a 10-year follow-up on evolution, risk factors, and prognostic significance. *Diabetes Care*, Nov; 23(11): 1672–1678. PMID: 11092291.

Wu YC, Buckner BR, Zhu M, Cavanagh HD, and DM Robertson. 2012. Elevated IGFBP3 levels in diabetic tears: a negative regulator of IGF-1 signaling in the corneal epithelium. *The Ocular Surface*, Apr; 10(2): 100–107. DOI: 10.1016/j.jtos.2012.01.004.

Xu KP, Li Y, Ljubimov AV, and FS Yu. 2009. High glucose suppresses epidermal growth factor receptor/ phosphatidylinositol 3-kinase/Akt signaling pathway and attenuates corneal epithelial wound healing. *Diabetes*, May; 58(5): 1077–1085. DOI: 10.2337/db08-0997.

Ye H, and Y Lu. 2015. Corneal bullous epithelial detachment in diabetic cataract surgery. *Optometry and Vision Science*, Jul; 92(7): e161–e164. DOI: 10.1097/OPX.0000000000000616.

Zhu X-f, Peng J-j, Zou H-d, Fu j, Wang W-w, Xu X, and X Zhang. 2012. Prevalence and risk factors of idiopathic epiretinal membranes in Beixinjing Blocks, Shanghai, China. *PLoS ONE*, 7(12): e51445 Dec. 10. https://doi.org/10.1371/journal.pone.0051445.

Zivkovic-Marinkov E, Milisavljevic D, Stankovic, Zivic M, and M Bojanovic. 2016. Is there a direct correlation between the duration and the treatment of type 2 diabetes mellitus and hearing loss? *Hippokratia*, Jan–Mar; 20(1): 32–37. PMCID: PMC5074394.

Zou C, Wang S, Huang F, and YA Zhang. 2012. Advanced glycation end products and ultrastructural changes in corneas of long-term streptozotocin-induced diabetic monkeys. *Cornea*, Dec; 31(12): 1455–1459. DOI: 10.1097/ICO.0b013e3182490907.

6 On the Importance of Monitoring Blood Sugar and Other "Vital Signs"

He who knows others is wise; he who knows himself is enlightened.

Lao Tzu

6.1 THE IMPORTANCE OF REGULAR AND COMPREHENSIVE TESTING

Type 2 diabetes is generally attributed to the consequences of insulin resistance. This disorder has both causes and consequences. In other words, there are conditions that aggravate diabetes and, in turn, there are conditions that it aggravates. The "Complementary" management of diabetes must take into consideration both of these sets of conditions—cause and consequence—because insulin resistance is not the only factor of concern. This approach to the management of diabetes is not generally advocated, by clinicians, and that oversight may create additional complications for diabetes sufferers.

For instance, without regard for cause or consequence, Type 2 diabetes is closely linked to hypertension, elevated serum low-density lipoprotein (LDL) cholesterol and triglycerides, chronic systemic inflammation, macrovascular complications often manifesting as peripheral artery disease (PAD), low thyroid function (Wu. 2000), microvascular complications, and hearing and vision impairments, including higher risk of cataracts (Li, Wan, and Zhao. 2014), kidney stones (Torricelli, De, Gebreselassie et al. 2014), and even unexplained fatigue (Fritschi, and Quinn. 2010). Aside from routine—and occasionally not-so-routine—clinical tests, there are also self-administered tests of the magnitude of markers of some of these dysfunctions that can help with health monitoring and self-management.

The focus of this chapter is mainly on some of the tests that that shed light on glycemic and related cardiovascular status that can be self-administered. In a following chapter, complementary/integrative management strategies to counter dysfunction are proposed, and these can be implemented with the usual caveat that the implementation be done under the supervision of a qualified healthcare provider: Intervention in any medical disorder must always be done with medical supervision for a number of reasons, not the least being possible adverse interaction with medications being taken.

6.2 SELF-MONITORING OF BLOOD GLUCOSE

Self-monitoring of blood glucose is widely recognized as an important factor in effective diabetic self-management (Rodbard, Blonde, Braithwaite et al. 2007). The website, *Diabetes Self-Management*, gives the following advice regarding self-testing blood sugar level: "Unlike some other diseases that rely primarily on professional medical treatment, diabetes treatment requires active participation by the person who has it. Monitoring your blood sugar level on a regular basis and analyzing the results is believed by many to be a crucial part of the treatment equation" (Abma. May 21, 2015. https://www.diabetesselfmanagement.com/managing-diabetes/blood-glucose-management/blood -glucose-monitoring-when-to-check-and-why/; accessed 5.31.17).

When first diagnosed with diabetes, it is usually recommended to patients by their healthcare provider that they purchase a blood sugar meter (glucometer), and they may be told how and when to use it, and what numbers are desirable targets.

The recommendations may depend not only on age, gender, and state of overall health but also on the healthcare provider's understanding of what guidelines and criteria are appropriate because American diabetes-related health authorities have published slightly different recommendations regarding goals for blood sugar levels.

The following information is summarized from instructions in the journal of the American Diabetes Association (ADA), *Clinical Diabetes*, titled "Self-monitoring of blood glucose" (No authors listed. 2002).

Self-monitoring of blood glucose entails using a home glucose meter (glucometer) to check and track blood sugar levels. Being able to check blood sugar levels on a day-to-day basis can greatly improve diabetes control. Today's meters can measure blood sugar quickly and easily. There are more than 20 different meters that can be purchased in pharmacies and online. They vary in size, shape, test time, and memory features and a healthcare provider can recommend specific features to look for. Most meters now require only a very small drop of blood, and this makes testing less painful than it was in the past, and some meters can now use blood from the forearm or the thigh instead of the fingertip.

While the ADA recommends that all people with diabetes who are treated with insulin check their blood sugar, for people whose diabetes is not treated with insulin, checking blood sugar is still very helpful in deciding which medicine works best, and how much may be needed, and when over the day.

For persons who do not use insulin, how often to check blood sugar levels depends on how well the condition is controlled. If blood sugar is very well controlled, it may only be necessary to check once in a while. However, if blood sugar is not in the target range, checking more often can provide information about how to get the diabetes under better control. Most people quickly learn to use the meter and to record their results in a logbook or use their meter memory function to record results.

The value of "structured" self-monitoring is illustrated in a study published in the journal *Diabetes Care*. The purpose of the study was to determine the effectiveness of structured blood glucose testing in poorly controlled non–insulin-treated Type 2 diabetes (A1c greater or less than 7.5%). A1c is detailed below.

The participants were drawn from primary care practices in the United States. There was an active control group with enhanced usual care, or a structured testing group with enhanced usual care, and at least quarterly use of structured self-monitoring of blood glucose. Structured testing group patients and physicians were trained to collect/interpret 7-point glucose profiles, over three consecutive days.

A1c and HbA1c are interchangeable terms; Hb stands for hemoglobin.

After 12 months, there was a significantly greater reduction in mean HbA1c in the structured testing group compared to the active control group. Significantly, more patients in the structured testing group received a treatment change recommendation at the month 1 visit than did the active control group patients, regardless of the patient's initial baseline HbA1c level. Both the structured testing group and active control group patients displayed improvements in general well-being.

The investigators concluded that appropriate use of structured self-monitoring of blood glucose significantly improves glycemic control and facilitates more timely/aggressive treatment changes in non–insulin-treated Type 2 diabetes, without decreasing greater well-being (Polonsky, Fisher, Schikman et al. 2011).

The study that preceded the one cited above, the preliminary trial, was sponsored by the pharmaceutical company Hoffman-LaRoche, Ltd. The glucometer used by the participants was the Accu-Chek 360° Diabetes Management System with software. The Accu-Chek 360° Diabetes Management System delivers features that are designed to help make storing, accessing, and reviewing diabetes information simple, fast, and convenient. It has a user-friendly platform and easy-to-navigate design for use with a pc (http://www.roche.com/products/product-details.htm?productId=66d04c29-9932 -4f24-8de8-f275567cfbf7; accessed 6.2.17; Polonsky, Fisher, Schikman et al. 2010).

6.2.1 Choosing a Glucometer

The Mayo Clinic offers guidelines for choosing a suitable glucometer. See http://www.mayoclinic .org/diseases-conditions/diabetes/in-depth/blood-glucose-meter/art-20046335 (accessed 6.1.17).

Many types of blood glucose meters are available, ranging from basic models to more advanced meters with multiple features and options.

The cost of blood glucose meters and test strips varies, as does health insurance reimbursement coverage for the meter device, the test strips, and the lancets.

When using the glucometer, one usually first inserts a test strip into the meter device. Then, blood is drawn by a (clean-) finger prick with a special needle called a *lancet*. The drop of blood is applied to the test strip, and then there is a very brief period during which the meter measures the glucose content, and then a blood glucose reading appears on the screen.

Visiting the website http://thecornerinthemiddle.com/home-blood-glucose-test/ (accessed 6.2.17) provides access to numerous links to different types of commercially available glucometers.

When used and stored properly, glucometers generally tend to remain accurate in glucose measurement. Meters vary in price, and so do also lancets and test strips, but there are many to choose from online. Some meters are easier to use than others, and some meters and test strips are more comfortable and easy to hold than others. In some glucometers, the numbers on the screen are easier to read than in others. Another consideration is how big a drop of blood is required for a "reading."

Some glucometers have more advanced information storage and analysis software to track the time and date of a test, the result, and trends over time; with some meters, one can even download blood glucose readings to a computer, or mobile device, then e-mail the test results to a healthcare provider.

Lancing the finger to obtain a drop of blood is unpleasant, and it could lead to infrequent monitoring, and even noncompliance. Although finger pricks presently remain the gold standard for blood sugar monitoring, researchers are developing products designed to be "ouch"-less. They are not presently available to consumers.

6.2.2 BLOOD GLUCOSE TARGET CRITERIA

The *Diabetes Self-Management* website offers the following healthy blood sugar criteria. Self-testing values obtained by the use of a glucometer can be compared to the appropriate values shown.

Fasting:	
Normal range for a person without diabetes	70–99 mg/dL (3.9–5.5 mmol/L)
Official ADA-recommended range for someone with diabetes	80–130 mg/dL (4.5–7.2 mmol/L)
Two hours after meals:	
Normal for person without diabetes	Less than 140 mg/dL (7.8 mmol/L)
Official ADA recommendation for someone with diabetes	Less than 180 mg/dL (10.0 mmol/L)
HbA1c:	
Normal for person without diabetes	Less than 5.7%
Official ADA recommendation for someone with diabetes	7.0% or less

These blood sugar limits are for normal blood glucose levels before and after meals and recommended HbA1c levels for people with and without diabetes (based on https://www.diabetesself management.com/managing-diabetes/blood-glucose-management/blood-sugar-chart/, dated March 7, 2017, accessed 6.2.17).

6.2.2.1 HbA1c

One of the reasons for regular blood glucose level monitoring is to detect the dangerous and all too common fluctuations or swings in blood levels of glucose, especially "postprandial spikes." It is, however, desirable to determine the trend in blood glucose levels over time and the HbA1c test is routinely performed to determine that trend.

The HbA1 (*complex*) is formed when the glucose in the blood binds irreversibly (glycates) to hemoglobin. Hb is the symbol for hemoglobin and HbA1c is a component of hemoglobin to which glucose binds over time. HbA1c is also commonly referred to as "glycated" or "glycosylated hemoglobin." The HbA1c is given in percentage units in the United States, and in mmol/mol units in other countries.

The higher the glucose level in the blood, the more of it that binds to hemoglobin. Therefore, HbA1c values are proportional to the amount of glucose in the blood, over time. Hemoglobin remains glycated for the lifespan of the red blood cell, about 90 to 120 days and, therefore, the HbA1c test reflects an average blood glucose control—usually for the past 2 to 3 months.

Because red blood cells in the human body survive for 8–12 weeks before renewal, measuring glycated hemoglobin can be used to reflect average blood glucose levels over that duration, thus providing a useful longer-term gauge of blood glucose control. If blood sugar levels were elevated in recent weeks, HbA1c would also be elevated. Table 6.1 shows acceptable values for HbA1c.

The normal range for HbA1c for persons without diabetes is between 4% and 5.6%. HbA1c levels between 5.7% and 6.4% predict a higher chance of getting diabetes. Levels of 6.5%, or more, indicate diabetes.

By measuring HbA1c, clinicians can get an overall picture of what average blood sugar levels have been over a period of weeks, even months. For people with diabetes, this is important as the higher the HbA1c, the greater the risk of developing diabetes-related complications.

In fact, as reported in the journal *Diabetes Care*, the ADA recommended that HbA1c, with a cutoff point at a level greater than or equal to 6.5%, be the criterion for diagnosing diabetes as an alternative to fasting plasma glucose (FPG ≥7.0 mmol/L)–based criteria (Nathan, Balkau, Bonora et al. 2009).

The levels of HbA1c are strongly correlated with those of fasting blood glucose (Khan, Sobki, and Khan. 2007), and therefore, fasting blood glucose, 2-h post-glucose load plasma glucose, and oral glucose tolerance tests are recommended for the diagnosis of diabetes only if HbA1c testing is not possible due to unavailability of the assay, patient factors that preclude its interpretation, and during pregnancy (Herman, and Fajans. 2010).

According to a report in the journal *Biomarker Insights*, HbA1c is an important indicator of long-term glycemic control that not only provides a reliable measure of chronic hyperglycemia but also correlates well with the risk of long-term diabetes complications. Elevated HbA1c has also been regarded as an independent risk factor for coronary heart disease and stroke in people with or without diabetes.

Furthermore, HbA1c is not only a useful marker of long-term glycemic control but also a good predictor of lipid profile: monitoring HbA1c could have additional benefits of identifying those with diabetes that are at a greater risk of cardiovascular complications (Khan, Sobki, and Khan. 2007). Elevated HbA1c has been shown to be a marker of increased blood viscosity (Leiper, Lowe, Anderson et al. 1984), thus lowering red blood cell flexibility and increasing the tendency to aggregate (Watala, Witas, Olszowska et al. 1992; Sherwani, Khan, Ekhzaimy et al. 2016).

Finally, as noted in Chapter 3, hypertension is about twice as frequent in persons with Type 2 diabetes, than it is in those without it.

Formation of HbA1c is implicated in many adverse effects on the vascular endothelium, which leads to the development of hypertension in diabetes. As previously noted also, nitric oxide (NO)–dependent vasodilatation is an important factor in the maintenance and regulation of peripheral vascular tone. A study published in the *International Journal of Biomedical Science* aimed to determine the relationship between HbA1c, serum NO, and mean arterial blood pressure. The data in this study were collected from a group of persons who had diabetes and hypertension, and from a control group with diabetes but normal blood pressure.

A significant difference was found between the two groups in calculated glycosylated hemoglobin (cHbA1c), normalized mean arterial blood pressure (MAPn), and NO levels; there was a positive correlation between cHbA1c and MAPn, and there was a negative correlation between NO and MAPn and between glycosylated hemoglobin (HbA1c) and NO.

The investigators concluded that as the severity of diabetes increases, blood pressure rises mainly due to the significant decrease in available NO (Manju, Mishra, Toora et al. 2014).

TABLE 6.1

American Heart Association (AHA) Monitoring Your Blood Pressure at Home Pressure Categories Chart

Blood Pressure Category	Systolic mmHg (Upper Number)		Diastolic mmHg (Lower Number)
Normal	Less than 120	and	Less than 80
Elevated	120–129	and	Less than 80
High blood pressure (Hypertension) Stage 1	130–139	or	80–89
High blood pressure (Hypertension) Stage 2	140 or higher	or	90 or higher
Hypertension crisis (consult your doctor immediately)	Higher than 180	and/or	Higher than 120

Source: American Heart Association. *Treatment of High Blood Pressure.* With permission.

6.2.3 HBA1C TEST UNITS

Devices that assess HbA1c can be purchased online, but the manufacturer and retailer often make it clear that, while not forbidden to do so by law, they are not intended for home-use self-testing. For example, there is the "A1CNow glycated hemoglobin–HbA1c–hemoglobin A1C Multi-test system 20 tests" (Bayer). It has the following information on their website:

> The Hemoglobin A1C Test provides healthcare professionals with a fast and easy way to obtain accurate A1C results. This innovative technology enables clinicians to communicate face-to-face with patients about their diabetes. With just a fingerstick, the information is available to control diabetes in minutes, not days. The A1C blood test only requires a small blood sample to show accurate results. This small portable device can be used in multiple exam rooms and requires minimal training for use. Results are available five minutes after sticking the patient. (See the Walmart website for "A1CNow glycated hemoglobin - HbA1c - hemoglobin A1C Multi-test system 20 tests.") This unit apparently works pretty much like a home-use conventional glucometer, but some of its components need to be refrigerated.

Some units carry the designation "CLIA Waived," and this means that a CLIA test has been reviewed by the Food and Drug Administration (FDA) and Centers for Medicare and Medicaid Services. This defines the device as meant to be a simple laboratory examination and a procedure that is cleared by the FDA for home use; that it employs methodologies that are so simple and accurate so as to render the likelihood of erroneous results negligible; or that it poses no reasonable risk of harm to the user if the test is performed incorrectly (https://www.healthchecksystems.com /A1CNow_Multi_Test.cfm).

CLIA refers to the Clinical Laboratory Improvement Amendments of 1988. These are US federal regulatory standards that apply to all clinical laboratory testing performed on humans in the United States, except clinical trials and basic research.

6.2.4 How Often to Test?

It is recommended that if one has Type 2 diabetes and is using diabetes medications and insulin, one should perhaps test three or four times a day. In the case of Type 2 diabetes, using medications, and having trouble achieving good control, testing two or four times a day is recommended. If one has Type 2 diabetes and managing with diet/exercise only, there is no specific recommendation.

Recommendations vary depending on each person's situation. Many people like to do a "fasting test" when they wake up, as a gauge to start the day. If they are concerned about meal planning, they may opt to do a "preprandial" and "postprandial" test (before the meal and 2 h after), so as to do a "before-and-after" comparison.

One may test before exercise to determine that glucose is at a healthy level.

Unfortunately, health insurance companies often cover only one or two test strips a day for people with Type 2 diabetes, and this may not be sufficient. However, in some cases, insurance companies will cover more strips if a physician writes a prescription for more strips.

Health authorities generally endorse frequent monitoring regardless of type of diabetes, or method of treatment, but one study reported finding little value in monitoring for people with Type 2 diabetes who are not taking insulin (Farmer, Wade, French et al. 2009).

6.2.5 Fasting Readings, the Dawn Phenomenon

A fasting blood sugar reading, taken first thing in the morning before eating breakfast or drinking anything, gives a starting point for the day and helps to determine what happened overnight. The American College of Endocrinology recommends a target for fasting levels below 110 mg/dL, while the Joslin Diabetes Center and the ADA recommend a range of 80 to 130 mg/dL.

Readings exceeding these values may be due to the *dawn phenomenon*. Very high blood glucose in the early morning may be due to the release of certain hormones in the middle of the night. The body can make counter-regulatory hormones that work against the action of insulin. These hormones, including glucagon, epinephrine, growth hormone, and cortisol, raise blood glucose levels when needed by signaling the liver to release more glucose and by inhibiting glucose utilization throughout the body.

There is a surge in the amount of growth hormone the body releases in the middle of the night, followed by a surge in cortisol that effectively drives up glucose production in the liver. In people with Type 2 diabetes, whose liver may not respond to insulin well enough to stop glucose production, changes in glucose metabolism during sleep can have a profound effect on morning blood glucose levels. Typically, the blood glucose level rises between 4 a.m. and 8 a.m.

6.2.6 The Somogyi Effect

The *Somogyi effect*, also known as the "rebound" effect, occurs when blood glucose levels drop too low. Then, the body sometimes reacts by releasing counter-regulatory hormones, such as glucagon and epinephrine, to signal the liver to convert its stores of glycogen into glucose, raising blood glucose levels. This can result in a period of high blood sugar following an episode of hypoglycemia.

The *Somogyi effect* is most likely to occur following an episode of nighttime hypoglycemia resulting in high blood sugar levels in the morning. People who wake up with high blood sugar should check their blood glucose levels in the middle of the night (e.g., around 3 a.m.). If their blood sugar level is falling, or low, at that time, they should alert their healthcare provider with a view to implementing strategies of increasing food intake or lowering insulin dose in the evening.

6.2.7 Checking After Meals

Premeal monitoring is a critical tool in diabetes management but sometimes postmeal readings are needed. For example, postmeal readings are beneficial when a person's fasting and premeal readings are in acceptable range, but HbA1c level is high. Postmeal, or postprandial, readings are also important to assess a person's response to short-acting meds that are taken just before meals, or to the dose and timing of rapid-acting insulin given before meals.

If one chooses to monitor after the meal, timing begins at the start of the meal. Some people with diabetes monitor 1 h after the start of meals in an effort to find their peak blood sugar level and then work to prevent spikes above certain levels. However, the experts say that is not a good idea, and that there isn't any clinical, peer-reviewed, data to support monitoring at 1 h. The after-meal blood sugar goals for nonpregnant adults published by major diabetes organizations now specify that the levels should be measured 2 h after the start of a meal.

What should blood sugar level be 2 h after meals? As of 2015, American Association of Clinical Endocrinologists guidelines call for the tightest control, with 2-h readings below 140 mg/dL (Handelsman, Bloomgarden, Grunberger et al. 2015). The Joslin Diabetes Center and the ADA suggest postmeal readings below 180 mg/dL.

6.3   ARTERIAL BLOOD PRESSURE AND CHRONIC HYPERGLYCEMIA

From a practical point of view, it is not important to determine whether hypertension contributes to the onset of diabetes or whether diabetes contributes to the onset of hypertension. In any case, these two conditions are strongly linked and the combination is especially hazardous to health.

The aim of a study published in the *Journal of Hypertension* was to determine whether there exists a gender-specific association between blood pressure levels and incident Type 2 diabetes mellitus in a representative population sample.

The data were collected from several thousand men and women aged 25 to 74 years, who participated in one of the three Monitoring Trends and Determinants on Cardiovascular Diseases Augsburg (Germany) surveys between 1984 and 1995, and who were free of diabetes at baseline.

It was found that higher blood pressure levels were associated with older age, higher body mass index (BMI), a higher prevalence of dyslipidemia, and a lower prevalence of regular smoking (and high alcohol consumption by men only). Compared to individuals with normal blood pressure, the hazard ratios of incident diabetes were associated with an optimal blood pressure and high normal blood pressure, and hypertension were 0.67, 1.76, and 1.93 for men and 0.74, 1.07, and 2.05 for women. The association was present in the subgroup with low BMI as well as in the group with high BMI, supporting the assumption that blood pressure may contribute to the manifestation of Type 2 diabetes, independent of BMI.

The authors concluded that established hypertension was significantly associated with incident Type 2 diabetes in men and women from the general population, whereas high normal blood pressure significantly increased the risk of diabetes in men only (Meisinger, Döring, and Heier. 2008).

A study titled "Blood pressure lowering in type 2 diabetes: a systematic review and meta-analysis" appeared in the *Journal of the American Medical Association* in 2015. It aimed to determine the associations between blood pressure–lowering treatment and vascular disease in Type 2 diabetes.

The investigators reported that each 10 mmHg of lower systolic blood pressure was associated with a significantly lower risk of mortality; absolute risk reduction in events per 1000 patient-years and cardiovascular events; and absolute risk reduction in coronary heart disease, stroke, and retinopathy.

The authors concluded that in patients with Type 2 diabetes, lowering blood pressure is associated with decreased mortality and other clinical outcomes, with lower risk reduction observed among those with baseline blood pressure of 140 mmHg and higher (Emdin, Rahimi, Neal et al. 2015).

The standard blood pressure target currently recommended is less than 130/80 mmHg for the general population of people with elevated blood pressure. However, another study published in *Cochrane Database of Systematic Reviews*, concerning blood pressure targets for people with Type 2 diabetes, aimed to determine whether achieving targets lower than the standard target will reduce mortality and morbidity in those with elevated blood pressure and diabetes.

The authors concluded that at the present time, evidence from randomized trials does not support blood pressure targets lower than the standard targets in people with elevated blood pressure and diabetes (Arguedas, Leiva, and Wright. 2013). That being said….

6.3.1 SELF-MONITORING BLOOD PRESSURE

The American Heart Association (AHA) recommends home monitoring for all people with high blood pressure. In choosing a home blood pressure monitor, the AHA recommends an automatic, cuff-style, bicep (upper-arm) monitor because wrist and finger monitors yield less reliable readings.

When selecting a blood pressure monitor, it is essential to determine that the cuff fits the arm. It is also recommended that the home user bring the instrument to the next appointment with a healthcare provider to calibrate it with a conventional aneroid sphygmomanometer.

6.3.1.1 On Using a Home Blood Pressure Monitor

The following recommendations to the user are intended to ensure proper use of the unit:

*   Be still.
*   Don't smoke, drink caffeinated beverages, or exercise within 30 min before measuring blood pressure.
*   Sit with your back straight and supported (on a dining chair, rather than a sofa). The feet should be flat on the floor, and the legs should not be crossed. The arm with the cuff should be supported on a flat surface (such as a table) with the upper part of the arm at heart level.
*   Make sure that the middle of the cuff is placed directly above the eye of the elbow (check the monitor instructions for an illustration, or have a healthcare provider demonstrate use).
*   Measure at the same time every day (it is important to take the readings at the same time each day, such as morning and evening, or as the healthcare professional recommends).

An illustration of blood pressure self-measurement positioning with a self-inflatable cuff can be found online. For instance:

*   http://drrajivdesaimd.com/2014/10/02/self-measurement-of-blood-pressure-smbp/
*   https://jamanetwork.com/journals/jama/fullarticle/2643764 (available also in Spanish)

It is advisable to take two or three readings, 1 min apart, at each measure session and record the results using a printable or online tracker. If the monitor has built-in memory to store readings, it can be taken to the next appointment with a healthcare provider. Some monitors may also allow uploading readings to a secure website after registering profile (http://www.heart.org/HEARTORG /Conditions/HighBloodPressure/KnowYourNumbers/Monitoring-Your-Blood-Pressure-at-Home _UCM_301874_Article.jsp#.WTNHrOQ2zcs; accessed 6.4.17)

6.3.1.2 "Know Your Numbers"

In general, people with atrial fibrillation, or other arrhythmias, may be poor candidates for home monitoring because in such cases, home blood pressure devices may not give accurate readings. Also, several studies have shown that it is normal to have blood pressure variation between the right and the left arm: A difference of 10 mmHg, or less, is considered normal and is not a cause for concern.

In November 2017, health authorities lowered the cutoff range to 130/80, as noted above. This new criterion is controversial.

6.3.2 PERIPHERAL AND MICROVASCULATURE ARTERIAL BLOOD VESSEL DISEASE—THE ANKLE–BRACHIAL (BLOOD PRESSURE) INDEX

The ankle–brachial pressure index, or ankle–brachial index (ABI), is the ratio of the blood pressure at the ankle to the blood pressure in the upper arm (brachium). Compared to the arm, lower blood pressure in the leg suggests blocked arteries due to PAD.

Because chronic hyperglycemia jeopardizes endothelium function and NO formation, it may result in damage to ordinary distal arterial blood vessels as well as to micro blood vessels throughout the body. "Distal" blood vessels are defined here as those in the extremities, that is, feet and hands. This kind of impairment is commonly known as PAD, for which there is a high risk in diabetes, and it is technically defined as "atherosclerotic occlusive disease of lower extremities."

People with PAD are at increased risk of heart attack, stroke, and death (No authors listed. 2003; Thiruvoipati, Kielhorn, and Armstrong. 2015). However, the damage of diabetes to blood vessels is not limited to the extremities, as noted in a report in *PLoS ONE*: The aim of the study cited was to determine whether PAD indicated by abnormally low or high ABI is associated with different stages of diabetic retinopathy in patients with Type 2 diabetes.

Men and women patients with Type 2 diabetes who underwent ABI measurement in an outpatient clinic were enrolled in the study. PAD was defined as ABI less than 0.9 or greater than or equal to 1.3 in either leg. Diabetic retinopathy was classified as nondiabetic retinopathy, nonproliferative diabetic retinopathy, and proliferative diabetic retinopathy stages.

The prevalence of ABI less than 0.9 or greater than or equal to 1.3 in either leg was 3.0%. Analysis showed that proliferative diabetic retinopathy was associated with abnormal ABI, whereas nonproliferative diabetic retinopathy was not. Furthermore, the presence of coronary artery disease, cerebrovascular disease, and declining kidney function in patients without diuretics use was associated with abnormal ABI in patients with proliferative diabetic retinopathy.

This study on Type 2 diabetes patients demonstrated that PAD was associated with proliferative diabetic retinopathy and, therefore, the ABI test was recommended for this population at risk (Chen, Hsiao, Huang et al. 2015).

6.3.2.1 The ABI Self-Test

The ABI test for peripheral vascular disease consists of blood pressure readings in the arms compared to readings in the ankles. It can be done at home and, while it may not be quite as accurate as if it were done in the office of a healthcare provider, if sufficient care is taken, it may be quite adequate.

The website Diabetes Self-Management makes the following recommendations: The ABI test takes about 20 to 30 min. First, the person lies down for about 10 min to equalize the effect of gravity on blood pressure in the arms and legs. Then, a blood pressure cuff is used to measure blood pressure in the arms and at the ankles. Systolic blood pressure at the ankles, lower than that in the arms, may be taken as evidence of possible peripheral vascular disease (https://www.diabetesselfmanagement.com/diabetes-resources/definitions/ankle-brachial-index/; accessed 6.4.17).

Using an electronic self-inflating cuff—in a supine position (lying down, face up), the blood pressure cuff is placed and inflated near the artery in the arm or in the leg as shown in Figure 6.1. The ABI is the ratio of the blood pressure in the lower legs to that in the arms, and it is calculated by dividing the systolic blood pressure at the ankles by the systolic blood pressures in the arms (Al-Qaisi, Nott, King et al. 2009).

Inflation is allowed to cycle, and when it ends, the blood pressure reading is recorded. This procedure is followed for the right and left arm and leg. The index is calculated as follows:

$$\text{ABPI}_{\text{Leg}} = \frac{P_{\text{Leg}}}{P_{\text{Arm}}},$$

where P_{Leg} is the systolic blood pressure of *dorsalis pedis* or posterior tibial arteries and P_{Arm} is the highest of the left and right arm brachial systolic blood pressure.

The higher of two systolic readings of the left and right arm brachial artery is generally used in the assessment. The pressures in each foot posterior *tibial* artery and *dorsalis pedis* artery are measured with the higher of the two values used as the ABI for that leg (Fried. 2014; McDermott, Criqui, Liu et al. 2000).

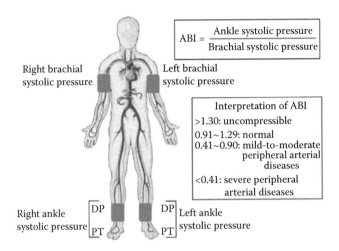

FIGURE 6.1 Measurement of the ABI. DP indicates dorsalis pedis artery, PT is posterior tibial artery. (From Li, Wang, Zhang et al. 2013. Why is ABI effective in detecting vascular stenosis? Investigation based on Multibranch Hemodynamic Model. *The Scientific World Journal*, 2013. With permission.)

Generally, ABI scores are interpreted as follows:

- Less than 0.40 = severe obstruction
- 0.41–0.70 = moderate obstruction
- 0.71–0.90 = mild obstruction
- Greater than 0.90 = normal
- Greater than 1.3 = elevated, incompressible vessels

(For further details, see No authors listed [2012])

There is also an ABI chart for direct determination of ABI: go to https://www.vitalitymedical .com/pdf/summitdoppler-lifedop-abi-calculation-chart.pdf (accessed 2.5.18). One can determine ABI by finding the appropriate arm (brachial) blood pressure in the column on the left and the corresponding leg (brachial) blood pressure in the row at the top of the chart. The column/row intersection is the ABI.

Studies have shown the sensitivity of the ABI to be about 90%, with a corresponding 98% specificity for detecting serious abnormal narrowing in major leg arteries, defined by angiogram (Bernstein, and Fronek. 1982). The ABI typically reported in published clinical studies is not obtained with an automated blood pressure cuff but rather with a sphygmomanometer, or other medical-grade blood pressure device, and systolic pressure is determined with the help of a Doppler device.

The journal *Archives of Cardiovascular Diseases* reported a study titled "Accuracy of ABI using an automatic blood pressure device to detect peripheral artery disease in preventive medicine." The authors concluded that the correlations between the automatic and Doppler methods were good in left and right legs.

In participants with an abnormal automatic index, correlations with Doppler indexes were good in both legs. In terms of detecting an abnormal index in a routine preventive examination, the automatic method had good sensitivity (92%), specificity (98%), positive predictive value (86%), negative predictive value (99%), and accuracy (97%) compared with the Doppler method.

Good results were obtained in participants with an abnormal index with regard to agreement and concordance with the Doppler method (Benchimol, Pillois, Benchimol et al. 2009).

There are, however, concerns about the trustworthiness of the index in certain clinical conditions where, for instance, there may be significant hardening of the arteries, and in some cases, in diabetes. However, they do not detract from the present message that ABI has shown to be a useful index to the severity of conditions that impair endothelial function, especially conditions such as Type 2 diabetes.

A study titled "Ankle-arm index as a marker of atherosclerosis in the Cardiovascular Health Study" was conducted by the Cardiovascular Heart Study (CHS) Collaborative Research Group and published in the journal of the AHA, *Circulation*.

An inverse response relationship was found between the ABI (here labeled "ankle-arm index") and the cardiovascular risk factors, and subclinical and clinical cardiovascular disease among older adult participants. The lower the ABI, the greater the risk of cardiovascular disease. However, it was also the case that even those who are asymptomatic but have modest reductions in the ABI (0.8 to 1.0) appear to be at increased risk of cardiovascular disease (Newman, Siscovick, Manolio et al. 1993).

Another study in the journal *Angiology* aimed to determine the link between high ABI and cardiovascular disease, and PAD in Chinese patients with Type 2 diabetes. The ABI was measured, and foot inspection was performed in these outpatients.

Compared to the normal ABI group, it was found that the high ABI (greater than 1.3) group had a higher prevalence of cardiovascular disease and PAD, but lower than the low ABI (less than or equal to 0.9) group. High ABI was an independent risk factor for the development of cardiovascular disease and PAD.

It was also determined that the optimal cutoff of high ABI to predict cardiovascular disease and PAD was 1.43 and 1.45, respectively. The odds ratio of high ABI for cardiovascular disease and PAD was 2.25 and 6.97, respectively, after adjusting for other confounding risk factors (Li, Zeng, Liu et al. 2015).

6.3.2.2 The ABI in Diabetes

Although only a very small sample of studies are cited here for evidence-based support of the value of the ABI in substantiating micro- and macrovascular problems and cardiovascular hazard, it is clear that the ABI yields valuable information specific to Type 2 diabetes.

The aim of a study published in the journal of the Czech Society of Internal Medicine (*Vnitrni Lekarstvi*) was to determine the association between the low ABI (less than 0.9) and the cardiovascular risk in Type 2 diabetes men and women patients.

An ABI below 0.9 was found in older men with higher elevated coronary calcium score, higher total cholesterol, and higher total homocysteine, by comparison with those with an ABI lower than or equal to 0.9. Many cardiovascular risk factors correlated positively with low ABI (below 0.9), and it was independently associated with age, smoking, LDL cholesterol level, total homocysteine, and coronary calcium score.

Low ABI (below 0.9) predicted ischemic stroke in Type 2 diabetes patients and manifest cardiovascular disease in the following 3 years. Curiously, no correlation was found between ABI and the high-sensitivity C-reactive protein (hsCRP) (Nussbaumerová, Rosolová, Ferda et al. 2011).

A study published in the journal *International Angiology* was titled "ABI in a type 2 diabetic population with proliferative retinopathy: associated risk factors and complications." The study examined low ABI in a Type 2 diabetes population with proliferative retinopathy. Participants with an ABI, measured with a Doppler device, shown to be less than 0.9, were diagnosed with peripheral vascular disease. The exclusion criterion was medial coronary artery calcification.

The average age and diabetes duration were 65 ± 9.7 years and 18.6 ± 9.1 years, respectively. ABI below 0.9 was associated with increasing age, diabetes duration, higher total and LDL cholesterol, higher erythrocyte sedimentation rate (ESR is the rate at which red blood cells settle at the bottom of a test tube in 1 h), and lower eGFR. Sedimentation rate is a nonspecific measure of inflammation; eGFR is the estimated kidney glomerular filtration rate, which tells how well the kidneys are working. It is based on the blood level of creatinine, a by-product of muscle function. BMI, waist index, fasting plasma glucose, and HbA1c were significantly lower in patients with peripheral vascular disease.

The investigators concluded that increasing age, total cholesterol levels, and vibration perception threshold, together with declining renal function and lower BMI, are independent predictors of peripheral vascular disease in a Type 2 diabetes population with advanced microvascular disease (Magri, Calleja, Buhagiar et al. 2012). The vibration perception threshold is a test for loss of cutaneous sensitivity, and it is also correlated with BMI in Type 2 diabetes (Shen, Liu, Zeng et al. 2012).

As previously noted, there is a strong link between Type 2 diabetes and atherosclerosis, and there is a strong link also between both atherosclerosis and Type 2 diabetes, and systemic inflammation. It is particularly interesting, therefore, that a study published in the *Journal of Clinical and Diagnostic Research* addressed the strength of the link between the ABI in Type 2 diabetes and the hsCRP test providing a marker of systemic inflammation.

The study aimed to compare the ABI and the hsCRP in Type 2 diabetes patients between 45 and 60 years old, to comparable healthy participants, and to determine the association of serum hsCRP with ABI in the Type 2 diabetes patients and in the healthy participants.

The serum hsCRP levels were determined by conventional laboratory methods and the ABI values were determined with the NICOLET VERSALAB Doppler unit. It was found that the ABI was significantly low, and the serum hsCRP was significantly elevated in the Type 2 diabetic patients, compared to comparable values in the healthy participants. There was also a significant inverse relationship between ABI and hsCRP in the Type 2 diabetes patients that was not observed in the healthy participants.

These data led to the conclusion that since elevated serum hsCRP is a key element in Type 2 diabetes patients, inflammation may play an important role in the pathogenesis of atherosclerosis (Thejaswini, Roopakala, Dayananda et al. 2013).

6.3.2.3 The ABI and Microalbuminuria

The ADA recommends an annual microalbuminuria test for people between the ages of 12 and 70 who have been diagnosed with Type 1 or Type 2 diabetes. This is also known as the albumin-to-creatinine ratio test or the urine albumin test. Microalbuminuria is a subtle increase in the urinary excretion of the protein albumin that cannot be detected by a conventional assay. In diabetes, microalbuminuria is an early sign of diabetic kidney disease: The normal urinary albumin is less than 30 mg per 24 h, and 300 mg or more of urinary albumin per day is considered gross albuminuria.

According to a report in the journal *Diabetes Care*, albuminuria has also been shown to predict cardiovascular outcomes in diabetic populations and that reducing it leads to reduced risk of adverse kidney and cardiovascular events (Basi, Fesler, Mimran et al. 2008; Brenner, Cooper, de Zeeuw et al. 2001; Lewis, Hunsicker Clarke et al. 2001; Parving, Lehnert, Brochner-Mortensen et al. 2001; Ibsen, Olsen, Wachtell et al. 2005).

A study reported in the *Iranian Journal of Kidney Diseases* aimed to determine the value of the ABI for predicting microalbuminuria in Type 2 diabetic patients.

Measurement of ABI with color Doppler ultrasonography was carried out on patients with Type 2 diabetes. An ABI of less than 0.9 was defined as the predictive marker for atherosclerosis. Microalbuminuria and risk factors of atherosclerosis were compared in the patients on the basis of their ABI. The mean ABI was 1.1 ± 0.2, and 20% had an abnormal ABI (less than 0.9). A significant correlation was found between ABI and microalbuminuria.

The investigators concluded that the ABI is a reliable noninvasive assay of peripheral and cardiovascular complications and also early-stage nephropathy in diabetic patients (Makhdoomi, Mohammadi, Yekta et al. 2013).

6.3.2.4 ABI Alerts to Postprandial Elevated Lipids

The focus on abnormal postprandial status in diabetes is commonly on hyperglycemia, even though its connection to atherosclerosis is well documented. A review in the *World Journal of Diabetes* reports that PAD, as it is manifested as intermittent claudication, or critical limb ischemia, or identified by an ABI less than 0.9, is observed to be present in at least one in every four patients with Type 2 diabetes.

Several reasons explain PAD in diabetes: hyperglycemia, smoking, and hypertension, and the dyslipidemia that accompanies Type 2 diabetes, including increased triglyceride levels and reduced high-density lipoprotein (HDL) cholesterol concentrations, all seem to contribute to this association.

Postprandial lipidemia has come to the forefront as a result of more recent studies showing that nonfasting triglycerides predict the onset of arteriosclerotic cardiovascular disease better than fasting measurements do. Also, postprandial particle markers such as apolipoprotein B-48 (apo B-48) makes it easier and simpler to examine the postprandial phenomenon.

Nevertheless, relatively few studies have evaluated the role of postprandial triglycerides in the development of PAD and Type 2 diabetes. The purpose of the following review was to examine the epidemiology and risk factors of PAD in Type 2 diabetes, focusing on the role of postprandial triglycerides and particles (Valdivielso, Ramírez-Bollero, and Pérez-López. 2014).

In fact, a study published in the *International Journal of Clinical Chemistry* (*Clinica Chimica Acta*), previously conducted by the same team of investigators, aimed to determine the potential of apo B-48 to establish the presence of subclinical PAD: The participants were patients with Type 2 diabetes and healthy control participants free of clinical cardiovascular disease.

The principal outcome measures were to be the presence of subclinical PAD as evidenced by the ABI, and the intestinal particles measured as the concentration of apo B-48 at fasting and 4 h after a mixed breakfast.

It was found that no control participants had subclinical PAD. One-fifth of the diabetic patients had subclinical PAD. The levels of apo B-48, both fasting and postprandial, were only significantly raised in the diabetic patients who had PAD. The diabetic patients without vascular disease had apo B-48 concentrations similar to that of the controls.

The analysis also showed that only smoking and postprandial B-48 levels, in addition to diabetes, were independently associated with PAD. On the other hand, PAD, but not diabetes, was associated with the fasting and postprandial levels of apo B-48.

It was therefore concluded that apo B-48 levels might be a marker of occult PAD in patients suffering from Type 2 diabetes and that subclinical PAD should therefore be considered in studies on postprandial lipidemia involving patients with diabetes (Valdivielso, Puerta, Rioja et al. 2010).

6.4 CHRONIC HYPERGLYCEMIA AND LIPID PROFILE

Lipid profile or "lipid panel" is a set of blood test values that serves as an initial broad medical screening tool for abnormalities in lipids, such as cholesterol and triglycerides. An undesirable lipid profile is a common feature of Type 2 diabetes.

According to a report in the journal *Nature Reviews Endocrinology*, the major features of diabetic dyslipidemia are as follows:

- Elevated total cholesterol
- High plasma triglyceride concentration
- Low HDL cholesterol concentration
- Higher concentration of small dense LDL cholesterol particles

The website *Lab Test Online* (https://labtestsonline.org/understanding analytes/lipid/tab/test/) lists the following criteria:

LDL cholesterol:
- Optimal: Less than 100 mg/dL (2.59 mmol/L); for those with known disease (ASCVD or diabetes), less than 70 mg/dL (1.81 mmol/L) is optimal.
- Near/above optimal: 100–129 mg/dL (2.59–3.34 mmol/L).
- Borderline high: 130–159 mg/dL (3.37–4.12 mmol/L).
- High: 160–189 mg/dL (4.15–4.90 mmol/L).
- Very high: Greater than 190 mg/dL (4.90 mmol/L).

Total cholesterol:
- Desirable: Less than 200 mg/dL (5.18 mmol/L)
- Borderline high: 200–239 mg/dL (5.18 to 6.18 mmol/L)
- High: 240 mg/dL (6.22 mmol/L) or higher

HDL cholesterol:
- Low level, increased risk: Less than 40 mg/dL (1.0 mmol/L) for men and less than 50 mg/dL (1.3 mmol/L) for women
- Average level, average risk: 40–50 mg/dL (1.0–1.3 mmol/L) for men and 50–59 mg/dL (1.3–1.5 mmol/L) for women
- High level, less than average risk: 60 mg/dL (1.55 mmol/L) or higher for both men and women

Fasting triglycerides:
- Desirable: Less than 150 mg/dL (1.70 mmol/L)
- Borderline high: 150–199 mg/dL (1.7–2.2 mmol/L)
- High: 200–499 mg/dL (2.3–5.6 mmol/L)
- Very high: Greater than 500 mg/dL (5.6 mmol/L)

Non-HDL cholesterol:
- Optimal: Less than 130 mg/dL (3.37 mmol/L)
- Near/above optimal: 130–159 mg/dL (3.37–4.12 mmol/L)
- Borderline high: 160–189 mg/dL (4.15–4.90 mmol/L)
- High: 190–219 mg/dL (4.9–5.7 mmol/L)
- Very high: Greater than 220 mg/dL (5.7 mmol/L)

The lipid changes associated with diabetes are said to be due to increased free fatty acid flux secondary to insulin resistance.

The prevalence of elevated serum cholesterol is not increased in patients with diabetes, but mortality from coronary heart disease increases exponentially as a function of serum cholesterol levels. However, lowering cholesterol with statins may reduce diabetic patients' relative cardiovascular risk (Mooradian. 2009).

The aim of a study of dyslipidemia reported in the *Indian Journal of Pharmaceutical Science* was to determine the lipid profile of Type 2 diabetic and age-/gender-matched healthy participants, and its association to fasting plasma glucose in clinically diagnosed diabetic participants. The fasting plasma glucose and lipid profiles were compiled for both diabetic and healthy volunteers. The blood samples were analyzed for fasting plasma glucose, total cholesterol, triglycerides, HDL cholesterol, LDL cholesterol, and very low density lipoprotein cholesterol. The levels of HDL cholesterol and LDL cholesterol were found to be significantly low in diabetics, and participants with lower LDL cholesterol were on statins.

Despite lower lipid values, the risk ratio for diabetics was significantly higher. There was a significant difference between fasting plasma glucose, lipid parameters, and risk ratios in the two groups.

Diabetic participants with lower HDL cholesterol and higher total cholesterol have a higher risk ratio, pointing to the need of non-statin HDL-raising medications in order to decrease their predisposition to cardiovascular disorders. Thus, the study points to an altered pattern of lipid profile with fasting plasma glucose in diabetics and their increased risk of cardiovascular disorders (Khadke, Harke, Ghadge et al. 2015).

The importance of regular testing cannot be overestimated: A report in the journal *Atherosclerosis. Supplement* informs us that

Patients with Type 2 diabetes have an atherogenic lipid profile which greatly increases their risk of coronary heart disease (CHD) compared with people without diabetes. The largest disparity in lipid levels among people with, and those without diabetes, occurs for high-density lipoprotein cholesterol (HDL-C) and triglycerides: triglycerides tend to be markedly higher and HDL-C moderately lower in patients with diabetes, in contrast to the negligible difference observed in low-density lipoprotein cholesterol (LDL-C) and total cholesterol. However, patients with Type 2 diabetes are more likely to have the atherogenic form of LDL-C than people without diabetes, as well as low HDL-C, which restricts reverse cholesterol transport, and may also be associated with increased lipid oxidation. Among patients who have suffered a myocardial infarction, increased LDL-C is apparent in early adulthood, whereas a detectable difference in HDL-C levels becomes increasingly apparent with age and most pronounced after age 60 years, compared with healthy controls. It should be noted that evidence indicates that the increased risk of macrovascular complications of Type 2 diabetes begins long before the onset of clinical hyperglycemia. Therefore, despite successful reduction of LDL-C with statin therapy, patients continue to be at increased risk for coronary heart disease if their HDL-C levels remain suboptimal, in part due to persistence of enhanced lipid exchange. (From Windler E. 2005. *Atherosclerosis. Supplement*, Sep; 6(3): 11–14. With permission.)

6.4.1 Cholesterol Self-Testing

Cholesterol self-test kits are available online for purchase by consumers. Enter: "home cholesterol self test kit." One can purchase one of these test kits for home use and track lipids levels. One can purchase an analyzer and a few test strips may (or they may not) be included. The test strips are usually expensive and they are not reusable. In addition, few units seem to measure small particle cholesterol.

Unlike glucometers and test strips, most health insurance plans, including Medicare, do not reimburse any part of the cost of cholesterol self-test kits.

6.5 THYROID DYSFUNCTION AND TYPE 2 DIABETES

Type 2 diabetes is frequently present in patients with hypertension, atherosclerosis, coronary heart disease, kidney disease, PAD, macro- and microvasculature impairment, endothelium impairment, vision loss, thyroid dysfunction, and even cataract formation.

The complete list includes other less well-known conditions such as periodontitis, a gum disease, usually attributed to poor oral hygiene and, parenthetically, widely recognized to be a risk for diabetes and heart disease. In fact, one of the most often cited culprits in periodontitis is *Staphylococcus aureus*, a common resident in gum epithelial tissue (Colombo, Barbosa, Higashi et al. 2013). A report in the *Danish Medical Journal* finds that diabetes is strongly associated with an increased risk of *S. aureus* (Smit. 2017).

However, a study published in the journal *Circulation* that reported finding many varieties of bacteria, including *Chlamydia*, and various types of *Staphylococcus*, in atherosclerotic plaques, reported that it could not be concluded that their presence indicated causality. In fact, they concluded that "bacterial agents could have secondarily colonized atheromatous lesions and could act as an additional factor accelerating disease progression" (Ott, El Mokhtari, Musfeldt et al. 2006).

It is rarely mentioned that Type 2 diabetes is linked to thyroid dysfunction, that thyroid dysfunction needs to be addressed, and that there exists a self-administered test for that condition that can be done at home.

The journal *Clinical Diabetes* published a comprehensive report in 2000, titled "Thyroid disease and diabetes." The report tells us that diabetic patients have a higher prevalence of thyroid disorders compared with the nondiabetic population. In fact, thyroid disease in the general population is about 6.6%.

6.5.1 How Thyroid Dysfunction May Affect Persons with Chronic Hyperglycemia

The presence of thyroid dysfunction may affect diabetes by worsening glycemic control and in some cases requiring increased insulin. It entails an underlying increased hepatic gluconeogenesis, rapid gastrointestinal glucose absorption, and increased insulin resistance.

The pituitary gland produces the thyroid-stimulating hormone (TSH), which signals the thyroid gland to release the hormone thyroxine, also known as T4 because it has four iodine molecules. The T4 has to be converted to triiodothyronine (T3) because T3 is the active thyroid hormone.

The TSH level in blood reveals how much the pituitary gland is signaling the thyroid gland to release T4. If TSH levels are abnormally high—a normal level for TSH being 0.4 milliunits per liter (mU/L) to 4.0 mU/L—it could mean that the thyroid is underactive. TSH levels are inversely related to thyroid hormone level.

The aim of a study published in the journal *Diabetes Research* was to determine the prevalence of abnormal TSH concentrations in patients with Type 2 diabetes using a sensitive immunometric assay. The study population consisted of men and women with Type 2 diabetes aged 40 to 93 years and hospitalized because of poor diabetic control or recent-onset diabetes (mean HbA1c value = 9.6% ± 2.2%).

All patients with TSH values outside the normal range (0.45 to 3.66 mU/L in that particular study) had an FT4 assay and thyroid microsomal autoantibody assay performed on the same specimen of serum. The FT4 assay is a measure of free (unbound) T4 circulating in the blood.

It was found that high TSH concentrations were observed in 31.4% of the patients. Subclinical hypothyroidism (high TSH, normal FT4) was most common (48.3%), followed by subclinical hyperthyroidism (low TSH, normal FT4) (24.2%) and by definite hypothyroidism (high TSH, low FT4) (23.1%). Definite hyperthyroidism (low TSH, raised FT4) was found in 4.4% of the patients.

None of the patients with low TSH values had increased FT3 concentrations. T3 is the active form of the thyroid hormone. The prevalence of abnormal thyroid function test results was significantly higher in women than in men (40.9% vs. 19.8%) and in insulin-treated patients than in those receiving oral hypoglycemic agents (37.3% vs. 23.1%). Thirty-three percent of the patients with abnormal thyroid function test results showed evidence of thyroid autoimmunity (titer of thyroid microsomal autoantibodies greater than 250 U/L). Five thyroid microsomal antibody-negative patients had non-autoimmune thyroid diseases, seven had nonthyroidal illnesses other than diabetes, and four were receiving drugs known to affect the hypothalamic-–pituitary–thyroid axis.

Twenty-seven thyroid microsomal autoantibody-negative patients with abnormal TSH values (17 with subclinical hypothyroidism and 10 with subclinical hyperthyroidism), who were not receiving drugs known to affect TSH secretion and were free of diseases other than diabetes, were retested after 2 months of adequate treatment of diabetes with oral hypoglycemic agents or insulin. TSH concentrations decreased in all but one patient with initial subclinical hypothyroidism and increased in all patients with initial subclinical hyperthyroidism. These changes were coupled with a significant fall of glycated hemoglobin values.

The authors concluded that in view of the transient changes in TSH release, the diagnosis of thyroid dysfunction in Type 2 diabetics should be delayed until improvement of the metabolic status (Celani, Bonati, and Stucci. 1994).

Thyroid dysfunction appears to be common in diabetic patients, and it can produce significant metabolic disturbances. Therefore, regular screening for thyroid abnormalities in all diabetic patients is recommended to allow early treatment of subclinical thyroid dysfunction. A sensitive serum TSH assay is the screening test of choice. In Type 2 diabetes patients, a TSH assay is recommended at the time of diagnosis and then repeated at least every 5 years (Wu. 2000).

The detection of thyroid dysfunction in connection with Type 2 diabetes is not restricted to the population of the United States: A study conducted in Buenos Aires, Argentina, and reported in the journal *Medicina* aimed to investigate the prevalence of thyroid dysfunction in patients with Type 2 diabetes. Clinical and laboratory evaluation was performed on outpatients at the Endocrinology Diabetes and Nutrition Center in Concepcion City, Tucuman, Argentina.

Thyroid dysfunction was classified as clinical hypothyroidism with TSH greater than 4.20 mUI/mL and FT4 less than 0.93 ng/dL; subclinical hypothyroidism with TSH greater than 4.20 mUI/mL and free T4 less than 0.93 to 1.70 ng/dL. Subclinical hyperthyroidism was considered with TSH less than 0.27 mUI/mL and free T4 was in normal range (0.93 to 1.70 ng/dL), and clinical hyperthyroidism was considered with TSH less than 0.27 mUI/mL and free T4 greater than 1.70 mUI/mL. Autoimmunity was diagnosed with anti-TPO greater than 34 U/mL. Anti-thyroid autoantibodies (anti-TPO) are antibodies targeted against one or more components on the thyroid.

Thyroid dysfunction prevalence in Type 2 diabetes patients was 48%. In participants who denied prior thyroid dysfunction, the prevalence was 40%, and 45% had subclinical hypothyroidism.

The investigators concluded that early detection of thyroid dysfunction in patients with Type 2 diabetes should be performed routinely, given the high rate of newly diagnosed cases and increased cardiovascular risk associated with undiagnosed thyroid dysfunction (Centeno Maxzud, Gómez Rasjido, Fregenal et al. 2016).

A study published in the *Journal of Diabetes Research* cited evidence that hypothyroidism is more frequent in the elderly with diabetes and noted that an adaptation of TSH levels to age should be considered in thyroid function assessment. In particular, some antidiabetes drugs reportedly interfere with TSH levels. Therefore, the authors proposed to determine the prevalence of undiagnosed hypothyroidism in patients with diabetes and the influence of antidiabetes drugs.

Participants 60 years and older, some with diabetes, were enrolled in the study. They were compared according to diabetes treatment to persons without diabetes: TSH, FT4, antithyroperoxidase, fasting glucose, and HbA1c were measured.

It was found that 6.4% of patients with diabetes had hypothyroidism, a higher prevalence compared with persons without diabetes (5.1%), but lower than observed in many other studies. The use of an age-specific TSH reference interval (RI) could explain this difference.

Patients taking metformin had slightly lower TSH than those not on metformin, indicating that metformin doses may have influenced TSH levels.

The authors concluded that the use of a specific TSH RI could avoid the misdiagnosis of hypothyroidism in the elderly with diabetes. Patients on metformin, as a single drug, had lower TSH than those using other medications and those persons who do not have diabetes (Fontes, de Fatima dos Santos Teixeira, and Vaisman. 2016).

Parenthetically, a study published in the *Canadian Medical Association Journal* also reported that metformin is associated with an increased incidence of low TSH levels in Type 2 diabetes patients with treated hypothyroidism, but not in euthyroid patients (Fournier, Yin, Yu et al. 2014). "Euthyroid sick syndrome" is a condition characterized by low serum levels of thyroid hormones in patients with nonthyroid systemic illness.

6.5.2 The Barnes Test—A Simple Self-Test for Low Thyroid Function

There are many reasons why one may have low thyroid function. In normal circumstances, and baring tangible medical evidence of even minimal thyroid dysfunction, it could simply be inadequate dietary intake of iodine. However, as shown above, there is a link between Type 2 diabetes and thyroid dysfunction, and it is not clear which "causes" which: Does thyroid dysfunction contribute to hyperglycemia, or does hyperglycemia contribute to thyroid dysfunction? From a practical point of view, it doesn't matter. However, as noted above, because of the higher incidence of thyroid dysfunction in people with Type 2 diabetes, it might be wise to try to find out if there is low thyroid function if one suffers from diabetes.

A routine TSH test can readily reveal thyroid deficiency. Basal metabolic rate is the rate at which the body uses energy while at rest to keep vital functions going, such as breathing and keeping warm. Assuming that one is not on medication(s) that would directly affect these measures, consistently low body temperature (below 98.0°F) and low pulse rate (below 65) may be an indication of low thyroid function.

The Barnes basal temperature test is a simple, do-it-at-home self-test. It is reasonably accurate and requires only a digital thermometer.

The test:

- When awakening in the morning, and before rising, note the basal body temperature and make a record of it. Using an ear thermometer such as the Braun Thermoscan Ear Thermometer, for example, is the quickest and simplest way to do that. Repeat this procedure each morning for 5 days. Keep in mind that a woman's body temperature varies with the different phases of the menstrual cycle. The second and third days of the menstrual cycle are when the most accurate/reliable basal body temperature can be obtained.
- If the basal temperature consistently runs below 98.0°F, one may have hypothyroidism and it is recommended that he or she consults a physician.

The healthy adult body should hold about 15 to 20 mg of iodine, and 70% to 80% is stored in the thyroid gland. The daily intake requirement during adult life is about 150 µg. The body conserves only about 10% to 20% of iodine consumed in daily diet; the rest is excreted from the body.

There are many possible reasons for thyroid deficiency. Hashimoto's thyroiditis, an autoimmune inflammation of the thyroid gland, is actually the most common form of thyroid disorder in the United States. Therefore, supplementing dietary iodine is not invariably medically sound, so it should not be undertaken without express direction by and with supervision of a qualified healthcare provider, as there may be contraindication. Excess amounts of iodine intake can induce hyperthyroidism, aggravating Hashimoto's thyroiditis. Furthermore, there may be other causes of lower body core temperature and depressed metabolism that need to be detected and some, perhaps, can be treated.

6.5.2.1   Factors That Can Affect Body Core Temperature

The *Japanese Journal of Geriatrics* reported that age is one of the most important factors in changes in energy metabolism. The basal metabolic rate decreases almost linearly with age since skeletal musculature, which consumes the largest part of energy in the normal human body, decreases and the percentage of fat tissue rises. It is shown that the decrease in muscle mass, relative to total body mass, may be wholly responsible for the age-related decreases in basal metabolic rate (Shimokata, and Kuzuya. 1993). However, there may also be other reasons.

A study published in the journal *Gerontology* reports that the body temperature of older men and women is lower than that of younger people. However, the report gives no quantitative information (Blatteis. 2012) and, as is so common in this type of study, there is no mention of screening for conditions known to lower body temperature that may not be present across the board in the elderly. One of these conditions is body weight.

Another study is that reported in the *Journal of Clinical Nursing* aimed to determine whether body temperature changes in the elderly. Axillary (armpit) body temperatures in older participants (average age, 77.2) in a nursing home ranged from 95.3°F to 97.6°F (35.1°C to 36.4°C). The mean temperature of those aged 65 to 74 was higher than that of those aged 75 to 84 (Güneş, and Zaybak. 2008).

Does body weight affect body temperature? The biological inability to create sufficient core body heat could be linked to obesity. According to a study reported in the journal *Chronobiology International*, there is "Evidence of a diurnal thermogenic handicap in obesity." The study found that obesity is associated with a significant reduction of body core temperature during daytime hours. In other words, the reduced ability of obese people to spend energy as heat, compared to lean individuals, could result in long-term weight gain of about 4.5 lb per year, depending on the lifestyle (Grimaldi, Provini, Pierangeli et al. 2015).

Keeping that in mind, and assuming that supplementation with dietary iodine is safe, success should be seen in just a few days in the form of normalizing basal body temperature.

Supplementing the diet with iodine, described in a later chapter of this book, has been found effective where the cause is iodine deficiency, but one needs to be careful not to take too much of it, too quickly, for that is not good for the thyroid either: too much iodine can also result in hyperthyroidism.

6.6 DIABETES AND KIDNEY STONES

Diabetes is a major risk factor for kidney stones. This relationship has been detailed in a previous chapter but elements of it are reiterated here because they are relevant to understanding the testing/ monitoring devices that are available. Type 2 diabetes is associated with excessively low (meaning acidic) urine pH, which increases the risk for formation of uric acid kidney stones (nephrolithiasis). A study published in the *Clinical Journal of the American Society of Nephrology* reports that the overly acidic urine in patients with Type 2 diabetes persists even after controlling for dietary factors, body size, and age. The lower pH is due to a combination of greater net acid secretion and lower use of ammonia buffers in patients with diabetes, which predisposes them to uric acid stone formation (Maalouf, Cameron, Moe et al. 2010).

Kidney stones are bits of grit formed from minerals in the kidneys or the bladder; they can be terribly painful, block urine flow, and damage the kidneys. Many start out small, like grains of sand; they may hurt, but they will pass by themselves. When they get larger than about 4 mm (about 0.2 inches) in diameter, they can get stuck in the ureters, the passageways that carry the urine from the kidneys to the bladder; then, they can become agonizing, cause infection, and block urine in the kidney. This is a very serious complication.

Kidney stones can form from several different minerals. The two main categories are calcium oxalate and uric acid. People with diabetes have higher rates of both, and much higher rates for the uric acid kind, because their urine tends to be more acidic. One study at the Mayo Clinic followed 3500 patients, for 20 years, and concluded that those with diabetes developed 40% more uric acid kidney stones than those without diabetes. The low pH has also been implicated in metabolic syndrome (Maalouf, Cameron, Moe et al. 2007).

The American Society of Nephrology reports that insulin resistance has something to do with it because high levels of insulin in the blood are associated with acid urine (Li, Klett, Littleton et al. 2014). The body makes buffers, of course, such as ammonia, to neutralize the acid, but insulin resistance seems to lower the production of ammonia, and, adding to that, there is evidence of involvement of the liver.

It is reported in the *World Journal of Gastroenterology*, that perhaps as many as 30% of patients with cirrhosis have diabetes. The article suggests that perhaps Type 2 diabetes, in the absence of obesity and hypertriglyceridemia, may be a risk factor for chronic liver disease (Garcia-Compean, Jaquez-Quintana, Gonzalez-Gonzalez et al. 2009).

The journal *European Urology* featured a study aimed to determine what associations exist among the presence and severity of Type 2 diabetes, glycemic control and insulin resistance, and kidney stone disease. The study consisted of an analysis of all adult participants in the 2007 to 2010 National Health and Nutrition Examination Survey.

A history of kidney stone disease was obtained by self-report. Type 2 diabetes was defined by (a) self-reported history, (b) Type 2 diabetes–related medication usage, and (c) reported diabetic comorbidity.

Insulin resistance was estimated using fasting plasma insulin levels and the homeostasis model assessment of insulin resistance definition. Glycemic control was determined by using HbA1c and fasting plasma glucose levels.

It was found that persons with fasting plasma glucose levels of 100 to 126 and greater than 126 mg/ dL had increased odds of kidney stone disease (odds ratio [OR], 1.28 and 2.29, respectively). There were similar results for persons with HgbA1c 5.7% to 6.4% and equal to or greater than 6.5% (OR, 1.68 and 2.82), respectively. When adjusting for patient factors, a history of Type 2 diabetes, the use of insulin, fasting plasma insulin, and HgbA1c were significantly associated with kidney stone disease (Weinberg, Patel, Chertow et al. 2014).

A study titled "Type-2 diabetes and kidney stones: impact of diabetes medications and glycemic control" was published in the journal *Urology*. The investigators aimed to evaluate the impact of diabetic medications and glycemic control on the urine pH, 24-h urine stone risk profile, and stone composition.

A study published in the journal *Urology* reported reviewing a database of Type 2 diabetes patients with kidney stones. Data from Type 2 diabetic patients with stone disease were collected; 20.5% of them were assigned to the insulin group, and 79.5% were assigned to the antihyperglycemics group.

Patients were further assigned to one of two groups depending on whether their diabetic medication was insulin or oral antihyperglycemic. Urine collection and stone composition were compared.

In a subgroup analysis, patients on thiazolidinediones (i.e., pioglitazone) were compared with patients on other oral antihyperglycemics.

Analysis of the data showed male gender and insulin therapy to be ameliorating factors of low urine pH, whereas HbA1c level was inversely related to the urine pH (OR, −0.066). There were no significant differences in other 24-h urine stone risk parameters or stone composition between the groups.

The investigators concluded that urine pH is inversely related to HbA1c level and that insulin therapy is associated with higher urine pH than oral antihyperglycemic agents, despite higher HbA1c. This suggested that insulin may modify urine pH independent of glycemic control (Torricelli, De, Gebreselassie et al. 2014).

Finally, the *Journal of the American Society of Nephrology* published a report titled "Type 2 diabetes increases the risk for uric acid stones." The authors contended that an increased prevalence of kidney stones has been reported in patients with diabetes. Because insulin resistance, characteristic of the metabolic syndrome and Type 2 diabetes, results in lower urine pH through impaired kidney ammonia production, and because a low urine pH is the main factor of uric acid stone formation, it was hypothesized that Type 2 diabetes should favor the formation of uric acid stones.

Therefore, the distribution of the main stone components was analyzed in a series of 2464 stones from a group of patients with Type 2 diabetes and another group without Type 2 diabetes.

The proportion of uric acid stones was 35.7% in patients with Type 2 diabetes and 11.3% in patients without Type 2 diabetes. The proportion of patients with Type 2 diabetes was significantly higher among uric acid than among calcium stone formers (27.8% vs. 6.9%). Analysis identified Type 2 diabetes as the strongest factor that was independently associated with the risk for uric acid stones (OR, 6.9).

The authors concluded that the strong link of Type 2 diabetes to uric acid stone formation should be added to the list of factors associated with insulin resistance. Therefore, the authors suggest that patients with uric acid stones, especially if overweight, should be screened for the presence of Type 2 diabetes or components of the metabolic syndrome (Daudon, Traxer, Conort et al. 2006).

Having established by a sample of representative research reports that Type 2 diabetes results in a urine pH that favors kidney stone formation, it might be advisable for any diabetes sufferer to avail himself or herself of simple ways to monitor it.

6.6.1 URINE pH AND NEPHROLITHIASIS IN TYPE 2 DIABETES

Nephrolithiasis is the process of forming a kidney stone, or a stone lower down in the urinary tract. According to a report in the *Journal of the American Society of Nephrology*, Type 2 diabetes is a risk factor for stone formation (nephrolithiasis) and uric acid stones in particular. In the study cited in that publication, the aim was to identify the metabolic features that raise the risk of uric acid nephrolithiasis in patients with Type 2 diabetes.

Three groups of participants were recruited in an outpatient study: those patients who have Type 2 diabetes and are not stone formers, patients who do not have diabetes and are uric acid stone formers, and healthy volunteers. Participants provided a fasting blood sample and a single 24-h urine collection for stone risk analysis.

It was found that 24-h urine volume, and total uric acid, did not differ among the three groups. Patients with Type 2 diabetes and small stones had lower 24-h urine pH than healthy volunteers.

Urine pH was inversely correlated with both body weight and 24-h urine sulfate in all groups. Urine pH remained significantly lower in patients with Type 2 diabetes and small stones than that of healthy volunteers.

The main risk factor for uric acid nephrolithiasis in patients with Type 2 diabetes was found to be low urine pH (Cameron, Maalouf, Adams-Huet et al. 2006). We are cautioned again in a subsequent report in the *Clinical Journal of the American Society of Nephrology* that the overly acidic urine in patients with Type 2 diabetes persists after controlling for dietary factors, body size, and age. The lower pH is due to a combination of greater net acid excretion and lower levels of ammonia buffers in patients with diabetes, which predisposes them to uric acid urolithiasis (Maalouf, Cameron, Moe et al. 2010).

6.6.2 Measuring Urine pH

The pH scale ranges from 0 (very acid) to 14 (very base or alkaline). The midpoint of the scale is 7 (neutral). The pH is a logarithmic scale—that is, a difference of 1 pH unit is a 10-times greater difference. Normally, blood pH is 7.4, which is slightly alkaline (or basic).

Many enzymes that facilitate chemical reactions in the body function only in a narrow range of pH. Therefore, any significant change (at or below 7, or over 7.7) means almost certain death. A series of buffers and compensation mechanisms keep the pH of blood in the healthy body from wandering too far from 7.4. Because the blood constantly circulates throughout the body, it can usually compensate any changes in pH in any of our organs (e.g., our muscles during intense exercise).

The lungs actually preserve a portion of the CO_2 needed to maintain proper pH, but they eliminate most of it—about 75%. The kidneys provide a secondary protection of the pH, eliminating acid in urine, but more slowly. Carbon dioxide dissolved in water can react with the water to form carbonic acid. In blood, this reaction is accelerated by the enzyme carbonic anhydrase. Carbonic acid can in turn give up a hydrogen ion to become bicarbonate. Most of the carbon dioxide in blood is in the form of bicarbonate. The result is that an increase in CO_2 concentrations will slightly decrease blood pH, making it slightly more acidic, while a decrease in CO_2 concentrations will make it slightly less acidic.

Several means of testing the pH of urine are readily available to consumers. For instance, one of the simplest is the pH test strip unit. A selection of such units can be found on a number of websites, for instance, GOOGLE images, "urinary pH test strips."

A small piece of the paper strip is dipped briefly into a receptacle holding fresh urine and the color matched to the color code gives an approximate pH value. Alternatively, a pH meter can be dipped briefly into a receptacle holding urine and it will show a numerical pH value. A number of pH meters are available to consumers for purchase online. They vary in sensitivity and cost: https://www.google.com/search?source=hp&ei=9-15WveIDoHv5gLvyJrgDA&q=ph+meters+for+sale&oq=pH+meters&gs_l=psy-ab.1.1.0l10.1442.3798.0.6906.9.7.0.2.2.0.93.547.7.7.0....0...1c.1.64.psy-ab..0.9.563...0i131k1j0i10k1.0.0nMbjGRDXoU.

An alkaline pH favors the crystallization of calcium- and phosphate-containing stones, whereas an acidic urine pH promotes uric acid or cystine stones. The three major risk factors for stones formation are low urine pH (less than 5.5), low urine volume, and elevated levels of uric acid in the urine (hyperuricosuria).

The *Journal of the Medical Association of Thailand* reports a study of "Serum and urinary uric acid levels in healthy people subjects and in patients with urolithiasis." Serum uric acid and 24-h urine uric acid levels were determined in patients with urolithiasis and in healthy volunteers. The normal volunteers' serum and urinary uric acid levels were as follows:

- Men: 6.0–6.4 mg/dL, 619.4–683.7 mg/day
- Women: 4.6–4.8 mg/dL, 531.5–589.6 mg/day

Patients with urolithiasis showed significantly higher levels of serum uric acid:

- 8.0 ± 0.3 mg/dL, compared with healthy volunteers
- 5.5 ± 0.1 mg/dL, but showed no difference in urinary uric acid levels compared with healthy volunteers

The 24-h urine pH of healthy volunteers showed a range of

- pH: 5.1–7.0

The patients with urolithiasis had a range of

- pH: 4.6–7.0 (Sila-On, Pavaro, Nuchpramool. 1991)

The laboratory reference ranges for uric acid are as follows:

- Men: 2.5–8 mg/dL
- Women: 1.9–7.5 mg/dL

Elevations of uric acid greater than 4 mg/dL should be considered a "red flag" in those patients at risk for cardiovascular disease and diabetes (Hayden, and Tyagi. 2004).

6.7 TESTING NO AVAILABILITY TO SUPPORT HEALTHY ENDOTHELIUM FUNCTION

It was shown in previous chapters that a healthy endothelium is essential to healthy cardiovascular and heart function. It was also shown that there is a link between Type 2 diabetes and impaired endothelium-derived NO formation, a key to healthy cardiovascular and heart function. While it is not clear which comes first, impaired endothelium or diabetes, nevertheless the consequences of NO unavailability are clearly risky.

A study reported in the journal *Diabetes* found that in Type 2 diabetes patients, NO was lower than in control participants. In patients with nephropathy, intravascular NO synthesis from L-arginine is decreased (Tessari, Cecchet, Cosma et al. 2010).

Researchers reported in the *International Journal of Applied and Basic Medical Research* that serum NO was observed to be significantly low in diabetic participants as compared to control participants, along with differences in other biochemical parameters. In this study, the Griess reaction was used for indirect assay of stable decomposition products in serum (serum nitrite and nitrate levels) as an index of NO generation (Ghosh, Sherpa, Bhutia et al. 2011). (For more on the Griess reaction used in the analysis of nitrite and nitrate in biological fluids, see Tsikas. 2007.)

The nutritional recommendations in the succeeding chapters encourage a diet rich in nitrates that ensure adequate substrate for NO formation: L-arginine is likely one of the main sources of NO in human nutrition; dietary nitrates found in many foods are rich NO donors.

6.7.1 NOx Self-Test

The HumanN® (formerly NEOGENIS LABS) Nitric Oxide Indicator Strips provide a simple and inexpensive way to assess the levels of NO in the body (see: https://www.humann. com/products/). It should be noted that, by convention, nitric oxide is designated NO. However, in research, NO is rarely measured directly as a volume of gas. Instead, its presence is usually inferred from a reliable but indirect reaction measure. Unless NO is observed directly, it should be designated NOx. This rule is, however, largely ignored.

Dr. N. S. Bryan (adjunct assistant professor at Baylor College of Medicine in the Department of Molecular and Human Genetics) pioneered the use of salivary nitrite as a marker of human NO status. Up to now, "*... there have not been any new developments in the use of NO biomarkers in the clinical setting for diagnostic or prognostic utility. In fact, NO status is still not part of the standard blood chemistry routinely used for diagnostic purposes. This is simply unacceptable given the critical nature of NO in many disease processes and new technologies should be developed in Humans,*" says Dr. Bryan. He proposes sampling salivary nitrite as an accurate representation of total body NO production/availability (personal communication).

HumanN is a leader in NO research, and they invented the world's first standard noninvasive salivary NO test strip that can be used to assess one's NO levels at home: N-O Indicator Strips (https://www.humann.com/products/nitric-oxide-indicator-strips/) (Figure 6.2, below). Utilizing one's saliva, it is quick and easy to conduct the test: Saliva is applied to a strip, and its coloration is then compared to a color code on the side of the strips container.

The test strip assesses total body NO availability by the level of NOx in salivary nitrite. If one consumes a nitrate-rich diet, that is, beets, green leafy vegetables, and so on (see Chapters 2 and 13), but lacks the proper oral nitrate-reducing bacteria, then there may be no increase in salivary nitrite, resulting in NO deficiency. If, on the other hand, one has the right oral nitrate-reducing bacteria but does not eat sufficient nitrate-enriched vegetables, then the test strip will also reflect low NOx availability because the body is not getting enough nitrate from the diet to convert to nitrite. Only 5% of the nitrate is reduced to nitrite in saliva.

Directions are given on the website, https://www.humann.com/products/nitric-oxide-indicator-strips/. It is suggested that the user place a drop of saliva on the indicator strip first thing in the morning, before eating and drinking anything. Then, compare the indicator strip with the accompanying color chart on the N-O Indicator Strip packaging. Results are practically instantaneous, and one can tell at a glance if he or she is getting sufficient NO-activating nutrients from the diet.

Results are easy to read by comparing the test strip coloration to the four color-coded reading indicators on the package. The more NO in the body, the deeper red the indicator pad will appear.

Note: When using the Test Strips, a high (NEO Optimal) reading may or may not invariably indicate the concentration of available endothelium-derived NO. The "reading" could also be confounded by a number of factors including recently consuming high–L-arginine foods including meats, fish,

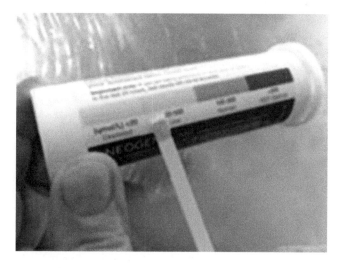

FIGURE 6.2 HumanN N-O Strips are used to assess nitrite levels in saliva as an index of NOx availability. (With permission.)

nuts, or beans, and/or high-nitrate foods including green leafy vegetables, beans, beets, or carrots, or if one is suffering from a lung, bowel, or other forms of inflammatory disease. Immune system cells go into overdrive production of NO in serious infections and inflammation—potentially fatally in the case of septicemia.

On the other hand, a low reading may be a clear indication that endothelial NO formation is simply inadequate. To ensure the proper use of the test, it is therefore very important to follow the instructions that accompany the test strips.

The use of such a test strip provides *"feedback"*—knowledge of results—insofar as it may help to determine sooner the positive outcome of one's attention to daily nutrition.

Because of the implication for the health risks, hypertension, atherosclerosis, cardiovascular and heart disease, and diabetes, the value of discovering that one has a LOW NO reading cannot be underestimated. Such a reading may be interpreted to mean that one's diet may be low in the food stuffs that are used in the body to form NO.

The nutrition program proposed in Chapter 8 is based on the most recent information about the beneficial impact of a Mediterranean Diet plan to promote endothelial NO formation. Using the NO Test Strips is the easiest way to track the availability of NO in the body, and it can help in making food choices to maintain desirable levels. Adequate NO formation is very important to lowering the free radical and ROS load. Reducing this load is the key to improving and maintaining cardiovascular and metabolic health in the face of Type 2 diabetes.

Certain vegetables in daily diet are our principal source of nitrate. Much of the nitrate in foods is actively taken up by the salivary glands as we consume the foods and concentrated in saliva. Bacteria in the mouth then reduce salivary nitrate to nitrite. Continuously swallowing nitrite in saliva forms different nitrogen compounds in the stomach and, in particular, NO. This is the second "pathway" for forming NO and it is called the "enterosalivary circulation of nitrate" (Lundberg, Carlström, Larsen et al. 2011; Lundberg, Gladwin, and Weitzberg. 2015; Lundberg, Weitzberg, and Gladwin. 2008).

Inorganic nitrate in foods is rapidly absorbed in the small intestine. Much of the circulating nitrate is eventually excreted in the urine, but up to 25% is actively extracted by the salivary glands and concentrated in saliva. Bacteria in the mouth effectively reduce nitrate to nitrite by the action of enzymes, leading to a thousand-fold higher concentrations of nitrite in saliva than in plasma.

In the acidic stomach, nitrite is spontaneously decomposed to form NO and other nitrogen compounds that regulate important physiological functions. Nitrate and the remaining nitrite are absorbed from the intestine into the circulation and can convert to NO in blood and tissues (Lundberg, Gladwin, Ahluwalia et al. 2009).

It is possible to determine one's NO availability level indirectly as a function of the concentration of nitrite in saliva because it has been shown that (a) consuming nitrate actually raises NO availability in the body (McKnight, Smith, Drummond et al. 1997) and (b) salivary nitrate and nitrite levels reflect the amount ingested.

In a study published in the journal *Food and Cosmetics Toxicology*, volunteers consumed vegetables and vegetable juices with high concentrations of nitrate. Levels of nitrate and nitrite concentrations in saliva were determined for up to 7 h at intervals of 30 or 60 min: First, the amount of nitrate secreted by the salivary glands increased directly with the amount of nitrate ingested. Second, nitrite concentration in saliva correlated directly with salivary nitrate content, indicating a direct relationship between the salivary nitrite concentrations and the amounts of nitrate ingested in the diet (Spiegelhalder, Eisenbrand, and Preussmann. 1976).

The results of this, and similar studies, support the use of salivary nitrite assay to estimate NO availability.

Disclaimer: The authors have no commercial interest in the HumanN nitric oxide saliva test strips, nor are they in any way commercially involved with any other products of that company.

REFERENCES

Al-Qaisi M, Nott DM, King DH, and S Kaddoura. 2009. Ankle brachial pressure index (ABPI): an update for practitioners. *Vascular Health and Risk Management*, 5, 833–841. PMCID: PMC2762432.

Arguedas JA, Leiva V, and JM Wright. 2013. Blood pressure targets for hypertension in people with diabetes mellitus. *Cochrane Database of Systematic Reviews*, Oct 30; (10): CD008277. DOI: 10.1002/14651858 .CD008277.pub2.

Basi S, Fesler P, Mimran A, and JB Lewis. 2008. Microalbuminuria in Type 2 diabetes and hypertension. A marker, treatment target, or innocent bystander? *Diabetes Care*, Feb; 31(Supplement 2): S194–S201. https://doi.org/10.2337/dc08-s249.

Benchimol D, Pillois X, Benchimol A, Houitte A, Sagardiluz P, Tortelier L, and J Bonnet. 2009. Détection de l'artériopathie des membres inférieurs en médecine préventive par la détermination de l'index de pression systolique à l'aide d'un tensiomètre automatique [Accuracy of ankle-brachial index using an automatic blood pressure device to detect peripheral artery disease in preventive medicine]. *Archives of Cardiovascular Diseases*, 102, 519–524.

Bernstein EF, and A Fronek. 1982. Current status of non-invasive tests in the diagnosis of peripheral arterial disease. *Surgical Clinics of North America*, 62, 473–487.

Blatteis CM. 2012. Age-dependent changes in temperature regulation—a mini review. *Gerontology*, Nov; 58(4): 289–295. DOI: 10.1159/000333148.

Brenner BM, Cooper ME, de Zeeuw D, Keane WF, Mitch WE, Parving HH, Remuzzi G, Snapinn SM, Zhang Z, Shahinfar S, and RENAAL Study Investigators. 2001. Effects of losartan on renal and cardiovascular outcomes in patients with type 2 diabetes and nephropathy. *New England Journal of Medicine*, Sep 20; 345(12): 861–869. DOI: 10.1056/NEJMoa011161.

Cameron MA, Maalouf NM, Adams-Huet B, Moe OW, and K Sakhaee. 2006. Urine composition in type 2 diabetes: predisposition to uric acid nephrolithiasis. *Journal of the American Society of Nephrology*, May; 17(5): 1422–1428. DOI: 10.1681/ASN.2005121246.

Celani MF, Bonati ME, and N Stucci. 1994. Prevalence of abnormal thyrotropin concentrations measured by a sensitive assay in patients with type 2 diabetes mellitus. *Diabetes Research*, 27(1): 15–25. PMID: 7648793.

Centeno Maxzud M, Gómez Rasjido L, Fregenal M, Arias Calafiore F, Córdoba Lanus M, D'Urso M, and H Luciardi. 2016. Prevalence of thyroid dysfunction in patients with type 2 diabetes mellitus [article in Spanish]. *Medicina* (B Aires), 76(6): 355–358. PMID: 27959843.

Chen SC, Hsiao PJ, Huang JC, Lin KD, Hsu WH, Lee YL, Lee MY, Chang JM, and SJ Shin. 2015. Abnormally low or high Ankle-Brachial Index is associated with proliferative diabetic retinopathy in Type 2 diabetic mellitus patients. *PLoS ONE*, Jul 31; 10(7): e0134718. DOI: 10.1371/journal.pone.0134718.

Colombo AV, Barbosa GM, Higashi D, di Micheli G, Rodrigues PH, and MRL Simionato. 2013. Quantitative detection of *Staphylococcus aureus*, *Enterococcus faecalis* and *Pseudomonas aeruginosa* in human oral epithelial cells from subjects with periodontitis and periodontal health. *Journal of Medical Microbiology*, 62, 1592–1600 DOI: 10.1099/jmm.0.055830-0.

Daudon M, Traxer O, Conort P, Lacour B, and P Jungers. 2006. Type 2 diabetes increases the risk for uric acid stones. *Journal of the American Society of Nephrology*, Jul: 17(7): 2026–2033. DOI: 10.1681/ASN .2006030262 JASN July.

Emdin CA, Rahimi K, Neal B, Callender T, Perkovic V, and A Patel. 2015. Blood pressure lowering in type 2 diabetes: a systematic review and meta-analysis. *Journal of the American Medical Association*, Feb 10; 313(6): 603–615. DOI: 10.1001/jama.2014.18574.

Farmer AJ, Wade AN, French DP, Simon J, Yudkin P, Gray A, Craven A, Goyder L, Holman RR, Mant D, Kinmonth AL, and HA Neil HA (DiGEM Trial Group and 44 collaborators). 2009. Blood glucose self-monitoring in type 2 diabetes: a randomised controlled trial. *Health Technology Assessment*, Feb; 13(15): iii–iv, ix–xi, 1–50. DOI: 10.3310/hta13150.

Fontes R, de Fatima dos Santos Teixeira P, and M Vaisman. 2016. Screening of undiagnosed hypothyroidism in elderly persons with diabetes according to age-specific reference intervals for serum thyroid stimulating hormone and the impact of antidiabetes drugs. *Journal of Diabetes Research*, 2016: 1417408. DOI: 10.1155/20 16/1417408.

Fournier JP, Yin H, Yu OH, and L Azoulay. 2014. Metformin and low levels of thyroid-stimulating hormone in patients with type 2 diabetes mellitus. *Canadian Medical Association Journal*, Oct 21; 186(15): 1138–1145. DOI: 10.1503/cmaj.140688.

Fried R. 2014. *Erectile Dysfunction as a Cardiovascular Impairment*. Academic Press/Elsevier Science.

Fritschi C, and L Quinn. 2010. Fatigue in patients with diabetes: a review. *Journal of Psychosomatic Research*, Jul; 69(1): 33–41. DOI: 10.1016/j.jpsychores.2010.01.021.

Garcia-Compean D, Jaquez-Quintana JO, Gonzalez-Gonzalez JA, and H Maldonado-Garza. 2009. Liver cirrhosis and diabetes: risk factors, pathophysiology, clinical implications and management. *World Journal of Gastroenterology*, Jan; 15(3): 280–288. Published online 2009 Jan 21. DOI: 10.3748/wjg.15.280.

Ghosh A, Sherpa ML, Bhutia Y, Pal R, and S Dahal. 2011. Serum nitric oxide status in patients with type 2 diabetes mellitus in Sikkim. *International Journal of Applied & Basic Medical Research*, Jan–Jun; 1(1): 31–35. DOI: 10.4103/2229-516X.81977.

Grimaldi D, Provini F, Pierangeli G, Mazzella N, Zamboni G, Marchesini G, and P Cortelli. 2015. Evidence of a diurnal thermogenic handicap in obesity. *Chronobiology International*, Oct; 32 (2): 299–302. DOI: 10.3109/07420528.

Güneş UY, and A Zaybak. 2008. Does the body temperature change in older people? *Journal of Clinical Nursing*, Sep; 17(17): 2284–2287. DOI: 10.1111/j.1365-2702.2007.02272.x.

Handelsman Y, Bloomgarden ZT, Grunberger G, Umpierrez G, Zimmerman RS, Bailey TS, Blonde L, Bray GA, Cohen AJ, Dagogo-Jack S, Davidson JA, Einhorn D, Ganda OP, Garber AJ, Garvey WT, Henry RR, Hirsch IB, Horton ES, Hurley DL, Jellinger PS, Jovanovič L, Lebovitz HE, LeRoith D, Levy P, McGill JB, Mechanick JI, Mestman JH, Moghissi ES, Eric A. Orzeck EA, Pessah-Pollack R, Rosenblit PD, Vinik AI, Wyne K, and F Zangeneh. 2015. American Association of Clinical Endocrinologists and American College of Endocrinology—clinical practice guidelines for developing a diabetes mellitus comprehensive care plan—2015. AACE/ACE Diabetes Guidelines. *Endocrinology Practice*, 21(Suppl 1).

Hayden MR, and SC Tyagi. 2004. Uric acid: a new look at an old risk marker for cardiovascular disease, metabolic syndrome, and type 2 diabetes mellitus: the urate redox shuttle. *Nutrition and Metabolism* (Lond), Oct 19; 1(1): 10. DOI: 10.1186/1743-7075-1-10.

Herman WH, and SS Fajans. 2010. Hemoglobin A1c for the diagnosis of diabetes: practical considerations. *Polskie Archiwum Medycyny Wewnetrznej*, 120(1–2): 37–40. PMID: 20150843.

Ibsen H, Olsen MH, Wachtell K, Borch-Johnsen K, Lindholm LH, Mogensen CE, Dahlof B, Devereux RB, de Faire U, Fyhrquist F, Julius S, Kjeldsen SE, Lederballe-Pedersen O, Nieminen MS, Omvik P, Oparil S, and Y Wan. 2005. Reduction in albuminuria translates to reduction in cardiovascular events in hypertensive patients: losartan intervention for endpoint reduction in hypertension study. *Hypertension*, Jan; 45:198–202. https://doi.org/10.1161/01.HYP.0000154082.72286.2a.

Khadke S, Harke S, Ghadge A, Kulkarni O, Bhalerao S, Diwan A, Pankaj M, and A Kuvalekar. 2015. Association of fasting plasma glucose and serum lipids in Type 2 diabetics. *Indian Journal of Pharmaceutical Science*, Sep–Oct; 77(5): 630–634. PMCID: PMC4700719.

Khan HA, Sobki SH, and SA Khan. 2007. Association between glycaemic control and serum lipids profile in type 2 diabetic patients: HbA1c predicts dyslipidaemia. *Clinical and Experimental Medicine*, Mar; 7(1): 24–29. DOI: 10.1007/s10238-007-0121-3.

Leiper JM, Lowe GD, Anderson J, Burns P, Cohen HN, Manderson WG, Forbes CD, Barbenel JC, and AC MacCuish. 1984. Effects of diabetic control and biosynthetic human insulin on blood rheology in established diabetics. *Diabetes Research*, May; 1(1): 27–30. PMID: 6397284.

Lewis EJ, Hunsicker LG, Clarke WR, Berl T, Pohl MA, Lewis JB, Ritz E, Atkins RC, Rohde R, and I Raz. 2001. Renoprotective effect of the angiotensin-receptor antagonist irbesartan in patients with nephropathy due to type 2 diabetes. *New England Journal of Medicine*, Sept; 345(12): 851–860. DOI: 10.1056/NEJ Moa011303.

Li H, Klett DE, Littleton R, Elder JS, and JD Sammon. 2014. Role of insulin resistance in uric acid nephrolithiasis. *World Journal of Nephrology*, Nov 6; 3(4): 237–242. Published online 2014 Nov 6. DOI: 10.5527/wjn.v3.i4.237.

Li L, Wan X-h, and G-h Zhao. 2014. Meta-analysis of the risk of cataract in type 2 diabetes. *BMC Ophthalmology*, 201414:94. DOI: 10.1186/1471-2415-14-94.

Li Q, Zeng H, Liu F, Shen J, Li L, Zhao J, Zhao J, and W Jia. 2015. High Ankle-Brachial Index indicates cardiovascular and peripheral arterial disease in patients with Type 2 diabetes. *Angiology*, Nov; 66(10): 9189–9124. DOI: 10.1177/000331971557 3657.

Li X, Wang L, Zhang C, Li S, Pu F, Fan Y, and D Li D. 2013. Why is ABI effective in detecting vascular stenosis? Investigation based on multibranch hemodynamic model. *Scientific World Journal*, https://openi.nlm.nih.gov/detailedresult.php?img= PMC3780660_TSWJ2013-185691.001&req=4.

Lundberg JO, Carlström M, Larsen FJ, and E Weitzberg. 2011. Roles of dietary inorganic nitrate in cardiovascular health and disease. *Cardiovascular Research*, Feb 15; 89(3): 525–532. DOI: 10.1093/cvr/cvq325.

Lundberg JO, Gladwin MT, Ahluwalia A, Benjamin N, Bryan NS, Butler A, Cabrales P, Fago A, Feelisch M, Ford PC, Freeman BA, Frenneaux M, Friedman J, Kelm M, Kevil CG, Kim-Shapiro DB, Kozlov AV, Lancaster JR Jr, Lefer DJ, McColl K, McCurry K, Patel RP, Petersson J, Rassaf T, Reutov VP, Richter-Addo GB, Schechter A, Shiva S, Tsuchiya K, van Faassen EE, Webb AJ, Zuckerbraun BS, Zweier JL, and E Weitzberg. 2009. Nitrate and nitrite in biology, nutrition and therapeutics. *Nature Chemical Biology*, Dec; 5(12): 865–869. DOI: 10.1038/nchembio.260.

Lundberg JO, Gladwin MT, and E Weitzberg. 2015. Strategies to increase nitric oxide signalling in cardiovascular disease. *Nature Reviews. Drug Discovery*, Sep; 14(9): 623–641. DOI: 10.1038/nrd4623.

Lundberg JO, Weitzberg E, and MT Gladwin. 2008. The nitrate-nitrite-nitric oxide pathway in physiology and therapeutics. *Nature Reviews. Drug Discovery*, Feb; 7(2): 156–167. DOI: 10.1038/nrd2466.

Maalouf NM, Cameron MA, Moe OW, Adams-Huet B, and K Sakhaee. 2007. Low urine pH: a novel feature of the metabolic syndrome. *Clinical Journal of the American Society of Nephrology*, Sep; 2(5): 883–888. DOI: 10.2215/CJN.00670207.

Maalouf NM, Cameron MA, Moe OW, and K Sakhaee. 2010. Metabolic basis for low urine pH in Type 2 diabetes. *Clinical Journal of the American Society of Nephrology*, Jul; 5(7): 1277–1281. DOI: 10.2215/CJN.08331109.

Magri CJ, Calleja N, Buhagiar G, Fava S, and J Vassallo. 2012. Ankle-brachial index in a type 2 diabetic population with proliferative retinopathy: associated risk factors and complications. *International Angiology*, Apr; 31(2):134–141. PMID: 22466978.

Makhdoomi K, Mohammadi A, Yekta Z, Aghasi MR, Zamani N, and S Vossughian. 2013. Correlation between ankle-brachial index and microalbuminuria in type 2 diabetes mellitus. *Iranian Journal of Kidney Diseases*, May; 7(3): 204209. PMID: 23689152.

Manju M, Mishra S, Toora BD, Vijayakumar and R Vinod. 2014. Relationship between glycosylated hemoglobin, serum nitric oxide and mean arterial blood pressure. *International Journal of Biomedical Science*, Dec; 10(4): 252–257. PMCID: PMC4289699.

McDermott MM, Criqui MH, Liu K, Guralnik JM, Greenland P, Martin GJ, and W Pearce. 2000. Lower ankle/brachial index, as calculated by averaging the dorsalis pedis and posterior tibial arterial pressures, and association with leg functioning in peripheral arterial disease. *Journal of Vascular Surgery*, 32, 1164–1171. DOI: 10.1067/mva.2000.108640.

McKnight GM, Smith LM, Drummond RS, Duncan CW, Golden M, and N Benjamin. 1997. Chemical synthesis of nitric oxide in the stomach from dietary nitrate in humans. *Gut*, Feb; 40(2): 211–214. PMCID: PMC1027050.

Meisinger C, Döring A, and M Heier. 2008. Blood pressure and risk of type 2 diabetes mellitus in men and women from the general population: the Monitoring Trends and Determinants on Cardiovascular Diseases/Cooperative Health Research in the Region of Augsburg Cohort Study. *Journal of Hypertension*, Sep; 26(9): 1809–1815. DOI: 10.1097/HJH.0b013e328307c3e9.

Mooradian AD. 2009. Dyslipidemia in type 2 diabetes mellitus. *Nature Reviews Endocrinology*, Mar; 5: 150–159. DOI: 10.1038/ncpendmet1066.

Nathan DM, Balkau B, Bonora E, Borch-Johnsen K, Buse JB, Colagiuri S, Davidson MB, DeFronzo R, Genuth S, Holman RR, Ji L, Kirkman S, Knowler WC, Schatz D, Shaw J, Sobngwi E, Steffes M, Vaccaro O, Wareham N, Zinman B, and R Kahn. 2009. International Expert Committee report on the role of the A1C assay in the diagnosis of diabetes. *Diabetes Care*, Jul; 32(7): 1327–1334. DOI: 10.2337/dc09-9033.

Newman AB, Siscovick DS, Manolio TA, Polak J, Fried LP, Borhani NO, and SK Wolfson. 1993. Ankle-arm index as a marker of atherosclerosis in the Cardiovascular Health Study. Cardiovascular Heart Study (CHS) Collaborative Research Group. *Circulation*, 88, 837–845. https://doi.org/10.1161/01.CIR.88.3.837.

No authors listed. 2003. Peripheral arterial disease in people with diabetes. *Diabetes Care*, Dec; 26(12): 3333–3341. PMID: 14633825.

No authors listed. 2002. Self-monitoring of blood glucose, *Clinical Diabetes*, Jan; 20(1): 48–48. https://doi.org/10.2337/diaclin.20.1.48.

No authors listed. 2012. Ankle brachial index, quick reference guide for clinicians. *Journal of Wound Ostomy and Continence Nursing*. 39(2S): S21–S29.

Nussbaumerová B, Rosolová H, Ferda J, Sifalda P, Sípová I, and F Sefrna. 2011. The ankle brachial index in type 2 diabetes [article in Czech]. *Vnitrni Lekarstvi* (journal of the Czech Society of Internal Medicine). Mar; 57(3): 299–305.

Ott SJ, El Mokhtari NE, Musfeldt M, Stephan Hellmig S, Freitag S, Rehman A, Kühbacher T, Nikolaus S, Namsolleck P, Blaut M, Hampe J, Sahly H, Reinecke A, Haake N, Günther R, Krüger D, Lins M, Herrmann G, Fölsch UR, Simon R, and S Schreiber. 2006. Detection of diverse bacterial signatures in atherosclerotic lesions of patients with coronary heart disease. *Circulation*, 113:929–937. DOI: 10.1161 /CIRCULATIONAHA.105.579979.

Parving HH, Lehnert H, Brochner-Mortensen J, Gomis R, Andersen S, and P Arner. 2001. The effect of irbesartan on the development of diabetic nephropathy in patients with type 2 diabetes. *New England Journal of Medicine*, Sep; 345(12): 870–878. DOI: 10.1056/NEJMoa011489.

Polonsky W, Fisher L, Schikman C, Hinnen D, Parkin C, Jelsovsky Z, Amstutz L, Schweitzer M, and R Wagner. 2010. The value of episodic, intensive blood glucose monitoring in non-insulin treated persons with Type 2 Diabetes: design of the Structured Testing Program (STeP) study, a cluster-randomised, clinical trial [NCT00674986]. BMC Family Practice. 2010 May 18;11:37. DOI: 10.1186/1471-2296-11-37.

Polonsky WH, Fisher L, Schikman CH, Hinnen DA, Parkin CG, Jelsovsky Z, Petersen B, Schweitzer M, and RS Wagner. 2011. Structured self-monitoring of blood glucose significantly reduces A1C levels in poorly controlled, noninsulin-treated Type 2 diabetes. Results from the Structured Testing Program study. *Diabetes Care*, Feb; 34(2): 262–267. DOI: 10.7860/JCDR/2012/4854.2667.

Rodbard HW, Blonde L, Braithwaite SS, Brett EM, Cobin RH, Handelsman Y, Hellman R, Jellinger PS, Jovanovic LG, Levy P, Mechanick JI, Zangeneh F; and AACE Diabetes Mellitus Clinical Practice Guidelines Task Force. 2007. American Association of Clinical Endocrinologists medical guidelines for clinical practice for the management of diabetes mellitus. *Endocrinology Practice*, May–Jun;13 Suppl 1:1–68. DOI: 10.4158/EP.13.S1.1.

Shen J, Liu F, Zeng H, Wang J, Zhao J-G, Zhao J, Lu F-D, and W-P Jia. 2012. Vibrating perception threshold and body mass index are associated with abnormal foot plantar pressure in Type 2 diabetes outpatients. *Diabetes Technology and Therapeutics*, Nov; 14(11): 1053–1059. DOI: 10.1089/dia.2012.0146.

Sherwani S, Khan HA, Ekhzaimy A, Masood A, and MK Sakharkar. 2016. Significance of HbA1c test in diagnosis and prognosis of diabetic patients. *Biomarker Insights*. 2016; 11: 95–104. DOI: 10.4137/BMI.S38440.

Shimokata H, and F Kuzuya. 1993. Aging, basal metabolic rate, and nutrition [article in Japanese]. *Japanese Journal of Geriatrics* (Nihon Ronen Igakkai Zasshi), Jul; 30(7): 572–576. PMID: 8361073.

Sila-On A, Pavaro U, W Nuchpramool. 1991. Serum and urinary uric acid levels in healthy subjects and in patients with urolithiasis. *Journal of the Medical Association of Thailand*, Aug; 74(8): 352–357. PMID: 1791385.

Smit J. 2017. Community-acquired *Staphylococcus aureus* bacteremia: studies of risk and prognosis with special attention to diabetes mellitus and chronic heart failure. *Danish Medical Journal*, May; 64(5). pii: B5379. PMID: 28552097.

Spiegelhalder, B, Eisenbrand G, and R Preussmann. 1976. Influence of dietary nitrate on nitrite content of human saliva: possible relevance to in vivo formation of N-nitroso compounds. *Food and Cosmetics Toxicology*, 14(6): 545–548. PMID: 1017769.

Tessari P, Cecchet D, Cosma A, Vettore M, Coracina A, Millioni R, Iori E, Puricelli L, Avogaro A, and M Vedovato. 2010. Nitric oxide synthesis is reduced in subjects with Type 2 diabetes and nephropathy. *Diabetes*, Sep; 59(9): 2152–2159. DOI: 10.2337/db09-1772.

Thejaswini KO, Roopakala MS, Dayananda G, Chandrakala SP, and KM Prasanna Kumar. 2013. A study of association of Ankle Brachial Index (ABI) and the Highly Sensitive C-Reactive Protein (hsCRP) in Type 2 diabetic patients and in normal subjects. *Journal of Clinical and Diagnostic Research*, Jan; 7(1): 46–50. DOI: 10.7860/JCDR/2012/4854.2667.

Thiruvoipati T, Kielhorn CE, and EJ Armstrong. 2015. Peripheral artery disease in patients with diabetes: Epidemiology, mechanisms, and outcomes. *World Journal of Diabetes*, Jul 10; 6(7): 961–969. Published online 2015 Jul 10. DOI: 10.4239/wjd.v6.i7.961.

Torricelli FC, De S, Gebreselassie S, Li I, Sarkissian C, and M Monga. 2014. Type-2 diabetes and kidney stones: impact of diabetes medications and glycemic control. *Urology*, Sep; 84(3): 544–548. DOI: 10.1016/j.urology.2014.02.074.

Tsikas D. 2007. Analysis of nitrite and nitrate in biological fluids by assays based on the Griess reaction: appraisal of the Griess reaction in the L-arginine/nitric oxide area of research. *Journal of Chromatography. B, Analytical Technologies in the Biomedical and Life Sciences*, May; 851(1–2): 51–70. DOI: 10.1016/j.jchromb .2006.07.054.

Valdivielso P, Puerta S, Rioja J, Alonso I, Ariza MJ, Sánchez-Chaparro MA, Palacios R, and P González-Santos. 2010. Postprandial apolipoprotein B48 is associated with asymptomatic peripheral arterial disease: a study in patients with type 2 diabetes and controls. *International Journal of Clinical Chemistry* (*Clinica Chimica Acta*), Mar; 411(5–6): 433–437. DOI: 10.1016/j.cca.2009.12.022.

Valdivielso P, Ramírez-Bollero J, and C Pérez-López. 2014. Peripheral arterial disease, type 2 diabetes and postprandial lipidaemia: is there a link? *World Journal of Diabetes*, Oct 15; 5(5): 577–585. Published online 2014 Oct 15. DOI: 10.4239/wjd.v5.i5.577.

Watala C, Witas H, Olszowska L, and W Piasecki. 1992. The association between erythrocyte internal viscosity, protein non-enzymatic glycosylation and erythrocyte membrane dynamic properties in juvenile diabetes mellitus. *International Journal of Experimental Pathology*, Oct; 73(5): 655–663. PMCID: PMC2002015.

Weinberg AE, Patel CJ, Chertow GM, and JT Leppert. 2014. Diabetic severity and risk of kidney stone disease. *European Urology*, Jan; 65(1): 0.1016/j.eururo.2013.03.026. DOI: 10.1016/j.eururo.2013.03.026.

Windler E. 2005. What is the consequence of an abnormal lipid profile in patients with type 2 diabetes or the metabolic syndrome? *Atherosclerosis. Supplement*, Sep; 6(3): 11–14. DOI: 10.1016/j.atherosclerosissup .2005.06.003.

Wu P. 2000. Thyroid disease and diabetes. *Clinical Diabetes*, 18(1): 38; http://journal.diabetes.org/clinicaldiabetes /v18n12000/pg38.htm.

7 Advanced Glycation End Products—A Special Hazard in Diabetes

7.1 WHAT ARE ADVANCED GLYCATION END PRODUCTS—"AGEs"?

"AGE" stands for advanced glycation end product. "Glycation" means to combine with glucose, that is, sugar. AGEs are carbohydrates, lipids, or proteins that are combined with glucose. AGEs may occur naturally to a lesser extent in our body as we age; however, according to a report in the journal *Dermatoendocrinology*, they are formed in high amounts in diabetes (Gkogkolou, and Böhm. 2012). The emphasis in this chapter is on those that occur to a greater extent in "prepared" foods we consume.

AGEs are harmful by-products of common food preparation methods such as frying, and they are more likely to be present in certain food categories such as meats.

Unfortunately, the combination of high AGE-potential foods and an AGE-promoting cooking method is very popular in the United States, and these AGEs are particularly damaging for people with Type 2 diabetes.

Most people, even those who have read about Type 2 diabetes and otherwise informed themselves about it, probably have never heard of "advanced glycation end products." Yet, AGEs are found in various concentrations in many if not most of our common prepared food—including those we ourselves prepare. It is not surprising that Americans, with few exceptions, haven't heard about AGEs.

Many health authorities issue advice, "tips" as it were, to those with Type 2 diabetes. Consider the following from the Mayo Clinic:

1. Get more physical activity.
2. Get plenty of fiber.
3. Go for whole grains.
4. Lose extra weight.
5. Skip fad diets and just make healthier choices (http://www.mayoclinic.org/diseases-conditions /type-2-diabetes/in-depth/diabetes-prevention/art-20047639; accessed May 19, 2017).

Sound advice, but shouldn't there be a number 6, avoid those AGEs?

Most foods we eat nowadays come to us as the "end product" of preparation, that is, cooking in some way. It could be just plain heating, or boiling, or frying, or broiling or roasting, or whatever. For instance, "cuisine" is about end product. We generally gravitate to cuisine for the taste of the end product, and not usually because we look forward to a particular molecular distortion of food constituents.

The journal *Molecular Nutrition and Food Research* tells us that AGEs form in the late stages of the so-called Maillard reaction in foods and biological systems. The Maillard reaction, named after the French chemist Louis-Camille Maillard who first described it in 1912, is a chemical reaction that he observed between amino acids and reducing sugars that gives browned food its distinctive flavor. But there is more, as seared steaks, pan-fried dumplings, cookies, and other kinds of biscuits, breads, toasted marshmallows, and many other foods undergo this reaction during preparation.

The reaction is a form of nonenzymatic browning that typically proceeds rapidly when heating foods from about 280°F to 330°F (140°C to 165°C). In practical terms, these end products are mostly formed by the reactions of reducing sugar or the degradation products of carbohydrates, proteins, and lipids.

It has emerged recently that some AGEs, in concentration, may be harmful to the body, and they may possibly cause or aggravate various kinds of diseases, especially diabetes and kidney disorder, through the function of the AGE receptor (RAGE) (Chuyen. 2006).

AGEs affect nearly every type of cell and molecule in the body and are implicated in causing the blood vessel damage complications of diabetes. Under certain conditions such as the oxidative stress caused by hyperglycemia (high blood sugar) in patients with diabetes and elevated serum lipids, AGEs formation can rise beyond ordinary levels and then become particularly harmful.

There is considerable evidence that significant amounts of dietary AGEs (dAGEs) aggravate Type 2 diabetes and also contribute to the formation of atherosclerosis and kidney disease (Uribarri, Woodruff, Goodman et al. 2010).

AGEs are implicated in the glycation of low-density lipoprotein (LDL) cholesterol, that is, the bonding of a sugar molecule to a protein or lipid molecule without enzymatic regulation, which can promote its oxidation, thus forming reactive oxygen species (ROS) (Prasad, Bekker, and Tsimikas. 2012).

In addition, AGEs can induce cross-linking of collagen, which can cause blood vessel stiffening and entrapment of LDL particles in the artery walls. Cross-linking collagen is a characteristic of the aging skin (Yamaguchi, Woodley, and Mechanic. 1988).

Substantial evidence of a direct association between dietary AGE intake and markers of systemic inflammation such as C-reactive protein was found in a large group of healthy people (Uribarri, Cai, Sandu et al. 2005). However, while AGEs are probably best kept to a minimum in the diet, it is not clear just how harmful they are in healthy adults. A study reported in *The Journal of Nutrition* aimed to compare the effects of a diet high or low in AGEs on endothelial function, circulating AGEs, inflammatory mediators, and receptors for AGEs on circulating cells in healthy adults. It is the only study that database research found that contradicts Uribarri, Cai, Sandu et al. (2005) and similar studies cited above.

A dietary intervention was conducted for 6 weeks with healthy adults, 50 to 69 years old, that compared isocaloric, food-equivalent diets that were prepared at either high or mild temperatures. The isocaloric diet is a moderate-carbohydrate, moderate-fat diet that allows dieters to eat whatever they want as long as they consume the same amount of carbohydrates, proteins, and fats as daily food equivalents.

Based on the markers observed, after 6 weeks of dietary intervention, a high- or low-AGE diet had no significant impact on peripheral arterial tonometry, a noninvasive method to measure endothelial dysfunction, or on any inflammatory mediators in healthy middle-aged to older adults (Semba, Gebauer, Baer et al. 2014).

AGEs can bind to the receptor for advanced glycation end-products, causing oxidative stress as well as inflammation in endothelial cells (Di Marco, Gray and Jandeleit-Dahm. 2013).

There are basic strategies to reduce the impact of AGEs: by preventing their formation, by breaking cross-links after they are formed, and by preventing their detrimental effects. These will be detailed later in this chapter.

7.1.1 ARE AGEs, THE "MISSING LINK"?

In 2012, the author of a report in the *Proceedings of the National Academy of Sciences USA* cited research by Cai, Ramdas, Zhu et al. 2012, appearing in the same journal: "In a series of elegant and convincing experiments in mice, Cai et al. now may have found a possible 'missing link.'"

They demonstrated that AGEs are responsible for inducing an inflammatory state, which, in turn, leads to the development of insulin resistance and hyperglycemia" (Poretsky. 2012).

Indeed, Cai, Ramdas, Zhu et al. 2012, proposed on the basis of research evidence that chronic consumption of AGEs actually promotes insulin resistance (IR) and Type 2 diabetes. In one study, the mechanisms involved in these outcomes were assessed in four generations of mice fed isocaloric diets with or without AGEs. The mice manifested increased adiposity and premature insulin resistance marked by severe deficiency of advanced AGE glycation receptor 1 and of survival factor sirtuin 1 (SIRT1) in white adipose tissue, skeletal muscle, and liver. Sirtuin 1 expression is a response to caloric restriction due to food shortage.

In fact, it was shown in a study comparing diabetic patients to nondiabetic participants, published in the journal *Diabetes Care*, that restricting advanced glycation end production improves insulin resistance in Type 2 diabetes (Uribarri, Cai, Ramdas et al. 2011).

This chapter will first look at the formation of AGEs, then their targets, and then follow up with strategies to avoid and/or reduce their adverse effects, strategies that are particularly suited to the needs of patients with Type 2 diabetes.

7.2   AGES IN COMMONLY CONSUMED FOODS

AGEs can form naturally in the body and they can form in foods, as previously noted. They are present in uncooked animal-derived foods, but cooking, especially grilling, broiling, roasting, searing, and frying, results in the formation of new AGEs and accelerates their production (O'Brien, and Morrissey. 1989; Goldberg, Cai, Peppa et al. 2004). A wide variety of foods in modern diets are exposed to cooking or thermal processing for reasons of safety and convenience, as well as to enhance flavor, color, and appearance. Modern diet is a substantial source of AGEs (Goldberg, Cai, Peppa et al. 2004).

It had previously been assumed that dAGEs are poorly absorbed, and therefore, their potential role in human health and disease was largely ignored. However, recent studies clearly show that not only are dAGEs absorbed but they also contribute significantly to the body's AGE pool (Koschinsky, He, Mitsuhashi et al. 1997; He, Sabol, Mitsuhashi et al. 1999; Cai, He, Zhu et al. 2008).

AGEs are formed mostly from glucose–protein or glucose–lipid interactions, and they strongly promote the complications of diabetes and they accelerate aging. The *Journal of the American Dietetic Association* featured a report in 2004 titled "Advanced glycoxidation end products in commonly consumed foods" (the terms glycoxidation and glycation are interchangeable). The focus of that article was to determine the AGE content of commonly consumed foods and to evaluate the effects of various methods of food preparation on AGE production.

Two hundred fifty foods were tested for their content of a common AGE marker— $N(\varepsilon)$-(carboxymethyl)lysine, CML for short, using conventional laboratory enzyme-linked assay methods. Lipid and protein AGEs were represented in units of AGEs per gram of food (U/g). Keep in mind the term CML representing a marker, evidence as it were of the presence of AGEs. It will come up again.

Foods of the fat group showed the highest content with an average of 100 ± 19 kU/g. High values were also observed for the meat and meat-substitute group, 43 ± 7 kU/g. The carbohydrate group contained the lowest values of AGEs, 3.4 ± 1.8 kU/g.

The amount of AGEs present in all food categories was related to cooking temperature, length of cooking time, and presence of moisture: Broiling (437°F or 225°C) and frying (350.6°F or 177°C) resulted in the highest levels of AGEs, followed by roasting (350.6°F or 177°C) and boiling (212°F or 100°C).

The authors of the report concluded that diet can be a significant environmental source of AGEs, constituting a chronic risk factor for cardiovascular and kidney damage (Goldberg, Cai, Peppa et al. 2004). In fact, a report in the *Journal of Food Science* and Technology cautions about the rise in consumption of commercial processed food products. The authors contend that as modern diets are largely heat processed, they are more prone to contain high levels of AGEs.

The authors conclude that the emerging evidence of the adverse effects of AGEs makes it necessary to find therapies to inhibit AGEs (Sharma, Kaur, Thind et al. 2015). But, what constitutes a "high" AGEs concentration?

7.2.1 Levels in Some Common Foods

The *Journal of the American Dietetic Association* published a report that significantly expands the available dAGE database, validates the testing methodology, and compares cooking procedures and inhibitory agents on new dAGE formation. In addition, the report introduces practical approaches for reducing dAGE consumption in daily life.

It is reported in that publication that dry heat promotes new dAGE formation by more than 10 to 100 times above the uncooked state—across food categories.

As previously noted, animal-derived foods that are high in fat and protein are generally AGE rich and prone to new AGE formation by cooking. In contrast, carbohydrate-rich foods such as vegetables, fruits, whole grains, and milk contain relatively few AGEs, even after cooking.

The formation of new dAGEs during cooking can be prevented by the AGE inhibitory compound aminoguanidine and significantly reduced by cooking with moist heat, using shorter cooking time, cooking at lower temperature, and by the use of acidic ingredients such as lemon juice or vinegar. Aminoguanidine is an investigational drug for the treatment of diabetic kidney disease, but it is no longer under development as a medication.

The new dAGE database (shown below) may be a valuable instrument for estimating dAGE intake and for guiding food choices to reduce dAGE intake.

The formation of AGEs is part of normal metabolism, but if excessively high levels of AGEs are reached in tissues and in blood circulation, they can become harmful (Ulrich, and Cerami. 2001). The health hazard created by AGEs is that they tend to promote oxidative stress and inflammation by binding with cell surface receptors, or cross-linking with body proteins, altering their structure and function (Eble, Thorpe, and Baynes. 1983; Vlassara. 2001; Schmidt, Yan, Wautier et al. 1999).

Studies in healthy people show that dAGEs directly correlate with circulating AGEs as well as with markers of oxidative stress (Uribarri, Cai, Peppa et al. 2007). Moreover, restriction of dAGEs in patients with diabetes (Vlassara, Cai, Crandall et al. 2002) or kidney disease (Uribarri, Peppa, Cai et al. 2003) as well as in healthy people also reduces markers of oxidative stress and inflammation (Vlassara, Cai, Goodman et al. 2009).

As indicated in the opening paragraph of this section, but with some elaboration at this point, the aims of a study reported in the *Journal of the American Dietetic Association* were to add to the existing dAGE database by more than twofold, to validate the methods used to test AGEs in food, to examine different procedures and reagents on new dAGE formed, and to introduce practical methods to reduce the consumption of dAGEs in daily life (Uribarri, Woodruff, Goodman et al. 2010; https://www.ncbi.nlm.nih.gov/pmc/articles/PMC3704564/; accessed May 23, 2017).

The AGE content of food samples was obtained during the period 2003 to 2008 when foods were selected for their frequency of consumption on 3-day food records collected from healthy participants in the Upper East Side and East Harlem, in Manhattan, New York, New York. These foods therefore represent foods and culinary techniques typical of a Northeastern American multiethnic urban population.

The foods were obtained from the cafeteria of The Mount Sinai Hospital or from local restaurants or supermarkets, or were prepared in the General Clinical Research Center at the Mount Sinai School of Medicine, New York, New York.

The foods were cooked conventionally, including boiling (212°F or 100°C), broiling (437°F or 225°C), deep frying (356°F or 180°C), oven frying (446°F or 230°C), and roasting (350.6°F or

177°C), unless otherwise stated in the database (see Table 7.1, available also online at www.ada journal.org).

Cooking time varied as described in the database. Test procedures such as marinating, application of differing heating conditions, or cooking foods in different fats or oils are also described in the database. The abbreviations in the table are explained at the end.

Although Table 7.1 is an excellent guide to the amounts of AGEs that may be reasonably expected in common foods, it has limited generalizability due in large part to the likely geographic/regional bias and other constraints on the sampling of foods included.

Concerning the metabolic fate of glyoxal, the large majority is enzymatically converted into glycolate by a glutathione (GSH)-dependent glyoxalase system, which comprises two isozymes differing for tissue and subcellular localization (Mannervik. 2008). When GSH is depleted, as happens in many oxidative-based disorders, other enzymes including aldehyde reductase, aldose reductase, carbonyl reductase, aldehyde dehydrogenase, and 2-oxoaldehyde dehydrogenase can contribute to the glyoxal metabolism (Shangari, Bruce, Poon et al. 2003).

Finally, several lines of evidence have revealed that glyoxal catabolism could be involved in oxalate formation as suggested, for example, by studies on diabetes sufferers showing that they have increased levels of both plasma glyoxal and urinary oxalate (Eisner, Porten, Bechis et al. 2010). Such a pathway is catalyzed by glycolate oxidase and lactate dehydrogenase, involves glycolate as a key oxidized intermediate, and may influence calcium oxalate stone formation (Lange, Wood, Knight et al. 2012).

In fact, the journal *Molecular and Cell Biochemistry* reported the investigation of the role of GSH on kidney mitochondrial integrity and function during the stone-forming process in the hyperoxaluric state in male Wistar rats. Hyperoxaluria was induced by feeding ethylene glycol (EG) in drinking water. GSH was depleted by administering buthionine sulfoximine (BSO), a specific inhibitor of GSH biosynthesis. Glutathione monoester (GME) was administered for supplementing GSH. BSO treatment alone, or along with EG, depleted mitochondrial GSH by 40% and 51%, respectively.

A significant elevation was observed in lipid peroxidation and oxidation of protein thiols. Mitochondrial oxalate binding was enhanced by 74%, and 129% in BSO and BSO + EG treatment, respectively.

By comparison, ethylene glycol treatment produced only a 33% increase in mitochondrial oxalate binding. Significant alteration in calcium homeostasis was seen following BSO and BSO + EG treatment.

The investigators proposed that this may be due to altered mitochondrial integrity and function as evidenced from decreased activities of mitochondrial inner membrane marker enzymes, succinate dehydrogenase and cytochrome c oxidase, and respiratory control ratio and enhanced NADH oxidation by mitochondria in these two groups.

NADH oxidation and oxalate deposition in the kidney correlated negatively with mitochondrial GSH depletion. GME supplementation restored normal levels of GSH and maintained mitochondrial integrity and function, as a result of which oxalate deposition was prevented despite hyperoxaluria.

These results suggest that mitochondrial dysfunction resulting from GSH depletion could be a contributing factor in the development of calcium oxalate stones (Muthukumar, and Selvam. 1998).

7.2.1.1 AGE Lowering Factor

The *Journal of the American Dietetic Association* study cited above also reports that a low or acidic pH arrests AGE development: New AGE formation in cooked meat was tested after exposure to acidic solutions (marinades) of lemon juice or vinegar. Samples from lean beef were marinated in acidic solutions of either lemon or vinegar for 1 h before cooking.

TABLE 7.1
The AGE Content of 549 Foods, Based on Carboxymethyllysine Content

Food Item	AGE[a] (kU/100 g)	Serving Size (g)	AGE (kU/Serving)
		AGE Content	
Fats			
Almonds, blanched slivered (Bazzini's Nut Club, Bronx, New York)	5473	30	1642
Almonds, roasted	6650	30	1995
Avocado	1577	30	473
Butter, whipped[b]	26,480	5	1324
Butter, sweet cream, unsalted, whipped (Land O'Lakes, St Paul, Minnesota)	23,340	5	1167
Cashews, raw (Bazzini's Nut Club)	6730	30	2019
Cashews, roasted	9807	30	2942
Chestnut, raw	2723	30	817
Chestnut, roasted, in toaster oven 350°F for 27 min	5353	30	1606
Cream cheese, Philadelphia soft (Kraft, Northfield, Illinois)	10,883	30	3265
Cream cheese, Philadelphia original (Kraft)	8720	30	2616
Margarine, tub	17,520	5	876
Margarine, tub, I Can't Believe it's Not Butter (Unilever, Rotterdam, The Netherlands)	9920	5	496
Margarine, tub, Smart Balance (CFA Brands, Heart Beat Foods, Paramus, New Jersey)	6220	5	311
Margarine, tub, Take Control (Unilever Best Foods)	4000	5	200
Mayonnaise	9400	5	470
Mayonnaise, imitation (Diet Source, Novartis Nutrition Group, East Hanover, New Jersey)	200	5	10
Mayonnaise, low fat (Hellman's, Unilever Best Foods)	2200	5	110
Olive, ripe, large (5 g)	1670	30	501
Peanut butter, smooth, Skippy (Unilever)	7517	30	2255
Peanuts, cocktail (Planters, Kraft)	8333	30	2500
Peanuts, dry roasted, unsalted (Planters, Kraft)	6447	30	1934
Peanuts, roasted in shell, salted (Frito-Lay, Plano, Texas)	3440	30	1032
Pine nuts (pignolias), raw (Bazzini's Nut Club)	11,210	30	3363
Pistachios, salted (Frito Lay)	380	30	114
Pumpkin seeds, raw, hulled (House of Bazzini, Bronx, New York)	1853	30	556
Soybeans, roasted and salted (House of Bazzini)	1670	30	501
Sunflower seeds, raw, hulled (House of Bazzini)	2510	30	753
Sunflower seeds, roasted and salted (House of Bazzini)	4693	30	1408
Tartar Sauce, creamy (Kraft)	247	15	37
Walnuts, roasted	7887	30	2366
Fat, Liquid			
Cream, heavy, ultra-pasteurized (Farmland Dairies, Fairlawn, New Jersey)	2167	15	325
Oil, canola	9020	5	451
Oil, corn	2400	5	120

(*Continued*)

TABLE 7.1 (CONTINUED)
The AGE Content of 549 Foods, Based on Carboxymethyllysine Content

Food Item	AGE Content		
	AGE[a] (kU/100 g)	Serving Size (g)	AGE (kU/Serving)
Fat, Liquid			
Oil, cottonseed (The B Manischewitz Company, Cincinnati, Ohio)	8520	5	426
Oil, diaglycerol, Enova (ADM Kao LLC, Decatur, Illinois)	10,420	5	521
Oil, olive	11,900	5	595
Oil, olive, extra virgin, first cold pressed (Colavita, Linden, New Jersey)	10,040	5	502
Oil, peanut (Planters)	11,440	5	572
Oil, safflower (The Hain Celestial Group, Inc., Melville, New York)	3020	5	151
Oil, sesame (Asian Gourmet)	21,680	5	1084
Oil, sunflower (The Hain Celestial Group, Inc.)	3940	5	197
Salad dressing, blue cheese (Kraft)	273	15	41
Salad dressing, caesar (Kraft)	740	15	111
Salad dressing, French (H. J. Heinz Co, Pittsburgh, Pennsylvania)	113	15	17
Salad dressing, French, lite (Diet Source, Novartis Nutr Corp)	0	15	0
Salad dressing, Italian (Heinz)	273	15	41
Salad dressing, Italian, lite (Diet Source, Novartis Nutr Corp)	0	15	0
Salad dressing, thousand island (Kraft)	187	15	28
Meats and Meat Substitutes			
Beef			
Beef, bologna	1631	90	1468
Beef, corned brisket, deli meat (Boar's Head, Sarasota, Florida)	199	90	179
Beef, frankfurter, boiled in water, 212°F, 7 min	7484	90	6736
Beef, frankfurter, broiled 450°F, 5 min	11,270	90	10,143
Beef, ground, boiled, marinated 10 min w/ lemon juice	1538	90	1384
Beef, ground, pan browned, marinated 10 min w/ lemon juice	3833	90	3450
Beef, ground, 20% fat, pan browned	4928	90	4435
Beef, ground, 20% fat, pan/cover	5527	90	4974
Beef, hamburger (McDonald's Corp, Oak Brook, Illinois)	5418	90	4876
Beef, hamburger patty, olive oil 180°F, 6 min	2639	90	2375
Beef, meatball, potted (cooked in liquid), 1 h[c]	4300	90	3870
Beef, meatball, w/ sauce[c]	2852	90	2567
Beef, meatloaf, crust off, 45 min	1862	90	1676
Beef, raw	707	90	636
Beef, roast[b]	6071	90	5464
Beef, salami, kosher (Hebrew National, ConAgra Foods, Omaha, Nebraska)	628	90	565

(Continued)

TABLE 7.1 (CONTINUED)

The AGE Content of 549 Foods, Based on Carboxymethyllysine Content

Food Item	AGE Content		
	AGE[a] (kU/100 g)	Serving Size (g)	AGE (kU/Serving)
Meats and Meat Substitutes			
Beef			
Beef, steak, broiled[c]	7479	90	6731
Beef, steak, grilled 4 min, George Foreman grill (Salton Inc., Lake Forest, Illinois)	7416	90	6674
Beef, steak, microwaved, 6 min	2687	90	2418
Beef, steak, pan fried w/ olive oil	10,058	90	9052
Beef, steak, raw	800	90	720
Beef, steak, strips, 450°F, 15 min[c]	6851	90	6166
Beef, steak, strips, stir fried with 1 T canola oil, 15 min	9522	90	8570
Beef, steak, strips, stir fried without oil, 7 min	6973	90	6276
Beef, stewed, shoulder cut[c]	2230	90	2007
Beef, stewed[b]	2657	90	2391
Beef, stewed (mean)	2443	90	2199
Poultry			
Chicken, back or thigh, roasted then BBQ[b]	8802	90	7922
Chicken, boiled in water, 1 h	1123	90	1011
Chicken, boiled with lemon	957	90	861
Chicken, breast, skinless, roasted with BBQ sauce[c]	4768	90	4291
Chicken, breast, skinless, breaded[b]	4558	90	4102
Chicken, breast, skinless, breaded, reheated 1 min[b]	5730	90	5157
Chicken, breast, boiled in water[c]	1210	90	1089
Chicken, breast, breaded, deep fried, 20 min	9722	90	8750
Chicken, breast, breaded, oven fried, 25 min, with skin[c]	9961	90	8965
Chicken, breast, breaded/pan fried[c]	7430	90	6687
Chicken, breast, grilled/George Foreman grill (Salton Inc.)	4849	90	4364
Chicken, breast, pan fried, 13 min, high[c]	4938	90	4444
Chicken, breast, pan fried, 13 min high/microwave 12.5 s[c]	5417	90	4875
Chicken, breast, poached, 7 min, medium heat[c]	1101	90	991
Chicken, breast, potted (cooked in liquid), 10 min medium heat[c]	2480	90	2232
Chicken, breast, roasted, 45 min with skin[c]	6639	90	5975
Chicken, breast, skinless, microwave, 5 min	1524	90	1372
Chicken, breast, skinless, poached, 15 min	1076	90	968
Chicken, breast, skinless, raw	769	90	692
Chicken, breast, steamed in foil, 15 min, medium heat[c]	1058	90	952
Chicken, breast, strips, stir fried with canola oil, 7 min	4140	90	3726
Chicken, breast, strips, stir fried without oil, 7 min	3554	90	3199
Chicken, breast, with skin, 450°F, 45 min[c]	8244	90	7420
Chicken, breast, skinless, broiled, 450°F, 15 min	5828	90	5245
Chicken, crispy (McDonald's[d])	7722	90	6950
Chicken, curry, cube skinless breast, panfry10 min, broiled 12 min[c]	6340	90	5706

(Continued)

TABLE 7.1 (CONTINUED)
The AGE Content of 549 Foods, Based on Carboxymethyllysine Content

Food Item	AGE Content		
	AGE[a] (kU/100 g)	Serving Size (g)	AGE (kU/Serving)
Meats and Meat Substitutes			
Poultry			
Chicken, curry, cube skinless breast, steam 10 min, broiled 12 min[c]	5634	90	5071
Chicken, dark meat, broiled, inside, 450°F, 15 min	8299	90	7469
Chicken, fried, in olive oil, 8 min	7390	90	6651
Chicken, ground, dark meat with skin, raw[c]	1223	90	1101
Chicken, ground, dark w/ skin, pan fried, w/ canola oil, 2.5 min, high heat[c]	3001	90	2701
Chicken, ground, white meat, pan fried, no added fat, 5 min, high heat[c]	1808	90	1627
Chicken, ground, white meat, pan fried, with oil	1647	90	1482
Chicken, ground, white meat, raw	877	90	789
Chicken, kebab, cubed skinless breast, pan fried, 15 min[c]	6122	90	5510
Chicken, leg, roasted[b]	4650	90	4185
Chicken, loaf, roasted[c]	3946	90	3551
Chicken, loaf, roasted, crust off[c]	1420	90	1278
Chicken, meat ball, potted (cooked in liquid), 1 h	1501	90	1351
Chicken, nuggets, fast food (McDonald's[d])	8627	90	7764
Chicken, potted (cooked in liquid) with onion and water	3329	90	2996
Chicken, roasted[c]	6020	90	5418
Chicken, selects (McDonald's)	9257	90	8331
Chicken, skin, back or thigh, roasted then BBQ[b]	18,520	90	16,668
Chicken, skin, leg, roasted[b]	10,997	90	9897
Chicken, skin, thigh, roasted[b]	11,149	90	10,034
Chicken, thigh, roasted[b]	5146	90	4631
Turkey, burger, pan fried with cooking spray, 5 min, high heat[c]	7968	90	7171
Turkey, burger, pan fried with cooking spray, 5 min, high heat, microwaved 13.5 s, high heat[c]	8938	90	8044
Turkey, burger, pan fried with 5 mL canola oil, 3.5 min, high heat[c]	8251	90	7426
Turkey, ground, grilled, crust	6351	90	5716
Turkey, ground, grilled, interior	5977	90	5379
Turkey, ground, raw	4957	90	4461
Turkey, burger, broiled	5366	90	4829
Turkey, breast, roasted	4669	90	4202
Turkey, breast, smoked, seared[c]	6013	90	5412
Turkey, breast, steak, skinless, marinated w/orange juice, broiled[c]	4388	90	3949
Pork			
Bacon, fried 5 min no added oil	91,577	13	11,905
Bacon, microwaved, 2 slices, 3 min	9023	13	1173
Ham, deli, smoked	2349	90	2114

(Continued)

TABLE 7.1 (CONTINUED)
The AGE Content of 549 Foods, Based on Carboxymethyllysine Content

| | AGE Content | | |
Food Item	AGE[a] (kU/100 g)	Serving Size (g)	AGE (kU/Serving)
Meats and Meat Substitutes			
Pork			
Liverwurst (Boar's Head)	633	90	570
Pork, chop, marinated w/balsamic vinegar, BBQ[b]	3334	90	3001
Pork, chop, raw, marinated w/balsamic vinegar[b]	1188	90	1069
Pork, chop, pan fried, 7 min	4752	90	4277
Pork, ribs, roasted, Chinese take out	4430	90	3987
Pork, roast, Chinese take out	3544	90	3190
Sausage, beef and pork links, pan fried	5426	90	4883
Sausage, Italian, raw[b]	1861	90	1675
Sausage, Italian, BBQ[b]	4839	90	4355
Sausage, pork links, microwaved, 1 min	5943	90	5349
Lamb			
Lamb, leg, boiled, 30 min	1218	90	1096
Lamb, leg, broiled, 450°F, 30 min	2431	90	2188
Lamb, leg, microwave, 5 min	1029	90	926
Lamb, leg, raw	826	90	743
Veal			
Veal, stewed	2858	90	2572
Fish/Seafood			
Crabmeat, fried, breaded (take out)	3364	90	3028
Fish, loaf (gefilte), boiled 90 min	761	90	685
Salmon, Atlantic, farmed, prev. frozen, microwaved, 1 min, high heat[c]	954	90	859
Salmon, Atlantic, farmed, prev. frozen, poached, 7 min, medium heat[c]	1801	90	1621
Salmon, Atlantic, farmed, prev. frozen, steamed, 10 min, medium heat[c]	1212	90	1091
Salmon, Atlantic, farmed, prev. frozen, steamed in foil, 8 min, medium heat[c]	1000	90	900
Salmon, breaded, broiled 10 min	1498	90	1348
Salmon, broiled with olive oil	4334	90	9301
Salmon, canned pink (Rubenstein, Trident Seafoods, Seattle, Washington)	917	90	825
Salmon, fillet, boiled, submerged, 18 min	1082	90	974
Salmon, fillet, broiled	3347	90	3012
Salmon, fillet, microwaved	912	90	821
Salmon, fillet, poached	2292	90	2063
Salmon, pan fried in olive oil	3083	90	2775
Salmon, raw, previously frozen	517	90	465
Salmon, raw	528	90	475
Salmon, smoked	572	90	515
Scrod, broiled 450°F, 30 min	471	90	424
Shrimp frozen dinner, microwaved 4.5 min	4399	90	3959

(Continued)

TABLE 7.1 (CONTINUED)
The AGE Content of 549 Foods, Based on Carboxymethyllysine Content

Food Item	AGE[a] (kU/100 g)	Serving Size (g)	AGE (kU/Serving)
		AGE Content	
Meats and Meat Substitutes			
Fish/Seafood			
Shrimp, fried, breaded (take out)	4328	90	3895
Shrimp, marinated raw[b]	1003	90	903
Shrimp, marinated, grilled on BBQ[b]	2089	90	1880
Trout, baked, 25 min	2138	90	1924
Trout, raw	783	90	705
Tuna, patty, chunk light, broiled, 450°F, 30 min	747	90	672
Tuna, broiled, with soy, 10 min	5113	90	4602
Tuna, broiled, with vinegar dressing	5150	90	4635
Tuna, fresh, baked, 25 min	919	90	827
Tuna, loaf (chunk light in recipe), baked 40 min	590	90	531
Tuna, canned, chunk light, w/ water	452	90	407
Tuna, canned, white, albacore, w/ oil	1740	90	1566
Whiting, breaded, oven fried, 25 min[c]	8774	90	7897
Cheese			
Cheese, American, low fat (Kraft)	4040	30	1212
Cheese, American, white, processed	8677	30	2603
Cheese, brie	5597	30	1679
Cheese, cheddar	5523	30	1657
Cheese, cheddar, extra sharp, made with 2% milk (Cracker Barrel, Kraft)	2457	30	737
Cheese, cottage, 1% fat (Light & Lively, Kraft)	1453	30	436
Cheese, feta, Greek, soft	8423	30	2527
Cheese, mozzarella, reduced fat	1677	30	503
Cheese, parmesan, grated (Kraft)	16,900	15	2535
Cheese, Swiss, processed[b]	4470	30	1341
Cheese, Swiss, reduced fat (Alpine Lace, Alpine Lace Brands, Inc, Maplewood, New Jersey)	4743	30	1423
Soy			
Bacon bits, imitation, Bacos (Betty Crocker, General Mills, Minneapolis, Minnesota)	1247	15	187
Meatless jerky, Primal Strips (Primal Spirit Inc., Moundsville, West Virginia)	1398	90	1258
Soy burger, Boca burger, 400°F, 8 min—4 each side[c] (BOCA Foods Co, Madison, Wisconsin)	130	30	39
Soy burger, Boca burger, microwaved, 1.5 min[c] (BOCA Foods Co)	67	30	20
Soy burger, Boca burger, skillet, cook spray, 5 min[c] (BOCA Foods Co)	100	30	30
Soy burger, Boca burger, skillet, w/ 1 tsp olive oil, 5 min[c] (BOCA Foods Co)	437	30	131
Soy burger, Boca burger (BOCA Foods Co) (mean)	183	30	55
Tofu, broiled	4107	90	3696

(Continued)

TABLE 7.1 (CONTINUED)
The AGE Content of 549 Foods, Based on Carboxymethyllysine Content

	AGE Content		
Food Item	AGE[a] (kU/100 g)	Serving Size (g)	AGE (kU/Serving)
Meats and Meat Substitutes			
Soy			
Tofu, raw	788	90	709
Tofu, soft, raw	488	90	439
Tofu, sautéed, inside	3569	90	3212
Tofu, sautéed, outside	5877	90	5289
Tofu, sautéed (mean)	4723	90	4251
Tofu, soft, boiled 5 min, +2 min to return to boil[c]	628	90	565
Tofu, soft, boiled 5 min, +2 min, + soy sauce, sesame oil[c]	796	90	716
Eggs			
Egg, fried, one large	2749	45	1237
Egg white powder (Deb-El Products, Elizabeth, New Jersey)	1040	10	104
Egg white, large, 10 min	43	30	13
Egg white, large, 12 min	63	30	19
Egg yolk, large, 10 min	1193	15	179
Egg yolk, large, 12 min	1680	15	252
Egg, omelet, pan, low heat, cooking spray, 11 min[c]	90	30	27
Egg, omelet, pan, low heat, corn oil, 12 min[c]	223	30	67
Egg, omelet, pan, low heat, margarine, 8 min[c]	163	30	49
Egg, omelet, pan, low, butter, 13 min[c]	507	30	152
Egg, omelet, pan, low, olive oil, 12 min[c]	337	30	101
Egg, poached, below simmer, 5 min[c]	90	30	27
Egg, scrambled, pan, high, butter, 45 s[c]	337	30	101
Egg, scrambled, pan, high, cooking spray, 1 min[c]	117	30	35
Egg, scrambled, pan, high, corn oil, 1 min[c]	173	30	52
Egg, scrambled, pan, high, margarine, 1 min[c]	123	30	37
Egg, scrambled, pan, high, olive oil, 1 min[c]	243	30	73
Egg, scrambled, pan, med-low, butter, 2 min[c]	167	30	50
Egg, scrambled, pan, med-low, cooking spray, 2 min[c]	67	30	20
Egg, scrambled, pan, med-low, corn oil, 1.5 min[c]	123	30	37
Egg, scrambled pan, med-low, margarine, 2 min[c]	63	30	19
Egg, scrambled, pan, med-low, olive oil, 2 min[c]	97	30	29
Carbohydrates			
Bread			
Bagel, small, Lender's[b]	133	30	40
Bagel, large[b]	107	30	32
Bagel, toasted[b]	167	30	50
Biscuit (Mc Donald's[d])	1470	30	441
Biscuit, refrigerator, oven-baked, 350°F, 17 min (Pillsbury Grands, General Mills)	1343	30	403
Biscuit, refrigerator, uncooked (Pillsbury Grands, General Mills)	823	30	247

(Continued)

TABLE 7.1 (CONTINUED)

The AGE Content of 549 Foods, Based on Carboxymethyllysine Content

Food Item	AGE Content		
	AGE[a] (kU/100 g)	Serving Size (g)	AGE (kU/Serving)
Carbohydrates			
Bread			
Bread, 100% whole wheat, center, toasted (Wonder, Interstate Bakeries, Inc., Irving, Texas)	83	30	25
Bread, 100% whole wheat, center (Wonder)	53	30	16
Bread, 100% whole wheat, top crust (Wonder)	73	30	22
Bread, 100% whole wheat, top crust, toasted (Wonder)	120	30	36
Bread, Greek, hard	150	30	45
Bread, Greek, hard, toasted	607	30	182
Bread, Greek, soft	110	30	33
Bread, pita	53	30	16
Bread, white, Italian, center (Freihoffer's, Bimbo Bakeries, Horsham, Pennsylvania)	23	30	7
Bread, white, Italian, center, toasted (Freihoffer's)	83	30	25
Bread, white, Italian, crust (Freihoffer's)	37	30	11
Bread, white, Italian, top crust, toasted (Freihoffer's)	120	30	36
Bread, white, slice (Rockland Bakery, Nanuet, New York)	83	30	25
Bread, white, slice, toasted (Rockland Bakery)	107	30	32
Bread, whole wheat, slice (Rockland Bakery)	103	30	31
Bread, whole wheat, slice, toasted, slice (Rockland Bakery)	137	30	41
Croissant, butter (Starbucks, Seattle, Washington)	1113	30	334
Roll, dinner, inside	23	30	7
Roll, dinner, outside	77	30	23
Breakfast Cereals			
Bran flakes, from raisin bran (Post, Kellogg Co, Battle Creek, Michigan)	33	30	10
Cinnamon Toast Crunch (General Mills)	1100	30	330
Corn Flakes (Kellogg's)	233	30	70
Corn Flakes, Honey Nut (Kellogg Co)	320	30	96
Corn Flakes, Sugar Frosted (Kellogg Co)	427	30	128
Corn Pops (Kellogg's)	1243	30	373
Cream of Wheat, instant, prepared (Nabisco, East Hanover, New Jersey)	108	175	189
Cream of Wheat, instant, prepared with honey (Nabisco)	189	175	331
Fiber One (General Mills)	1403	30	421
Froot Loops (Kellogg Co)	67	30	20
Frosted Mini Wheats (Kellogg Co)	210	30	63
Granola, Organic Oats & Honey (Cascadian Farms, Small Planet Foods, Minneapolis, Minnesota)	427	30	128
Life, mean (Quaker Oats, Chicago, Illinois)	1313	30	394
Puffed Corn Cereal (Arrowhead Mills, The Hain Celestial Group, Inc.)	100	30	30
Puffed Wheat	17	30	5
Rice Krispies (Kellogg Co)	2000	30	600

(Continued)

TABLE 7.1 (CONTINUED)
The AGE Content of 549 Foods, Based on Carboxymethyllysine Content

Food Item	AGE Content		
	AGE[a] (kU/100 g)	Serving Size (g)	AGE (kU/Serving)
Carbohydrates			
Breakfast Cereals			
Oatmeal, instant, dry (Quaker Oats)	13	30	4
Oatmeal, instant, prepared (Quaker Oats)	14	175	25
Oatmeal, instant, prepared with honey (Quaker Oats)	18	175	31
Breakfast Foods			
French toast, Aunt Jemima, frozen, microwaved 1 min (Pinnacle Foods)	603	30	181
French toast, Aunt Jemima, frozen, 10 min at 400°F (Pinnacle Foods Corp)	850	30	255
French toast, Aunt Jemima, frozen, not heated (Pinnacle Foods Corp, Cherry Hill, New Jersey)	263	30	79
French toast, Aunt Jemima frozen, toaster medium-1 cycle (Pinnacle Foods)	613	30	184
Hotcakes (McDonald's[d])	243	30	73
Pancake, from mix	823	30	247
Pancake, frozen, toasted (General Mills)	2263	30	679
Pancake, homemade	973	30	292
Waffle, frozen, toasted (Kellogg Co)	2870	30	861
Grains/Legumes			
Beans, red kidney, raw	116	100	116
Beans, red kidney, canned	191	100	191
Beans, red kidney, cooked 1 h	298	100	298
Pasta, cooked 8 min	112	100	112
Pasta, cooked 12 min	242	100	242
Pasta, spiral[b]	245	100	245
Rice, white, quick cooking, 10 min	9	100	9
Rice, Uncle Ben's white, cooked, 35 min (Mars, Inc., Houston, Texas)	9	100	9
Rice, white, pan-toasted 10 min, cooked 30 min	32	100	32
Starchy Vegetables			
Corn, canned	20	100	20
Potato, sweet, roasted 1 h	72	100	72
Potato, white, boiled 25 min	17	100	17
Potato, white, roasted 45 min, with 5 mL oil/serving[c]	218	100	218
Potato, white, French fries (McDonald's[d])	1522	100	1522
Potato, white, French fries, homemade	694	100	694
Potato, white, French fries, in corn oil, held under heat lamp[b]	843	100	843
Potato, white, hash browns (McDonald's[d])	129	100	129
Crackers/Snacks			
Breadsticks, Stella D'oro hard (Brynwood Partners, Greenwich, Connecticut)	127	30	38

(Continued)

TABLE 7.1 (CONTINUED)
The AGE Content of 549 Foods, Based on Carboxymethyllysine Content

Food Item	AGE Content		
	AGE[a] (kU/100 g)	Serving Size (g)	AGE (kU/Serving)
Carbohydrates			
Crackers/Snacks			
Chex mix, traditional (General Mills, Inc.)	1173	30	352
Chips, corn, Doritos (Frito Lay)	503	30	151
Chips, corn, Harvest Cheddar Sun Chips (Frito-Lay)	1270	30	381
Chips, Platanitos, plantain (Plantain Products Co, Tampa, Florida)	370	30	111
Chips, potato (Frito Lay)	2883	30	865
Chips, potato, baked original potato crisps (Frito Lay)	450	30	135
Combos, nacho cheese pretzel (M & M Mars, McLean, Virginia)	1680	30	504
Cracker, chocolate Teddy graham (Nabisco)	1647	30	494
Cracker, Pepperidge Farms Goldfish, cheddar (Campbell Soup Co, Camden, New Jersey)	2177	30	653
Cracker, Keebler honey graham (Kellogg Co)	1220	30	366
Cracker, Old London melba toast (Nonni's Food Co, Tulsa, Oklahoma)	903	30	271
Cracker, oyster	1710	30	513
Cracker, rice cake, corn (Taanug)	137	30	41
Cracker, saltine, hospital (Alliant)	937	30	281
Cracker, Keebler sandwich, club + cheddar (Kellogg Co)	1830	30	549
Cracker, toasted wheat	917	30	275
Cracker, wheat, round	857	30	257
Cracker, KA-ME rice crunch, plain (Liberty Richter, Bloomfield, New Jersey)	917	30	275
Popcorn, air popped, with butter	133	30	40
Popcorn, Pop Secret microwaved, fat free, no added fat (General Mills)	33	30	10
Pretzel, minis (Snyder's of Hanover, Hanover, New Jersey)	1790	30	537
Pretzel, Q rolled	1883	30	565
Pretzel, stick	1600	30	480
Pretzel (mean)	1757	30	527
Veggie Booty (Robert's American Gourmet, Seacliff, New York)	983	30	295
Cookies, Cakes, Pies, Pastries			
Bar, granola, chocolate chunk, soft (Quaker)	507	30	152
Bar, Nutrigrain, apple cinnamon (Kellogg's)	2143	30	643
Bar, Rice Krispies Treat (Kelloggs)	1920	30	576
Bar, granola, peanut butter and choc chunk, hard (Quaker)	3177	30	953
Cake, angel food, Danish Kitchen (Sam's Club, Bentonville, Arkansas)	27	30	8
Cookie, biscotti, vanilla almond (Starbucks)	3220	30	966
Cookie, chocolate chip, Chips Ahoy (Nabisco)	1683	30	505

(Continued)

TABLE 7.1 (CONTINUED)
The AGE Content of 549 Foods, Based on Carboxymethyllysine Content

	AGE Content		
Food Item	AGE[a] (kU/100 g)	Serving Size (g)	AGE (kU/Serving)
Carbohydrates			
Cookies, Cakes, Pies, Pastries			
Cookie, Greek wedding, nut cookie	960	30	288
Cookie, meringue, homemade	797	30	239
Cookie, Keebler oatmeal raisin (Kellogg Co)	1370	30	411
Cookie, Oreo (Nabisco)	1770	30	531
Cookie, Nilla vanilla wafer (Nabisco)	493	30	148
Croissant, chocolate (Au Bon Pain, Boston, Massachusetts)	493	30	148
Danish, cheese (Au Bon Pain)	857	30	257
Donut, glazed devil's food cake (Krispy Kreme, Winston-Salem, North Carolina)	1407	30	422
Donut, chocolate iced, crème filled (Krispy Kreme)	1803	30	541
Fruit pop, frozen (Dole, Westlake Village, California)	18	60	11
Fruit roll up, sizzlin' red (General Mills)	980	30	294
Gelatin, Dole strawberry (Nestle, Minneapolis, Minnesota)	2	125	2
Gelatin, Dole strawberry, sugar free (Nestle)	1	125	1
Ice cream cone, cake (Haagen Dazs, Oakland, California)	147	30	44
Ice cream cone, sugar (Haagen Dazs)	153	30	46
Muffin, bran (Au Bon Pain)	340	30	102
Pie, apple, individual, baked (McDonald's[d])	637	30	191
Pie, crust, frozen, baked per pkg, mean Mrs. Smith's Dutch Apple Crumb and Pumpkin Custard (Kellogg Co)	1390	30	417
Pie, Mrs. Smith's Dutch apple crumb, deep dish, apple filling (Kellogg Co)	340	30	102
Pie, Mrs. Smith's Dutch apple crumb, deep dish, crumbs (Kellogg Co)	1030	30	309
Pie, Mrs. Smith's Dutch apple crumb, deep dish, crust (Kellogg Co)	1410	30	423
Pie, Mrs. Smith's Dutch apple crumb, deep dish, pie (Kellogg Co)	893	30	268
Pie, Mrs. Smith's pumpkin custard, bake it fresh, original recipe, crust (Kellogg Co)	1373	30	412
Pie, Mrs. Smith's pumpkin custard, bake it fresh, original recipe, custard (Kellogg Co)	617	30	185
Pie, Mrs. Smith's pumpkin custard, bake it fresh, original recipe, pie (Kellogg Co)	880	30	264
Pop tart, microwave-3 s high power (Kellogg Co)	243	30	73
Pop tart, microwave-6 s medium high power (Kellogg's)	210	30	63
Pop tart, not heated (Kellogg Co)	133	30	40
Pop tart, toaster-low, 1 cycle (Kellogg Co)	260	30	78
Scone, cinnamon (Starbucks)	790	30	237
Sorbet, Edy's strawberry (Dryer's, Oakland, California)	2	125	3
Sweet roll, cinnamon swirl roll (Starbucks)	907	30	272

(Continued)

TABLE 7.1 (CONTINUED)
The AGE Content of 549 Foods, Based on Carboxymethyllysine Content

	AGE Content		
	---	---	---
Food Item	AGE[a] (kU/100 g)	Serving Size (g)	AGE (kU/Serving)
Carbohydrates			
Fruits			
Apple, baked	45	100	45
Apple, Macintosh	13	100	13
Banana	9	100	9
Cantaloupe	20	100	20
Coconut cream, Coco Goya cream of coconut (Goya, Secaucus, New Jersey)	933	15	20
Coconut milk, leche de coco (Goya)	307	15	140
Coconut, Baker's Angel Flake, sweetened (Kraft)	590	30	177
Dates, Sun-Maid California chopped (Sun-Maid, Kingsburg, California)	60	30	18
Fig, dried	2663	30	799
Plums, Sun-Maid dried pitted prunes (Sun-Maid)	167	30	50
Raisin, from Post Raisin Bran (Kellogg Co)	120	30	36
Vegetables (Raw Unless Specified Otherwise)			
Carrots, canned	10	100	10
Celery	43	100	43
Cucumber	31	100	31
Eggplant, grilled, marinated with balsamic vinegar[b]	256	100	256
Eggplant, raw, marinated with balsamic vinegar[b]	116	100	116
Green beans, canned	18	100	18
Portabella mushroom, raw, marinated with balsamic vinegar[b]	129	100	129
Onion	36	100	36
Tomato	23	100	23
Tomato sauce (Del Monte Foods, San Francisco, California)	11	100	11
Vegetables, grilled (broccoli, carrots, celery)	226	100	226
Vegetables, grilled (pepper, mushrooms)	261	100	261
Other Carbohydrates			
Sugar, white	0	5	0
Sugar substitute, aspartame as Canderel (Merisant, Chicago, Illinois)	0	5	0
Liquids			
Milk and Milk Products			
Cocoa packet, Swiss Miss, prepared (ConAgra Foods)	262	250	656
Cocoa packet, Swiss Miss sugar-free, prepared (ConAgra Foods)	204	250	511
Ice cream, America's Choice vanilla (The Great Atlantic and Pacific Tea Co, Montvale, New Jersey)	34	250	84
Milk, fat-free (hospital)	1	250	2
Milk, Lactaid fat free (McNeil Nutritionals, Fort Washington, Pennsylvania)	10	250	26
Milk, fat free (Tuscan Dairy Farms, Burlington, New Jersey)	2	250	4

(Continued)

TABLE 7.1 (CONTINUED)
The AGE Content of 549 Foods, Based on Carboxymethyllysine Content

| | AGE Content | | |
Food Item	AGE[a] (kU/100 g)	Serving Size (g)	AGE (kU/Serving)
	Liquids		
	Milk and Milk Products		
Milk, fat free, with A and D	0	250	1
Milk, fat free, with A and D (microwaved, 1 min)	2	250	5
Milk, fat free, with A and D (microwaved, 3 min)	34	250	86
Milk, soy (Imagine Foods, The Hain Celestial Group)	31	250	77
Milk, whole (4% fat)	5	250	12
Pudding, instant chocolate, fat-free, sugar-free, prepared	1	120	1
Pudding, instant chocolate, skim milk	1	120	1
Pudding, Hunt Wesson snack pack, chocolate (ConAgra Foods)	17	120	20
Pudding, Hunt Wesson snack pack, vanilla (ConAgra Foods)	13	120	16
Yogurt, cherry (Dannon, White Plains, New York)	4	250	10
Yogurt, vanilla (Dannon)	3	250	8
	Fruit Juice		
Juice, apple	2	250	5
Juice, cranberry	3	250	8
Juice, orange	6	250	14
Juice, orange, from fresh fruit	0	250	1
Juice, orange, with calcium	3	250	8
	Vegetable Juice		
Vegetable juice, V8 (Campbell Soup Co)	2	250	5
Other carbohydrate liquids			
Fruit pop, frozen (Dole)	18	60	11
Honey	7	15	1
Sorbet, strawberry (Edy's)	2	125	3
Syrup, caramel, sugar free	0	15	0
Syrup, dark corn	0	15	0
Syrup, pancake, lite	0	15	0
	Combination Foods and Solid Condiments		
	Combination Foods		
Bacon Egg Cheese Biscuit (McDonald's[d])	2289	100	2289
Bacon, Egg and Cheese McGriddles (McDonald's[d])	858	100	858
Big Mac (McDonald's[d])	7801	100	7801
Casserole, tuna	233	100	233
Cheeseburger (McDonald's[d])	3402	100	3402
Chicken McGrill (McDonald's[d])	5171	100	5171
Corned beef hash, canned, microwaved 2 min, high power (Broadcast)	1691	100	1691
Corned beef hash, canned, stove top, medium heat, 12 min (Broadcast)	2175	100	2175

(Continued)

TABLE 7.1 (CONTINUED)
The AGE Content of 549 Foods, Based on Carboxymethyllysine Content

	AGE Content		
Food Item	AGE[a] (kU/100 g)	Serving Size (g)	AGE (kU/Serving)
Combination Foods and Solid Condiments			
Combination Foods			
Corned beef hash, canned, unheated (Broadcast)	1063	100	1063
Double Quarter Pounder With Cheese (McDonald's[d])	6283	100	6283
Filet-O-Fish (McDonald's[d])	6027	100	6027
Gnocchi, potato/flour/Parmesan cheese, 3 min	535	100	535
Gnocchi, potato/flour/Parmesan cheese, 4.5 min	2074	100	2074
Hot Pocket, bacon, egg, cheese, oven, 350°F, 20 min (Nestle)	1695	100	1695
Hot Pocket-bacon, egg, cheese, microwaved 1 min (Nestle)	846	100	846
Hot Pocket-bacon, egg, cheese, frozen-not heated (Nestle)	558	100	558
Hummus, commercial	733	100	733
Hummus, with garlic and scallions	884	100	884
Hummus, with vegetables	487	100	487
Hummus (mean)	701	100	701
Macaroni and cheese[b]	2728	100	2728
Macaroni and cheese, baked[c]	4070	100	4070
Pasta primavera	959	100	959
Pesto, with basil (Buitoni, Nestle)	150	100	150
Pizza, thin crust	6825	100	6825
Salad, Italian pasta[c]	935	100	935
Salad, lentil potato[c]	123	100	123
Salad, tuna pasta[c]	218	100	218
Sandwich, cheese melt, open faced[c]	5679	100	5679
Sandwich, toasted cheese	4333	100	4333
Soufflé, spinach[c]	598	100	598
Timbale, broccoli[c]	122	100	122
Taramosalata (Greek style caviar spread)	678	100	678
Veggie burger, California burger, 400°F, 8 min-4 each side (Amy's Kitchen, Petaluma, California)	198	100	198
Veggie burger, California burger, skillet, with spray, 5 min (Amy's)	149	100	149
Veggie burger, California burger, skillet, with 1 tsp olive oil, 5 min (Amy's)	374	100	374
Veggie burger, California burger, microwave, 1 min (Amy's)	68	100	68
Won ton, pork, fried (take out)	2109	100	2109
Ziti, baked	2795	100	2795
Condiments			
Ginger, crystallized	490	100	49
Candy, Hershey Special Dark Chocolate (The Hershey Co, Hershey, Pennsylvania)	1777	30	533
Candy, M & M's, milk chocolate (Mars)	1500	30	450
Candy, Reese's Peanut Butter Cup (The Hershey Co)	3440	30	1032
Candy, Raisinets (Nestle)	197	30	59

(Continued)

TABLE 7.1 (CONTINUED)
The AGE Content of 549 Foods, Based on Carboxymethyllysine Content

	AGE Content		
Food Item	AGE[a] (kU/100 g)	Serving Size (g)	AGE (kU/Serving)
Combination Foods and Solid Condiments			
Condiments			
Candy, Snickers (Nestle)	263	30	79
Pickle, bread and butter	10	30	3
Soups, Liquid Condiments, and Miscellaneous Liquids			
Soups			
Soup, beef bouillon	0.40	250	1
Soup, chicken bouillon	1.20	250	3
Soup, College Inn chicken broth (Del Monte)	0.80	250	2
Soup, chicken noodle (Campbell Soup Company)	1.60	250	4
Soup, couscous and lentil (Fantastic World Foods, Edison, New Jersey)	3.60	250	9
Soup, Knorr vegetable broth (Unilever)	1.60	250	4
Soup, summer vegetable[c]	1.20	250	3
Condiments			
Ketchup	13.33	15	2
Mustard	0.00	15	0
Pectin	80.00	15	12
Soy sauce	60.00	15	9
Vinegar, balsamic	33.33	15	5
Vinegar, white	40.00	15	6
Miscellaneous			
SoBe Adrenaline Rush (South Beach Beverage Co, Norwalk, Connecticut)	0.40	250	1
Budweiser Beer (Anheuser-Busch, St Louis, Missouri)	1.20	250	3
Breast milk, fresh	6.67	30	2
Breast milk, frozen	10.00	30	3
Coca Cola, classic (The Coca-Cola Co, Atlanta, Georgia)	2.80	250	7
Coffee, with milk and sugar	2.40	250	6
Coffee, drip method	1.60	250	4
Coffee, heating plate >1 h	13.60	250	34
Coffee, Taster's Choice instant (Nestle)	4.80	250	12
Coffee, instant, decaf (mean Sanka [Kraft] and Taster's Choice)	5.20	250	13
Coffee, Spanish	4.80	250	12
Coffee, with milk	6.80	250	17
Coffee, with sugar	7.60	250	19
Coke	6.40	250	16
Coke, Diet (The Coca-Cola Company)	1.20	250	3
Coke, Diet 2008 (The Coca-Cola Company)	4.00	250	10
Coke, Diet plus (The Coca-Cola Company)	1.60	250	4
Enfamil, old (Mead Johnson Nutritional, Glenview, Illinois)	486.67	30	146

(Continued)

TABLE 7.1 (CONTINUED)

The AGE Content of 549 Foods, Based on Carboxymethyllysine Content

Food Item	AGE Content		
	AGE[a] (kU/100 g)	Serving Size (g)	AGE (kU/Serving)
Soups, Liquid Condiments, and Miscellaneous Liquids			
Miscellaneous			
Gelatin, Dole strawberry (Nestle)	1.60	125	2
Gelatin, Dole strawberry, sugar free (Nestle)	0.80	125	1
Glucerna (Abbott Nutrition, Columbus, Ohio)	70.00	250	175
Malta (Goya)	1.20	250	3
NOFEAR Super Energy Supplement (Pepsico, Purchase, New York)	0.40	250	1
Pepsi, diet (Pepsico)	2.80	250	7
Pepsi, diet MAX (Pepsico)	3.20	250	8
Pepsi, diet, caffeine free (Pepsico)	2.40	250	6
Pepsi, regular (Pepsico)	2.40	250	6
Resource (Nestle)	72.00	250	180
Rum, Bacardi Superior, 80 proof (Miami, Florida)	0.00	250	0
Sprite (The Coca-Cola Company)	1.60	250	4
Sprite, diet (The Coca-Cola Company)	0.40	250	1
Tea, apple (RC Bigelow, Inc., Fairfield, Connecticut)	0.40	250	1
Tea, Lipton Tea bag (Unilever)	2.00	250	5
Tea, Lipton Tea bag, decaf (Unilever)	1.20	250	3
Vodka, Smirnoff, 80 proof (Diageo, London, UK)	0.00	250	0
Whiskey, Dewar's White Label (Dewar's, Perthsire, UK)	0.40	250	1
Wine, pinot grigio (Cavit Collection, Port Washington, New York)	32.80	250	82
Wine, pinot noir (Cavit Collection)	11.20	250	28

Source: From Uribarri, Woodruff, Goodman et al. 2010. Advanced glycation end products in foods and a practical guide to their reduction in the diet. *Journal of the American Dietetic Association*, Jun; 110(6): 911–916.e12. With permission.

[a] AGEs were assessed as carboxymethyllysine by enzyme-linked immunosorbent assay.

[b] MSC, Mount Sinai Hospital cafeteria.

[c] CRC, Mount Sinai Hospital Clinical Research Center.

[d] All McDonald's products were purchased in New York, New York, before July 2008.

7.2.1.2 Some Guidelines

A number of other findings and conclusions from the above study are worth noting. For instance: Higher-fat and aged cheeses, such as full-fat American and parmesan, contain more dAGEs than lower-fat cheeses such as reduced-fat mozzarella, 2% milk cheddar, and cottage cheese. Whereas cooking is known to drive the generation of new AGEs in foods, it is interesting to note that even uncooked, animal-derived foods such as cheeses can contain large amounts of dAGEs. High-fat spreads, including butter, cream cheese, margarine, and mayonnaise, were also among the foods highest in dAGEs, followed by oils and nuts.

Keeping the degree of heating constant, the type of cooking fat that was used led to different amounts of dAGEs. For instance, scrambled eggs prepared with a cooking spray, margarine, or oil had approximately 50% to 75% less dAGEs than if cooked with butter. In comparison to the meat and fat groups, the carbohydrate group generally contained lower amounts of AGEs. This may be due to the often higher water content, or higher level of antioxidants and vitamins in these foods, which may diminish new AGE formation.

Grains, legumes, breads, vegetables, fruits, and milk were among the lowest items in dAGE, unless they were prepared with added fats. For instance, biscuits had more than 10 times the amount of dAGEs than is commonly found in low-fat breads, rolls, or bagels.

Nonfat milk had significantly lower dAGEs than whole milk. Whereas heating increased the dAGE content of milk, the values were modest and remained low relative to those of cheeses. Likewise, milk-related products with a high moisture index such as yogurt, pudding, and ice cream were also relatively low in AGEs. However, hot cocoa made from a dehydrated concentrate contained significantly higher amounts of AGEs.

Preparation of common foods under varying conditions of water and heat had a different effect on dAGE content. For example, scrambled eggs prepared in an open pan over medium-low heat had about one-half the dAGEs of eggs prepared in the same way but over high heat. Poached or steamed chicken had less than one-fourth the dAGEs of roasted or broiled chicken.

In all food categories, exposure to higher temperatures and lower moisture levels coincided with higher dAGE levels for equal weight of food as compared to foods prepared at lower temperatures or with more moisture. Thus, frying, broiling, grilling, and roasting yielded more dAGEs compared to boiling, poaching, stewing, and steaming. Microwaving did not raise dAGE content to the same extent as other dry heat cooking methods for the relatively short cooking times (6 min or less) that were tested.

A safe and optimal dAGE intake intended to prevent disease and complications has not yet been firmly established; however, in animal studies, a reduction of dAGE by 50% of the usual intake is associated with reduced levels of oxidative stress, less deterioration of insulin sensitivity, less loss of kidney function with age, and longer life span (Cai, He, Zhu et al. 2008).

7.2.1.3 How Much AGE-ing Do We Actually Do?

According to the study cited above, data on dAGE intakes in the general population is limited. However, it was recently estimated that in a cohort of healthy adults from the New York City area, the average dAGE intake was about 14,700 ± 680 AGE kU/day (Uribarri, Cai, Peppa et al. 2007). These data could tentatively be used to define a high- or low-AGE diet, depending on whether the estimated daily AGE intake is significantly greater or less than 15,000 kU/day.

People who consume a diet rich in grilled or roasted meats, fats, and highly processed foods could achieve a dAGE intake in excess of 20,000 kU/day. Conversely, those who regularly consume lower-meat meals prepared with moist heat (such as soups and stews) as part of a diet rich in plant foods could realistically consume half the daily intake seen in this cohort.

As previously noted, reducing dAGE may be especially important for people with diabetes because it has been shown that they generate more endogenous AGEs than do those without diabetes (Huebschmann, Regensteiner, Vlassara et al. 2006). That also holds true for people with kidney disease, because they have impaired AGE clearance from the body (Koschinsky, He, Mitsuhashi et al. 1997).

7.2.1.4 A Diet Low in dAGEs Can Improve Insulin Sensitivity

In 2014, the journal *Diabetes Care* reported a Danish study titled "Consumption of a diet low in AGEs for 4 weeks improves insulin sensitivity in overweight women." It held that because high-heat cooking of food induces the formation of AGEs thought to impair glucose metabolism in Type 2 diabetic patients, high intake of fructose might additionally affect endogenous formation of AGEs. Therefore, an intervention study was undertaken to determine whether the addition of fructose, or of cooking methods that influence the AGE content of food, affected insulin sensitivity in overweight individuals.

TABLE 7.2
High- and Low-AGE Meals and Snacks

	High-AGE			Low-AGE		
Meal	Recipe Name	Servings[a]	Provided Food Product in Total	Recipe Name	Servings[a]	Provided Food Product in Total
Breakfast	Fried eggs and bacon	1	15 Eggs (Danaeg Denmark)	Boiled eggs and bacon	1	15 Eggs (Danaeg Denmark)
	Muesli Meal	4	4 × 500 g Crüsli (Quark)	Oatmeal	4	2 × 1 kg Oats (7 mornings, Denmark)
Lunch	Fried sausages	1	[b]	Boiled sausages	1	[b]
	Fried chicken breast	1	4 × 1 Chicken breast without skin ~ 125 g (Lantmännen Danpo A/S, Denmark)	Boiled chicken breast	1	4 × 1 Chicken breast without skin ~ 125 g (Lantmännen Danpo A/S, Denmark)
Dinner	Bread cod fillet with baked potatoes and vegetables	1	4 × 2 Cod fillets of ~150 g (Royal, Greenland A/S, Denmark)	Steamed cod fillet with vegetables and boiled potatoes	1	4 × 2 Cod fillets of ~150 g (Royal, Greenland A/S, Denmark
	Fried chicken breast with rice in curry sauce	1	4 × 2 Chicken breast without skin ~ 125 g (Lantmännen Danpo A/S, Denmark)	Pasta salad with boiled chicken	1	4 × 2 Chicken breast without skin ~ 125 g (Lantmännen Danpo A/S, Denmark)
	Pizza with fried chicken	1	4 × 2 Chicken breast without skin ~ 125 g (Lantmännen Danpo A/S, Denmark)	Pita bread with boiled chicken	1	4 × 2 Chicken breast without skin ~ 125 g (Lantmännen Danpo A/S, Denmark)
	Fried salmon with vegetables and rice	1	4 × 2 Salmon fillets ~100 g (Rolyal Greenland, A/S, Denmark)	Salmon soup with tomatoes and crust-free bread	1	4 × 2 Salmon fillets ~100 g (Rolyal Greenland, A/S, Denmark)
	Fried meatballs with baked potatoes and vegetables	1	4 × 250 g Minced pork meat 8–12% fat (Danish Crown A/S, Denmark)	Pasta with tomato meat sauce	1	4 × 250 g Minced pork meat 8–12% fat (Danish Crown A/S, Denmark)
	Fried noodles with fried minced meat and vegetables	1	4 × 250 g Minced pork meat 8–12% fat (Danish Crown A/S, Denmark)	Pasta with tomato meat sauce	1	4 × 250 g Minced pork meat 8–12% fat (Danish Crown A/S, Denmark

(*Continued*)

TABLE 7.2 (CONTINUED)
High- and Low-AGE Meals and Snacks

| Meal | High-AGE | | | Low-AGE | | |
	Recipe Name	Servings[a]	Provided Food Product in Total	Recipe Name	Servings[a]	Provided Food Product in Total
	Pork chops with bruschetta bread and baked tomatoes	1	4 × 2 Pieces of pork chops ~125 g (Danish Crown A/S, Denmark)	Pork with coconut milk, boiled vegetables and rice	1	4 × 2 Pieces of pork chops ~125 g (Danish Crown A/S, Denmark)
Snack	Tortilla chips	125 g	4 × 125 g (Urtekram, Denmark)	Rice cakes	100 g	4 × 125 g (Urtekram, Denmark)
	Cashew nuts	75 g	4 × 75 g (SystemFrugt, Denmark)	Pistachio nuts	80 g	4 × 80 g (Trend, Denmark)
	Oat biscuits	c	300 g (MyChoice, Denmark)	Muffins	c	300 g (Dancake, Denmark)
	Oreo biscuits	c	2 × 154 g (Kraft, Denmark)	Sponge cake	c	2 × 160 g (Karen Volf, Denmark)

Source: From Mark, Poulsen, Andersen et al. 2014. Consumption of a diet low in Advanced Glycation End Products for 4 weeks improves insulin sensitivity in overweight women. *Diabetes Care*, Jan; 37: 88–95. With permission.

[a] Number of servings per week.

[b] Had to be purchased by the volunteers.

[c] Optional.

Overweight women participants were assigned to follow either a high- or low-AGE diet for 4 weeks, together with consumption of either fructose or glucose drinks. Glucose and insulin concentrations were measured after fasting and 2 h after an oral glucose tolerance test. Participants were evaluated before and after the intervention.

Homeostasis model assessment of insulin resistance (HOMA-IR) and insulin sensitivity index were calculated. Dietary and urinary AGE concentrations were evaluated by liquid chromatography tandem mass spectrometry to estimate AGE intake and excretion. The Homeostatic model assessment (HOMA) is a method for assessing β-cell function and insulin resistance from basal (fasting) glucose and insulin or C-peptide concentrations.

The dietary intervention procedure entailed the following general procedure: The volunteers received oral and written instructions on how to comply with either high-AGE or low-AGE diets. Both diets resembled habitual Danish food intake and were similar in nutrient quality, but differed in cooking methods. The instructions included thorough guidance on cooking methods, a food choice list, and predefined recipes for mandatory meals. The high-AGE group was instructed to fry, bake, roast, or grill their foods; to consume toasted bread with a crust; and to choose foods with a high content of AGEs based on the food choice list.

The low-AGE group was instructed to boil or steam their food, to consume bread without a crust, and to choose foods with low content of AGEs based on the food choice list. The food choice list contained examples of foods commonly available in Denmark to be chosen as "preferred," "accepted," or "not allowed."

The predefined recipes shown in Table 7.2 (their Table 1) included one, four, and seven weekly breakfast, lunch, and dinner recipes, respectively. Additionally, the volunteers were instructed to consume four weekly portions of muesli or oatmeal in the high-AGE and low-AGE groups, respectively.

The volunteers were provided with all the meat and fish for the predefined dinner meals; most of the meat and fish for the predefined lunch meals; and all the necessary eggs, corn oil for cooking, and snacks. The remaining foods were purchased and consumed freely, but in compliance with the food choice list.

Snacks other than the ones provided were not allowed. The volunteers were instructed to keep their habitual meal portion sizes and not attempt changes in body weight.

The investigators reported that when adjusted for changes in anthropometric measures during the intervention, the low-AGE diet decreased urinary AGEs, fasting insulin concentrations, and HOMA-IR, compared with the high-AGE diet. Addition of fructose did not affect any outcomes.

The investigators concluded that diets with high AGE content may increase the development of insulin resistance, and that AGEs can be reduced by adjustment of cooking methods, but that it is unaffected by moderate fructose intake (Mark, Poulsen, Andersen et al. 2014).

7.3 WEIGHT LOSS DIET CAUTION

Weight loss diets that are higher in protein and fat and lower in carbohydrates are popular for the management of weight loss, diabetes, and cardiovascular disease (Shai, Schwarzfuchs, Henkin et al. 2008; Kirk, Graves, Craven et al. 2008; Miller, Erlinger, and Appel. 2006; De Souza, Swain, Appel et al. 2008; Swain, McCarron, Hamilton et al. 2008). However, this type of dietary pattern may substantially raise dAGE intake and thus contribute to health problems over the long term. On the other hand, it has been reported in the Chilean medical journal *Nutricion Hospitalaria* that a low-calorie Mediterranean diet reduces AGEs (Rodríguez, Leiva Balich, Concha et al. 2015).

7.4 AGES IMPAIR ENDOTHELIUM FUNCTION

Impairment of endothelium function, and thus decreased formation of endothelium-derived nitric oxide (NO), is a well-established basis for the numerous health hazards that face diabetes sufferers. With that in mind, the rest of this chapter is devoted to establishing the adverse impact of AGEs on endothelium function and its immediate consequences.

Normal endothelial cells form the enzyme endothelial nitric oxide synthase (eNOS), which plays a critical role in NO production and maintaining the endothelial functions, including regulation of vascular tone, inhibition of coagulation, thrombosis, suppression of inflammatory cell adhesion and migration, and angiogenesis. Endothelium-derived NO, synthesized from the amino acid L-arginine via eNOS by the cells of the endothelium, is a major mediator of endothelium-dependent vasorelaxation as noted in a previous chapter.

Endothelial dysfunction has largely been attributed to alterations of endothelium-dependent vasorelaxation. Many cardiovascular risk factors induce endothelial dysfunction through impairment of the eNOS–NO system, which likely explains their promotion of the development of atherosclerosis.

It has been suggested that AGEs and derivatives form at an accelerated rate in diabetes, and they promote the development of endothelial dysfunction in diabetic patients by binding to its receptor, RAGE, triggering the production of proinflammatory cytokines and chemokines, inducing oxidative stress, and thereby reducing NO production (Huebschmann, Regensteiner, Vlassara et al. 2006).

Cytokines are substances such as interferon, interleukin, and growth factors that are secreted by certain cells of the immune system. Chemokines are particular cytokines with functions that include attracting white blood cells to sites of infection.

Endothelium damage has also been reported in induced diabetes in mice, in a report in the *Chinese Journal of Natural Medicine*: A high-AGE diet in diabetic mice damaged the pancreas, heart, and kidneys and caused structural changes in endothelial cells and in the kidneys. Eventually, it contributed to the high AGE levels in serum and kidneys, high levels of reactive oxygen species (ROS) and low levels of superoxide dismutase (SOD) in serum, heart, and kidneys. The authors concluded that the high-AGE diet seriously damaged the endothelium in the diabetic mice (Lv, Lv, Dai et al. 2016).

7.4.1   AGEs Impair the Formation of eNOS, the Key to NO Formation

A study reported in the journal *Cardiovascular Diabetology* aimed to identify the cellular mechanisms by which AGEs aggravate endothelial dysfunction in human coronary artery endothelial cells (HCAECs). Plasma levels of AGE peptides (AGE-p) were obtained from diabetic patients with or without coronary artery atherosclerosis. Endothelial function was tested by brachial artery flow-mediated vasodilation (FMD).

It was found that the level of AGE-p was inversely associated with FMD in diabetic patients with coronary artery atherosclerosis, meaning that as the levels of AGE-p went up, FMD decreased.

After exposure to AGEs, the human coronary artery endothelial cells showed significant reductions of eNOS and cellular NO levels, whereas free radical (superoxide anion) production was significantly increased.

AGEs significantly decreased mitochondrial membrane potential, catalase, and superoxide dismutase (SOD) activities, whereas it increased NADPH oxidase activity. Treatment of the cells with antioxidants effectively blocked these effects induced by AGEs. Both catalase and SOD are very important enzymes that protect cells from oxidative damage by ROS.

It was concluded that AGEs cause endothelial dysfunction by a mechanism associated with decreased eNOS expression and increased oxidative stress in human coronary artery endothelial cells (Ren, Ren, Wei et al. 2017).

7.4.2   AGEs Also Target Kidneys

A study published in the *American Journal of Kidney Diseases* was conducted on long-term dialysis patients to determine the effects of dietary AGEs on renal function. Dietary AGE intake was estimated by means of dietary records and questionnaires, and sera were obtained for measurement of two well-characterized AGEs, CML and MG (methylglyoxal) derivatives. CML is $N(6)$-carboxymethyllysine, also known as $N(\varepsilon)$-(carboxymethyl)lysine, an AGE. It has been the most commonly used marker for AGEs in food analysis.

Although no correlation was observed with nutrient intake (protein, fat, saturated fat, or carbohydrate), both serum CML and MG levels correlated with blood urea nitrogen and serum albumin levels.

The authors concluded that dietary AGE content, independently of other diet constituents, is an important contributor to excess serum AGE levels in patients with kidney failure. Moreover, the lack of correlation between serum AGE levels and dietary protein, fat, and carbohydrate intake indicates that a reduction in dietary AGE content can be obtained safely without compromising the content of necessary nutrients (Uribarri, Peppa, Cai et al. 2003a; 2003b).

Another study published in the *Clinical Journal of the American Society of Nephrology* aimed to examine the association of AGE accumulation and endothelial dysfunction in chronic kidney disease.

The study evaluated ambulatory patients without diabetes and with different stages of chronic kidney disease, compared with gender- and age-matched healthy participants. Fasting blood was obtained for measurement of advanced AGEs and mRNA receptor for AGE expression in peripheral blood mononuclear cells. mRNA is "messenger RNA," a subtype of RNA that carries a translation of the DNA code to other parts of the cell for processing into proteins. Endothelial function was assessed by post-occlusive reactive hyperemia. This is a method that measures the increase in blood flow in an arterial vessel after arterial compression to momentarily stop blood flow.

Sera were pooled and passed through affinity columns to separate AGE-rich fractions, which were incubated with human aortic endothelial cells, with or without blockade of receptor for AGEs, to measure their effect on eNOS formation.

Kidney filtration rate correlated with serum AGEs, mRNA receptor for AGEs levels, and post-occlusive reactive hyperemia. Serum AGEs correlated with receptor for AGEs and inversely with post-occlusive reactive hyperemia. AGE-rich fractions from chronic kidney disease sera suppressed eNOS expression of human aortic endothelial cells compared to sera from healthy participants, an effect overturned by blockade of the receptor for Advanced Glycation End-products (RAGE).

The authors concluded that they demonstrated for the first time that there is an excess AGE burden and *in vivo* endothelial dysfunction in patients with chronic kidney disease. Endothelial dysfunction in chronic kidney disease may be partly mediated by AGE-induced inhibition of eNOS through the receptor for AGEs activation (Linden, Cai, He et al. 2008).

7.5 TIPS FOR REDUCING AGES

Tips to reduce AGE levels include choosing different cooking methods: Rather than using dry, high heat for cooking, stew, poach, boiling, and steam. Cooking with moist heat, at lower temperatures and for shorter periods of time, all help keep AGE production low.

In addition, cooking meat with acidic ingredients, such as vinegar, tomato juice, or lemon juice, can reduce AGE production by up to 50%. Cooking over ceramic surfaces rather than directly on metal can also reduce AGE production. Slow cookers are thought to be one of the healthiest ways to cook food.

Limit foods known to be high in AGEs: Fried foods and highly processed foods contain higher levels of AGEs. Certain foods, such as animal foods, also tend to be higher in AGEs. These include meat (especially red meat), certain cheeses, fried eggs, butter, cream cheese, margarine, mayonnaise, oils, and nuts. Try eliminating or limiting these foods and instead choose whole, fresh, and natural foods, which are naturally lower in AGEs. For example, foods such as fruits, vegetables, and whole grains have lower levels, even after cooking.

Eat a high-antioxidant diet.

7.6 ETHNIC AND OTHER FOLKLORE-BASED NUTRACEUTICALS AS ANTI-AGE STRATEGIES

In the last few decades, "Traditional Medicine" has gained global interest. Many studies have now shown that dietary supplementation with functional foods or nutraceuticals, local to various indigenous regions worldwide, hold antiglycation and antioxidant constituents, and they may be a safe and simple complement to traditional therapies targeting diabetic complications.

In laboratory studies, natural antioxidants, such as vitamin C and quercetin, have been shown to hinder AGE formation (Grzebyk, and Piwowar. 2016). In addition, animal model studies have shown that some natural plant phenols can prevent the adverse health effects of AGEs. These include curcumin, found in turmeric, and resveratrol, found in the skins of dark fruits like grapes, blueberries, and raspberries (Mizutani, Ikeda, and Yamori. 2000; Tang, and Chen. 2014).

An antioxidant diet rich in fruits, vegetables, herbs, and spices may help protect against the damaging effects of AGEs on the body. There are numerous other reports of various plant-derived substances that reduce AGEs. Here follows a small sample of these.

7.6.1 Australian Petalostigma banksii and Petalostigma pubescens

Australian medicinal plants collected from the Kuuku I'yu (Northern Kaanju) homelands, Cape York Peninsula, Queensland, Australia, were investigated to determine their therapeutic potential. Extracts were tested for inhibition of protein glycation and key enzymes relevant to the management of hyperglycemia and hypertension. The inhibitory activities were further correlated with the antioxidant activities.

Extracts of the leaves of *P. banksii* and *P. pubescens* showed the strongest inhibition of α-amylase with IC50 values of 166.50 ± 5.50 µg/mL and 160.20 ± 27.92 µg/mL, respectively. The *P. pubescens* leaf extract was also the strongest inhibitor of α-glucosidase with an IC50 of 167.83 ± 23.82 µg/mL. This ability of *P. pubescens* to inhibit α-glucosidase is noteworthy, because the antidiabetic efficacy of the prescription medication acarbose is based on the ability to inhibit that same enzyme, thereby slowing down the rate at which certain dietary carbohydrates will be digested and absorbed, and such slowing down, in turn, results in lower peaks of insulin (better insulin tolerance).

The IC50 is the concentration of an inhibitor at which point the response (or binding) is reduced by half.

Testing for the antiglycation potential of the extracts showed that *P. banksii* root and fruit extracts had IC50 values of 34.49 ± 4.31 µg/mL and 47.72 ± 1.65 µg/mL, respectively, which were significantly lower than other extracts. The inhibitory effect on α-amylase and α-glucosidase and the antiglycation potential of the extracts did not correlate with the total phenolic, total flavonoid, FRAP, or DPPH.

For AGE inhibition, IC50 values ranged from 266.27 ± 6.91 µg/mL to 695.17 ± 15.38 µg/mL (Deo, Hewawasam, Karakoulakis et al. 2016). The FRAP assay is a method for assessing "antioxidant power" by reduction of ferric to ferrous ion at low pH.

7.6.2 Yucatan Cassia fistula, Piper auritum, Ehretia tinifolia, Manilkara zapota, and Ocimum campechianum

Ethanol extracts from nine plants used to treat diabetes, hypertension, and obesity in Yucatecan traditional medicine were tested for their anti-AGE and free radical scavenging activities. Significant activity against vesperlysine and pentosidine-like AGE was detected in the root extract of *C. fistula* and the leaf extract of *P. auritum*.

Traditional preparations and the ethanolic extracts of *E. tinifolia*, *M. zapota*, *O. campechianum*, and *P. auritum* showed significant activity in the DPPH reduction assay. Results suggest that the metabolites responsible for the detected radical-scavenging activity are different from those involved in inhibiting AGE formation (Dzib-Guerra, Escalante-Erosa, García-Sosa et al. 2016). DPPH is a common antioxidant assay.

7.6.3 Sida cordifolia, Plumbago zeylanica, Tribulus terrestris, Glycyrrhiza glabra, and Rosa indica

Twenty-six medicinal plants commonly found in different regions of the Arabian Peninsula were evaluated for their protein antiglycation activity by using standard assay and incubation procedures.

Five of twenty-six medicinal plants, *S. cordifolia*, *P. zeylanica*, *T. terrestris*, *G. glabra*, and *R. indica*, were active against *in vitro* protein glycation with IC50 values between 0.408 and 1.690 mg/mL. *G. glabra* L. was found to be the most effective (IC50 = 0.408 ± 0.027 mg/mL), followed by *R. indica* (IC50 = 0.596 ± 0.0179 mg/mL) and *S. cordifolia* L. IC50 = 0.63 ± 0.009 mg/mL).

The antioxidant potential of these plant extracts was also determined by using DPPH, iron chelation, and superoxide anion radical scavenging assays.

S. cordifolia exhibited strong antioxidant activity in both DPPH and superoxide anion radical scavenging assays (IC50 = 0.005 ± 0.0004 mg/mL and 0.078 ± 0.002 mg/mL, respectively), followed by *R. indica* (IC50 = 0.023 ± 0.0005 mg/mL and 0.141 ± 0.003 mg/mL, respectively) (Siddiqui, Rasheed, Saquib et al. 2016).

7.6.4 AGED GARLIC

The *Journal of Nutrition* reports an examination of aged garlic extract compounds with combined antiglycation and antioxidant properties for their therapeutic potential. It was suggested that these inhibit the formation of AGEs *in vitro* and formation of glycation-derived free radicals. *S*-allylcysteine, a key component of aged garlic, is a potent antioxidant and can inhibit AGE formation (Ahmad, and Ahmed. 2006).

7.6.5 TOMATO PASTE IS ANTI AGE-ING

An article in the journal *Bioscience, Biotechnology, and Biochemistry* tells us that a water-soluble and low-molecular-weight fraction (SB) was obtained from tomato paste. The effects of that SB on the formation of AGEs in protein glycation were studied by conventional laboratory assay methods using the anti-AGE antibody after incubating protein with sugar.

The results suggest that the low-molecular-weight fraction (SB) contained an antioxidant, rutin, which showed potent inhibitory activity. The results also suggest that rutin chiefly contributed to inhibiting the formation of AGEs and that other compounds in SB may also have been related to the activity (Kiho, Usui, Hirano et al. 2004).

7.6.6 HOLLY EXTRACT INHIBITS AGE FORMATION

Ilex paraguariensis, or holly, is the only living species in a genus of some 400 to 600 other species that have become extinct. The species are evergreen trees, shrubs, and climbers from tropics to temperate zones worldwide.

A study appearing in the journal *Fitoterapia* aimed to test polyphenol-rich *I. paraguariensis* extracts for the ability to inhibit formation of AGEs and to compare the potency of these extracts with green tea and with the standard antiglycation agent aminoguanidine.

The test was conducted on bovine serum albumin by glycation with methylglyoxal. A dose-dependent effect that reached 40% at 20 μL/mL of extract was demonstrated.

The results showed that there is a significant, dose-dependent effect of water extracts of *I. paraguariensis* on formation of AGE adducts on a protein model, *in vitro*, whereas green tea displayed no significant effect. The inhibition of AGE formation was comparable to that obtained by using millimolar concentrations of the standard antiglycation agent, aminoguanidine (Lunceford, and Gugliucci. 2005).

7.6.7 FROM INDONESIA AND MALAYSIA: *CLITORIA TERNATEA*

C. ternatea, commonly known as Asian pigeonwings, butterfly pea, cordofan pea, and Darwin pea, is a plant species belonging to the *Fabaceae* family.

A study published in the journal *BMC Complementary and Alternative Medicine* aimed to determine the antiglycation activity of *C. ternatea* extract (CTE) by assessing its inhibitory effect on fructose-induced formation of AGEs and protein oxidation.

The aqueous extract of CTE was measured for the content of total phenolic compounds, flavonoid, and anthocyanin by the Folin–Ciocalteu assay, by conventional laboratory methods.

The results revealed that the content of total phenolics, flavonoids, and total anthocyanins in CTE was 53 ± 0.34 mg gallic acid equivalents/gram dried extract, 11.2 ± 0.33 mg catechin equivalents/g dried extract, and 1.46 ± 0.04 mg cyanidin-3-glucoside equivalents/gram dried extract, respectively.

CTE (0.25–1.00 mg/mL) significantly inhibited the formation of AGEs in a concentration-dependent manner, and it also markedly reduced the levels of fructosamine, as well as the oxidation of protein by the mechanism of decreasing protein carbonyl content and preventing free thiol depletion.

In the DPPH radical scavenging activity and SRSA, CTE had IC50 values of 0.47 ± 0.01 mg/mL and 0.58 ± 0.04 mg/mL and the FRAP and TEAC values of CTE were 0.38 ± 0.01 mmol $FeSO_4$ equivalents/mg dried extract and 0.17 ± 0.01 mg trolox equivalents/mg dried extract. However, CTE proved to be a weak scavenger of hydroxyl radical and a weak antioxidant iron chelator.

The investigators concluded that CTE has strong antiglycation and antioxidant properties and might have therapeutic potentials in the prevention of AGE-mediated diabetic complications (Chayaratanasin, Barbieri, Suanpairintr et al. 2015).

An excellent review of data for 42 plants/constituents studied for antiglycation activity is presented in an article in the journal *Current Diabetes Reviews*: It concerns some commonly used medicinal plants that possess antiglycation activity and details their active ingredients, mechanism of action, and therapeutic potential (Elosta, Ghous, and Ahmed. 2012).

7.6.8 GSH SUPPLEMENTS

Glutathione (GSH) is a complex amino acid that serves as a highly potent scavenger of free radicals. It is a catalyst for some of the enzymes that break down AGEs. In laboratory models of hyperoxaluria, supplements of GSH protected the kidneys from the oxalate stone formation that was abundant in the control animals.

Thus, a tentative case could be made that patients (diabetic or not) who have a tendency to form oxalate stones in the urinary tract might want to consider supplementing with GSH. However, clinical experience suggests that only the "reduced" form of GSH should be ingested, because taking an oxidized GSH preparation will require "reduction," thus stressing the body's antioxidant reserves (Muthukumar, and Selvam. 1998).

7.7 A NOTE ON GLUCOSEPANE AND TYPE 2 DIABETES

Glucosepane, the most common AGE, is an irreversible, covalent lysine–arginine protein cross-linking product derived from D-glucose. There is no agent known that can break it down. It appears 10 to 1000 times more often in human tissue than any other cross-linking AGE (Monnier, Mustata, Biemel et al. 2005; Furber. 2006). Covalent protein cross-links irreversibly link proteins together in the extracellular matrix of tissues.

The extracellular matrix is the noncellular component present within all tissues and organs, and it not only provides essential physical scaffolding for the cellular constituents but also initiates crucial biochemical signals that are required for tissue morphogenesis, differentiation, and homeostasis.

The journal *Clinical Chemistry and Laboratory Medicine* published a study titled "Glucosepane: a poorly understood advanced glycation end product of growing importance for diabetes and its complications." The investigators report that AGE formation in diabetes makes them "potential culprits of diabetic complications," and in particular, retinopathy, nephropathy, and neuropathy.

The investigators review studies on AGE formation in two skin biopsies obtained near the close-out of the Diabetes Control and Complications Trial, one of which was processed in 2011 for assay of novel AGEs. The results of these analyses show that while several AGEs are associated and predict complication progression, the glucose/fructose–lysine/glucosepane AGE axis is one of the most robust markers for microvascular disease, especially diabetic retinopathy—despite adjustment for past or future average glycemia (Monnier, Sun, Sell et al. 2014).

The Journal of Biological Chemistry published an excellent review linking glucosepane to both diabetes and senescence (Sell, Biemel, Reihl et al. 2005).

REFERENCES

Ahmad MS, and N Ahmed. 2006. Antiglycation properties of aged garlic extract: possible role in prevention of diabetic complications. *Journal of Nutrition*, Mar; 136(3 Suppl): 796S–799S. PMID: 16484566.

Cai W, He JC, Zhu L, Chen X, Zheng F, Striker GE, and H Vlasara. 2008. Oral glycotoxins determine the effects of calorie restriction on oxidant stress, age-related diseases, and lifespan. *American Journal of Pathology*, Aug; 173(2): 327–336. DOI: 10.2353/ajpath.2008.080152.

Cai W, Ramdas M, Zhu L, Chen X, Striker GE, and H. Vlassara. 2012. Oral advanced glycation end products (AGEs) promote insulin resistance and diabetes by depleting the antioxidant defenses AGE receptor-1 and sirtuin 1. *Proceedings of the National Academy of Sciences USA*, Sep; 109(39): 15888–15893. DOI: 10.1073/pnas.120 5847109.

Chayaratanasin P, Barbieri MA, Suanpairintr N, and S Adisakwattana. 2015. Inhibitory effect of *Clitoria ternatea* flower petal extract on fructose-induced protein glycation and oxidation-dependent damages to albumin in vitro. *BMC Complementary and Alternative Medicine*, Feb 18; 15:27. DOI: 10.1186/s12906-015-0546-2.

Chuyen NV. 2006. Toxicity of the AGEs generated from the Maillard reaction: on the relationship of food-AGEs and biological-AGEs. *Molecular Nutrition and Food Research*, Dec; 50(12):1140–1149. DOI: 10.1002/mnfr.200600144.

De Souza RJ, Swain JF, Appel LH, and FM Sacks. 2008. Alternatives for macronutrient intake and chronic disease: A comparison of the Omni-Heart diets with popular diets and with dietary recommendations. *American Journal of Clinical Nutrition*, Jul;88(1): 1–11. PMCID: PMC2674146.

Deo P, Hewawasam E, Karakoulakis A, Claudie DJ, Nelson R, Simpson BS, Smith NM, and SJ Semple. 2016. In vitro inhibitory activities of selected Australian medicinal plant extracts against protein glycation, angiotensin converting enzyme (ACE) and digestive enzymes linked to type II diabetes. *BMC Complementary and Alternative Medicine*, Nov; 16(1): 435. DOI: 10.1186/s12906-016-1421-5.

Di Marco E, Gray SP, and K Jandeleit-Dahm. 2013. Diabetes alters activation and repression of pro- and anti-inflammatory signaling pathways in the vasculature. *Frontiers in Endocrinology*, Jan; 4: 68. DOI:10.3389/fendo.2013.00068.

Dzib-Guerra WD, Escalante-Erosa F, García-Sosa K, Derbré S, Blanchard P, Richomme P, and LM Peña-Rodríguez. 2016. Anti-advanced glycation end-product and free radical scavenging activity of plants from the Yucatecan flora. *Pharmacognosy Research*, Oct–Dec; 8(4): 276–280. DOI: 10.4103/0974-8490.188883.

Eble AS, Thorpe SR, and JW Baynes. 1983. Nonenzymatic glucosylation and glucose-dependent cross-linking of protein. *The Journal of Biological Chemistry*, Aug; 258(15): 9406–9412. PMID: 6409904.

Eisner BH, Porten SP, Bechis SK, and MI Stoller.2010. Diabetic kidney stone formers excrete more oxalate and have lower urine pH than nondiabetic stone formers. *Journal of Urology*, Jan; 183(6): 2244–2248. DOI: 10.1016/j.juro.2010.02.007.

Elosta A, Ghous T, and N. Ahmed. 2012. Natural products as anti-glycation agents: possible therapeutic potential for diabetic complications. *Current Diabetes Reviews*, Jan; 8(2): 92–108. DOI: 10.2174/157339912799424528.

Furber JD. 2006. Extracellular glycation crosslinks: *Prospects for removal. Rejuvenation Research*, 9(2): 274–278. DOI:10.1089/rej.2006.9.274.

Gkogkolou P, and M Böhm. 2012. Advanced glycation end products. Key players in skin aging? *Dermatoendocrinology*, Jul 1; 4(3): 259–270. DOI: 10.4161/derm.22028.

Goldberg T, Cai W, Peppa M, Dardaine V, Baliga BS, Uribarri J, and H Vlassara. 2004. Advanced glycoxidation end products in commonly consumed foods. *Journal of the American Dietetic Association*, Aug; 104(8): 1287–1291. DOI: 10.1016/j.jada.2004. 05.214.

Grzebyk E, and A Piwowar. 2016. Inhibitory actions of selected natural substances on formation of advanced glycation endproducts and advanced oxidation protein products. *BMC Complementary and Alternative Medicine*, Sept: 16: 381. DOI: 10.1186/s12906-016-1353-0.

He C, Sabol J, Mitsuhashi T, and H Vlassara. 1999. Dietary glycotoxins: Inhibition of reactive products by aminoguanidine facilitates renal clearance and reduces tissue sequestration. *Diabetes*, Jun; 48: 1308–1315. PMID: 10342821.

Huebschmann AG, Regensteiner JG, Vlassara H, and JEB Reusch. 2006. Diabetes and advanced glycoxidation end products. *Diabetes Care*, Jun; 29(6): 1420–1432. DOI: 10.2337/dc05-2096.

Kiho T, Usui S, Hirano K, Aizawa K, and T Inakuma. 2004. Tomato paste fraction inhibiting the formation of advanced glycation end-products. *Bioscience, Biotechnology, and Biochemistry*, Jan; 68(1): 200–205. DOI: 10.1271/bbb.68.200.

Kirk JK, Graves DE, Craven TE, Lipkin EW, Austin M, and KL Margolis. 2008. Restricted-carbohydrate diets in patients with type 2 diabetes: A meta-analysis. *Journal of the American Dietetic Association*, Jan; 108(1): 91–100. DOI: 10.1016/j.jada.2007.10.003.

Koschinsky T, He CJ, Mitsuhashi T, Bucala R, Liu C, Bueting C, Heitmann K, and H Vlassara. 1997. Orally absorbed reactive advanced glycation end products (glycotoxins): an environmental risk factor in diabetic nephropathy. *Proceedings of the National Academy of Sciences USA*, Jun; 94: 6474–6479. PMCID: PMC21074.

Lange JN, Wood KD, Knight J, Assimos DG, and RP Holmes. 2012. Glyoxal formation and its role in endogenous oxalate synthesis. *Advances in Urology*, 2012: 819202. DOI: 10.1155/2012/819202.

Linden E, Cai W, He JC, Xue C, Li Z, Winston J, Vlassara H, and J Uribarri. 2008. Endothelial dysfunction in patients with chronic kidney disease results from advanced glycation end products (AGE)-mediated inhibition of endothelial nitric oxide synthase through RAGE activation. *Clinical Journal of the American Society of Nephrology*, May; 3(3): 691–698. DOI: 10.2215/CJN.04291007.

Lunceford N, and A Gugliucci. 2005. *Ilex paraguariensis* extracts inhibit AGE formation more efficiently than green tea. *Fitoterapia*, Jul; 76(5): 419–427. DOI: 10.1016/j.fitote.2005.03.021.

Lv X, Lv GH, Dai GY, Sun HM, and HQ Xu. 2016. Food-advanced glycation end products aggravate the diabetic vascular complications via modulating the AGEs/RAGE pathway. *Chinese Journal of Natural Medicine*, Nov; 14(11): 844–855. DOI: 10.1016/S1875-5364(16)30101-7.

Mannervik B. 2008. Molecular enzymology of the glyoxalase system. *Drug Metabolism and Drug Interactions*, 2008; 23(1–2): 13–27.

Mark AB, Poulsen MW, Andersen S, Andersen JM, Bak MJ, Ritz C, Holst JJ, Nielsen J, de Courten B, Dragsted LO, and SG Bugel. 2014. Consumption of a diet low in advanced glycation end products for 4 weeks improves insulin sensitivity in overweight women. *Diabetes Care*, Jan; 37: 88–95. DOI: 10.2337/dc13-0842. http://care.diabetesjournals.org/content/diacare/37/1/88.full.pdf.

Miller ER, Erlinger TP, and LJ Appel. 2006. The effects of macronutrients on blood pressure and lipids: an overview of the DASH and OmniHeart trials. *Current Atherosclerosis Reports*, Nov;8(6): 460–465. PMID: 17045071.

Mizutani K, Ikeda K, and Y Yamori. 2000. Resveratrol inhibits AGEs-induced proliferation and collagen synthesis activity in vascular smooth muscle cells from stroke-prone spontaneously hypertensive rats. *Biochemical and Biophysical Research Communication*, Jul; 274(1): 61–67. DOI: 10.1006/bbrc.2000.3097.

Monnier VM, Mustata GT, Biemel KL, Reihl O, Lederer MO, Zhenyu D, and DR Sell. 2005. Cross-linking of the extracellular matrix by the maillard reaction in aging and diabetes: an update on "a puzzle nearing resolution." *Annals of the New York Academy of Sciences*, 1043: 533–544. DOI: 10.1196/annals.1333.061.

Monnier VM, Sun W, Sell DR, Fan X, Nemet I, Genuth S. 2014. Glucosepane: a poorly understood advanced glycation end product of growing importance for diabetes and its complications. *Clinical Chemistry and Laboratory Medicine*, Jan; 52(1): 21–32. DOI: 10.1515/cclm-2013-0174.

Muthukumar A, and R Selvam, 1998. Role of glutathione on renal mitochondrial status in hyperoxaluria. *Molecular and Cell Biochemistry*, Aug; 185(1–2): 77–84.

O'Brien J, and PA Morrissey. 1989. Nutritional and toxicological aspects of the Maillard browning reaction in foods. *Critical Reviews in Food Science and Nutrition*, 28(3): 211–248. DOI: 10.1080/10408398909527499.

Poretsky L. 2012. Looking beyond overnutrition for causes of epidemic metabolic disease. *Proceedings of the National Academy of Sciences USA*, 2012 Sep 25; 109(39): 15537–15538. DOI: 10.1073/pnas.1213503109.

Prasad A, Bekker P, and S Tsimikas. 2012. Advanced glycation end products and diabetic cardiovascular disease. *Cardiology in Review*, Aug; 20(4): 177–183. doi:10.1097/CRD.0b013e318244e57c. PMID 22314141.

Ren X, Ren L, Wei Q, Shao H, Chen L, and N Liu. 2017. Advanced glycation end-products decreases expression of endothelial nitric oxide synthase through oxidative stress in human coronary artery endothelial cells. *Cardiovascular Diabetology*, 201716:52 DOI: 10.1186/s12933-017-0531-9.

Rodríguez JM, Leiva Balich L, Concha MJ, Mizón C, Bunout Barnett D, Barrera Acevedo G, Hirsch Birn S, Jiménez Jaime T, Henríquez S, Uribarri J, and MP de la Maza Cave. 2015. Reduction of serum advanced glycation end-products with a low calorie Mediterranean diet. *Nutricion Hospitalaria*. Jun; 31(6): 2511–2517. DOI: 10.3305/nh.2015.31.6.8936.

Schmidt AM, Yan SD, Wautier JL, and D Stern. 1999. Activation of receptor for advanced glycation end products: a mechanism for chronic vascular dysfunction in diabetic vasculopathy and atherosclerosis. *Circulation Research*, Mar; 84(5): 489–497. PMID: 10082470.

Sell DR, Biemel KM, Reihl O, Lederer MO, Strauch CM, and VM Monnier. 2005. Glucosepane is a major protein cross-link of the senescent human extracellular matrix. Relationship with diabetes. *The Journal of Biological Chemistry*, Jan: 280; 12310–12315. DOI: 10.1074/jbc.M500733200 April 1, 2005.

Semba RD, Gebauer SK, Baer DJ, Sun K, Turner R, Silber HA, Talegawkar S, Ferrucci L, and JA Novotny. 2014. Dietary intake of advanced glycation end products did not affect endothelial function and inflammation in healthy adults in a randomized controlled trial. *The Journal of Nutrition*, Jul; 144(7): 1037–1042. DOI: 10. 3945/jn.113.189480.

Shai IS, Schwarzfuchs D, Henkin Y, Shahar DR, Witkow S, Greenberg I, Golan R, Fraser D, Bolotin A, Vardi H, Tangi-Rozental O, Zuk-Ramot R, Sarusi B, Brickner D, Schwartz Z, Sheiner E, Marko R, Katorza E, Thiery J, Fiedler GM, Blüher M, Stumvoll M, and MJ Stampfer. 2008. Dietary Intervention Randomized Controlled Trial (DIRECT) Group. Weight loss with a low-carbohydrate, Mediterranean, or low-fat diet. *New England Journal of Medicine*, Jan; 359(1): 229–241. PMID: 20050018.

Shangari N, Bruce WR, Poon R, and PJ O'Brien. 2003. Toxicity of glyoxals—role of oxidative stress, metabolic detoxification and thiamine deficiency. *Biochemical Society Transactions*, Dec; 31(P1–6): 1390–1393.

Sharma C, Kaur A, Thind SS, Singh B, and S Raina. 2015. Advanced glycation end-products (AGEs): an emerging concern for processed food industries. *Journal of Food Science and Technology*, Dec; 52(12): 7561–7576. DOI: 10.1007/s13197-015-1851-y.

Siddiqui MA, Rasheed S, Saquib Q, Al-Khedhairy AA, Al-Said MS, Musarrat J, and MI Choudhary. 2016. In-vitro dual inhibition of protein glycation, and oxidation by some Arabian plants. *BMC Complementary and Alternative Medicine*, Aug; 16: 276. DOI: 10.1186/s12906-016-1225-7.

Swain JF, McCarron PB, Hamilton EF, Sacks FM, and LJ Appel. 2008. Characteristics of the diet patterns tested in the optimal macronutrient intake trial to prevent heart disease (OmniHeart): options for a heart-healthy diet. *Journal of the American Dietetic Association*, Feb;108(2): 257–265. DOI: 10.1016/j.jada.2007.10.040.

Tang Y, and A Chen. 2014. Curcumin eliminates the effect of advanced glycation end-products (AGEs) on the divergent regulation of gene expression of receptors of AGEs by interrupting leptin signaling. *Laboratory Investigation*, May; 94(5): 503–516. DOI: 10.1038/labinvest.2014.42.

Ulrich P, and A Cerami. 2001. Protein glycation, diabetes, and aging. *Recent Progress in Hormone Research*, 56: 1–21. PMID: 11237208.

Uribarri J, Cai W, Peppa M, Goodman S, Ferruci L, Striker G, and H Vlassara. 2007. Circulating glycotoxins and dietary advanced glycation end-products: two links to inflammatory response oxidative stress, and aging. *Journal of Gerontology. Series A, Biological Sciences and Medical Sciences*, April; 62(4): 427–433. PMCID: PMC2645629.

Uribarri J, Cai W, Ramdas M, Goodman S, Pyzik R, Chen X, Zhu L, Striker GE, and H Vlassara. 2011. Restriction of advanced glycation end products improves insulin resistance in human type 2 diabetes: potential role of AGER1 and SIRT1. *Diabetes Care*, Jul; 34(7): 1610–1616. DOI: 10.2337/dc11-0091.

Uribarri J, Cai W, Sandu O, Peppa M, Goldberg T, and H Vlassara. 2005. Diet-derived advanced glycation end products are major contributors to the body's AGE pool and induce inflammation in healthy subjects. *Annals of the New York Academy of Sciences*, Jun; 1043: 461–466. DOI: 10.1196/annals.1333.052.

Uribarri J, Peppa M, Cai W, Goldberg T, Lu M, Baliga S, Vassalotti JA, and H Vlassara. 2003a. Dietary glycotoxins correlate with circulating advanced glycation end product levels in renal failure patients. *American Journal of Kidney Diseases*, Sep; 42(3): 532–538. PMID: 12955681.

Uribarri J, Peppa M, Cai W, Goldberg T, Lu M, He C, and H Vlassara. 2003b. Restriction of dietary glycotoxins reduces excessive advanced glycation end products in renal failure patients. *Journal of the American Society of Nephrology*, Mar; 14(3): 728–731. PMID: 12595509.

Uribarri J, Woodruff S, Goodman S, Cai W, Chen X, Pyzik R, Yong A, Striker GE, and H Vlassara. 2010. Advanced glycation end products in foods and a practical guide to their reduction in the diet. *Journal of the American Dietetic Association*, Jun; 110(6): 911–916.e12. DOI:10.1016/j.jada.2010.03.018.

Vlassara H, Cai W, Crandall J, Goldberg T, Oberstein R, Dardaine V, Peppa M, and EJ Rayfield. 2002. Inflammatory mediators are induced by dietary glycotoxins: a major risk factor for diabetic angiopathy. *Proceedings of the National Academy of Sciences USA*. Nov; 99:15596–15601. DOI: 10.1073/pnas.242407999.

Vlassara H, Cai W, Goodman S, Pyzik R, Yong A, Zhu L, Neade T, Beeri M, Silverman JM, Ferrucci L, Tansman L, Striker GE, and J Uribarri. 2009. Protection against loss of innate defenses in adulthood by low AGE intake: role of a new anti-inflammatory AGE-receptor-1. *Journal of Clinical Endocrinology and Metabolism*, Nov; 94(11): 4483–4491. DOI: 10.1210/jc.2009-0089.

Vlassara H. 2001. The AGE-receptor in the pathogenesis of diabetic complications. *Diabetes/Metabolism Research and Reviews*, Nov–Dec; 17(6): 436–443. PMID: 11757079.

Yamaguchi M, Woodley DT, and GL Mechanic. 1988. Aging and cross-linking of skin collagen. *Biochemical and Biophysical Research Communication*, 1988 Apr; 152(2): 898–903. PMID: 3130057.

8 General Nutritional Considerations for Chronic Hyperglycemia— Type 2 Diabetes

A man can eat his dinner without understanding exactly how food nourishes him.

C.S. Lewis

8.1 HOW TO AVOID AGE-ING

The previous chapter detailed the health hazards of advanced glycation end products (AGEs) that may accumulate in the body in large part as a consequence of certain types of food preparation. AGEs are especially harmful to persons with diabetes and they compound the effects of hyperglycemia to jeopardize endothelium function and therefore cardiovascular and heart health. In a sense, this information represents what we know is harmful and should be avoided. However, it does not tell us what is healthful eating—an issue in diabetes.

The American Diabetes Association (ADA) has gone to great lengths to offer nutrition guidance, and their website, *Recipes for Healthy Living*, offers meal plan guidance:

They propose that breakfast, lunch, dinner, and two snacks per day meal plans should be balanced to include about eight servings of fruits and vegetables in almost every meal and snack. The diet should deliver about 1550–1650 calories per day depending on age, gender, activity level, and whether or not weight loss is a goal. The calories should be distributed throughout the day between the meals and the two snacks.

The guidelines also suggest a "moderate" (about 45%) carbohydrate intake, amounting to about 45 to 60 g, spread throughout the day; limiting trans fat as much as possible (less than 10%), and emphasizing healthy or "good" fat sources; cholesterol should be kept to no more than 300 mg/day; more than 25 g of dietary fiber per day is desirable—preferably from plant-based foods such as whole grains, fruit, vegetables, nuts, seeds, and beans.

The daily sodium intake is said.

Finally, the ADA guidelines suggest some simple ways to reducing the sodium in the daily diet to no more than 2300 mg/day, by learning what foods are major sources of sodium, making wise food choices, and controlling portion sizes (see Recipes for Healthy Living: http://www.diabetes .org/mfa-recipes/about-our-meal-plans.html; accessed 2.23.18).

These guidelines are based on the compilation of data collected over countless hours of clinical and laboratory research, and they constitute the best of what is conventionally known about an ideal diet for persons with diabetes.

There is one drawback: these guidelines are difficult for most people to implement… consistently. Furthermore *The Review of Diabetic Studies* featured an interesting report titled "Eating behavior among Type 2 diabetic patients: a poorly recognized aspect in a poorly controlled disease." The authors of the report contend that nutrition intervention is essential in Type 2 diabetes and that dietary management requires eating behavior changes in connection with meal planning, food selection, food preparation, dinning out, portion control, and appropriate responses to eating challenges.

It is clear that diabetes patients encounter difficulties in complying with a dietary regime. They may exhibit restrictive eating behaviors, express feelings of deprivation, and some may believe that rigid dietary control is the only way to a proper diet and weight management. In addition, pressure to conform to nutritional recommendations may cause diabetes sufferers to be more likely to engage in dietary underreporting.

Binge eating (difficulty restraining) and body dissatisfaction frequently occur among these patients. Health professionals, therefore, need to take into account these difficulties in their collaboration with the patients in order to improve the effectiveness of nutrition intervention. The author (Yannakoulia. 2006) makes a number of salient points, some of which appear below:

First, little of daily human food choice and intake is directly determined by the chemical composition of foods, and the physiological characteristics of the individual; it is mostly influenced by events tangential to these factors such as perceptions, beliefs, and responses to cues. There are global rules that operate on human eating behavior that apply to food choice and intake that depend on food availability, existing eating habits, and also learning and individual beliefs and expectations such as cognitive influences and meanings (Mela. 1999).

Second, healthful eating can result in low HbA1c levels, and it may be positively related to specific food habits such as limiting the amount of high-sugar foods and smaller portion sizes, eating only an occasional dessert, reducing high-fat foods and eating low-fat foods, eating regularly and planning meals, eating large amounts of vegetables, and limiting specific carbohydrates. In contrast, healthful eating is inversely related to eating at buffets, fast-food, and large-chain restaurants; choosing high-fat menu selections; and eating high-fat sources of protein. Deviations in prescribed eating patterns, particularly skipping breakfast and snack additions and deletions, are also associated with poor metabolic control (Schmidt, Rost, McGill, et al. 1994).

Third, adopting new food habits is not an easily achieved goal: Diabetic patients encounter many educational, environmental, psychological, and lifestyle difficulties in accommodating disease management (Snoek. 2000). Barriers to dietary adherence include complications with daily life, such as eating out, social events, temptations, need for food planning, need for constant self-care, denial of the severity of the disease, poor understanding of diet-disease associations, misinformation, lack of appropriate social support, and time constraints (Brown, Pope, Hunt et al. 1998; Travis. 1997; Schlundt, Rea, Kline et al. 1994; El-Kebbi, Bacha, Ziemer et al. 1996).

Persons with Type 2 diabetes also encounter difficulties with following food exchange systems and express their need for revised dietary strategies that would incorporate appropriate education on how to make healthy food choices (El-Kebbi, Bacha, Ziemer et al. 1996).

Fourth, food consumption is often accompanied by feelings of fear, guilt and anger, whereas diet compliance elicits aversive and restrictive attitudes. Thoughts of dietary deprivation have also been reported (Schlundt, Rea, Kline et al. 1994; Samuel-Hodge, Headen, Skelly et al. 2000). It should be noted that the more "restrictive" or rigid the eating practices, such as eliminating sugar, limiting carbohydrate-containing foods, and decreasing total dietary fat, were far more frequently described by persons with diabetes as an important element of diabetes dietary management, compared to the more flexible eating patterns of portion control and regular eating (Savoca, and Miller. 2001).

Fifth, high underreporting rates have been found among patients with Type 2 diabetes (Martin, Tapsell, Denmeade et al. 2003; Samuel-Hodge, Fernandez, Henriquez-Roldan et al. 2004). In particular, Samuel-Hodge, Fernandez, Henriquez-Roldan et al. (2004) concluded that, because diabetic underreporters actually reported diets closely matching the currently recommended diet for diabetes, it seems plausible that they were more likely to report what they should be eating, rather than what they were eating. There is much more to this, and for further details, see Yannakoulia (2006).

In most cases, attention to diet is paramount, but there is evidence that it will not successfully substitute for antidiabetes medication in well-established disease. *The Cochrane Database of*

Systematic Reviews published a report titled "Dietary advice for treatment of type 2 diabetes in adults." The authors tell us that "While initial dietary management immediately after formal diagnosis is an 'accepted' cornerstone of treatment of type 2 diabetes, a formal and systematic overview of its efficacy and method of delivery is not currently available." Therefore they aimed to assess the effects of type and frequency of different types of dietary advice for adults with Type 2 diabetes.

The investigators reported a comprehensive search of The Cochrane Library, MEDLINE, EMBASE, CINAHL, AMED, and bibliographies and contacted relevant experts. All randomized controlled trials of 6 months or longer, where dietary advice was the main intervention, were selected. Thirty-six articles reporting a total of 18 trials following 1467 participants were included. Dietary approaches assessed in this review were low-fat/high-carbohydrate diets, high-fat/low-carbohydrate diets, low-calorie (1000 kcal/day) and very-low-calorie (500 kcal/day) diets and modified fat diets.

Two trials compared the ADA exchange diet with a standard reduced fat diet and five studies assessed low-fat diets versus moderate-fat or low-carbohydrate diets. Two studies assessed the effect of a very-low-calorie diet versus a low-calorie diet. Six studies compared dietary advice with dietary advice plus exercise, and three other studies assessed dietary advice versus dietary advice plus behavioral approaches. The studies all measured weight and measures of glycemic control, although not all studies reported these in the articles published.

Other outcomes measured in these studies included mortality, blood pressure, serum cholesterol (including low-density lipoprotein [LDL] and high-density lipoprotein [HDL] cholesterol), serum triglycerides, maximal exercise capacity, and compliance.

The results suggested that adoption of regular exercise is a good way to promote better glycemic control in Type 2 diabetic patients; however, all of these studies were thought to be at high risk of bias. Therefore, the investigators concluded that there are no high-quality data on the efficacy of the dietary treatment of Type 2 diabetes; however, the data available indicate that the adoption of exercise appears to improve glycated hemoglobin at 6 and 12 months (Nield, Moore, Hooper et al. 2007).

The bottom line is that in most cases, diet cannot substitute for medication in treatment of Type 2 diabetes, but in studies cited later in this chapter, it is clear that a poor diet can certainly undermine medication treatment.

It may be preferable for diabetes sufferers, for the reasons cited above, to adopt an integrative intervention nutrition plan that comes closest to meeting their specific needs without actually drawing their attention to the fact that, in so doing, they are actually battling a very serious disease. Drawing attention to that very fact may be one reason why the diabetes population seems to sabotage what is otherwise valuable advice in the many diabetes diet books currently on the bookstore shelves.

The most innocuous and perhaps least threatening diet—or challenging, for that matter—yet a diet with evidence-based benefits for persons with Type 2 diabetes, is the Mediterranean diet plan.

8.2 THE MEDITERRANEAN DIET PLAN

Anyone who regularly monitors blood glucose between meals, and early in the morning, must be drawn to the inescapable conclusion that the body is basically a sugar conversion machine: Sugar is extracted in various proportions from just about everything eaten. This leaves the average consumer with a (false) sense that unless laboratory-grade weights and measuring equipment are a fixture in the kitchen, then there is little chance of attaining success at meeting guidelines. There is another approach.

In terms of dietary food constituents and proportions, the recipes recommended by the ADA have much in common with the American Heart Association Heart Healthy diet—previously known as the Prudent Diet—as for instance, "How to Eat Healthy without 'Dieting'" (http://healthyfor good.heart.org/eat-smart/articles/how-to-eat-healthy-without-dieting; accessed 7.25.17). These and similar diets also have one thing in common, they are very much like the Mediterranean diet plan known to be cardiovascular and heart protective and beneficial to persons with Type 2 diabetes.

Since there is typically nothing starkly medical about the Mediterranean diet plan, it may seem perhaps a little less daunting to implement it, as it may not conjure up concerns about heart health, cholesterol levels, or meeting blood sugar level criteria.

The Mediterranean diet, developed by Dr. Ancel Keys (1904–2004) in 1958, in connection with the *Seven Countries Study*, examined the relationship between dietary pattern and the prevalence of coronary heart disease in Greece, Italy, Spain, South Africa, Japan, and Finland. The Mediterranean diet is beneficial because of its low energy (calories); low glycemic index; high fiber content; high L-arginine; high nitrates; high levels of polyphenolics, anthocyanidins, and other antioxidants; and activation of sirtuin 1 (Chatzianagnostou, Del Turco, Pingitore et al. 2015).

The Mediterranean diet consists largely of

- Minimal processed foods
- Olive oil as the principal fat, replacing other fats and oils (including butter and margarine), total fat ranging from less than 25% to over 35% of energy, with saturated fat no more than 7% to 8% of energy (calories)
- Daily consumption of low to moderate amounts of cheese and yogurt
- Twice-weekly consumption of fish and poultry (up to 7 eggs per week)
- Fresh fruit as the typical daily dessert
- Red meat limited to a maximum of 12 to 16 ounces (340 to 450 g) per month
- Moderate consumption of wine

It is beyond the scope of this book, limited as it is to evidence-based benefits of an integrative approach to blood glucose control, to detail a diet plan illustrated with recipes. However, there are many of them readily available on the Internet. For instance:

- Gaples Institute for Integrative Cardiology: http://www.gaplesinstitute.org/the-heart-of-the -dash-and-mediterranean-diets-fruit-and-vegetables/
- Oldways: https://oldwayspt.org/recipes?gclid=EAIaIQobChMIpYawwt-k1QIVUUwNCh3Vw gG6EAAYASAAEgJNevD_BwE
- Allrecipes: http://allrecipes.com/recipes/16704/healthy-recipes/mediterranean-diet/
- Dr. Axe: https://draxe.com/mediterranean-diet-recipes/
- EatingWell: http://www.eatingwell.com/recipes/18314/cuisines-regions/mediterranean/
- Mayo Clinic: http://www.mayoclinic.org/healthy-lifestyle/nutrition-and-healthy-eating/in -depth/mediterranean-diet-recipes/art-20046682
- Olive Oils from Spain: https://www.oliveoilsfromspain.org/recipes?gclid=EAIaIQobCh MIpYawwt-k1QIVUUwNCh3VwgG6EAMYASAAEgIkEfD_BwE
- MyGreekDish.com: http://www.mygreekdish.com/

The following sections detail the science-based evidence that the Mediterranean diet plan is a beneficial nutritional support in diabetes and diabetes-related cardiovascular and heart disorders. However, it needs to be emphasized that, while adherence to a Mediterranean diet plan regimen can improve long-term outcome as part of integrative glycemia control, it is not to be taken as a substitute for prescription antihyperglycemia medication(s).

Many studies—only a sample is cited here—show the benefits of the Mediterranean diet as part of an integrative treatment program. However, no science-based study supports any nutrition plan as an alternative to medication(s) in most cases of established Type 2 Diabetes.

8.3   THE MEDITERRANEAN DIET PLAN AS INTEGRATIVE INTERVENTION IN TYPE 2 DIABETES

In 2015, the journal *BMJ Open* reported a study titled "A journey into a Mediterranean diet and type 2 diabetes: a systematic review with meta-analyses." The objective of the analyses was to summarize evidence of the efficacy of a Mediterranean diet on the management of Type 2 diabetes and prediabetic states.

The study consisted of a systematic review of all meta-analyses and randomized controlled trials that compared the Mediterranean diet to a control diet on the treatment of Type 2 diabetes and prediabetic states. Electronic searches were carried out up to January 2015; trials were included for meta-analyses if they had a control group treated with another diet, if they were of at least 6 months duration, and if they had at least 30 adult participants with or at risk for Type 2 diabetes.

The interventions chosen focused on dietary patterns that were described as using a "Mediterranean" dietary pattern, and the outcome measures were glycemic control, cardiovascular risk factors, and remission from the metabolic syndrome.

A *de novo* meta-analysis of three long-term randomized controlled trials of the Mediterranean diet, and glycemic control of diabetes, favored the Mediterranean diet as compared to simply lower-fat diets.

Another such meta-analysis of two long-term randomized controlled trials showed a 49% increased probability of remission from the metabolic syndrome.

Five meta-analyses showed a favorable effect of Mediterranean diet on body weight, total cholesterol, and HDL cholesterol compared to other diets. Two meta-analyses demonstrated that higher adherence to the Mediterranean diet reduced the risk of future diabetes by between 19% and 23%, respectively.

The investigators concluded that the Mediterranean diet was associated with better glycemic control and reduced cardiovascular risk factors than control diets, such as simply lower-fat diets (Esposito, Maiorino, Bellastella et al. 2015).

Another systematic review titled "Effect of Mediterranean Diet in diabetes control and cardiovascular risk modification" was published in the journal *Frontiers in Public Health*. The review was based on comprehensive search of multiple electronic databases such as MEDLINE, Google Scholars, PubMed, and the Cochrane central register data, until May 2014. Cross-sectional, prospective, and controlled clinical trials were included, which looked at the associations between the Mediterranean diet and indices of diabetes control such HbA1c, fasting glucose, and homeostasis model assessment, in addition to cardiovascular and peripheral vascular outcomes.

It was found that most of the studies showed favorable effects of the Mediterranean diet on glycemic control although some controversy remains regarding issues, such as obesity (Sleiman, Al-Badri, and Azar. 2015).

Could adherence to a Mediterranean diet plan be sufficient for glycemic control in Type 2 diabetes, or are meds necessary? This question was addressed in a study published in the *Annals of Internal Medicine*.

The aim of the study was to compare the effects of a low-carbohydrate Mediterranean-style or a low-fat diet on the need for antihyperglycemic drug therapy in patients with newly diagnosed Type 2 diabetes. The study was conducted on overweight patients with newly diagnosed Type 2 diabetes who were never treated with antihyperglycemic drugs, and who had hemoglobin HbA1c levels less than 11%. They were assigned a Mediterranean-style diet with less than 50% of daily calories from carbohydrates, or a low-fat diet with less than 30% of daily calories from fat.

After 4 years, 44% of patients in the Mediterranean-style diet group, and 70% in the low-fat diet group, required treatment (hazard ratio = 0.63, hazard ratio adjusted for weight change = 0.70).

Participants assigned to the Mediterranean-style diet lost more weight, and they experienced greater improvements in some glycemic control and coronary risk measures than did those assigned to the low-fat diet: Compared to a low-fat diet, a low-carbohydrate, Mediterranean-style diet led to more favorable changes in glycemic control and coronary risk factors, but only delayed the need for antihyperglycemic drug therapy in overweight patients with newly diagnosed Type 2 diabetes (Esposito, Maiorino, Ciotola et al. 2009).

In 2014, the journal *Annals of Internal Medicine* published a study titled "Prevention of diabetes with Mediterranean diets: a subgroup analysis of a randomized trial." The aim of the study was to determine whether dietary changes, without calorie restriction, also protect from diabetes in the context of a plan to assess the efficacy of Mediterranean diets for the primary prevention of diabetes in the Prevención con Dieta Mediterránea trial, from October 2003 to December 2010 (median follow-up, 4.1 years).

Participants were men and women without diabetes who were at high cardiovascular risk. They were randomly assigned and stratified by site, gender, and age, but not diabetes status to receive one of three diets: Mediterranean diet supplemented with extra virgin olive oil (EVOO), Mediterranean diet supplemented with nuts, or a control diet (advice on a low-fat diet). A control group received no intervention other than instructions to increase physical activity or lose weight.

During follow-up, new-onset cases of diabetes occurred in the Mediterranean diet supplemented with EVOO group at the rate of 16/1000 (hazard ratio = 0.60), in the Mediterranean diet supplemented with mixed nuts group at the rate of 18.7/1000 (hazard ratio = 0.82), and in the control diet groups at the rate of 23.6/1000, compared to the control group.

It was concluded that a Mediterranean diet enriched with EVOO, even without energy restrictions, reduced diabetes risk among persons with high cardiovascular risk (Salas-Salvadó, Bulló, Estruch et al. 2014).

The journal *Diabetic Medicine* reported a study of the relation between HbA1c and adherence to a Mediterranean-type diet, assessed by a 9-point scale that incorporated the salient characteristics of this diet (range of scores, 0 to 9, with higher scores indicating greater adherence).

Diabetic patients with the highest scores (6 to 9) had lower body mass index (BMI) and waist circumferences, a lower prevalence of the metabolic syndrome, and lower HbA1c and post-meal glucose levels than diabetic patients with the lowest scores (0 to 3).

Mean HbA1c and 2-h post-meal glucose concentrations were significantly lower in diabetic patients with high adherence to a Mediterranean-type diet than in those with low adherence.

In Type 2 diabetes, greater adherence to a Mediterranean-type diet is associated with lower HbA1c and post-meal glucose levels (Esposito, Maiorino, Di Palo et al. 2009). In a subsequent report, published in *Diabetes Research and Clinical Practice*, the investigators concluded that not only does adopting a Mediterranean diet help prevent Type 2 diabetes, but it also improves glycemic control and reduces cardiovascular risk in persons with established diabetes (Esposito, Maiorino, Ceriello et al. 2010).

A study to investigate the impact of a diet modeled on the traditional Cretan Mediterranean diet on metabolic control and vascular risk in Type 2 diabetes was published in the journal *Nutrition, Metabolism, and Cardiovascular Diseases*.

Participants 47 to 77 years old with Type 2 diabetes were to consume either the intervention diet *ad lib* or their usual diet for 12 weeks and then cross over to the alternate diet. Most of the meals and staple foods for the intervention diet were provided.

Lipids, glycemic variables, blood pressure, homocysteine, C-reactive protein, plasma carotenoids, and body composition (anthropometry and dual-energy x-ray absorptiometry) were assessed at baseline and at the end of both diet periods. Dietary adherence was monitored using plasma carotenoid and fatty acid analysis, complemented by diet diaries.

When on the Mediterranean intervention diet, glycosylated hemoglobin fell from 7.1% to 6.8%, and diet quality improved significantly: plant to animal food in grams/day ratio increased from 1.3 to 5.4; plasma lycopene and lutein/zeaxanthin increased by 36% and 25% respectively; plasma saturated and trans FAs decreased; and monounsaturated FAs increased, compared to the usual diet (Itsiopoulos, Brazionis, Kaimakamis et al. 2011).

The *Journal of Human Nutrition and Dietetics* reported an interesting study that concluded that the Mediterranean diet improves HbA1c but not fasting blood glucose, compared to alternative dietary strategies. The investigators conducted a systematic review and meta-analysis to determine whether a Mediterranean diet accomplished better glycemic control than other dietary interventions, irrespective of weight loss in participants. Electronic databases were searched for controlled trials of interventions that included all major components of the Mediterranean diet and were carried out in free-living individuals at high risk or diagnosed with Type 2 diabetes.

None of the interventions were found to be superior in lowering glucose parameters. However, the Mediterranean diet reduced HbA1c significantly better than all others except a Palaeolithic diet (Carter, Achana, Troughton et al. 2014).

8.3.1   THE MEDITERRANEAN DIET IS A RICH SOURCE OF NO DONOR NITRATES

Many studies of the beneficial effects of the Mediterranean diet—including some cited below—focus mostly on olive oil as an antiatherogenic food. However, medical science really only learned that the Mediterranean diet is beneficial when it became clear that its cornucopia of foods were a rich source of nitric oxide (NO) from two food groups that are antioxidant, support healthy blood vessel and heart function, and combat inflammation. In addition, the oleic acid found in olive oil, plentiful in the diet, can help reduce the damage to blood vessels caused by Type 2 diabetes (see below).

The two NO donor food groups are as follows:

- Group 1 foods include meats that are rich in L-arginine from which cells in the blood vessel lining the endothelium form NO (Palmer, Ashton, and Moncada. 1988).
- Group 2 foods are greens and beans (and beets), also rich in L-arginine, but most important, they are rich in nitrate (Lidder, and Webb. 2013), another source of NO.

Dietary source nitrate is metabolized to nitrite in the body to form NO. An article titled "Nitrate and nitrite in biology, nutrition and therapeutics," published in *Nature Chemical Biology*, in 2009, teaches the following about dietary nitrate:

Certain vegetables in the daily diet are our principal source of nitrate. Much of the nitrate in foods is actively taken up by the salivary glands as we consume the foods and is then concentrated in saliva. Bacteria in the mouth then reduce salivary nitrate to nitrite. Continuously swallowing nitrite in saliva forms different nitrogen compounds in the stomach and in particular, NO. This is the second "pathway" for forming NO, and it is called the "enterosalivary circulation of nitrate" (Lundberg, Gladwin, Ahluwalia et al. 2009; Lundberg, and Govoni. 2004).

8.3.1.1   The Enterosalivary Circulation Cycle

Inorganic nitrate in foods is rapidly absorbed in the small intestine. Much of the circulating nitrate is eventually excreted in the urine, but up to 25% is actively extracted by the salivary glands and concentrated in saliva. Bacteria in the mouth effectively reduce nitrate to nitrite by the action of enzymes, leading to thousand-fold higher concentrations of nitrite in saliva than in plasma. In the acidic stomach, nitrite is spontaneously decomposed to form NO and other nitrogen compounds that regulate important physiological functions. Nitrate and the remaining nitrite are absorbed from the intestine into the circulation and can convert to NO in blood and tissues (Lundberg, Gladwin, Ahluwalia et al. 2009).

It is possible to determine one's NO availability level indirectly as a function of the concentration of nitrite in saliva because it has been shown that (a) consuming nitrate actually raises NO availability in the body (McKnight, Smith, Drummond et al. 1997) and (b) salivary nitrate and nitrite levels reflect the amount ingested.

In a study published in the journal *Food and Cosmetics Toxicology*, volunteers consumed vegetables and vegetable juices with high concentrations of nitrate. Variations of nitrate and nitrite concentrations in saliva were determined for up to 7 h, at intervals of 30 or 60 min.

- First, the amount of nitrate secreted by the salivary glands increased directly with the amount of nitrate ingested.
- Second, nitrite concentration in saliva correlated directly with salivary nitrate content, indicating a direct relationship between the salivary nitrite concentrations and the amounts of nitrate ingested in the diet (Spiegelhalder, Eisenbrand, Preussmann. 1976).

The results of this, and similar studies, support the use of salivary nitrite assay to estimate NO availability (see Chapter 6).

The journal *Nutrition and Metabolism (Lond)* published a review titled "Beneficial effects of inorganic nitrate/nitrite in Type 2 diabetes and its complications." The investigators reviewed experimental and clinical studies investigating the effect of nitrate/nitrite administration on various aspects of Type 2 diabetes. They found studies that showed that altered metabolism of nitrate/nitrite and impaired NO pathway are linked to diabetes, contributing to its complications.

Consumption of dietary inorganic nitrate/nitrite has important beneficial properties, including regulation of glucose homeostasis and insulin signaling pathway, improvement of insulin resistance and vascular function, and hypotensive, hypolipidemic, anti-inflammatory, and antioxidative effects. The investigators concluded that dietary nitrate/nitrite could be a "compensatory fuel for a disrupted nitrate/nitrite/NO pathway and related disorders in diabetes" (Bahadoran, Ghasemi, Mirmiran et al. 2015).

8.4   IS TOASTING WITH WINE REALLY "TO YOUR HEALTH"?

There is little by way of carbohydrates in a glass of wine, but the calories in that glass of wine are not low. A glass of wine may have only 0.5 g of carbohydrates, but it may nevertheless yield 83 calories. Alcohol burns (is metabolized) faster than fat, protein, and carbohydrates, so even on a low carb diet, wine should not be a low carb drink of choice.

Health authorities often tout a "moderate" amount of wine to be a safe supplement to diet and a potential benefit in cardiovascular and heart disease. WebMD recommends a glass a day, with some *caveats* (http://www.webmd.com/food-recipes/features/wine-how-much-is-good-for-you#1; accessed 7.26.17). The argument in favor of wine often makes mention of the value of resveratrol as an antioxidant.

First, there is usually a negligible amount of resveratrol in a reasonable amount of wine consumed. Second, and perhaps more to the point, the resveratrol in commercially available wine is not in a beneficial form, because it is cis-resveratrol. Trans-resveratrol, which is the active form, is extremely fragile and it would not survive in that form in a bottle of wine, or when exposed for any time to light and air in a wine glass.

It could well be argued that the suggestion that one have a drink (wine usually) "in moderation" constitutes an unfortunate recommendation, and not all authorities agree. For instance: The purpose of a study published in the journal *Diabetic Medicine* was to evaluate the effects of dry and sweet wine on glycemic control in Type 2 diabetes. Diabetic patients consumed a light meal with either 300 mL of tap water, 300 mL of dry white wine, 300 mL of sweet white wine with ethanol added, or 300 mL of dry white wine with glucose added.

Similar glucose, insulin, and triglyceride responses were obtained in all four conditions, but there was a greater suppression of the free fatty acid levels in the three wine consumptions as compared to tap water.

The results indicated to the investigators that patients with well-controlled Type 2 diabetes can drink moderate amounts of dry or sweet wine with meals without risking acute deterioration of glycemic control (Christiansen, Thomsen, Rasmussen et al. 1993).

Another study published in the journal *Diabetes Care* went one step further. In this study, intended to examine the effect of moderate alcohol intake (with a meal) on glucose homeostasis in diabetic patients, the participants were given an aperitif before dinner, wine during the meal, and a drink after dinner (alcohol 1 g/kg)—or an equal amount of mineral water.

The participants in the study included Type 1 diabetes patients treated with insulin and Type 2 diabetes patients treated with diet alone, or with diet and oral drugs.

In Type 1 diabetes patients, blood glucose and insulin concentrations were virtually identical in both conditions. In Type 2 diabetes patients, alcohol slightly enhanced the meal-induced insulin secretion, resulting in lower blood glucose concentrations the next morning. No hypoglycemic glucose concentrations were observed in either group after alcohol ingestion.

The investigators concluded that moderate alcohol intake with a meal does not lead to hypo- or hyperglycemia in diabetes patients (Koivisto, Tulokas, Toivonen et al. 1993). On the other hand, a study published in the journal *Metabolism* reported (in the very title of the study) that "Ethanol with a mixed meal decreases the incretin levels early postprandially and increases postprandial lipemia in Type 2 diabetic patients." Incretin is a hormone that stimulates insulin secretion in response to meals. The two most important incretin hormones are glucagon-like peptide-1 (GLP-1) and glucose-dependent insulinotropic polypeptide (GIP). Lipemia is the presence in the blood of an abnormally high concentration of emulsified fat.

Supplementation of a fat-rich, mixed meal with alcohol in Type 2 diabetes patients suppressed GLP-1 early in the postprandial phase and increased the late triacylglycerol (triglyceride) responses compared with the two other meals. No significant differences in HDL cholesterol levels were seen. Isocaloric amounts of carbohydrate and alcohol suppressed equally the postprandial free fatty acid levels, but carbohydrate increased the postprandial glucose, GLP-1, and insulin levels the most.

Early in the postprandial phase, alcohol suppressed the incretin responses and increased the late postprandial triacylglycerol levels in Type 2 diabetes patients (Dalgaard, Thomsen, Rasmussen et al. 2004).

Furthermore, does drinking alcohol contribute to the development of diabetes? The aim of a study on middle-aged Swedish men and women, published in the journal *Diabetic Medicine*, was to investigate the influence of alcohol consumption and specific alcoholic beverages on the risk of developing prediabetes and Type 2 diabetes.

It was found that total alcohol consumption and binge drinking increased the risk of prediabetes and Type 2 diabetes in men (odds ratio [OR], 1.42 and 1.67, respectively), while low consumption decreased diabetes risk in women (OR, 0.41).

Men showed higher risk of prediabetes with high beer consumption (OR, 1.84) and of Type 2 diabetes with high consumption of spirits (OR, 2.03). Women showed a reduced risk of prediabetes with high wine intake (OR, 0.66) and of Type 2 diabetes with medium intake of both wine and spirits (OR, 0.46 and 0.55, respectively), whereas high consumption of spirits increased the risk of prediabetes risk (OR, 2.41).

The authors concluded that high alcohol consumption raises the risk of abnormal glucose regulation in men, whereas in women, the associations are more complex: decreased risk with low or medium intake and increased risk with high alcohol intake (Cullmann, Hilding, and Östenson. 2012).

8.5 ACTIVATING SIRTUIN 1 IMPROVES GLYCEMIA IN TYPE 2 DIABETES

Sirtuin 1, NAD (nicotinamide adenine dinucleotide)-dependent deacetylase sirtuin-1, is a protein that in humans is encoded by the SIRT1 gene (Frye. 1999). SIRT1 stands for sirtuin 1 (silent mating type information regulation 2 homolog), referring to the fact that its sirtuin homolog (the biological equivalent across species) in yeast (*Saccharomyces cerevisiae*) is Sir2. SIRT1 is an enzyme that deacetylates proteins that contribute to cellular regulation (reaction to stressors, longevity).

Sirtuin genes function as antiaging genes in yeast, in the worm *Caenorhabditis elegans*, and in fruit flies (*Drosphila*). In yeast, sirtuin proteins are known to regulate epigenetic gene silencing and to suppress recombination of rDNA. Studies suggest that the human sirtuins may function as intracellular regulatory proteins with mono-ADP-ribosyltransferase activity (https://www.ncbi.nlm.nih.gov/gene/23411).

Among seven mammalian sirtuins, SIRT1 has been the most extensively studied and has been demonstrated to play a critical role in all major metabolic organs and tissues. SIRT1 regulates glucose and lipid homeostasis in the liver, modulates insulin secretion in pancreatic islets, controls insulin sensitivity and glucose uptake in skeletal muscle, increases adiponectin expression in white adipose tissue, and controls food intake and energy expenditure in the brain.

The nicotinamide adenine dinucleotide (NAD) requirement for sirtuin function indicates a link between aging and metabolism, and a boost in sirtuin activity may in part explain how calorie restriction extends life span (NAD is a coenzyme found in all living cells). In a report in the *Cold Spring Harbor Symposia on Quantitative Biology*, Dr. L. Guarente asserts that SIRT1-mediated mitochondrial biogenesis may reduce the production of reactive oxygen species, thereby overcoming a possible cause of aging (Guarente. 2007).

A report, published in the journal *NATURE*, concluded that activating sirtuin 1 has beneficial effects on glucose balance and insulin sensitivity: sirtuin activators improve whole-body glucose balance and insulin sensitivity in adipose (fat) tissue, skeletal muscle, and liver. The investigators concluded that "SIRT1 activation is a promising new therapeutic approach for treating diseases of ageing such as type 2 diabetes" (Milne, Lambert, Schenk et al. 2007).

Investigators reporting in the *Journal of Diabetes Complications* noted the growing evidence that SIRT1 regulates glucose and lipid metabolism through its deacetylase activity. In their review, they summarized the recent progress in SIRT1 research with a particular focus on the role of SIRT1 in insulin resistance in different metabolic tissues: Activated SIRT1 seems to improve the insulin sensitivity of liver, skeletal muscle, and adipose tissues and protects the pancreatic β-cells.

These findings suggested to them that SIRT1 might be a new therapeutic target for the prevention of disease related to insulin resistance, such as metabolic syndrome and Type 2 diabetes (Cao, Jiang, Ma et al. 2016). Activation of sirtuin 1 can be accomplished by a diet consistent with the Mediterranean diet (Fried and Nezin. 2017). However, it is also possible to deactivate sirtuin 1 by diet:

A study titled "Oral advanced glycation endproducts (AGEs) promote insulin resistance and diabetes by depleting the antioxidant defenses AGE receptor-1 and sirtuin 1," published in the *Proceedings of the National Academy of Sciences USA*, concluded exactly that. The investigators pointed out that our contemporary "lifestyle" includes a preference for thermally processed foods high in AGEs that enhance appetite and cause overnutrition. Consequently, they proposed that regular consumption of AGEs promotes insulin resistance and Type 2 diabetes. The study was conducted on mice fed isocaloric diets with or without AGEs.

Mice fed AGEs manifested increased adiposity and premature insulin resistance marked by severe deficiency of anti-AGE advanced glycation receptor 1 and of survival factor sirtuin 1 (SIRT1) in white adipose tissue, skeletal muscle, and liver. Impaired glucose uptake was associated with marked changes in insulin receptor and a macrophage and adipocyte shift to a pro-oxidative stress/inflammatory phenotype. These features were absent in the control mice.

It was concluded that prolonged oral exposure to AGEs can deplete host defenses and SIRT1, raise basal oxidative stress/inflammation, and increase susceptibility to dysmetabolic insulin resistance (Cai, Ramdas, Zhu et al. 2012).

There are several ways to avoid deactivation of sirtuin 1 and to promote its activation. First, it can be done by caloric restriction or by the selection of foods that promote its activation (Fried and Nezin. 2017). Second, as noted above, by adhering to a Mediterranean diet plan. Most important is that the Mediterranean diet plan has been consistently shown to be effective in management and even prevention of Type 2 diabetes. This is corroborated in the following reviews:

An English-language review in the *Chinese Medical Journal* was based on electronic database on PubMed up to April 14, 2014. The studies selected had to match the following inclusion criteria: (1) randomized clinical trials and meta-analysis or systematic review, and (2) provide strong evidence for the diet as a way to prevent Type 2 diabetes and improve glycemic control and cardiovascular risk factors in diabetic patients.

Based on the analyses, the investigators concluded that adherence to the Mediterranean diet plan is inversely related to Type 2 diabetes and, in those so diagnosed, it plays an important role in management of the condition. The importance of the combination and interaction of Mediterranean diet components, such as fruits, vegetables, nuts, legumes, whole grains, fish, and moderate intakes of red wine, which contain essential nutrients and health-promoting properties, including high fibers, high magnesium, high antioxidant, and high monounsaturated fatty acids, was underscored. Interaction and combination of these essential nutrients and health-promoting properties were found to lower body weight, HbA1c, LDL, and oxidative stress and to improve HDL level, all beneficial for prevention and improved prognosis for persons with Type 2 diabetes (Khemayanto, and Shi. 2014).

Likewise, a study published in the *Journal of Research in Medical Sciences* reported a systematic review of databases from Cochrane Central Register of Controlled Trials databases, PubMed, Iran Medex, and MagIran, with the keywords "diabetes" and "dietary pattern."

The studies were concerned with diabetes, insulin resistance, metabolic syndrome, and dietary patterns. The major dietary patterns were "healthy," "Western," "Traditional," "Prudent," "unhealthy," "Mediterranean," "Modern," and "Dietary Approach to Stop Hypertension" (DASH) diets.

Comparison of the effects of different diets revealed that dietary patterns containing fiber-rich foods have a protective role in managing diabetes. "Healthy," "Mediterranean," "Pruden," and "DASH" dietary patterns were associated with lower risk of hyperglycemia (Maghsoudi, and Azadbakht. 2012).

8.6 MEDITERRANEAN DIET AND OBESITY

Obesity is closely linked to Type 2 diabetes. In fact, obesity is probably the most important factor in the development of insulin resistance, according to investigators at the Salk Institute for Biological Studies (Montminy. 2009). They attribute obesity to endoplasmic reticulum stress, which is induced by a high-fat diet and is overly activated in obese people. It appears to trigger abnormal glucose production in the liver, an important step on the path to insulin resistance. This is in sharp contrast to the physiology in nondiabetic people, where there is a "fasting switch" that activates glucose production only when blood glucose levels are low (e.g., during fasting).

It had been well established that obesity promotes insulin resistance through the inappropriate inactivation of a process called gluconeogenesis, where the liver creates glucose for fuel, and which ordinarily occurs only in times of fasting. Yet, not all obese people become insulin resistant, and insulin resistance occurs in nonobese individuals as well, leading Montminy and his colleagues to suspect that fasting-induced glucose production is only half the story.

When a cell starts to sense stress, a metaphoric "red light" signals slowing down the production of proteins. This process, which is known as the "endoplasmic reticulum stress response," is abnormally active in the liver of obese individuals, where it contributes to the development of hyperglycemia. The endoplasmic reticulum is a structure within the cell that functions as a protein factory.

Glucose production is activated by a transcriptional switch called CRTC2, which is normally outside the nucleus awaiting the signal to slip inside and perform its function. Once in the nucleus, CRTC2 links up with another protein, CREB, and together, they activate the genes necessary to increase glucose output.

In insulin-resistant mice, however, the CRTC2 switch appears to be set in the "ON" position, and the cells start to overproduce glucose. Surprisingly, when mimicking the conditions of ER stress in mice, CRTC2 moved to the nucleus but failed to activate gluconeogenesis. Instead, it activated another factor, ATF6a, along with genes for combating stress and returning cells to health: when endoplasmic reticulum stress signaling is abnormal, glucose output rises (Wang, Vera, Fischer et al. 2009).

The purpose of a study published in the *Journal of Nutrition* was to assess the relation between BMI and obesity, based on the level of adherence to the traditional Mediterranean diet (TMD). The participants were about 1500 Spanish men and about 1600 Spanish women, ranging in age from 25 to 74 years. A Mediterranean pattern diet score was created, including foods considered to be characteristic components of the TMD including vegetables, fruits, pulses, nuts, fish, meat, cereals, olive oil, and wine.

The obesity risk decreased in men and in women with increasing adherence to the traditional Mediterranean dietary pattern. Both gender participants in the top third of this score were less likely to be obese. These data suggest that BMI and obesity decrease as traditional Mediterranean dietary pattern score increases (Schroder, Marrugat, Vila et al. 2004).

During the period 2005 to 2007, elderly men and elderly women (mean age, 74 years) from eight Mediterranean Islands in Greece, and in Cyprus, participated in a study of clinical and dietary demographic characteristics reported in the *International Journal of Food Science and Nutrition*. The conventional MedDietScore was used to assess adherence to the Mediterranean dietary pattern.

The prevalence of diabetes, hypercholesterolemia, and hypertension was higher in the obese elderly than in the simply overweight, or in those with normal weight. It was found that a one-unit increase in the MedDietScore resulted in an 88% decrease in likelihood of being obese. The authors concluded that greater adherence to the Mediterranean diet may reduce the burden of obesity among elderly individuals (Tyrovolas, Bountziouka, Papairakleous et al. 2009).

In a study conducted in Naples, Italy, and published in the *Journal of the American Medical Association*, investigators found that after 2 years, women randomly assigned to an intervention group who received detailed advice on weight reduction through a low-energy Mediterranean-style diet consumed more foods rich in complex carbohydrates, monounsaturated fat, and fiber; had a lower ratio of omega-6 to omega-3 fatty acids; and had lower energy (calories), saturated fat, and cholesterol intake than a control group. Their BMI decreased and so did insulin resistance. The investigators also noted that there was a significant reduction in markers of blood vessel inflammation (Esposito, Pontillo, Di Palo et al. 2003).

It was reported in the journal *Nutrition, Metabolism, and Cardiovascular Diseases* that epidemiologic and interventional studies suggest that weight loss is the main driving force to reduce diabetes risk. Landmark clinical trials of lifestyle changes in subjects with prediabetes have shown that diet and exercise leading to weight loss consistently reduce the incidence of diabetes. However, it cannot be established from these studies whether dietary changes alone play a significant role in preventing diabetes.

In this report, the investigators reviewed epidemiologic and clinical trials evidence relating nutrients, foods, and dietary patterns to diabetes risk and the possible mechanisms involved: They describe the differential effects of carbohydrate and fat quantity and quality, and those of specific foods and whole diets. They found that most dietary components influencing diabetes risk have similar effects on biomarkers of cardiovascular risk and inflammation, and they concluded that there is no universal dietary strategy to prevent diabetes or delay its onset.

Nevertheless, they recommend maintaining ideal body weight, by adherence to the so-called Mediterranean dietary pattern rich in olive oil, fruits, and vegetables, including whole grains, pulses and nuts, low-fat dairy, and moderate alcohol consumption—mainly red wine—or the prudent diet. The latter is characterized by a higher intake of food groups that are generally recommended for health promotion, particularly plant-based foods, and a lower intake of red meat, meat products, sweets, high-fat dairy, and refined grains as the best strategy to decrease diabetes risk, especially if dietary recommendations take into account individual preferences, thus enabling long-time adherence (Salas-Salvadó, Martinez-González, Bulló et al. 2011).

8.7   MEDITERRANEAN DIET AND THE METABOLIC SYNDROME

Metabolic syndrome is a cluster of factors that raise the risk of coronary heart disease and other health problems, especially Type 2 diabetes. Five conditions, described below, are metabolic risk factors.

- A large waistline, also called abdominal obesity or "having an apple shape." Excess fat in the stomach area is a greater risk factor for heart disease, than excess fat in other parts of the body such as on the hips.
- A high triglyceride level (or one is on medicine to treat high triglycerides).
- A low HDL cholesterol level (or one is on medicine to treat low HDL cholesterol). A low HDL cholesterol level raises the risk of heart disease.
- High blood pressure (or one is on medicine to treat high blood pressure).
- High fasting blood sugar (or one is on medicine to treat high blood sugar). Mildly high blood sugar may be an early sign of diabetes (https://www.nhlbi.nih.gov/health/health-topics/topics/ms; accessed 7.28.17).

One can have any one of these risk factors by itself, but they tend to cluster. The presence of at least three metabolic risk factors forms the basis for the diagnosis of metabolic syndrome. There is mounting evidence that the Mediterranean diet could help fight metabolic syndrome (Giugliano, and Esposito. 2008).

Because the Mediterranean diet has long been associated with low cardiovascular disease risk in the adult population, investigators conducted a large-scale meta-analysis of epidemiological and clinical studies from databases such as PubMed, EMBASE, Web of Science, and the Cochrane Central Register of Controlled Trials until April 30, 2010. The study was reported in the *Journal of the American College of Cardiology*. The database covered about 534,900 participants.

Analysis showed that adherence to the Mediterranean diet was associated with reduced risk of metabolic syndrome and, in addition, results from clinical studies revealed the protective role of the Mediterranean diet on waist circumference, HDL cholesterol, triglycerides, systolic and diastolic blood pressure, and insulin/glucose. Results from epidemiological studies also confirmed those of the clinical trials (Kastorini, Milionis, Esposito et al. 2011).

In a study appearing in *The Journal of the American Medical Association*, patients with metabolic syndrome were assigned to follow either a Mediterranean diet or a Prudent low-fat diet for 2½ years. At the end of the study, while 86% of the patients in the control group still had metabolic syndrome, only 44% of those in the Mediterranean diet group still had metabolic syndrome. The Mediterranean diet group also had improvements in several risk factors:

- Body weight decreased by 8.8 lb in the Mediterranean diet group, compared to 2.6 lb in the low-fat control group.
- Endothelial function score improved in the Mediterranean diet group, but remained poor and unchanged in the low-fat control group.
- Inflammatory markers (hs-CRP) and insulin resistance decreased significantly in the Mediterranean diet group (Esposito, Marfella, Ciotola et al. 2004).

A prospective longitudinal cohort study, meaning a study that follows, over time, a group of similar individuals (cohorts) who differ with respect to certain factors under study, to determine how these factors affect rates of outcome, appeared in the journal *Diabetes Care*.

It reported an inverse relationship between adherence to a Mediterranean diet pattern and cumulative incidence of the metabolic syndrome. The results are consistent with previous findings of an inverse association between adherence to a Mediterranean diet and obesity, diabetes, insulin resistance, or hypertension. The "prospective" aspect of the study means that information about risk factors for the metabolic syndrome, food habits, and lifestyles was collected before the diagnosis of the disease (Tortosa, Bes-Rastrollo, Sanchez-Villegas et al. 2007).

8.8 MEDITERRANEAN DIET AND ELEVATED SERUM LIPIDS

A report in the *Journal of the CardioMetabolic Syndrome* points out that both the metabolic syndrome and Type 2 diabetes increase the risk of coronary heart disease and cardiovascular disease. The rise in prevalence of these disorders will result in a rise in the number of individuals with or at risk for cardiovascular disease. One major underlying cause of cardiovascular disease in patients with these disorders is a characteristic form of atherogenic dyslipidemia (Ginsberg and MacCallum. 2009).

A study on this subject, published in the journal *Archives of Internal Medicine*, aimed to assess the effect of the Mediterranean diet on lipoprotein oxidation. Men and women participants at high cardiovascular risk, ranging in age between 55 and 80 years, were recruited into a large clinical trial (the Prevención con Dieta Mediterránea Study) directed at testing the efficacy of the Mediterranean diet (TMD) on the primary prevention of coronary heart disease.

They were assigned to a low-fat diet, or one of two TMDs (TMD + virgin olive oil, or TMD + nuts). The TMD participants received nutritional education and either free virgin olive oil for all the family (1 L/week) or free nuts (30 g/day). Diets were *ad libitum*. Changes in oxidative stress markers were evaluated at 3 months.

After the 3-month interventions, mean oxidized LDL levels had decreased in the TMD + virgin olive oil and the TMD + nuts groups, without changes in the low-fat diet control group. The decrease in the levels of oxidized LDL levels in the TMD + virgin olive oil group was statistically significantly from that of the low-fat group. The decreases in malondialdehyde in the mononuclear cells of the TMD patients paralleled the decline of oxidized LDL. Malondialdehyde is a marker of oxidative stress. No changes from baseline in serum glutathione peroxidase activity were observed.

It was concluded that individuals at high cardiovascular risk who improved their diet by switching to a TMD pattern showed significant reductions in cellular lipid levels and LDL oxidation. The results provide further evidence to recommend the TMD as a useful tool against risk factors for cardiovascular and heart disease (Fitó, Guxens, Corella et al. 2007).

8.9 MEDITERRANEAN DIET AND HYPERTENSION

Diet has been reported to influence arterial blood pressure, and evidence indicates that, by lowering it, the Mediterranean diet reduces cardiovascular mortality. In fact, consuming olive oil alone, a major constituent of that diet, has been reported to reduce both systolic and diastolic blood pressure.

The *American Journal of Clinical Nutrition* reported a study titled "Olive oil, the Mediterranean diet, and arterial blood pressure: the Greek European Prospective Investigation into Cancer and Nutrition (EPIC) study." The objective of the study was to determine whether the Mediterranean diet, *per se*, and olive oil in particular reduce arterial blood pressure.

Arterial blood pressure and several sociodemographic, anthropometric, dietary, physical activity, and clinical variables were recorded at enrollment among participants in the Greek arm of the European Prospective Investigation into Cancer and Nutrition study. Of these participants, more than 20,000 had never been diagnosed with hypertension and were included in an analysis wherein systolic and diastolic blood pressure were correlated with possible predictors, including a 10-point score that reflects adherence to the Mediterranean diet and, alternatively, the individual components and olive oil.

It was found that the Mediterranean diet score was inversely related to both systolic and diastolic blood pressure. The intake of olive oil, vegetables, and fruit was inversely associated with both systolic and diastolic blood pressure, whereas intake of cereals, meat and meat products, and ethanol were linked to higher arterial blood pressure. It was also found that olive oil, combined with vegetables, has the dominant beneficial effect on arterial blood pressure in this population.

It was concluded that adherence to the Mediterranean diet is inversely related to arterial blood pressure, even though a beneficial component of the Mediterranean diet score—cereal intake—is positively related to arterial blood pressure. The amount of olive oil consumed, *per se*, is inversely related to both systolic and diastolic blood pressure (Psaltopoulou, Naska, Orfanos et al. 2004).

The *Journal of Hypertension* (2003) reported the prevalence, awareness, treatment, and control of hypertension in Greece, in a random sample of adults free of cardiovascular disease, and an evaluation of the association between hypertension status and adoption of the Mediterranean diet.

The prevalence of hypertension was 38.2% in men and 23.9% in women. The majority of men and women were untreated, and of those who were treated, only 34% had their blood pressure adequately controlled. Thus, overall, only 15% of the hypertensive population had their blood pressure well controlled.

Consumption of a Mediterranean diet was associated with a 26% lower risk of being hypertensive and with a 36% greater probability of having the blood pressure controlled. It was concluded that consumption of a Mediterranean type of diet seems to reduce rates of hypertension in the population (Panagiotakos, Pitsavos, Chrysohoou et al. 2003).

As previously noted, the endothelium is the cell inner lining of blood vessels that regulates their function in large part by forming NO. Hypertension and cardiovascular and heart disease have been linked to dysfunction of the endothelium/NO mechanism. In fact, one of the newer antihypertensive beta-blocker prescription medications, Bystolic (nebivolol), is a NO-potentiating medication (Weiss. 2006).

8.10   AVERTING PREMATURE AGING OF THE ENDOTHELIUM

The endothelial lining of blood vessels is subject to progressive age-related decline in its ability to synthesize the NO needed to control blood flow and blood pressure. As NO production declines with age, the risk of hypertension rises. In fact, by age 40, blood vessels can produce only about half the NO that they could produce when younger. And so, systolic blood pressure naturally rises and there is good reason to believe that it is because, simultaneously, NO formation by the endothelium is declining (Izzo, Levy, and Black. 2000). It is advisable therefore to prevent premature aging of the endothelium so as to preserve control of blood pressure. This can be accomplished with the Mediterranean diet.

NO performs many functions in the body and, for one, it delays the formation of atherosclerosis plaque in blood vessels. As the journal *Circulation Research* reported, age-related impairment in NO formation leads to cell senescence (Vasa, Breitschopf, Zeiher et al. 2000). However, the Mediterranean diet, rich in leafy vegetables that are high in nitrates, and other foods rich in the amino acid L-arginine, can actually reverse impairment in the formation of NO, thus protecting blood vessels and preventing premature cell senescence (Fried, and Edlen-Nezin. 2006; Lidder, and Webb. 2013; Chauhan, More, Mullins et al. 1996).

8.10.1   Mediterranean Diet, Endothelial Function, and Type 2 Diabetes

Endothelial dysfunction involves an imbalance between vasodilating and vasoconstricting substances produced by (or acting on) the endothelium (Deanfield, Donald, Ferri et al., 2005). It is causally linked to diabetes. In fact, the *Journal of the American College of Cardiology* published a study titled "The postprandial effect of components of the Mediterranean diet on endothelial function."

The investigators of the study describe the Mediterranean diet as containing olive oil, pasta, fruits, vegetables, fish, and wine, and contend that it is associated with an unexpectedly low rate of cardiovascular events: The Lyon Diet Heart Study found that a Mediterranean diet, which substituted omega-3 fatty acid–enriched canola oil for the traditionally consumed omega-9 fatty acid–rich olive oil, significantly reduced cardiovascular events.

Therefore, in their study, they fed healthy, normolipidemic participants five meals containing 900 kcal and 50 g of fat. Three meals contained different fat sources: olive oil, canola oil, and salmon. Two olive oil meals also contained antioxidant vitamins (C and E) or foods (balsamic vinegar and salad), and they measured serum lipoproteins, blood glucose, and brachial artery flow-mediated vasodilation (FMD), an index of endothelial function, before and 3 h after each meal.

The results showed that all five meals significantly raised serum triglycerides, but did not change other lipoproteins, or glucose, 3 h postprandially.

The olive oil meal reduced FMD by 31%, and an inverse correlation was noted between postprandial changes in serum triglycerides and FMD. The remaining four meals did not significantly reduce FMD.

The investigators concluded that the components of the Mediterranean diet beneficial to endothelial function appear to be antioxidant-rich foods, including vegetables, fruits, and their derivatives such as vinegar, along with omega-3–rich fish and canola oils (Vogel, Corretti, and Plotnick. 2000).

A study titled "Diabetes and the Mediterranean diet: a beneficial effect of oleic acid on insulin sensitivity, adipocyte glucose transport and endothelium-dependent vasoreactivity," published in the *Monthly Journal of the Association of Physicians*, focused on abnormalities in endothelial function and the increased cardiovascular risk in diabetic patients.

The study centered on the effect of an oleic acid–rich diet on insulin resistance and endothelium-dependent vasoreactivity in Type 2 diabetes: Type 2 diabetic patients were changed from their usual diet and treated for 2 months with an oleic acid–rich diet.

Insulin-mediated glucose transport was measured in isolated adipocytes. Fatty acid composition of the adipocyte membranes was determined by gas–liquid chromatography, and flow-mediated endothelium-dependent and -independent vasodilation were measured in the superficial femoral artery at the end of each dietary period.

The results showed a significant increase in serum oleic acid and a decrease in linoleic acid on the oleic acid–rich diet. Diabetic control was not different between the diets, but there was a small but significant decrease in fasting glucose/insulin on the oleic acid–rich diet.

Insulin-stimulated (1 ng/mL) glucose transport was significantly greater on the oleic acid–rich diet (0.56 ± 0.17 vs. 0.29 ± 0.14 nmol/10^5 cells/3 min), suggesting that the cells had improved insulin sensitivity.

Endothelium-dependent FMD was significantly greater on the oleic acid–rich diet ($3.90\% \pm 0.97\%$ vs. $6.12\% \pm 1.36\%$).

There was a significant correlation between adipocyte membrane oleic/linoleic acid and insulin-mediated glucose transport but no relationship between insulin-stimulated glucose transport and change in endothelium-dependent FMD. There was a significant positive correlation between adipocyte membrane oleic/linoleic acid and endothelium-dependent FMD.

Change from polyunsaturated to monounsaturated diet in Type 2 diabetes reduced insulin resistance and restored endothelium-dependent vasodilation, suggesting an explanation for the antiatherogenic benefits of a Mediterranean-type diet (Ryan, McInerney, Owens et al. 2000).

8.10.2 Mediterranean Diet, Incretin, and Type 2 Diabetes

It was noted in Chapter 1 that an incretin is a type of hormone that stimulates insulin secretion in response to meals. The two most important incretin hormones are GLP-1 and GIP. The incretin hormones are released from gut endocrine cells during meals. They potentiate glucose-induced insulin secretion and may be responsible for up to 70% of postprandial insulin secretion.

It was reported in the journal *Cardiovascular Diabetology* that the Mediterranean diet may confer some degree of protection from endothelial resistance to GLP-1 in Type 2 diabetes. According to the authors of the study, acute hyperglycemia worsens endothelial function and inflammation, due to resistance to GLP-1 action in Type 2 diabetes. Furthermore, it is thought that this impairment results from oxidative stress.

Because the Mediterranean diet, supplemented with olive oil, increases plasma antioxidant capacity, it was thought that its implementation might have a favorable effect on endothelial resistance to GLP-1, perhaps counteracting the effects of acute hyperglycemia on the resistance of the endothelium to the action of GLP-1.

In research on this subject, two groups of Type 2 diabetic patients participated in a study for 3 months. Group 1 followed a Mediterranean diet using olive oil, and a control group followed a low-fat diet.

Plasma antioxidant capacity, endothelial function, nitrotyrosine, 8-iso-PGF2a, interleukin-6 (IL-6), and intercellular adhesion molecule-1 (ICAM-1) levels were evaluated at baseline and at the end of the study. The effect of GLP-1 during a hyperglycemic clamp was also studied at baseline and at the end of the study.

The glucose clamp technique measures how well an individual metabolizes glucose or how sensitive an individual is to insulin (von Wartburg. 2007). The hyperglycemic clamp consists of quickly raising plasma glucose concentration to 125 mg/dL above basal levels by a continuous infusion of glucose. This hyperglycemic plateau is maintained by adjustment of a variable glucose infusion, based on the rate of insulin secretion and glucose metabolism.

Because the plasma glucose concentration is held constant, the glucose infusion rate is an index of insulin secretion and glucose metabolism. The hyperglycemic clamp is often used to assess insulin secretion capacity.

The results of the study showed that the Mediterranean diet increased plasma antioxidant capacity and improved basal endothelial function, nitrotyrosine, 8-iso-PGF2a, IL-6, and ICAM-1 levels compared to the control diet. The Mediterranean diet also reduced the adverse effects of acute hyperglycemia, induced by a hyperglycemic clamp, on endothelial function, nitrotyrosine, 8-iso-PGF2a, IL-6, and ICAM-1 levels. Furthermore, the Mediterranean diet improved the protective action of GLP-1 on endothelial function, nitrotyrosine, 8-iso-PGF2a, IL-6, and ICAM-1 levels, also increasing GLP-1–induced insulin secretion.

The investigators concluded that the Mediterranean diet, using olive oil, prevents the effect of acute hyperglycemia on endothelial function, inflammation, and oxidative stress, and improves the action of GLP-1, which may have a favorable effect on the management of Type 2 diabetes (Ceriello, Esposito, La Sala et al. 2014).

Note: Nitrotyrosine is a product of reactive nitrogen species and indicates cell damage, inflammation, and NO production. The prostaglandin 8-iso-PGF(2alpha) in urine is a reliable, noninvasive index of lipid peroxidation (Tacconelli, Capone, and Patrignani. 2010). IL-6 is an interleukin that acts as both a pro-inflammatory cytokine and an anti-inflammatory myokine. ICAM-1 plays an important role in adhesion phenomena involved in the immune response (Roy, Audette, and Tremblay. 2001).

In connection with the promotion of endothelium function, a number of studies report that GLP-1 may be an appropriate target for treatment of Type 2 diabetes. For instance, an article in the journal *Cardiovascular and Hematological Agents in Medicinal Chemistry* states that:

> Risk factors for endothelial dysfunction are numerous and include among others fasting and postprandial hyperglycemia and hyperlipidemia, hypertension, obesity, insulin resistance and inflammation. Many of these conditions can be improved by synthetic glucagon like peptide 1 (GLP-1) mimetics, or inhibitors of the main GLP-1 degrading enzyme dipeptidyl peptidase 4 (DPP-4). Acute increases in GLP-1 activity abolish endothelial dysfunction induced by high-fat meals or by hyperglycemia. Preliminary clinical studies also indicate that GLP-1 or GLP-1 agonists can improve endothelial function by direct action on endothelium. GLP-1 or GLP-1 mimetic effects appear to extend to both the conduit arteries and the microvasculature, and may depend on activation of endothelial GLP-1 receptors and downstream nitric oxide production (Koska. 2012. Cardiovascular and Hematological Agents in Medicinal Chemistry, Dec; 10(4): 295–308. With permission.)

This book is not about prescription medical treatment, but the reader may find it useful to note the following small sample of citations.

In favor:

- Incretin-based therapies for Type 2 diabetes mellitus: effects on insulin resistance. Grigoropoulou, Eleftheriadou, Zoupas et al. 2013. *Current Diabetes Review*, Sep; 9(5): 412–417.
- Focus on incretin-based therapies: targeting the core defects of Type 2 diabetes. Jellinger. 2011. *Postgraduate Medicine*, Jan; 123(1): 53–65.
- Incretin-based therapies in the management of Type 2 diabetes: rationale and reality in a managed care setting. Garber. 2010. *The American Journal, of Managed Care*, Aug; 16(7 Suppl): S187–S194.
- Distinguishing among incretin-based therapies. Glucose-lowering effects of incretin-based therapies. Campbell, Cobble, Reid et al. 2010. *The Journal of Family Practice*, Sep; 59(9 Suppl 1): S10–S19.

Against:
- GLP-1–Based therapy for diabetes: What you do not know can hurt you. Butler, Dry, and Elashoff. 2010. *Diabetes Care*, Feb; 33(2): 453–455.

REFERENCES

Bahadoran Z, Ghasemi A, Mirmiran P, Azizi F, and F Hadaegh. 2015. Beneficial effects of inorganic nitrate/nitrite in type 2 diabetes and its complications. *Nutrition and Metabolism (Lond)*, May; 12: 16. Published online 2015 May 16. DOI: 10.1186/s12986-015-0013-6.

Brown SL, Pope JF, Hunt AE, and NM Tolman. 1998. Motivational strategies used by dietitians to counsel individuals with diabetes. *The Diabetes Educator*, May–Jun; 24(3): 313–318. DOI: 10.1177/014572179802400305.

Butler PC, Dry S, and R Elashoff. 2010. GLP-1–Based therapy for diabetes: What you do not know can hurt you. *Diabetes Care*, Feb; 33(2): 453–455. DOI: 10.2337/dc09-1902.

Cai W, Ramdas M, Zhu L, Chen X, Striker GE, and H Vlassara. 2012. Oral advanced glycation endproducts (AGEs) promote insulin resistance and diabetes by depleting the antioxidant defenses AGE receptor-1 and sirtuin 1. *Proceedings of the National Academy of Sciences USA*, Sep 25; 109(39): 15888–15893. DOI: 10.1073/pnas.1205 847109.

Campbell RK, Cobble ME, Reid TS, and ME Shomali. 2010. Distinguishing among incretin-based therapies. Glucose-lowering effects of incretin-based therapies. *The Journal of Family Practice*, Sep; 59(9 Suppl 1): S10–S19. PMID: 20824235.

Cao Y, Jiang X, Ma H, Wang Y, Xue P, and Liu Y. 2016. SIRT1 and insulin resistance. *Journal of Diabetes Complications*, Jan–Feb; 30(1): 178–183. DOI: 10.5604/17322693.1136379.

Carter P, Achana F, Troughton J, Gray LJ, Khunti K, MJ Davies. 2014. A Mediterranean diet improves HbA1c but not fasting blood glucose compared to alternative dietary strategies: a network meta-analysis. *Journal of Human Nutrition and Dietetics*, Jun; 27(3): 280–297. DOI: 10.1111/jhn.12138.

Ceriello A, Esposito K, La Sala L, Pujadas G, De Nigris V, Testa R, Bucciarelli L, Rondinelli M, and S Genovese. 2014. The protective effect of the Mediterranean diet on endothelial resistance to GLP-1 in type 2 diabetes: a preliminary report. *Cardiovascular Diabetology*, 13: 140. Published online 2014 Nov 19. DOI: 10.1186/s12933-014-0140-9.

Chatzianagnostou K, Del Turco S, Pingitore A, Sabatino L, and C Vassalle. 2015. The Mediterranean lifestyle as a non-pharmacological and natural antioxidant for healthy aging. *Antioxidants* (Basel), Dec; 4(4): 719–736. DOI: 10.3390/antiox4040719.

Chauhan A, More RS, Mullins PA, Taylor G, Petch C, and PM Schofield. 1996. Aging-associated endothelial dysfunction in humans is reversed by L-arginine. *Journal of the American College of Cardiology*, Dec; 28(7):1796–1804. PMID: 8962569.

Christiansen C, Thomsen C, Rasmussen O, Balle M, Hauerslev C, Hansen C, and K Hermansen. 1993. Wine for type 2 diabetic patients? *Diabetic Medicine*, Dec; 10(10): 958- 961. PMID: 8306592.

Cullmann M, Hilding A, and CG Östenson. 2012. Alcohol consumption and risk of pre-diabetes and type 2 diabetes development in a Swedish population. *Diabetic Medicine*, Apr; 29(4): 441–452. DOI: 10 .1111/j.1464-5491.2011.03450.x.

Dalgaard M, Thomsen C, Rasmussen BM, Holst JJ, and K Hermansen. 2004. Ethanol with a mixed meal decreases the incretin levels early postprandially and increases postprandial lipemia in type 2 diabetic patients. *Metabolism*, Jan; 53(1): 77–83. PMID: 14681846.

Deanfield J, Donald A, Ferri C, Giannattasio C, Halcox J, Halligan S, Lerman A, Mancia G, Oliver JJ, Pessina AC, Rizzoni D, Rossi GP, Salvetti A, Schiffrin EL, Taddei S, and DJ Webb, and the Working Group on Endothelin and Endothelial Factors of the European Society of Hypertension. 2005. Endothelial function and dysfunction. Part I: Methodological issues for assessment in the different vascular beds: a statement by the Working Group on Endothelin and Endothelial Factors of the European Society of Hypertension. *Journal of Hypertension*, Jan; 23(1): 7–17. PMID: 15643116.

El-Kebbi IM, Bacha GA, Ziemer DC, Musey VC, Gallina DL, Dunbar V, and LS Phillips. 1996. Diabetes in urban African Americans. V. Use of discussion groups to identify barriers to dietary therapy among low-income individuals with non-insulin-dependent diabetes mellitus. *The Diabetes Educator*, Sept–Oct; 22(5): 488–492. DOI: 10.1177/014572179602200508.

Esposito K, Maiorino MI, Bellastella G, Chiodini P, Panagiotakos D, and D Giugliano. 2015. A journey into a Mediterranean diet and type 2 diabetes: a systematic review with meta-analyses. *BMJ Open* (*British Medical Journal Open*), Aug; 5(8): e008222. DOI: 10.1136/bmjopen-2015-008222.

Esposito K, Maiorino MI, Ceriello A, and D Giugliano. 2010. Prevention and control of type 2 diabetes by Mediterranean diet: a systematic review. *Diabetes Research & Clinical Practice*, Aug; 89(2): 97–102. DOI: 10.1016/j.diabres.2010.04.019.

Esposito K, Maiorino MI, Ciotola M, Di Palo C, Scognamiglio P, Gicchino M, Petrizzo M, Saccomanno F, Beneduce F, Ceriello A, and D Giugliano. 2009. Effects of a Mediterranean-style diet on the need for antihyperglycemic drug therapy in patients with newly diagnosed type 2 diabetes: a randomized trial. *Annals of Internal Medicine*, Sep; 151(5): 306–314. PMID: 19721018.

Esposito K, Maiorino MI, Di Palo C, D Giugliano and the Campanian Postprandial Hyperglycemia Study Group. 2009. Adherence to a Mediterranean diet and glycaemic control in Type 2 diabetes mellitus. *Diabetic Medicine*, Sep; 26(9): 900–907. DOI: 10.1111/j.1464-5491.2009.02798.x.

Esposito K, Marfella R, Ciotola M, Di Palo C, Giugliano F, Giugliano G, D'Armiento M, D'Andrea F, and D Giugliano. 2004. Effect of a Mediterranean-style diet on endothelial dysfunction and markers of vascular inflammation in the metabolic syndrome. *The Journal of the American Medical Association*, Sept; 292(12):1440–1446. DOI: 10.1001/jama.292.12.1440.

Esposito, K, Pontillo, A, Di Palo C, Giuliano G, Masella M, Marfella R, and D Giugliano. 2003. Effect of weight loss and lifestyle changes on vascular inflammatory markers in obese women: a randomized trial. *Journal of the American Medical Association*, 289(14): 1799–1804. DOI: 10.1001/jama .289.14.1799.

Fitó M, Guxens M, Corella D, Sáez G, Estruch R, de la Torre R, Francés F, Cabezas C, López-Sabater Mdel C, Marrugat J, García-Arellano A, Arós F, Ruiz-Gutierrez V, Ros E, Salas-Salvadó J, Fiol M, Solá R, and MI Covas and the PREDIMED Study Investigators. 2007. Effect of a traditional Mediterranean diet on lipoprotein oxidation: a randomized controlled trial. *Archives of Internal Medicine*, Jun 11; 167(11): 1195–1203. DOI: 10.1001/archinte.167.11.1195.

Fried R, and L Edlen-Nezin. 2006. *Great Food/Great Sex*. New York: Ballantine Books.

Fried R, and L Nezin. 2017. *Evidence-Based Proactive Nutrition to Slow Cellular Aging*. Boca Raton, FL: CRC Press/Taylor & Francis Group Publishers.

Frye RA. 1999. Characterization of five human cDNAs with homology to the yeast SIR2 gene: Sir2-like proteins (sirtuins) metabolize NAD and may have protein ADP-ribosyltransferase activity. *Biochemical and Biophysical Research Communication*, Jun; 260(1): 273–279. DOI: 10.1006/bbrc.1999.0897.

Garber AJ. 2010. Incretin-based therapies in the management of type 2 diabetes: rationale and reality in a managed care setting. *The American Journal, of Managed Care*, Aug; 16(7 Suppl): S187–S194. PMID: 20809667.

Ginsberg HJN, and PR MacCallum. 2009. The obesity, metabolic syndrome, and Type 2 diabetes mellitus pandemic: Part I. Increased cardiovascular disease risk and the importance of atherogenic dyslipidemia in persons with the metabolic syndrome and Type 2 diabetes mellitus. *Journal of the Cardio Metabolic Syndrome*, Spring; 4(2): 113–119. DOI: 10.1111/j.1559-4572.2008.00044.x.

Giugliano D, and K Esposito. 2008. Mediterranean diet and metabolic diseases. *Current Opinion in Lipidology*, Feb; 19(1):63–68. DOI: 10.1097/MOL.0b013e3282f2fa4d.

Grigoropoulou P, Eleftheriadou I, Zoupas C, Diamanti-Kandarakis E, and N Tentolouris N. 2013. Incretin-based therapies for type 2 diabetes mellitus: effects on insulin resistance. *Current Diabetes Review*, Sep; 9(5): 412–417. PMID: 23855508.

Guarente L. 2007. Sirtuins in aging and disease. *Cold Spring Harbor Symposia on Quantitative Biology*, 72: 483–488. DOI: 10.1101/sqb.2007.72.024.

Itsiopoulos C, Brazionis L, Kaimakamis M, Cameron M, Best JD, O'Dea K, and K Rowley. 2011. Can the Mediterranean diet lower HbA1c in type 2 diabetes? Results from a randomized cross-over study. *Nutrition, Metabolism, and Cardiovascular Diseases*, Sep; 21(9): 740–747. DOI: 10.1016/j.numecd.2010.03.005.

Izzo JL, Levy D and HR Black. 2000. Clinical advisory statement. Importance of systolic blood pressure in older Americans. *Hypertension*, May; 35:1021–1024. PMID: 10818056.

Jellinger PS. 2011. Focus on incretin-based therapies: targeting the core defects of type 2 diabetes. *Postgraduate Medicine*, Jan; 123(1): 53–65. DOI: 10.3810/pgm.2011.01. 2245.

Kastorini C-M, Milionis HJ, Esposito K, Giugliano D, Goudevenos JA, and DB Panagiotakos. 2011. The effect of Mediterranean diet on metabolic syndrome and its components. A meta-analysis of 50 studies and 534,906 individuals. *Journal of the American College of Cardiology*, Mar; 57(11): 1299–1313. DOI: 10.1016/j.jacc. 2010. 09.073.

Khemayanto H, and B Shi. 2014. Role of Mediterranean diet in prevention and management of type 2 diabetes. *Chinese Medical Journal (Engl)*, 127(20): 3651–3656. PMID: 25316244.

Koivisto VA, Tulokas S, Toivonen M, Haapa E, and R Pelkonen. 1993. Alcohol with a meal has no adverse effects on postprandial glucose homeostasis in diabetic patients. *Diabetes Care*, Dec; 16(12): 1612–1614. PMID: 8299457.

Koska J. 2012. Incretins and preservation of endothelial function. *Cardiovascular and Hematological Agents in Medicinal Chemistry*, Dec; 10(4): 295–308. PMID: 22827294.

Lidder S, and AJ Webb. 2013. Vascular effects of dietary nitrate (as found in green leafy vegetables and beet-root) via the nitrate–nitrite–nitric oxide pathway. *British Journal of Clinical Pharmacology*, Mar; 75(3): 677–696. DOI: 10.1111/j.1365-2125.2012. 04420.x.

Lundberg JO, and M Govoni. 2004. Inorganic nitrate is a possible source for systemic generation of nitric oxide. *Free Radical Biology & Medicine*, Aug 1; 37(3): 395–400. DOI: 10.1016/j.freeradbiomed.2004.04.027.

Lundberg JO, Gladwin MT, Ahluwalia A, Benjamin N, Bryan NS, Butler A, Cabrales P, Fago A, Feelisch M, Ford PC, Freeman BA, Frenneaux M, Friedman J, Kelm M, Kevil CG, Kim-Shapiro DB, Kozlov AV, Lancaster JR Jr, Lefer DJ, McColl K, McCurry K, Patel RP, Petersson J, Rassaf T, Reutov VP, Richter-Addo GB, Schechter A, Shiva S, Tsuchiya K, van Faassen EE, Webb AJ, Zuckerbraun BS, Zweier JL, and E Weitzberg. 2000. Nitrate and nitrite in biology, nutrition and therapeutics. *Nature Chemical Biology*, Dec; 5(12): 865–869. DOI: 10.1038/nchembio.260.

Maghsoudi Z, and L Azadbakht. 2012. How dietary patterns could have a role in prevention, progression, or management of diabetes mellitus? Review on the current evidence. *Journal of Research in Medical Sciences*, Jul; 17(7): 694–709. PMCID: PMC3685790.

Martin GS, Tapsell LC, Denmeade S, and MJ Batterham. 2003. Relative validity of a diet history interview in an intervention trial manipulating dietary fat in the management of Type II diabetes mellitus. *Preventive Medicine*, Apr; 36(4):420–428. PMID: 12649050.

McKnight GM, Smith LM, Drummond RS, Duncan CW, Golden M, and N Benjamin. 1997. Chemical synthesis of nitric oxide in the stomach from dietary nitrate in humans. *Gut*, Feb; 40(2): 211–214. PMCID: PMC1027050.

Mela DJ. 1999. Food choice and intake: the human factor. *The Proceedings of the Nutrition Society*. Aug; 58(3): 513–521. PMID: 10604182.

Milne JC, Lambert PD, Schenk S, Carney DP, Smith JJ, Gagne DJ, Jin L, Boss O, Perni RB, Vu CB, Bemis JE, Xie R, Disch JS, Ng PY, Nunes JJ, Lynch AV, Yang H, Galonek H, Israelian K, Choy W, Iffland A, Lavu S, Medvedik O, Sinclair DA, Olefsky JM, Jirousek MR, Elliott PJ, and CH Westphal. 2007. Small molecule activators of SIRT1 as therapeutics for the treatment of type 2 diabetes. *Nature*, Nov; 450(7170): 712–716. DOI: 10.1038/nature06261.

Montminy M. 2009. The battle for CRTC2: how obesity increases the risk for diabetes Salk News. https://www.salk.edu/news-release/the-battle-for-crtc2-how-obesity-increases-the-risk-for-diabetes/; accessed 7.28.17.

Nield L, Moore HJ, Hooper L, Cruickshank JK, Vyas A, Whittaker V, and CD Summerbell. 2007. Dietary advice for treatment of type 2 diabetes mellitus in adults. *The Cochrane Database of Systematic Reviews*, Jul; (3): CD004097. DOI: 10.1002/14651858.CD004097.pub4.

Palmer RM, Ashton DS, and S Moncada. 1988. Vascular endothelial cells synthesize nitric oxide from L-arginine. *Nature*, Jun; 333(6174): 664–666. DOI: 10.1038/333664a0.

Panagiotakos DB1, Pitsavos CH, Chrysohoou C, Skoumas J, Papadimitriou L, Stefanadis C, and PK Toutouzas. 2003. Status and management of hypertension in Greece: role of the adoption of a Mediterranean diet: the ATTICA study. *Journal of Hypertension*, Aug; 21: 1483–1489. DOI: 10.1097/01.hjh.000 0084706.87421.7c.

Psaltopoulou T, Naska A, Orfanos P, Trichopoulos D, Mountokalakis T, and A Trichopoulou. 2004. Olive oil, the Mediterranean diet, and arterial blood pressure: the Greek European Prospective Investigation into Cancer and Nutrition (EPIC) study. *American Journal of Clinical Nutrition*, Oct; 80(4): 1012–1018. PMID: 15447913.

Roy J, Audette M, and MJ Tremblay. 2001. Intercellular adhesion molecule-1 (ICAM-1) gene expression in human T cells is regulated by phosphotyrosyl phosphatase activity. Involvement of NF-κB, Ets, and palindromic interferon-γ-responsive element-binding sites. *Journal of Biological Chemistry*, Jan; 276, 14553–14561. DOI: 10.1074/jbc.M005067200 May 4, 2001.

Ryan M, McInerney D, Owens D, Collins P, Johnson A, and GH Tomkin. 2000. Diabetes and the Mediterranean diet: a beneficial effect of oleic acid on insulin sensitivity, adipocyte glucose transport and endothelium-dependent vasoreactivity. *Monthly Journal of the Association of Physicians* (QJM), Feb; 93(2): 85–91. PMID: 10700478.

Salas-Salvadó J, Bulló M, Estruch R, Ros E, Covas MI, Ibarrola-Jurado N, Corella D, Arós F, Gómez-Gracia E, Ruiz-Gutiérrez V, Romaguera D, Lapetra J, Lamuela-Raventós RM, Serra-Majem L, Pintó X, Basora J, Muñoz MA, Sorlí JV, and MA Martínez-González MA. 2014. Prevention of diabetes with Mediterranean diets: a subgroup analysis of a randomized trial. *Annals of Internal Medicine*, Jan 7; 160(1): 1–10. DOI: 10.7326/M13-1725.

Salas-Salvadó J, Martinez-González MÁ, Bulló M, and E Ros. 2011. The role of diet in the prevention of type 2 diabetes. *Nutrition, Metabolism, and Cardiovascular Diseases*, Sep; 21 Suppl 2: B32–B48. DOI: 10.1016/j.numecd.2011.03.009.

Samuel-Hodge CD, Fernandez LM, Henriquez-Roldan CF, Johnston LF, and TC Keyserling. 2004. A comparison of self-reported energy intake with total energy expenditure estimated by accelerometer and basal metabolic rate in African-American women with type 2 diabetes. *Diabetes Care*, Mar; 27(3): 663–669. PMID: 14988282.

Samuel-Hodge CD, Headen SW, Skelly AH, Ingram AF, Keyserling TC, Jackson EJ, Ammerman AS, and TA Elasy. 2000. Influences on day-to-day self-management of type 2 diabetes among African-American women: spirituality, the multi-caregiver role, and other social context factors. *Diabetes Care*, Jul; 23(7): 928–933. PMID: 10895842.

Savoca M, and C Miller. 2001. Food selection and eating patterns: themes found among people with type 2 diabetes mellitus. *Journal of Nutrition Education*, Jul–Aug; 33(4): 224–233. PMID: 11953244.

Schlundt DG, Rea MR, Kline SS, and JW Pichert. 1994. Situational obstacles to dietary adherence for adults with diabetes. *Journal of the American Dietetic Association*, Aug; 94(8): 874–876. PMID: 8046181.

Schmidt LE, Rost KM, McGill JB, and JV Santiago. 1994. The relationship between eating patterns and metabolic control in patients with non-insulin-dependent diabetes mellitus (NIDDM). *The Diabetes Educator*, Jul–Aug; 20(4): 317–321. DOI: 10.1177/014572179402000410.

Schroder H, Marrugat J, Vila J, Covas MI, and R Elosua. 2004. Adherence to the traditional Mediterranean diet is inversely associated with body mass index and obesity in a Spanish population. *Journal of Nutrition*, Dec; 134(12): 3355–3361. PMID: 15570037.

Sleiman D, Al-Badri MR, and ST Azar. 2015. Effect of Mediterranean diet in diabetes control and cardiovascular risk modification. A systematic review. *Frontiers in Public Health*, Apr; 3: 69. Published online 2015 Apr 28. DOI: 10.3389/fpubh.2015.00069.

Snoek FJ. 2000. Barriers to good glycaemic control: the patient's perspective. *International Journal of Obesity and Related Metabolic Disorders*, Sep; 24 Suppl 3: S12–S20. PMID: 11063280.

Spiegelhalder B, Eisenbrand G, and R Preussmann. 1976. Influence of dietary nitrate on nitrite content of human saliva: possible relevance to in vivo formation of *N*-nitroso compounds. *Food and Cosmetics Toxicology*, 14(6): 545–548. PMID: 1017769.

Tacconelli S, Capone ML, and P Patrignani. 2010. Measurement of 8-iso-prostaglandin F2alpha in biological fluids as a measure of lipid peroxidation. *Methods in Molecular Biology*, 644: 165–178. DOI: 10.1007/978-1-59745-364-6_14.

Tortosa A, Bes-Rastrollo M, Sanchez-Villegas A, Basterra-Gortari FJ, Nuñez-Cordoba JM, and MA Martinez-Gonzalez. 2007. Mediterranean diet inversely associated with the incidence of metabolic syndrome: the SUN prospective cohort. *Diabetes Care*, Nov; 30(11): 2957–2959. DOI: 10.2337/dc07-1231.

Travis T. 1997. Patient perceptions of factors that affect adherence to dietary regimens for diabetes mellitus. *The Diabetes Educator*, mar-Apr; 23(2): 152–156. DOI: 10. 1177/014572179702300205.

Tyrovolas S, Bountziouka VN, Papairakleous Zeimbekis A, Anastassiou F, Gotsis E, Metallinos G, Polychronopoulos E, Lionis C, and D Panagiotakos. 2009. Adherence to the Mediterranean diet is associated with lower prevalence of obesity among elderly people living in Mediterranean islands: the MEDIS study. *International Journal of Food Science & Nutrition*, 60 (Suppl 6): 137–150. DOI: 10.1080/09 637480903130546.

Vasa M, Breitschopf K, Zeiher AM, and S Dimmeler. 2000. Nitric oxide activates telomerase and delays endothelial cell senescence. *Circulation Research*, Sept; 87 (7): 540–542. PMID: 11009557.

Vogel RA, Corretti MC, and GD Plotnick. 2000. The postprandial effect of components of the Mediterranean diet on endothelial function. *Journal of the American College of Cardiology*, Nov; 36(5): 1455–1460. PMID: 11079642.

von Wartburg L. 2007. What's a Glucose Clamp, anyway? *Diabetes Health*. http://www.diabeteshealth.com /whats-a-glucose-clamp-anyway/.

Wang Y, Vera L, Fischer WH, and M Montminy. 2009. The CREB coactivator CRTC2 links hepatic ER stress and fasting gluconeogenesis. *Nature 460*, Jul; 534–537. DOI:10.1038/nature08111.

Weiss R. 2006. Nebivolol: A novel beta-blocker with nitric oxide-induced vasodilatation. *Vascular Health Risk Management*, Sept; 2(3): 303–308. PMCID: PMC1993984.

Yannakoulia M. 2006. Eating behavior among Type 2 diabetic patients: a poorly recognized aspect in a poorly controlled disease. *The Review of Diabetic Studies*, Spring; 3(1): 11–16. DOI: 10.1900/RDS.2006.3.11.

9 Mode of Action of Selected Botanicals That Lower Blood Glucose

> If you are wise, you will mingle one thing with the other: not hoping without doubt, not doubting without hope.
>
> **Lucius Annaeus Seneca (4 BCE–65 CE)**

9.1 ANTIDIABETIC AGENTS FROM MEDICINAL PLANTS

Conventional prescription medications treat diabetes by improving insulin sensitivity, increasing insulin production, and/or decreasing the amount of glucose in the blood. Several herbal preparations are used to treat diabetes, but their reported hypoglycemic effects are complex and, in some cases, even paradoxical. The efficacy of hypoglycemic herbs is achieved by increasing insulin secretion, enhancing glucose uptake by adipose and muscle tissues, inhibiting glucose absorption from the intestine, and inhibiting glucose production from hepatocytes (Hui, Tang, and Go. 2009).

Plants with hypoglycemic potential mainly belong to the family Leguminoseae, Lamiaceae, Liliaceae, Cucurbitaceae, Asteraceae, Moraceae, Rosaceae, and Araliaceae. The most active plants are *Allium sativum*, *Gymnema sylvestre*, *Citrullus colocynthis*, *Trigonella foenum greacum*, *Momordica charantia*, and *Ficus bengalensis*.

A review published in the journal *Current Medicinal Chemistry* describes some new bioactive substances and isolated compounds from plants such as roseoside, epigallocatechin gallate, beta-pyrazol-1-ylalanine, cinchonain Ib, leucocyanidin 3-O-beta-d-galactosyl cellobioside, leucopelargonidin-3-O-α-L-rhamnoside, glycyrrhetinic acid, dehydrotrametenolic acid, strictinin, isostrictinin, pedunculagin, epicatechin, and christinin-A showing significant insulinomimetic and antidiabetic activity with more efficacy than conventional hypoglycemic agents.

In the majority of instances, the antidiabetic activity of medicinal plants is attributed to the presence of polyphenols, flavonoids, terpenoids, coumarins, and other constituents that show reduction in blood glucose levels (Jung, Park, Lee et al. 2006; Patel, Prasad, Kumar et al. 2012).

9.2 EVIDENCE-BASED INTEGRATIVE (ADJUNCTIVE) APPROACHES TO BLOOD GLUCOSE CONTROL

The adjunctive treatment of hyperglycemia, as described in this book, results for the most part from the therapeutic application of botanicals and botanical derivatives and extracts. Many of our modern treatments derive from botanicals, because plants constitute a multitude of biochemistry "laboratories" that owe their present existence to the success of their trial and error experiments in survival.

Many of the outcomes of their experiments turned out to be not only better nutrients but also powerful antioxidant defenses—from which *we* benefit today. Science historians know well that penicillin—obtained from a study of bacteria—was the outcome of a "failed experiment" by Sir Alexander Fleming, which inadvertently revealed that certain bacteria had not developed adequate defenses against micropredators. Nothing is perfect.

One advantage of adjunctive treatment with botanicals—in the wider sense of the term "botanicals"—is that they are complex and usually supply more than simply the laboratory-derived molecules that target hyperglycemia. The whole may be greater than the sum of its parts. It may also be different from the sum of its parts.

For instance, an α-glucosidase inhibitor such as White mulberry leaf extract that successfully lowers blood glucose levels also contains constituents that benefit the lipid profile and lower blood pressure as well, whereas a synthetic agent in this α-glucosidase category, such as acarbose (precose), will only lower blood glucose levels (by slowing down the digestion of certain carbohydrates).

It should be mentioned, however, that there is also a dark side to this story: Plants did not apparently have mankind "in mind" as they went about their business. Some of their constituents can be harmful (see berberine)—and some, deadly. *Caveat emptor.*

In some cases, botanical (herbal) products are phytosomes, advanced forms of herbal products that produce better results than conventional herbal extracts. Phytosomes are a complex of a natural active ingredient and a phospholipid—mostly lecithin. It is thought that phytosomes increase absorption of "conventional herbal extracts" or isolated active principles both topically and orally.

This chapter focuses on botanicals as integrative means of controlling blood glucose and supporting life functions that are adversely affected by hyperglycemia. The term "integrative" is chosen as an alternative to the term "alternative" because it is not intended that any of the following "treatments" or "natural" agents for blood sugar control should be substituted for medical treatments and interventions, absent medical supervision.

In the past, the term "complementary" might have been used but there is little requirement in the literature that complementary treatments be science-based. "Complementary" encompasses various support functions ranging from herbals to nutrition, to prayer.

Good medicine is based in the application of conventional science findings that advocate conventional remedies. Integrative medicine is also based in science but it integrates, into treatment, science-based remedies that are not a conventional part of contemporary medicine. For instance, whereas Chinese traditional medicine long knew that a tea brewed from the White Mulberry leaf lowered blood sugar, it was left to science to validate that claim by showing that one of its constituents (1-DNJ) is an α-glucosidase inhibitor that acts just like the prescription medication acarbose (Precose).

9.3 BOTANICALS THAT LOWER BLOOD GLUCOSE

In 2013, the journal *Evidence Based Complementary and Alternative Medicine* published a detailed review titled "Herbal therapies for Type 2 diabetes mellitus: chemistry, biology, and potential application of selected plants and compounds" (Chang, Lin, Bartolome et al. 2013). Much of it is either quoted or paraphrased below.

Long before what we now know as Western medicine, medicinal herbs were used to treat a wide variety of diseases. Now that Western medicine prevails over "traditional" forms of medicine, herbal medicines are often misinterpreted as being unscientific and anachronistic and, what's worse, useless.

However, it is clear that the use of medicinal herbs, alone or together with other herbs, can be a combination therapy because of the complexity of the phytochemicals and bioactivities in the plant: a single antidiabetic herb, for instance, with thousands of phytochemicals, may have multiple benefits by simultaneously targeting several metabolic pathways. In fact, one study published in the *Journal of Natural Medicine* supported this principle by demonstrating, in an animal model, that a combination therapy of orthodox medicine and herbal medicine exhibited a better (synergistic) effect than either medicine alone (Kaur, Afzal, Kazmi et al. 2013).

Medicinal herbs never faded from view and they still play a prominent role in human health care, particularly in Type 2 diabetes: In fact, more than 1200 different plants are considered to be remedies for diabetes (Marles, and Farnsworth. 1995; Habeck. 2003), and more than 400 plants, as well as 700 recipes and compounds, have been scientifically evaluated for treatment of Type 2 diabetes (Singh, Cumming, Manoharan et al. 2011). Some of these are described here.

As reported in the journal *Diabetologia*, metformin (now a first-line drug for treatment of Type 2 diabetes) was derived from an organic (biguanide) compound in French lilac (Oubré, Carlson, King et al. 1997).

In the Chang, Lin, Bartolome et al. (2013) review, the authors focused on scientific studies of selected glucose-lowering herbs and phytocompounds and their ability to target insulin resistance, beta-cell (β-cell) function, incretin-related pathways, and glucose (re)absorption (see Figure 9.1a and b).

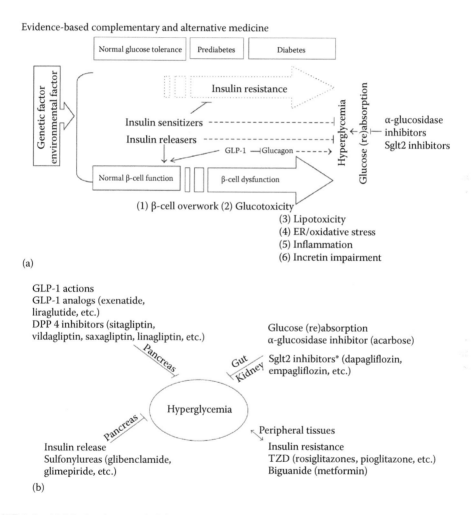

FIGURE 9.1 (a) Mechanisms underlying herbal therapies using antidiabetic plants and phytocompounds. different types of medicinal herbs can be classified based on their modes of action such as insulin resistance (type 1 herbs), β-cell function (type 2 herbs), glp-1 (type 3 herbs), and glucose (re)absorption (type 4 herbs). (b) The selected plants and compounds exert their antihyperglycemic effect through targeting one single mechanism (insulin resistance [type 1 herbs], β-cell function [type 2 herbs], glp-1 [type 3 herbs], or glucose [re] absorption [type 4 herbs]) or multiple mechanisms. (From Chang, Lin, Bartolome et al. 2013. *Evidence Based Complementary and Alternative Medicine*, vol. 2013, article no. 378657. With permission.)

9.4 SELECTED MEDICINAL HERBS AND COMPOUNDS BENEFICIAL IN TYPE 2 DIABETES

Instead of listing each extract/compound, the authors whose report is cited here select some plant chemicals and/or extracts with the ability to control blood glucose as well as to modulate at least one of the following mechanisms involved in insulin resistance: β-cell function, incretin-related pathways, and glucose (re)absorption. They discuss the chemical structure, antidiabetic activity and action in cells, animal models, and the results of administration of the plant extracts and compounds to patients with Type 2 diabetes (Chang, Lin, Bartolome et al. 2013).

The chemical and biological properties of the compounds discussed in this review are summarized in their Table 1: Active compounds and biological actions of antidiabetic herbs. The table lists the herbs, the name of the active compound, the chemical structure of that compound, the antidiabetic mechanism(s), and several references for each instance. To access the table, go to: https://www.hindawi.com/journals/ecam/2013/378657/tab1/.

9.5 HERBS AND COMPOUNDS THAT REGULATE INSULIN RESISTANCE

9.5.1 AMORFRUTINS AND LICORICE

Licorice, genus *Glycyrrhiza* (*Glycyrrhiza uralensis*), also known as Chinese licorice, is a flowering plant native to Asia. It is used as a sweetener and in traditional Chinese medicine, as an herbal medicine for a wide range of diseases. The ethanol extract of *G. uralensis* was found to reduce blood glucose, fat weight, and blood pressure in animal models (Mae, Kishida, Nishiyama et al. 2003).

Further, amorfrutins isolated from the licorice, *Glycyrrhiza foetida*, were found to bind to, and activate peroxisome proliferator-activated receptor gamma (PPAR-γ), a central player in glucose and lipid metabolism. These compounds lowered blood glucose, fat weight, and dyslipidemia, indicating that licorice and its active amorfrutins exert their antidiabetic function via the PPAR-γ pathway. The PPAR-γ receptor is a nuclear receptor highly expressed in adipose tissue, but also in the intestine, playing a key role in regulation of insulin resistance and inflammation.

In 2012, the *Proceedings of the National Academy of Sciences USA* published a report titled "Amorfrutins are potent antidiabetic dietary natural products." The investigators contend that the worldwide increase in the incidence of obesity and Type 2 diabetes requires new strategies for preventing and treating metabolic diseases. They point out that the nuclear receptor PPAR-γ plays a central role in lipid and glucose metabolism, but that current PPAR-γ-targeting drugs are characterized by undesirable side effects. They suggest that natural products from edible biomaterial could perhaps provide a structurally diverse resource to alleviate complex disorders via tailored nutritional intervention.

They identified a family of natural products, the amorfrutins, from edible parts of two botanicals, *G. foetida* and *Amorpha fruticosa*, as structurally new and powerful antidiabetics with unprecedented effects for a dietary molecule. Amorfrutins bind to and activate PPAR-γ, which results in selective gene expression and physiological profiles markedly different from activation by current synthetic PPAR-γ drugs.

In diet-induced obese and db/db mice, amorfrutin treatment strongly improved insulin sensitivity and other metabolic and inflammatory parameters without concomitant increase of fat storage or other unwanted side effects such as hepatoxicity. These results show that selective PPAR-γ activation by diet-derived ligands may constitute a promising approach to combat metabolic disease (Weidner, de Groot, Prasad et al. 2012).

9.5.2 *Dioscorea* Polysaccharides and *Dioscorea*

Dioscorea is a genus of over 600 species of flowering plants in the family Dioscoreaceae, native throughout the tropical and warm temperate regions of the world. The rhizome of *Dioscorea* (wild yam) is used as a traditional Chinese medicine for asthma, abscesses, chronic diarrhea, and ulcers (Kim, Jwa, Yanagawa et al. 2012).

Several studies on rodent models of diabetes have reported that *Dioscorea* extract improves glycemic control and insulin sensitivity (Kim, Jwa, Yanagawa et al. 2012; Lee, Hsu, and Pan. 2011; Hsu, Wu, Liu et al. 2007; Gao, Li, Jiang et al. 2007). *Dioscorea* extract reduced blood glucose in high-fat diet–induced diabetic rats (Kim, Jwa, Yanagawa et al. 2012). The antidiabetic mechanism of *Dioscorea* extract involves reduction of insulin resistance by diminution of the phosphorylation of extracellular signal–regulated kinase (ERK) and pS6K and increase of the phosphorylation of Akt and glucose transporter 4 (Glut4) (Kim, Jwa, Yanagawa et al. 2012).

Another study demonstrated that *Dioscorea* polysaccharides reduced insulin resistance mediated by inflammatory cytokines, as evidenced by the phosphorylation of insulin receptor substrate and Akt (Lee, Hsu, and Pan. 2011).

9.5.3 Anthocyanins and Blueberry

Blueberry (*Vaccinium* spp.) lowers systolic and diastolic blood pressure, reduces lipid oxidation, and improves insulin sensitivity, diabetes, diabetic complications, and digestion. In a study published in the journal *Phytomedicine* (Grace, Ribnicky, Kuhn et al. 2009), treatment in an animal model by gavage (500 mg/kg body weight) with a phenolic-rich extract, and an anthocyanin-enriched fraction formulated with Labrasol, lowered elevated blood glucose levels by 33% and 51%, respectively (Basu, and Lyons. 2011; DeFuria, Bennett, Strissel et al. 2009; Seymour, Tanone, Urcuyo-Llanes et al. 2011; Vuong, Benhaddou-Andaloussi, Brault et al. 2009). Labrasol is a self-emulsifying excipient used to improve the oral bioavailability of poorly water-soluble drugs.

Notably, blueberries contain powerful antioxidants that can neutralize free radicals that cause neurodegenerative disease, cardiovascular disease, and cancer (Grace, Ribnicky, Kuhn et al. 2009). Phenolics and anthocyanins were proposed as active compounds to treat diabetes and insulin resistance (Grace, Ribnicky, Kuhn et al. 2009).

A clinical study reported in the *Journal of Nutrition* showed that obese or Type 2 diabetes patients consuming 22.5 g of blueberry, twice a day for 6 weeks, reduced insulin resistance to a greater extent than those consuming a placebo.

At baseline (week 0), insulin sensitivity was measured in obese, nondiabetic, and insulin-resistant participants using a high-dose hyperinsulinemic–euglycemic clamp (insulin infusion of 120 mU [861 pmol] m^{-20} min^{-1}). Serum inflammatory biomarkers and adiposity were measured at baseline. At the end of the study, insulin sensitivity, inflammatory biomarkers, and adiposity were reassessed.

Participants were instructed to consume either a smoothie containing 22.5 g of blueberry bioactives, or a smoothie of equal nutritional value without added blueberry bioactives, twice daily for 6 weeks. Both groups were instructed to maintain their body weight by reducing *ad libitum* intake by an amount equal to the energy intake of the smoothies.

Participants' body weight was evaluated weekly, and 3-day food records were collected at baseline, the middle, and end of the study.

The mean increase in insulin sensitivity was greater in the blueberry group (1.7 ± 0.5 mg kg) than in the placebo group (0.4 ± 0.4 mg kg). Insulin sensitivity was enhanced in the blueberry group at the end of the study, without significant changes in adiposity, energy intake, and inflammatory biomarkers.

The authors concluded that dietary supplementation with bioactives from whole blueberries improved insulin sensitivity in obese, nondiabetic, and insulin-resistant participants [ClinicalTrials.gov NCT01005420] (Stull, Cash, Johnson et al. 2010).

9.5.4 ASTRAGALUS POLYSACCHARIDES AND ASTRAGALUS

Astragalus membranaceus is an important herb in traditional Chinese medicine. It has been used in a wide variety of herbal blends and "natural" remedies, including *Dang-gui buxue tang*, which is *A. membranaceus* paired with *Angelicae sinensis*.

The *A. membranaceus* root shows antioxidant, antidiabetic, antihypertensive, and immunomodulatory activities (Wu, and Chen. 2004). The extract of *A. membranaceus* was shown to treat diabetes and diabetic complications (Li, Cao, and Zeng. 2004). Moreover, treatment with *Astragalus* polysaccharides resulted in better glycemic control in diabetic rodents *via* an increase in insulin sensitivity (Liu, Wu, Mao et al. 2010; Mao, Yu, Wang et al. 2009; Zhao, Zhang, Ding et al. 2012).

The mode of action of *Astragalus* polysaccharides includes Akt activation and upregulation of Glut4, and inhibition of inflammation *via* the PTP1B/NF B pathway (Liu, Wu, Mao et al. 2010; Zhao, Zhang, Ding et al. 2012; Wu, Ou-Yang, Wu et al. 2005).

9.5.5 CINNAMON

Both common cinnamon (*Cinnamomum verum* and *Cinnamomum zeylanicum*) and cassia (*Cinnamomum aromaticum*), long used as food flavoring agents, and in drinks and medicines worldwide, have recently been studied in connection with diabetes and metabolic syndrome (Qin, Panickar, and Anderson. 2010). Cinnamon was shown to reduce blood glucose *via* reduction of insulin resistance and increase of hepatic glycogenesis (Qin, Panickar, and Anderson. 2010; Couturier, Qin, Batandier et al. 2011).

Cinnamon phenolics were proposed to be the active compounds in modulation of insulin signaling (Li, Liu, Wang et al. 2012; Qin, Dawson, Schoene et al. 2012; Subash Babu, Prabuseenivasan, and Ignacimuthu. 2007). Moreover, cinnamaldehyde showed antihyperglycemic and antihyperlipidemic effects on rodent models of diabetes (Li, Liu, Wang et al. 2012). This compound from cinnamon extract is thought of as a potential antidiabetic agent (Subash Babu, Prabuseenivasan, and Ignacimuthu. 2007). The molecular targets of cinnamon and cinnamaldehyde are unknown.

9.5.6 FENUGREEK

The seeds of fenugreek (*Trigonella foenum-graecum*) used as a food supplement are also known for improving metabolism and health (Basch, Ulbricht, Kuo et al. 2003). Animal studies have shown that extract of fenugreek seeds can lower blood glucose levels (Pavithran. 1994; Valette, Sauvaire, Baccou et al. 1984). Fenugreek is considered a promising agent for diabetes and its complications (Basch, Ulbricht, Kuo et al. 2003). The glucose-lowering action of this plant involves reduction of insulin resistance (Mohan, and Balasubramanyam. 2001).

Diosgenin, GII, galactomannan, trigoneosides, and 4-hydroxyisoleucine have been identified as the active antidiabetic compounds in fenugreek. However, little is known about the mechanisms of these compounds. Among them, diosgenin was shown to reduce adipocyte differentiation and inflammation, implying its action in reduction of insulin resistance (Uemura, Hirai, Mizoguchi et al. 2010).

The *Journal of the Association of Physicians of India* published a clinical study that aimed to evaluate the effects of *T. foenum-graecum* seeds on glycemic control and insulin resistance, as determined by the homeostasis model assessment (HOMA) model insulin resistance, in mild to moderate severity Type 2 diabetes.

Twenty-five newly diagnosed patients with Type 2 diabetes (fasting glucose less than 200 mg/dL) were randomly assigned to one of two groups: For two months, group 1 received 1 g/day of hydroalcoholic extract of fenugreek seeds, and group 2 received usual care (dietary control, exercise) and placebo capsules.

At baseline, both groups were similar in anthropometric and clinical variables. Oral glucose tolerance test (OGTT), lipid levels, fasting C-peptide, glycosylated hemoglobin, and HOMA model insulin resistance were also similar.

In group 1, at the end of 2 months, fasting blood glucose (148.3 ± 44.1 to 119.9 ± 25 vs. 137.5 ± 41.1 to 113.0 ± 36.0) and 2-h postglucose blood glucose (210.6 ± 79.0 to 181.1 ± 69 vs. 219.9 ± 41.0 to 241.6 ± 43) were not different from group 2. However, area under the curve (AUC) of blood glucose (2375 ± 574 vs. 2759 ± 274) and insulin (2492 ± 2536 vs. 5631 ± 2428) were significantly lower.

HOMA model–derived insulin resistance showed a significant decrease in percent β-cell secretion in the treated group (group 1), as compared to the control group (group 2) (86.3 ± 32 vs. 70.1 ± 52), and a significant increase in percent insulin sensitivity (112.9 ± 67 vs. 92.2 ± 57). Serum triglycerides decreased and high-density lipoprotein (HDL) cholesterol increased significantly in group 1 as compared to group 2.

The authors concluded that adjunctive use of fenugreek seeds improved glycemic control and decreased insulin resistance in mild Type 2 diabetic patients. A favorable effect on hypertriglyceridemia was also noted (Gupta, Gupta, and Lal. 2001).

9.5.7 LYCHEE

Lychee (*Litchi chinensis*) is an evergreen fruit tree. The seeds are known in Chinese herbal medicine for treatment of pain, gastrointestinal diseases, and others. Recently, lychee seed was reported to have antidiabetic activity in rats, and in human patients (Zhang, and Teng. 1986). Seed extract exerts its action through reduction of insulin resistance (Guo, Li, Pan et al. 2004). In addition, oligonol from lychee fruit showed antioxidative activity and, thus, protected the liver and kidney in Type 2 diabetes animal models (Noh, Park, and Yokozawa. 2011; Noh, Kim, Park et al. 2010).

Because of its significant integrative treatment potential for normalizing blood glucose and for reducing the damage of hyperglycemia to components of the eyes, the beneficial effects and active substances in lychee extract are detailed in Chapter 10.

9.6 HERBS AND COMPOUNDS THAT REGULATE CELL FUNCTION

Plant chemicals and/or extracts are listed here according to their impact on cells. Their chemical structures and antihyperglycemic activities and actions on cell function ([re]generation and survival) in cells, in animals, and in patients with Type 2 diabetes are discussed. The chemical and biological properties of the compounds discussed in this section are summarized in Chang, Lin, Bartolome et al. (2013) (*Evidence-Based Complementary and Alternative Medicine*, 2013: Article ID 378657 [http://dx.doi.org/10. 1155/2013/378657], Table 1, go to https://www.hindawi.com /journals/ecam/2013/378657/tab1/).

9.6.1 PAPAYA (*CARICA PAPAYA*) AND PANDAN (*PANDANUS AMARYLLIFOLIUS*)

The ethanol extracts of *P. amaryllifolius* and *C. papaya* reduced hyperglycemia in streptozotocin-treated mice. Histological staining data showed that these extracts significantly induced the regeneration of the pancreatic islet β-cells, which translated into reduced levels of blood glucose (Sasidharan, Sumathi, Jegathambigai et al. 2011). So far, no active components have been identified; however, the flavonoids, alkaloids, saponin, and tannin in both plants are thought to be bioactive phytochemicals (Sasidharan, Sumathi, Jegathambigai et al. 2011).

9.6.2 CONOPHYLLINE AND *TABERNAEMONTANA DIVARICATA*

Conophylline, a plant alkaloid present in *T. divaricata* or *Ervatamia microphylla*, facilitates differentiation and generation of pancreatic cells *in vitro* and *in vivo* (Kawakami, Hirayama, Tsuchiya et al. 2010; Kodera, Yamada, Yamamoto et al. 2009; Ogata, Li, Yamada et al. 2004).

The *International Journal of Biochemistry and Cell Biology* reported a study that aimed to determine whether there are agents that can induce differentiation of pancreatic progenitors to β-cells that would prove useful in developing a new therapeutic approach to treat diabetes. They screened various compounds using pancreatic AR42J cells, a model of pancreatic progenitor cells.

The investigators reported that conophylline, a vinca alkaloid extracted from leaves of a tropical plant *E. microphylla*, was effective in converting AR42J into endocrine cells. Conophylline reproduces the differentiation-inducing activity of activin A. Unlike activin A, however, conophylline does not induce apoptosis.

To induce differentiation of AR42J cells, conophylline increases expression of neurogenin-3 by activating p38 mitogen-activated protein kinase. Conophylline also induces differentiation in cultured pancreatic progenitor cells from fetal and neonatal rats. More importantly, conophylline is effective in reversing hyperglycemia in neonatal streptozotocin-treated rats, and both the insulin content and the β-cell mass are increased by conophylline. Histologically, conophylline increases the numbers of ductal cells positive for pancreatic–duodenal–homeobox protein-1 and islet-like cell clusters.

The investigators concluded that conophylline and related compounds are useful in inducing differentiation of pancreatic β-cells both *in vivo* and *in vitro* (Kojima, and Umezawa. 2006).

This phytochemical was also shown to decrease the fibrosis of pancreatic islet cells that is found in autoimmune or toxic diabetes (Saito, Yamada, Yamamoto et al. 2012). A crude extract of *T. divaricata* was shown to increase the level of blood insulin and reduce the level of blood glucose in streptozotocin-treated mice (Fujii, Takei, and Umezawa. 2009). These data imply a plausible role for conophylline and *T. divaricata* in improving β-cell function.

9.6.3 KINSENOSIDE

Kinsenoside, a major constituent of the jewel orchid (*Anoectochilus roxburghii*), exhibited hypoglycemic activity in streptozotocin-treated mice (Zhang, Cai, Ruan et al. 2007). This effect was partially attributed to β-cell repair and/or regeneration. However, the clinical potential of this compound in β-cell survival and regeneration awaits further investigation.

9.6.4 NYMPHAYOL

Nymphayol, a plant sterol, was initially isolated and identified from blue lotus (*Nymphaea stellata*). One study showed that this compound promoted the partial generation of pancreatic islet β-cells (Subash-Babu, Ignacimuthu, Agastian et al. 2009). In diabetic rats, oral administration of Nymphayol significantly lowered elevated blood glucose levels and increased the insulin concentration in serum. In addition, Nymphayol significantly increased the number of pancreatic islet β-cells (Subash-Babu, Ignacimuthu, Agastian et al. 2009). However, the impact of this compound on Type 2 diabetes patients is largely unknown.

9.6.5 SILYMARIN (MILK THISTLE)

Silymarin is a flavonoid mixture composed of silybin, silydianin, and silychristin, active components of the plant milk thistle (*Silybum marianum*) (Rui. 1991). Aside from antioxidant, anti-inflammatory, and hepatoprotective activities, the modes of action through which silymarin and/or milk thistle exert antidiabetic activity are not well understood, but it has nevertheless been shown to improve the glycemic profile (Huseini, Larijani, Heshmat et al. 2006; Hussain. 2007).

In a clinical study published in the *Journal of Medicinal Food*, silymarin was tested as an adjunct to glibenclamide (glyburide/USAN) therapy. The investigators held that oxidative stress rises postprandially as well as during long-term hyperglycemia in Type 2 diabetic patients with poor response to glibenclamide. Therefore, they undertook this study to evaluate the effects of the antioxidant flavonoid silymarin on long-term and postprandial glycemic and weight control in Type 2 diabetic patients treated with glibenclamide.

Type 2 diabetes patients previously maintained on 10 mg/day glibenclamide and diet control, but showing poor glycemic control, were assigned to one of three groups: the first two groups were treated with either 200 mg/day silymarin or placebo, as adjuncts to glibenclamide, and the third group was maintained on glibenclamide alone for 120 days.

Fasting and 4-h postprandial plasma glucose, glycated hemoglobin (HbA1c), and body mass index (BMI) were evaluated at baseline and after 120 days.

Compared to placebo, silymarin treatment significantly reduced both fasting and postprandial plasma glucose excursions, in addition to significantly reducing HbA1c levels and BMI after 120 days. No significantly different effects were observed for placebo compared to glibenclamide alone.

The authors concluded that adjunctive use of silymarin with glibenclamide improves the glycemic control targeted by glibenclamide during both fasting, and postprandially, and over the longer term, an effect that may be related to increased insulin sensitivity in peripheral tissues (Hussain. 2007).

Because milk thistle has shown strong evidence-based benefit in reducing HbA1c, it is detailed in Chapter 10.

9.6.6 POLYYNES AND *BIDENS PILOSA*

B. pilosa (a flowering plant in the aster family) is used as an herbal medicine for a variety of diseases. An aqueous ethanol extract of the aerial part of *B. pilosa* lowered blood glucose in db/db mice (mice genetically predisposed to rapidly develop diabetes) (Ubillas, Mendez, Jolad et al. 2000). Based on a bioactivity-guided identification, 2 polyynes, 3-β-D-glucopyranosyl-1-hydroxy-6(E)-tetradecene-8,10,12-triyne, and 2-β-D-glucopyranosyloxy-1-hydroxy-5(E)-tridecene-7,9,11-triyne were identified. Further, a mixture of both compounds significantly reduced blood glucose levels and food intake in the db/db mice (Ubillas, Mendez, Jolad et al. 2000). The term "polyynes" refers to any organic compound with alternating single and triple bonds.

Another study confirmed that water extracts of *B. pilosa*, at one dose and at multiple doses, significantly lowered fasting and postmeal hyperglycemia in db/db mice (Chien, Young, Hsu et al. 2009). The antihyperglycemic effect of *B. pilosa* was inversely correlated with an increase in serum insulin levels, suggesting that *B. pilosa* L. var. *radiata* acts to lower blood glucose *via* increased insulin production. Moreover, *B. pilosa* protected against islet atrophy in the mouse pancreas.

Despite the variation in the percentage of polyynes in different varieties, all displayed antidiabetic activity in db/db mice (Chien, Young, Hsu et al. 2009). Another polyyne isolated from *B. pilosa*, 2-β-D-glucopyranosyloxy-1-hydroxytrideca-5,7,9,11-tetrayne (cytopiloyne), showed better glycemic control than the previously mentioned polyynes (Li, Liu, Wang et al 2012).

The *B. pilosa* cytopiloyne derivative exerts antidiabetic function through regulation of β-cell function involving increased insulin expression/secretion and islet protection (Li, Liu, Wang et al 2012). Furthermore, cytopiloyne regulated β-cell function through a signaling cascade of calcium influx, diacylglycerol, and protein kinase C. Collectively, *B. pilosa* and its cytopiloyne derivatives can treat Type 2 diabetes by acting on β-cells. The data also suggest that combination therapy that targets multiple pathways involved in metabolism could be better remedies for Type 2 diabetes.

9.6.7 GYMNEMA SYLVESTRE

G. sylvestre is a woody climbing shrub native to India and Africa. The Hindi name, *gurmar*, means "destroyer of sugar." Its action enhances insulin secretion and (re)generation of pancreatic β-cells, as shown in rodents (Ramkumar, Lee, Krishnamurthi et al. 2009; Al-Romaiyan, King, Persaud et al. 2013). *G. sylvestre* increased plasma insulin and C-peptide levels, and decreased blood glucose concentrations in Type 2 diabetes patients.

The journal *Phytotherapy Research* published a report titled "A novel *Gymnema sylvestre* extract stimulates insulin secretion from human islets in vivo and in vitro." Its authors point out that, in India, extracts of *G. sylvestre* have been used for the treatment of Type 2 diabetes for centuries. They report the effects of a novel high-molecular-weight *G. sylvestre* extract, Om Santal Adivasi (OSA), on plasma insulin, C-peptide and glucose in a small cohort of patients with Type 2 diabetes.

Oral administration of OSA (1g/day for 60 days) induced significant increases in circulating insulin and C-peptide, associated with significant reductions in fasting and postprandial blood glucose. *In vitro* measurements with isolated human islets of Langerhans showed direct stimulatory effects of OSA on insulin secretion from human β-cells, consistent with an *in vivo* mode of action through enhancing insulin secretion. These *in vivo* and *in vitro* observations suggest that OSA may provide a potential alternative therapy for hyperglycemia (Al-Romaiyan, Liu, Asare-Anane et al. 2010).

9.7 HERBS AND COMPOUNDS THAT REGULATE GLUCAGON-LIKE PEPTIDE-1 HOMEOSTASIS

The chemical and biological properties of plants and phytochemicals that regulate glucagon-like peptide-1 (GLP-1) secretion and/or DPP-4 activity are summarized in a review titled "Herbal therapies for Type 2 diabetes mellitus: chemistry, biology, and potential application of selected plants and compounds," published in the journal *Evidence-Based Complementary and Alternative Medicine* (Chang, Lin, Bartolome et al. 2013). To access it, go to: https://www.hindawi.com/journals/ecam/2013/378657/tab1/.

9.7.1 FRUCTANS

A fructan is a polymer of fructose molecules. Fructans with a short chain length are known as fructooligosaccharides, and they occur in foods such as agave, artichokes, asparagus, leeks, garlic, onions, and wheat.

The American Diabetes Association established a link between high intake of soluble dietary fiber and improved hyperglycemia and insulin secretion in patients with Type 2 diabetes (Chandalia, Garg, Lutjohann et al. 2000). Inulins (Raftilose) are soluble dietary fibers made of short-chain fructans present in the roots of chicory, *Agave tequilana*, *Dasylirion* spp., and others.

A study reported in the *Journal of Endocrinology* showed that inulin-type fructans could prevent obesity, steatosis, and hyperglycemia. Moreover, the fermentation of fructans in the intestines of rats has been demonstrated to stimulate incretin secretion in the colon (Cani, Daubioul, Reusens et al. 2005; Kok, Morgan, Williams et al. 1998). In addition, 5-week feeding with inulin significantly slowed body weight gain, food intake, and blood glucose levels in C57BL/6J mice (Urías-Silvas, Cani, Delmée et al. 2008). An elevation of GLP-1 levels was observed in the portal vein and proximal colon (Urías-Silvas, Cani, Delmée et al. 2008). It remains unclear whether fructans can enhance incretin production in humans with Type 2 diabetes.

9.7.2 MONOUNSATURATED FATTY ACID

The journal *Diabetes Care* reported that epidemiological investigations have established an association between dietary fat and Type 2 diabetes (Thanopoulou, Karamanos, Angelico et al. 2003). However, fat was found to stimulate incretin secretion (Feinle, O'Donovan, Doran et al. 2003).

Decreases in gastric emptying, level of postprandial blood glucose and insulin, and an increase in plasma GLP-1 level were caused by ingesting fat before a carbohydrate meal in Type 2 diabetes patients, as reported in a study published in the *Journal of Clinical Endocrinology and Metabolism* (Gentilcore, Chaikomin, Jones et al. 2006). In another study, such patients took control meals, and control meals supplemented with olive oil (74% monounsaturated fatty acid) or butter (72% saturated fatty acid). In contrast to the control diet, both fat-rich meals induced a five- to sixfold increase in plasma GLP-1 and three- to fourfold increase in gastric inhibitory polypeptide (Thomsen, Storm, Holst et al. 2003).

However, no significant differences in the level of blood glucose, insulin, or fatty acids were observed. Data from humans and rodents suggest that fat, particularly unsaturated fatty acid, can stimulate GLP-1 secretion. GLP-1 increases insulin secretion in patients with Type 2 diabetes in a dose-dependent manner, and β-cell responsiveness to glucose may also be increased to normal levels with a low dose of GLP-1 infusion (Kjems, Holst, Vølund et al. 2003).

9.8 HERBS AND COMPOUNDS THAT REGULATE GLUCOSE ABSORPTION IN THE GUT

The chemical and biological properties of plants and phytochemicals regulating α-glucosidase activity discussed in this section are summarized in Chang, Lin, Bartolome et al. (2013) (*Evidence-Based Complementary and Alternative Medicine*, 2013: Article ID 378657 [http://dx.doi.org/10.1155/2013/378657], Table 1, go to https://www.hindawi.com/journals/ecam/2013/378657/tab1/).

9.8.1 SEROTONIN DERIVATIVES AND SAFFLOWER

A hydroalcoholic extract of safflower (*Carthamus tinctorius*) exhibited antidiabetic properties through enhancing insulin secretion in alloxan-induced diabetic rats (Asgary, Rahimi, Mahzouni et al. 2012). Two serotonin derivatives isolated from safflower seed were shown to suppress α-glucosidase activity to a greater degree than the positive control, acarbose. It will be recalled that acarbose is an FDA (Food and Drug Administration)-approved drug that inhibits the enzyme α-glucosidase, which is needed to break down a number of carbohydrate molecules. With fewer carbohydrates being broken down, fewer molecules of glucose are available to be absorbed, which in turn lowers blood glucose levels and makes fewer calls on the pancreas to secrete insulin.

In a study published in the journal *Phytotherapy Research*, the chemical components isolated from safflower seed (*C. tinctorius* L.) were evaluated as part of the search for naturally derived α-glucosidase inhibitors. The compounds active as α-glucosidase inhibitors were serotonin derivatives [e.g., N-p-coumaroyl serotonin (1) and N-feruloyl serotonin (2)]. These compounds showed a potent inhibitory activity; the 50% inhibitory concentration (IC50) values were calculated as 47.2 μm (1) and 99.8 μm (2), while that of the reference drugs acarbose and 1-deoxynojirimycin were evaluated as 907.5 μm and 278.0 μm, respectively. A lower IC50 value means that a given compound is more efficient at inhibiting a given enzyme than another compound with a higher number. Thus, the two plant compounds discussed above are far more efficient inhibitors of α-glucosidase than the two reference drugs.

Regarding the structure of the serotonin derivatives, the existence of the hydroxyl group at the 5-position in the serotonin moiety and the linkage of cinnamic acid and serotonin are essential for the respective α-glucosidase inhibitory activities of those plant derivatives.

These results are helpful for understanding the rationale for the use of safflower seed as a traditional medicine for the treatment of diabetes. Moreover, it could serve to develop medicinal preparations as supplements and functional foods for diabetes.

The investigators concluded that the serotonin compounds could be used as lead compounds for a new potential α-glucosidase inhibitor derived from the plant (Takahashi, and Miyazawa. 2012).

9.8.2 *Laminaria japonica* and *Ishige okamurae*—Japanese Kelp Seaweed

The journal *Phytotherapy Research* reports a study about a bioactivity-tailored isolation and detailed chemical characterization that was used to identify the antidiabetes compounds found in the *L. japonica* rhizoid.

Liquid chromatography/mass spectrometry (LC/MS), proton NMR, and carbon NMR spectra analyses demonstrated that the active compound was butyl-isobutyl-phthalate. Butyl-isobutyl-phthalate demonstrated a significant concentration-dependent, noncompetitive inhibitory activity against α-glucosidase *in vitro*, with an IC50 of 38 μm. *In vivo*, the ethyl acetate fraction and purified butyl-isobutyl-phthalate displayed a significant hypoglycemic effect in streptozocin-induced diabetic mice.

The investigators concluded that butyl-isobutyl-phthalate could be considered as an α-glucosidase inhibitor and developed as an important antidiabetes agent for Type 2 diabetes therapy (Bu, Liu, Zheng et al. 2010).

I. okamurae, an edible brown seaweed, has been shown to lower blood glucose in C57BL/-KsJ-db/db mice. It was reported in the journal *Diabetes Research and Clinical Practice* that its mode of action involves reduction of insulin resistance and regulation of the hepatic glucose metabolic enzymes (Min, Kim, Jeon et al. 2011).

Diphlorethohydroxycarmalol, a phlorotannin of *I. okamurae*, inhibits the activity of α-glucosidase and α-amylase. This compound also decreases postprandial blood glucose levels in streptozotocin-treated or normal mice (Heo, Hwang, Choi et al. 2009).

It was reported in an earlier chapter that there is a strong link between Type 2 diabetes and thyroid deficiency. In some cases, that problem can be traced to insufficient dietary iodine intake. For that reason, a later chapter will detail various forms of seaweed including kelp and their potential for supplementing iodine and supporting healthy thyroid function in people with diabetes.

9.9 HERBS AND COMPOUNDS WITH MULTIPLE ANTIDIABETIC ACTIONS

Some plants and plant compounds can target multiple metabolic pathways. The chemical and biological properties of the compounds discussed in this section are summarized in Chang, Lin, Bartolome et al. (2013) (*Evidence-Based Complementary and Alternative Medicine*, Vol. 2013: Article ID 378657 [http://dx.doi.org/10. 1155/2013/378657], Table 1, go to https://www.hindawi .com/journals/ecam/2013/378657/tab1/).

9.9.1 Berberine

Berberine was first isolated from *Berberis vulgaris*, also known as common barberry. European barberry, or simply barberry, is a shrub in the genus *Berberis*. It produces edible but sharply acidic berries that people in many countries eat as a tart and refreshing fruit. This compound has multiple functions ranging from inflammation inhibition to reduction of metabolic syndrome and related activities (Imanshahidi, and Hosseinzadeh. 2008).

The *Medical Science Monitor* reported a study of berberine to treat bacterial diarrhea that also showed it to lower blood glucose, which has been recently confirmed by many other studies.

Recent evidence suggests that the gut microbiota composition is associated with obesity and Type 2 diabetes, which are closely associated with a low-grade inflammatory state. The protective effect against diabetes of gut microbiota modulation with probiotics or antibiotics has been confirmed in recent observations.

Berberine has significant antimicrobial activity against several microbes through inhibiting the assembly function of "Filamenting temperature-sensitive mutant Z" (FtsZ) and halting bacterial cell division. FtsZ is a cell-division protein. Because berberine acts topically in the gastrointestinal tract and is poorly absorbed, berberine might modulate gut microbiota without systemic anti-infective activity. The authors hypothesized that gut microbiota modulation may be one mechanism of the antidiabetic effect of berberine (Han, Lin, and Huang. 2011).

In another study in an animal model of Type 2 diabetes, berberine decreased hyperglycemia, increased insulin resistance, stimulated pancreatic β-cell regeneration, and decreased lipid peroxidation (Chen, Zhang, and Huang. 2010; Kim, Lee, Cha et al. 2009; Lee, Kim, Kim et al. 2006).

Because of the strong link to blood glucose control, berberine will be detailed in the following chapter.

9.9.2 Bitter Melon

Bitter melon, the fruit of the plant *M. charantia* used in Ayurvedic medicine, is linked to the antidiabetic effect of extracts that can increase insulin secretion (Saxena, and Vikram. 2004). Modes of action of bitter melon and *M. charantia* include insulin secretion, inhibition of glucose reabsorption in the gut, preservation of islet cells and their functions, increase of peripheral glucose utilization, and suppression of gluconeogenic enzymes (Singh, Cumming, Manoharan et al. 2011). Of note, momorcharin and momordicin, isolated from *M. charantia* and its fruit, act to lower blood glucose, likely because they possess insulin-like chemical structures.

9.9.3 Capsaicin and Chili Pepper

Chili peppers, the fruits of the *Capsicum* plants, are commonly used as food and medicine. The extracts have insulinotropic action on cells (Islam, and Choi. 2008). Capsaicin, a pungent component of chili pepper, activates AMPK in 3T3-L1 preadipocytes (Hwang, Park, Shin et al. 2005). The data suggest that the chili pepper and its active ingredients prevent Type 2 diabetes by regulating insulin resistance. However, there is controversy about capsaicin to treat Type 2 diabetes: It may also contribute to diabetes by impairing insulin secretion (Gram, Ahrén, Nagy et al. 2007).

Chili is detailed in a following chapter, along with caveats.

9.9.4 Ginseng

Roots, berries, and/or leaves of ginseng (*Panax ginseng*) and North American ginseng (*Panax quinquefolius*) lower blood glucose, and they were found effective in the treatment of Type 2 diabetes both in humans and in animal models.

The journal *Diabetes* reported a study on an animal model to ascertain the antihyperglycemic and antiobesity effects of *P. ginseng* berry extract and its major constituent, *ginsenoside Re*, in obese diabetic C57BL/6J ob/ob mice in comparison to lean littermates. Animals received daily intraperitoneal injections of *P. ginseng* berry extract for 12 days.

On day 12, 150 mg/kg extract-treated ob/ob mice became normoglycemic (137 ± 6.7 mg/dL) and had significantly improved glucose tolerance. The overall glucose excursion during the 2-h intraperitoneal glucose tolerance test decreased by 46% compared to the vehicle-treated (mode of treatment) ob/ob mice.

The improvement in blood glucose levels in the extract-treated ob/ob mice was associated with a significant reduction in serum insulin levels in fed and fasting mice. A hyperinsulinemic–euglycemic clamp study revealed a more than twofold increase in the rate of insulin-stimulated glucose disposal in treated ob/ob mice (112 ± 19.1 vs. 52 ± 11.8 μmol kg^{-1} min^{-1} for the vehicle group).

In addition, the extract-treated ob/ob mice lost a significant amount of weight (from 51.7 ± 1.9 g on day 0 to 45.7 ± 1.2 on day 12 vs. vehicle-treated ob/ob mice), associated with a significant reduction in food intake and a very significant increase in energy expenditure and body temperature.

Treatment with the extract also significantly reduced plasma cholesterol levels in ob/ob mice. Additional studies demonstrated that *ginsenoside Re* plays a significant part in antihyperglycemic action. This antidiabetic effect of *ginsenoside Re* was not associated with body weight changes, suggesting that other constituents in the extract have distinct pharmacological mechanisms acting on energy metabolism (Attele, Zhou, Xie et al. 2002; see also Yun, Moon, Ko et al. 2004; Yoo, Lee, Lo et al. 2012).

The different parts of the plant are not equally effective as antihyperglycemic agents. This was shown in an animal model study titled "Anti-hyperglycemic effects of ginseng: comparison between root and berry" published in the journal *Phytomedicine*. The investigators compared the antihyperglycemic effect of *P. ginseng* root to that of the berry in ob/ob mice, which exhibit profound obesity and hyperglycemia that resemble human Type 2 diabetes.

The ob/ob mice had high baseline glucose levels (195 mg/dL). Ginseng root extract (150 mg/kg body weight) and ginseng berry extract (150 mg/kg body weight) significantly decreased fasting blood glucose to 143 ± 9.3 mg/dL and 150 ± 9.5 mg/dL on day 5, respectively, compared with the vehicle.

On day 12, although fasting blood glucose level did not continue to decline in the root group (155 ± 12.7 mg/dL), the berry group became normoglycemic (129 ± 7.3 mg/dL). Glucose tolerance was further evaluated using the intraperitoneal glucose tolerance test.

On the first day, basal hyperglycemia was exacerbated by intraperitoneal glucose load and failed to return to baseline after 120 min. After 12 days of treatment with ginseng root extract (150 mg/kg body weight), the AUC showed some decrease (9.6%). After 12 days of treatment with ginseng berry extract (150 mg/kg body weight), the AUC had decreased by 31.0%.

It was also observed that body weight did not change significantly after ginseng root extract (150 mg/kg body weight) treatment, but the same concentration of ginseng berry extract significantly decreased body weight. These data suggest that ginseng berry exhibits more potent antihyperglycemic activity than ginseng root, and only ginseng berry shows marked antiobesity effects in ob/ob mice (Dey, Xie, Wang et al. 2003).

Another study titled "American ginseng berry juice intake reduces blood glucose and body weight in ob/ob mice" published in the *Journal of Food Science* reported that after their animal subjects received daily berry juice 0.6 mL/kg or vehicle for 10 consecutive days, it was found that oral juice administration significantly lowered fasting blood glucose levels, and this effect continued for at least 10 days after termination of the treatment.

Data from intraperitoneal glucose tolerance tests demonstrated that there was a notable improvement in glucose tolerance in the juice-treated group as compared to the control group. In addition, the berry juice significantly reduced body weight. The investigators concluded that ginseng berry juice may have functional efficacy as a dietary supplement for patients with diabetes (Xie, Wang, Ni et al. 2007).

There are also clinical studies that reported that *P. ginseng* and North American ginseng improve glycemic control in Type 2 diabetes patients. For instance, the journal *Archives of Internal Medicine* published a study titled "American ginseng (*P. quinquefolius* L.) reduces postprandial glycemia in nondiabetic subjects and subjects with type 2 diabetes mellitus." The aim of the study was to determine whether American ginseng (*P. quinquefolius L*) affects postprandial glycemia in humans.

On four separate occasions, 10 nondiabetic participants with average age 34 ± 7 years and average BMI 25.6 ± 3 kg/m^2 and 9 participants with Type 2 diabetes with average age 62 ± 7 years, average BMI 29 ± 5 kg/m^2, and average glycosylated hemoglobin A1c 0.08 ± 0.005 were randomized to receive 3 g of ginseng, or placebo capsules, either 40 min before, or together with a 25-g oral glucose challenge.

The placebo capsules contained common flour and the quantity of carbohydrate and appearance matched the ginseng capsules. Only for participants with Type 2 diabetes was a capillary blood sample taken fasting, and then at 15, 30, 45, 60, 90, and 120 min after the glucose challenge.

In nondiabetic participants, no differences were found in postprandial glycemia between placebo and ginseng when administered together with the glucose challenge. However, when ginseng was taken 40 min before the glucose challenge, significant reductions were observed.

In participants with Type 2 diabetes, the same was true whether capsules were taken before or together with the glucose challenge. Reductions in area under the glycemic curve were 18% ± 31% for nondiabetic participants and 19% ± 22% and 22% ± 17% for participants with Type 2 diabetes administered before or together with the glucose challenge, respectively.

The investigators concluded that American ginseng lowered postprandial glycemia in both study groups. Furthermore, nondiabetic persons should take the ginseng with the meal to prevent unintended hypoglycemia (Vuksan, Sievenpiper, Koo et al. 2000). See also Vuksan, Sung, Sievenpiper et al. (2008), "Korean red ginseng (*Panax ginseng*) improves glucose and insulin regulation in well-controlled, type 2 diabetes: results of a randomized, double-blind, placebo-controlled study of efficacy and safety," published in the journal *Nutrition, Metabolism and Cardiovascular Diseases* [Jan; 18(1): 46–56; DOI: 10.1016/j.numecd.2006.04.003].

The study found that there was no change in the primary endpoint, HbA(1c), but the participants remained well controlled (HbA1c = 6.5%) throughout. The selected Korean red ginseng treatment also decreased 75-g OGTT plasma glucose indices by 8% to 11% as well as fasting plasma insulin and 75-g OGTT plasma insulin indices by 33% to 38%; and it increased fasting insulin sensitivity index (HOMA) and 75-g OGTT insulin sensitivity index by 33% compared with placebo (Vuksan, Sung, Sievenpiper et al. 2008).

It should be noted, however, that one study reported in the *Chinese Journal of Integrative Medicine* that neither of the ginsengs they investigated were found to have any antidiabetic effect (Kim, Shin, Lee et al. 2011).

This discrepancy in findings may be the result of known variations in concentration of the active ginsenosides in ginseng. That variability in constituents and concentration was reported in the journal *Diabetes Care* in a report titled "A systematic quantitative analysis of the literature of the high variability in ginseng (*Panax* spp.)." The glucose-lowering mechanisms of both ginsengs may involve a reduction in insulin resistance and an improvement in β-cell function (Lee, Kao, Liu et al. 2007; Lee, Lee, Park et al. 2009; Kim, and Kim. 2007; Wu, Luo, and Luo. 2007). It is well known in the literature on ginseng that, for any given strain of the plant, there can be great variations in the concentration of its active agents depending on geographical and climatological factors, such as the nature of the soil in which the plants were grown, and the growing conditions.

Ginsenosides are the primary constituents present in ginseng roots that are claimed to benefit health. Extracts of ginseng root have been shown to protect against apoptosis of the pancreatic β-cell line, Min-6 cells (Hye, and Kim. 2007). One study published in the journal *Evidence-Based Complementary and Alternative Medicine* proposed that ginseng alters mitochondrial function as well as the apoptosis cascades to ensure cell viability in pancreatic islet cells (Luo, and Luo. 2009). Moreover, ginsenosides from ginseng extracts were reportedly responsible for this protection *in vitro*: One study reported that ginsenoside Rh2 is an active compound that improves insulin resistance in fructose-rich chow-fed rats (Lee, Kao, Liu et al. 2007). In any case, *ginsenoside Re* was shown to possess antioxidant activity by upregulation of glutathione and malondialdehyde in kidney and/or eye (Cho, Chung, Lee et al. 2006). However, the *in vivo* protective role of the extracts, and ginsenosides within cells, remains to be further verified.

9.9.5 Turmeric (*Curcuma longa*)

Turmeric (*C. longa*) has been shown to increase postprandial serum insulin levels to maintain healthy blood glucose levels in healthy people. The *Nutrition Journal* reported a study that aimed to study the effect of *C. longa* on postprandial plasma glucose, insulin levels, and glycemic index in healthy participants. Healthy participants were given a standard 75-g OGTT together with capsules containing a placebo, or *C. longa*. Finger-prick capillary and venous blood samples were collected before and 15, 30, 45, 60, 90, and 120 min after the start of the OGTT to measure the glucose and insulin levels, respectively.

It was found that ingestion of 6 g of *C. longa* had no significant effect on the glucose response. However, the insulin level was significantly higher 30 min and 60 min after the OGTT that included *C. longa*.

The insulin AUC was also significantly higher after ingestion of *C. longa*, 15, 30, 90, and 120 min after the OGTT.

The investigators concluded that 6 g of *C. longa* increased postprandial serum insulin levels but did not seem to affect plasma glucose levels or glycemic index in healthy people. The results indicate that *C. longa* may favorably affect insulin secretion (Wickenberg, Ingemansson, and Hlebowicz. 2010).

Curcumin is a major constituent of the rhizomatous powder of turmeric (*C. longa*) and is commonly used as food and medicine in southern Asia. According to a report in the journal *Current Pharmaceutical Design*, the turmeric rhizome holds antioxidant, anti-inflammatory, antidiabetic, and immunomodulatory constituents (Meng, Li, and Cao. 2013). More important, curcumin has been shown to delay the onset of Type 2 diabetes.

The journal *Diabetes Care* reported a clinical study that aimed to determine the efficacy of curcumin in delaying development of Type 2 diabetes in the prediabetic population. This trial included participants with prediabetes who were to receive either curcumin or placebo capsules for 9 months. To assess the progress of diabetes after curcumin treatments, and to determine the number of participants progressing to the disease, changes in β-cell functions (HOMA-β, C-peptide, and proinsulin/insulin), insulin resistance (HOMA-IR), anti-inflammatory cytokine (adiponectin), and other parameters were monitored at baseline and at 3-, 6-, and 9-month visits during the course of intervention.

It was found that after 9 months of treatment, 16.4% of participants in the placebo group were diagnosed with Type 2 diabetes, whereas none were diagnosed with that disorder in the curcumin-treated group.

In addition, the curcumin-treated group showed a better overall function of β-cells, with higher HOMA-β (61.58 vs. 48.72) and lower C-peptide (1.7 vs. 2.17). The curcumin-treated group showed a lower level of HOMA-IR (3.22 vs. 4.04) and higher adiponectin (22.46 vs. 18.45) when compared with the placebo group.

The investigators concluded that a 9-month curcumin intervention in a prediabetic population significantly lowered the number of prediabetic individuals who eventually developed diabetes. In addition, the curcumin treatment appeared to improve overall function of β-cells with very minor adverse effects, with higher homeostatic measurement assessment (HOMA-β) and lower C-peptide. Also, the curcumin-treated group showed a lower level of HOMA insulin resistance.

Therefore, this study demonstrated that the curcumin intervention may be beneficial in a prediabetic population (Chuengsamarn, Rattanamongkolgul, Luechapudiporn et al. 2012).

As noted above, another clinical study published in the *Nutrition Journal* showed that ingestion of turmeric increased postprandial serum insulin levels in healthy subjects (Wickenberg, Ingemansson, and Hlebowicz. 2010). These data suggest that curcumin, a bioactive compound of turmeric, ameliorates Type 2 diabetes by regulating insulin resistance and β-cell function. Furthermore, as reported in a study published in the *International Journal of Food Sciences and Nutrition*, turmeric volatile oils inhibited α-glucosidase enzymes more effectively than the reference standard drug acarbose. Drying of rhizomes was found to enhance the inhibitory capacities of the volatile oils against α-glucosidase (IC50 = 1.32–0.38 μg/mL) and α-amylase (IC50 = 64.7–34.3 μg/mL). Ar-Turmerone, the major volatile component in the rhizome, also showed potent inhibition of α-glucosidase (IC50 = 0.28 μg) and α-amylase (IC50 = 24.5 μg) (Lekshmi, Arimboor, Indulekha et al. 2012). Overall, turmeric exerts antidiabetic actions likely by regulating insulin resistance, β-cell function, and gut absorption.

9.9.6 DICAFFEOYLQUINIC ACIDS, MATESAPONINS, AND YERBA MATE TEA

Yerba mate tea is made from the leaves of mate, *Ilex paraguariensis* (Aquifoliaceae), which is gaining popularity in South America. A study published in the journal *Phytomedicine* aimed to determine the effects of an aqueous extract of mate (pronounced ma-tay) on metabolic syndrome features in a metabolic syndrome model Tsumura Suzuki obese diabetic mouse.

Oral administration of mate (100 mg/kg) for 7 weeks induced significant decreases in body weight, BMI, and food intake in the mice. It significantly decreased the hyperglycemia by reducing fasting blood glucose level and increasing glucose uptake in glucose tolerance test. It also showed significant improvement in insulin sensitivity by increasing glucose uptake in the insulin tolerance test, increasing quantitative insulin sensitivity check index, and decreasing HOMA of insulin resistance index.

The results also showed significant effects of mate on hyperlipidemia by decreasing blood levels of triglycerides, nonesterified fatty acids, and total cholesterol. Moreover, mate significantly improved adiponectin levels and exhibited significant reduction in white adipose tissue weight, as well as adiposity index.

The investigators concluded that mate ameliorates metabolic syndrome by mechanisms involving increase of peripheral insulin sensitivity and cellular glucose uptake and by modulating the level of circulating lipid metabolites and adiponectin (Hussein, Matsuda, Nakamura et al. 2011). Mate also induces significant decreases in food intake and weight gain in high fat diet–fed ddY mice. Furthermore, 3,5-O-dicaffeoyl quinic acid and matesaponin 2, two major constituents of mate, significantly elevated serum GLP-1 levels in ddY mice. However, neither of them inhibited DPP-4 activity (Hussein, Matsuda, Nakamura et al. 2011).

Collectively, these findings suggest that mate, and probably its active compounds, act as an antidiabetic medicine through augmentation of GLP-1 production.

Nevertheless, a systematic review and meta-analysis of the effectiveness of yerba mate (and other supplements) for body weight reduction, reported in the journal *Obesity Reviews*, concluded otherwise: The reviewed studies provide some encouraging data, but no evidence beyond a reasonable doubt, that any specific dietary supplement is effective for reducing body weight. The only exceptions were *Ephedra sinica*- and ephedrine-containing supplements—which have been associated with an increased risk of adverse events (Pittler, Schmidt, and Erns. 2005). The other supplements in the analysis not previously mentioned were chitosan, chromium picolinate, *Garcinia cambogia*, glucomannan, guar gum, hydroxy-methylbutyrate, plantago psyllium, pyruvate, and yohimbe.

9.9.7 GINGER (*ZINGIBER OFFICINALE*) AND GINGEROL

Ginger (*Z. officinale*) extract has hypoglycemic and insulinotropic effects (Priya Rani, Padmakumari, Sankarikutty et al 2011; Fritsche, Larbig, Owens et al. 2010; Islam, and Choi. 2008). One clinical study reported in the journal *Plant Foods for Human Nutrition* that consumption of ginger powder, 3 g/day for 30 days, significantly reduced blood glucose and lipids in Type 2 diabetes patients (Andallu, Radhika, and Suryakantham. 2003).

On the other hand, another study reported in the journal *Prostaglandins Leukotrienes and Essential Fatty Acids* stated that consumption of ginger powder, 4 g/day for 3 months, did not alter blood sugar and lipids in patients with coronary artery disease (Bordia, Verma, and Srivastava. 1997). This discrepancy is thought to result from variation in chemical composition of different ginger preparations.

9.9.8 EPIGALLOCATECHIN-3-GALLATE AND CHINESE TEA

Chinese tea is made from the leaves and leaf buds of the *Camellia sinensis* species. One of the claimed health benefits of this tea is reduction of Type 2 diabetes risk and amelioration of the disease. Chinese green tea and oolong tea have also been shown to prevent and/or ameliorate Type 2 diabetes in humans (Iso, Date, Wakai et al. 2006; Hosoda, Wang, and Liao. 2003; Hayashino, Fukuhara, Okamura et al. 2011).

Epigallocatechin-3-gallate (EGCG) appears to have multiple antidiabetic properties including increasing insulin secretion, increasing insulin tolerance, decreasing gluconeogenesis, islet and β-cell protection, and protection against β-cell apoptosis mediated by islet amyloid polypeptide *in vitro* (Ortsater, Grankvist, Wolfram et al. 2012; Wolfram, Raederstorff, Preller et al. 2006; Waltner-Law, Wang, Law et al. 2002; Meng, Abedini, Plesner et al. 2010). EGCG was also reported to activate AMPK in adipocytes (Hwang, Park, Shin et al. 2005).

On the other hand, the purpose of a study published in the *British Journal of Nutrition* was to investigate the effect of dietary supplementation with EGCG on insulin resistance and associated metabolic risk factors in humans, because animal evidence indicates that green tea may modulate insulin sensitivity, with EGCG proposed as a likely health-promoting component.

Overweight or obese men, aged 40 to 65 years, were randomly assigned to take 400-mg capsules of EGCG, or the placebo lactose, twice daily for 8 weeks. Oral glucose tolerance testing and measurement of metabolic risk factors (BMI, waist circumference, percentage body fat, blood pressure, total cholesterol, low-density lipoprotein (LDL) cholesterol, HDL cholesterol, skin tags) were conducted pre- and postintervention. Mood was also evaluated weekly using the University of Wales Institute of Science and Technology mood adjective checklist.

It was found that EGCG treatment had no effect on insulin sensitivity, insulin secretion, or glucose tolerance, but did reduce diastolic blood pressure (mean change: placebo, 0.058 mmHg; EGCG, 2.68 mmHg). No significant change in the other metabolic risk factors was observed.

The authors concluded that regular intake of EGCG had no effect on insulin resistance, but it did result in a modest reduction in diastolic blood pressure. This antihypertensive effect may contribute to some of the cardiovascular benefits associated with habitual green tea consumption (Brown, Lane, Coverly et al. 2009).

9.9.9 SOYBEAN

Soy protein and isoflavonoids in soybeans improve insulin resistance and enhance insulin release (Kwon, Hong, Lee et al. 2007). Genistein, a key isoflavone in soybean, has been reported to treat obesity and diabetes. This compound was shown to preserve islet mass by increasing β-cell count, proliferation, and survival in the pancreas (Behloul, and Wu. 2013).

The authors of a study published in the journal *Applied Physiology, Nutrition, and Metabolism* contend that while peripheral insulin resistance is common during obesity and aging in mice and people, the progression to Type 2 diabetes is largely due to loss of β-cell mass and function through apoptosis (Fu, Gilbert, Pfeiffer et al. 2012).

The investigators had reported that the soy-derived isoflavone, genistein, can improve glycemic control and β-cell function in insulin-deficient diabetic mice. However, it was not known whether it can prevent β-cell loss and diabetes in Type 2 diabetes mice.

Their study therefore aimed to determine the effect of dietary supplementation of genistein in a nongenetic Type 2 diabetes mouse model: Nongenetic, middle-aged obese diabetic mice were fed a high-fat diet and a low dose of streptozotocin by injection. The effect of dietary supplementation of genistein on glycemic control and β-cell mass and function was then assessed.

It was found that dietary intake of genistein (250 mg·kg^{-1} diet) improved hyperglycemia, glucose tolerance, and blood insulin level in obese diabetic mice, whereas it did not affect body weight gain, food intake, fat deposit, plasma lipid profile, and peripheral insulin sensitivity.

Genistein increased the number of insulin-positive β-cell in islets, promoted islet β-cell survival, and preserved islet mass. The authors therefore concluded that dietary intake of genistein could prevent Type 2 diabetes by a direct protective action on β-cells without alteration of peripheral insulin sensitivity (Fu, Gilbert, Pfeiffer et al. 2012; see also Fu, Zhang, Zhen et al. 2010). Moreover, its antidiabetic mechanism involves activation of protein kinase A and ERK1/2 (Hwang, Park, Shin et al. 2005).

A review, published in the *American Journal of Clinical Nutrition*, reported that nutritional intervention studies performed in animals and humans suggest that soy protein associated with isoflavones and flaxseed rich in lignans improves glucose control and reduce insulin resistance. In animal models of obesity and diabetes, soy protein has been shown to reduce serum insulin and insulin resistance. In studies on humans, with or without diabetes, soy protein also appears to moderate hyperglycemia and reduce body weight, hyperlipidemia, and hyperinsulinemia, supporting its beneficial effects on obesity and diabetes. Most of these clinical trials were relatively brief and conducted on a small number of patients.

It is not clear, therefore, that the beneficial effects of soy protein and flaxseed are due to isoflavones (daidzein and genistein), lignans (matairesinol and secoisolariciresinol), or perhaps other components. Isoflavones and lignans appear to act through various mechanisms that modulate pancreatic insulin secretion, or through antioxidative actions. They may also act *via* estrogen receptor–mediated mechanisms.

Some of these actions have been shown *in vitro*, but the relevance of these studies to *in vivo* disease is not known. The diversity of cellular actions of isoflavones and lignans supports their possible beneficial effects on various chronic diseases. Further investigations are needed to evaluate the long-term effects of phytoestrogens on obesity and diabetes and their possible complications (Bhathena, and Velasquez. 2002).

A study published in the journal *Physiology and Behavior* reported that soybean has also been shown to promote the secretion of insulin as well as GLP-1 (Haberer, Tasker, Foltz et al. 2011).

A review published in the *Journal of Agricultural and Food Chemistry*, reported that glyceollins, a phytoalexin found in soybeans, may play an important role in glucose homeostasis by regulating glucose utilization in adipocytes, and improving β-cell function and survival. Glyceollins improved insulin-stimulated glucose uptake in 3T3-L1 adipocytes without activating the PPAR-γ agonist. They decreased triacylglycerol accumulation in adipocytes.

In addition, glyceollins slightly improved glucose-stimulated insulin secretion without palmitate treatment in Min6 cells, and they potentiated insulinotropic actions when 500 μM palmitate was used to induce β-cell dysfunction. This was associated with decreased β-cell apoptosis because of the reduction of endoplasmic reticulum stress, as determined by mRNA levels of XBP-1, ATF-4, ATF-6, and CHOP. Glyceollins also potentiated GLP-1 secretion to enhance insulinotropic actions in enteroendocrine cells.

The investigators concluded that glyceollins help normalize glucose homeostasis by potentiating β-cell function and survival and by improving glucose utilization in adipocytes (Park, Ahn, Kim et al. 2010).

Soybean and/or its active components can treat Type 2 diabetes by multiple pathways, mainly involving insulin resistance, β-cell function, and GLP-1 production.

9.9.10   *ALOE VERA*

Extract of *A. vera* was shown to reduce hyperglycemia in diabetic patients. A study appearing in the journal *Hormone Research* aimed to determine the efficacy of *A. vera* in lowering blood glucose. In the first part of the study, the participants were patients with non–insulin-dependent diabetes; in the second part, Swiss albino mice were made diabetic using alloxan.

In patients, during the ingestion of aloe, half a teaspoonful daily for 4 to 14 weeks, fasting serum glucose level fell in every patient from a mean of 273 ± 25 (SE) to 151 ± 23 mg/dL with no change in body weight.

Second part: In normal mice, both glibenclamide (10 mg/kg twice daily) and aloe (500 mg/kg twice daily) induced hypoglycemia after 5 days (71 ± 6.2 and 91 ± 7.6 mg/dL, respectively). Only glibenclamide was effective in the first 3 days in control animals (130 ± 7 mg/dL). In the diabetic mice, fasting plasma glucose was significantly reduced by glibenclamide and aloe after 3 days. Thereafter, only aloe was effective, and by day 7, the plasma glucose was 394 ± 22.0 mg/dL versus 646 ± 35.9 mg/dL in the controls and 726 ± 30.9 mg/dL in the glibenclamide-treated group.

It was concluded that aloe contains a hypoglycemic agent that lowers the blood glucose by as yet unknown mechanisms (Ghannam, Kingston, and Al-Meshaal. 1986).

Another report published in the journal *Phytomedicine* investigated the effect of oral administration of one tablespoonful of *A. vera* juice, twice a day, for at least 2 weeks, in patients with diabetes. It was found that blood sugar and triglyceride levels in the treated group declined.

The results suggest the potential of *A. vera* juice for use as an antidiabetic agent (Yongchaiyudha, Rungpitarangsi, Bunyapraphatsara et al. 1996).

Aloeresin A, an active compound of *A. vera*, inhibited α-glucosidase activity. *A. vera* and probably its active compounds exert their antidiabetic actions by inhibition of α-glucosidase and intestinal glucose absorption. In addition, extract of *A. vera* resulted in a reduction of hyperglycemia and insulin resistance (Pérez, Jiménez-Ferrer, Zamilpa et al. 2007; Jong-Anurakkun, Bhandari, Hong et al. 2008).

Can consumption of *A. vera* prevent diabetes? A study published in the journal *Metabolic Syndrome and Related Disorders* was based on the contention that numerous animal trials have reported positive effects of *A. vera* in *in vivo* models of diabetes, but there is little by way of controlled clinical trials in patients with prediabetes. Therefore, they aimed to determine the effect of aloe compared to placebo on fasting blood glucose, lipid profile, and oxidative stress in participants with prediabetes/metabolic syndrome.

This pilot study of two aloe products (UP780 and AC952) recruited patients with prediabetes over an 8-week period. Qualifying participants had impaired fasting glucose, or impaired glucose tolerance, and at least two other features of metabolic syndrome.

Parameters of glycemia, fasting glucose, insulin, HOMA, glycosylated hemoglobin (HbA1c), fructosamine, OGTT, and oxidative stress (urinary F2-isoprostanes) were measured along with lipid profile and high-sensitivity C-reactive protein levels before and after supplementation.

It was found that there were no significant baseline differences between groups. Compared to placebo, only the AC952 *A. vera* inner leaf gel powder resulted in significant reduction in total and LDL cholesterol levels, glucose, and fructosamine.

In the UP780 *A. vera* inner leaf gel powder standardized with 2% aloesin group, there were significant reductions in HbA1c, fructosamine, fasting glucose, insulin, and HOMA. Only the UP780 aloe group had a significant reduction in the F2-isoprostanes compared to placebo.

The investigators concluded that standardized aloe preparations may be an adjunctive strategy to reverse the impaired fasting glucose and impaired glucose tolerance observed in conditions of prediabetes/metabolic syndrome (Devaraj, Yimam, Brownell et al. 2013).

As a whole, *A. vera* and its active components may treat diabetes *via* inhibition of α-glucosidase activity (gut glucose absorption) and decrease of insulin resistance.

9.9.11 Resveratrol

Resveratrol is a stilbene compound, commonly found in plants and their products, that has been demonstrated to treat diabetes and related complications in animal models (Ramadori, Gautron, Fujikawa et al. 2009; Aribal-Kocatürk, Özelçi Kavas, and Iren Büyükkağnici. 2007).

For instance, a report in the journal *Free Radical Biology and Medicine* concludes that insulin and resveratrol synergistically prevented cardiac dysfunction in diabetes and this may be in parallel with activation of the insulin-mediated Akt/GLUT4 signaling pathway. Although activation of the protective signal (Akt/GLUT4) and suppression of the adverse markers (iNOS, nitrotyrosine, and superoxide anion) were simultaneously observed in insulin and resveratrol combination treatment, insulin counteracted the advantage of resveratrol in diabetic patients with acute heart attack (Huang, Huang, Deng et al. 2010). The *American Journal of Physiology* reports that resveratrol protects against cardiac dysfunction in Type 2 diabetes by inhibiting oxidative/nitrosative stress and improving NO availability.

It has also been shown that resveratrol enhances glucose-mediated insulin secretion in cells by activating SIRT1, one of the cellular targets of resveratrol. A report in the *Journal of Biological Chemistry* concluded that resveratrol markedly enhanced the glucose response of INS-1E cells and human islets. This effect was mediated by and fully dependent on active SIRT1, defining a new role for SIRT1 in the regulation of insulin secretion (Vetterli, Brun, Giovannoni et al. 2011).

Finally, a clinical study published in the journal *Nutrition Research* concluded that resveratrol can improve glycemic control in Type 2 diabetes patients: The authors hypothesized that oral supplementation of resveratrol would improve glycemic control and the associated risk factors in patients with Type 2 diabetes.

Patients with Type 2 diabetes were sought from Government Headquarters Hospital, Ootacamund, India. The patients were assigned to a control or an intervention group. The control group received only oral hypoglycemic agents, whereas the intervention group received resveratrol (250 mg/day) along with their oral hypoglycemic agents for a period of 3 months. Hemoglobin A(1c), lipid profile, urea nitrogen, creatinine, and protein were measured at the baseline and at the end of 3 months.

The results showed that supplementation of resveratrol for 3 months significantly improved the mean hemoglobin A(1c) (mean ± SD, 9.99 ± 1.50 vs. 9.65 ± 1.54), systolic blood pressure (mean ± SD, 139.71 ± 16.10 vs. 127.92 ± 15.37), total cholesterol (mean ± SD, 4.70 ± 0.90 vs. 4.33 ± 0.76), and total protein (mean ± SD, 75.6 ± 4.6 vs. 72.3 ± 6.2) in Type 2 diabetes patients.

No significant changes in body weight and HDL and LDL cholesterols were observed.

It was concluded that oral supplementation of resveratrol is effective in improving glycemic control and that it may possibly provide a potential adjunctive treatment for management of diabetes (Bhatt, Thomas, and Nanjan. 2012).

Resveratrol ameliorates Type 2 diabetes and complications by the regulation of insulin resistance and β-cell functions.

9.9.12 Coffee

Several recent studies have demonstrated an association between coffee consumption and improved glucose tolerance and insulin sensitivity, as well as a lower risk of Type 2 diabetes. The *Journal of the American Medical Association* published a review aimed at determining the validity of the assertion that epidemiological evidence suggests that higher coffee consumption may reduce the risk of Type 2 diabetes.

The authors searched MEDLINE through January 2005 and examined the reference lists of the retrieved articles. Because this review focused on studies of habitual coffee consumption and risk of Type 2 diabetes, they excluded studies of Type 1 diabetes, animal studies, and studies of short-term exposure to coffee or caffeine, leaving 15 epidemiological studies (cohort or cross-sectional).

Nine cohort studies of coffee consumption and risk of Type 2 diabetes, including 193,473 participants and 8394 incident cases of Type 2 diabetes, were identified and the summary relative risks (RRs) were calculated using a random-effects model. The RR of type 2 diabetes was 0.65 for the highest (more than or equal to 6, or more than or equal to 7 cups per day) and 0.72 for the second highest (4 to 6 cups per day) category of coffee consumption, compared to the lowest consumption category (0 or less than or equal to 2 cups per day). These associations did not differ substantially by gender, obesity, or geographic region (United States and Europe).

In the cross-sectional studies conducted in northern Europe, southern Europe, and Japan, higher coffee consumption was consistently associated with a lower prevalence of newly detected hyperglycemia, particularly postprandial hyperglycemia.

It was concluded that habitual coffee consumption is associated with a substantially lower risk of Type 2 diabetes (Van Dam, and Hu. 2005).

The active compound(s) and responsible target(s) are not known. However, research findings suggest that constituents other than caffeine are active in glycemic control and/or insulin sensitivity: A study on people who consumed caffeinated and decaffeinated coffee published in the *Nutrition Journal* found no difference in the risk of Type 2 diabetes and insulin sensitivity in those drinking either type of coffee after 8 weeks of consumption. However, it was concluded that although no changes in glycemia and/or insulin sensitivity were observed after 8 weeks of coffee consumption, improvements in adipocyte and liver function as indicated by changes in adiponectin and fetuin A concentrations may contribute to beneficial metabolic effects of long-term coffee consumption (Wedick, Brennan, Sun et al. 2011).

Coffee is one of the major sources of dietary antioxidants. Roasting at high temperature can convert chlorogenic acid into quinides, which are known to reduce blood glucose levels in animal models. Adequate coffee consumption seems to be beneficial in ameliorating Type 2 diabetes and its complications (Shearer, Farah, De Paulis et al. 2003).

REFERENCES

Al-Romaiyan A, King AJ, Persaud SJ, and PM Jones. 2013. A novel extract of *Gymnema sylvestre* improves glucose tolerance in vivo and stimulates insulin secretion and synthesis in vitro. *Phytotherapy Research*, Jul; 24(9): 1370–1376. DOI: 10.1002/ptr.4815

Al-Romaiyan A, Liu B, Asare-Anane H, Maity CR, Chatterjee SK, Koley N, Biswas T, Chatterji AK, Huang GC, Amiel SA, Persaud SJ, and PM Jones. 2010. A novel *Gymnema sylvestre* extract stimulates insulin secretion from human islets in vivo and in vitro. *Phytotherapy Research*, Sept; 24(9): 1370–1376. DOI: 10.1002/ptr.3125.

Andallu B, Radhika B, and V Suryakantham. 2003. Effect of aswagandha, ginger and mulberry on hyperglycemia and hyperlipidemia. *Plant Foods for Human Nutrition*, Sept; 58(3): 1–7. DOI: 10.1023/B:Q UAL.0000040352.23559.04.

Aribal-Kocatürk P, Özelçi Kavas G, and D Iren Büyükkağnici. 2007. Pretreatment effect of resveratrol on streptozotocin-induced diabetes in rats. *Biological Trace Element Research*, Sept; 118(3): 244–249. DOI: 10.1007/s12011-007-0031-y.

Asgary S, Rahimi P, Mahzouni P, and H Madani. 2012. Antidiabetic effect of hydroalcoholic extract of *Carthamus tinctorius* L. in alloxan-induced diabetic rats. *Journal of Research in Medical Sciences*, Apr; 17(4): 386–392. PMCID: PMC3526135.

Attele AS, Zhou YP, Xie JT, Wu JA, Zhang L, Dey L, Pugh W, Rue PA, Polonsky KS, and S Yuan. 2002. Antidiabetic effects of *Panax ginseng* berry extract and the identification of an effective component. *Diabetes*, 51(6): 1851–1858. PMID: 12031973.

Basch E, Ulbricht C, Kuo G, Szapary P, and M Smith. 2003. Therapeutic applications of fenugreek. *Alternative Medicine Review*, Feb; 8(1): 20–27. PMID: 12611558.

Basu A, and TJ Lyons. 2011. Strawberries, blueberries, and cranberries in the metabolic syndrome: clinical perspectives. *Journal of Agricultural and Food Chemistry*, Jun; 60(23): 5687–5692. DOI: 10.1021 /jf203488k.

Behloul N, and G Wu. 2013. Genistein: a promising therapeutic agent for obesity and diabetes treatment. *European Journal of Pharmacology*, Jan; 698(1–3): 31–38. PMID: 23178528 DOI: 10.1016/j .ejphar.2012.11.013.

Bhathena SJ, and MT Velasquez. 2002. Beneficial role of dietary phytoestrogens in obesity and diabetes. *American Journal of Clinical Nutrition*, Dec; 76(6): 1191–1201.

Bhatt JK, Thomas S, and MJ Nanjan. 2012. Resveratrol supplementation improves glycemic control in type 2 diabetes mellitus. *Nutrition Research*, Jul; 32(7): 537–541. DOI: 10.1016/j.nutres.2012.06.003.

Bordia A, Verma SK, and KC Srivastava. 1997. Effect of ginger (*Zingiber officinale* Rosc.) and fenugreek (*Trigonella foenumgraecum* L.) on blood lipids, blood sugar and platelet aggregation in patients with coronary artery disease. *Prostaglandins Leukotrienes and Essential Fatty Acids*, May; 56(5): 379–384. PMID: 9175175.

Brown AL, Lane J, Coverly J, Stocks J, Jackson S, Stephen A, Bluck L, Coward A, and H Hendrickx. 2009. Effects of dietary supplementation with the green tea polyphenol epigallocatechin-3-gallate on insulin resistance and associated metabolic risk factors: randomized controlled trial. *British Journal of Nutrition*, Mar; 101(6): 886–894. DOI: 10.1017/S0007114508047727.

Bu T, Liu M, Zheng L, Guo Y, and X Lin X. 2010. α-Glucosidase inhibition and the in vivo hypoglycemic effect of butyl-isobutyl-phthalate derived from the *Laminaria japonica* rhizoid. *Phytotherapy Research*, Nov; 24(11): 1588–1591. DOI: 10.1002/ptr.3139.

Cani PD, Daubioul CA, Reusens B, Remacle C, Catillon G, and NM Delzenne. 2005. Involvement of endogenous glucagon-like peptide-1 (7–36) amide on glycaemia-lowering effect of oligofructose in streptozotocin-treated rats. *Journal of Endocrinology*, Jun; 185(3): 457–465. DOI: 10.1677/joe.1.06100.

Chandalia M, Garg A, Lutjohann D, Von Bergmann K, Grundy SM, and LJ Brinkley. 2000. Beneficial effects of high dietary fiber intake in patients with type 2 diabetes mellitus. *The New England Journal of Medicine*, May; 342(19): 1392–1398. DOI: 10.1056/NEJM200005113421903.

Chang CLT, Lin Y, Bartolome AP, Chen Y-C, Chiu S-C, and W-C Yang. 2013. Herbal therapies for Type 2 diabetes mellitus: chemistry, biology, and potential application of selected plants and compounds. *Evidence Based Complementary and Alternative Medicine*, vol. 2013, article no. 378657, 33 pages. DOI: 10.1155/2013/378657.

Chen C, Zhang Y, and C Huang. 2010. Berberine inhibits PTP1B activity and mimics insulin action. *Biochemical and Biophysical Research Communications*, Jul; 397(3): 543–547. DOI: 10.1016/j.bbrc.2010.05.153.

Chien SC, Young PH, Hsu YJ, Chen CH, Tien YJ, Shiu SY, Li TH, Yang CW, Marimuthu P, Tsai LF, and WC Yang. 2009. Anti-diabetic properties of three common *Bidens pilosa* variants in Taiwan. *Phytochemistry*, Jul; 70(10): 1246–1254. DOI: 10.1016/j.phytochem.2009.07.011.

Cho WCS, Chung WS, Lee SKW, Leung AWN, Cheng CHK, and KKM Yue. 2006. Ginsenoside Re of *Panax ginseng* possesses significant antioxidant and antihyperlipidemic efficacies in streptozotocin-induced diabetic rats. *European Journal of Pharmacology*, Nov; 550(1–3): 173–179. https://doi.org/10.1016/j.ejphar.2006.08.056.

Chuengsamarn S, Rattanamongkolgul S, Luechapudiporn R, Phisalaphong C, and S Jirawatnotai. 2012. Curcumin extract for prevention of type 2 diabetes. *Diabetes Care*, Nov; 35(11): 2121–2127. DOI: 10.2337/dc12-0116.

Couturier K, Qin B, Batandier C, Awada M, Hininger-Favier I, Canini F, Leverve X, Roussel AM, and RA Anderson. 2011. Cinnamon increases liver glycogen in an animal model of insulin resistance. *Metabolism*, Nov; 60(11): 1590–1597. DOI: 10.1016/j.metabol.2011.03.016.

DeFuria J, Bennett G, Strissel KJ, Perfield JW 2nd, Milbury PE, Greenberg AS, and MS Obin. 2009. Dietary blueberry attenuates whole-body insulin resistance in high fat-fed mice by reducing adipocyte death and its inflammatory sequelae. *Journal of Nutrition*, Aug; 139(8): 1510–1516. DOI: 10.3945/jn.109.105155.

Devaraj S, Yimam M, Brownell LA, Jialal I, Singh S, and Q Jia. 2013. Effects of *Aloe vera* supplementation in subjects with prediabetes/metabolic syndrome. *Metabolic Syndrome and Related Disorders*. Feb; 11(1): 35–40. DOI: 10. 1089/met.2012.0066.

Dey L, Xie JT, Wang A, Wu J, Maleckar SA, and CS Yuan. 2003. Anti-hyperglycemic effects of ginseng: comparison between root and berry. *Phytomedicine*, 10(6–7): 600–605. DOI: 10.1078/094471103322331908.

Feinle C, O'Donovan D, Doran S, Andrews JM, Wishart J, Chapman IK, and M Horowitz. 2003. Effects of fat digestion on appetite, APD motility, and gut hormones in response to duodenal fat infusion in humans. *American Journal of Physiology. Gastrointestinal and Liver Physiology*, May; 284(5): G798–G807. DOI: 10.1152/ajpgi.00512.2002.

Fritsche A, Larbig M, Owens D, and HU Häring. 2010. Comparison between a basal-bolus and a premixed insulin regimen in individuals with type 2 diabetes-results of the GINGER study. *Diabetes, Obesity and Metabolism*, Feb; 12(2): 115–123. DOI: 10.1111/j.1463-1326.2009.01165.x.

Fu Z, Gilbert ER, Pfeiffer L, Zhang Y, Fu Y, and D Liu. 2012. Genistein ameliorates hyperglycemia in a mouse model of nongenetic type 2 diabetes. *Applied Physiology, Nutrition, and Metabolism*, Jun; 37(3): 480–488. DOI: 10.1139/h2012-005.

Fu Z, Zhang W, Zhen W, Hazel Lum, Jerry Nadler, Bassaganya-Riera J, Jia Z, Wang Y, Misra H, and D Liu. 2010. Genistein induces pancreatic β-cell proliferation through activation of multiple signaling pathways and prevents insulin-deficient diabetes in mice. *Endocrinology*, Jul; 151(7): 3026–3037. DOI: 10.1210/en.2009-1294.

Fujii M, Takei I, and K Umezawa. 2009. Antidiabetic effect of orally administered conophylline-containing plant extract on streptozotocin-treated and Goto-Kakizaki rats. *Biomedicine and Pharmacotherapy*, Feb; 63(10): 710–716. DOI: 10.1016/j. biopha.2009.01.006.

Gao X, Li B, Jiang H, Liu F, Xu D, and Z Liu. 2007. Dioscorea opposita reverses dexamethasone induced insulin resistance. *Fitoterapia*, Jan; 78(1): 12–15. Epub 2006 Sep 23. DOI: 10.1016/j.fitote.2006.09.015.

Gentilcore D, Chaikomin R, Jones KL, Russo A, Feinle-Bisset C, Wishart JM, Rayner CK, and M Horowitz. 2006. Effects of fat on gastric emptying of and the glycemic, insulin, and incretin responses to a carbohydrate meal in type 2 diabetes. *Journal of Clinical Endocrinology and Metabolism*, Jun; 91(6): 2062–2067. DOI: 10.1210/jc.2005-2644.

Ghannam N, Kingston M, and IA Al-Meshaal. 1986. The antidiabetic activity of aloes: preliminary clinical and experimental observations. *Hormone Research*, 24(4); 288–294. PMID: 3096865.

Grace MH, Ribnicky DM, Kuhn P, Poulev A, Logendra S, Yousef GG, Raskin I, and MA Lila. 2009. Hypoglycemic activity of a novel anthocyanin-rich formulation from lowbush blueberry, *Vaccinium angustifolium* Aiton. *Phytomedicine*, May; 16(5): 406–415. DOI: 10.1016/j.phymed.2009.02.018.

Gram DX, Ahrén B, Nagy I, Olsen UB, Brand CL, Sundler F, Tabanera R, Svendsen O, Carr RD, Santha P, Wierup N, and AJ Hansen. 2007. Capsaicin-sensitive sensory fibers in the islets of Langerhans contribute to defective insulin secretion in Zucker diabetic rat, an animal model for some aspects of human type 2 diabetes. *European Journal of Neuroscience*, Jan; 25(1): 213–223. DOI: 10.1111/j. 1460-9568.2006. 05261.x.

Guo J, Li L, Pan J, Qiu G, Li A, Huang G, and L Xu. 2004. Pharmacological mechanism of Semen Litchi on antagonizing insulin resistance in rats with type 2 diabetes. *Journal of Chinese Medicinal Materials* (*Zhong Yao Cai*), Jun; 27(6): 435–438. PMID: 15524300.

Gupta A, Gupta R, and B. Lal. 2001. Effect of *Trigonella foenum-graecum* (Fenugreek) seeds on glycaemic control and insulin resistance in type 2 diabetes mellitus: a double blind placebo controlled study. *Journal of Association of Physicians of India*, Nov; 49: 1057–1061.

Habeck M. 2003. Diabetes treatments get sweet help from nature. *Nature Medicine*, 9(10): 1228.

Haberer D, Tasker M, Foltz M, Geary N, Westerterp M, and W Langhans. 2011. Intragastric infusion of pea-protein hydrolysate reduces test-meal size in rats more than pea protein. *Physiology and Behavior*, 104(5): 1041–1047. https://doi.org/10. 1016/j.physbeh.2011.07.003.

Han J, Lin H, and W Huang. 2011. Modulating gut microbiota as an anti-diabetic mechanism of berberine. *Medical Science Monitor*, 17(7): RA164–RA167. PMCID: PMC3539561.

Hayashino Y, Fukuhara S, Okamura T, Tanaka T, and H Ueshima. 2011. High oolong tea consumption predicts future risk of diabetes among Japanese male workers: a prospective cohort study. *Diabetic Medicine*, Jul; 28(7): 805–810. DOI: 10.1111/j. 1464-5491.2011.03239.x.

Heo SJ, Hwang JY, Choi JI, Han JS, Kim HJ, and YJ Jeon. 2009. Diphlorethohydroxycarmalol isolated from *Ishige okamurae*, a brown algae, a potent α-glucosidase and α-amylase inhibitor, alleviates postprandial hyperglycemia in diabetic mice. *European Journal of Pharmacology*, Aug; 615(1–3): 252–256. DOI: 10.1016/j.ejphar.2009.05.017.

Hosoda K, Wang F, and ML Liao. 2003. Antihyperglycemic effect of oolong tea in type 2 diabetes. *Diabetes Care*, Jun; 26(6): 1714–1718. PMID: 12766099.

Hsu JH, Wu YC, Liu IM, and JT Cheng. 2007. Dioscorea as the principal herb of Die-Huang-Wan, a widely used herbal mixture in China, for improvement of insulin resistance in fructose-rich chow-fed rats. *Journal of Ethnopharmacology*, Jul; 112(3): 577–584. DOI: 10.1016/j.jep.2007.05.013.

Huang JP, Huang SS, Deng Y, Chang CC, Day YJ, and LM Hung. 2010. Insulin and resveratrol act synergistically, preventing cardiac dysfunction in diabetes, but the advantage of resveratrol in diabetics with acute heart attack is antagonized by insulin. *Free Radical Biology and Medicine*, Dec; 49(11): 1710–1721. DOI: 10.1016/j. freeradbiomed.2010.08.032.

Hui H, Tang G, and VLW Go. 2009. Hypoglycemic herbs and their action mechanisms. *Chinese Medicine*, Jun; 4: 11. DOI: https://doi.org/10.11 86/1749-8546-4-11.

Huseini HF, Larijani B, Heshmat R, Fakhrzadeh H, Radjabipour B, Toliat T, and M Raza. 2006. The efficacy of *Silybum marianum* (L.) Gaertn. (silymarin) in the treatment of type II diabetes: a randomized, double-blind, placebo-controlled, clinical trial. *Phytotherapy Research*, Dec; 20(12): 1036–1039. DOI: 10.1002/ptr.1988.

Hussain SAR. 2007. Silymarin as an adjunct to glibenclamide therapy improves long-term and postprandial glycemic control and body mass index in type 2 diabetes. *Journal of Medicinal Food*, Sept; 10(3): 543–547. DOI: 10. 1089/jmf.2006.089.

Hussein GM, Matsuda H, Nakamura S, Akiyama T, Tamura K, and M Yoshikawa. 2011. Protective and ameliorative effects of mate (*Ilex paraguariensis*) on metabolic syndrome in TSOD mice. *Phytomedicine*, Dec; 19(1): 88–97. DOI: 10.1016/j.phymed.2011.06.036.

Hwang JT, Park IJ, Shin JI, Lee YK, Lee SK, Baik HW, Ha J, and OJ Park. 2005. Genistein, EGCG, and capsaicin inhibit adipocyte differentiation process via activating AMP-activated protein kinase. *Biochemical and Biophysical Research Communications*, Dec; 338(2): 694–699. DOI: 10.1016/j .bbrc.2005.09.195.

Hye YK, and K Kim. 2007. Protective effect of ginseng on cytokine-induced apoptosis in pancreatic β-cells. *Journal of Agricultural and Food Chemistry*, Mar; 55(8): 2816–2823. DOI: 10.1021/jf062577r.

Imanshahidi M, and H Hosseinzadeh. 2008. Pharmacological and therapeutic effects of *Berberis vulgaris* and its active constituent, berberine. *Phytotherapy Research*, Aug; 22(8): 999–1012. DOI: 10.1002/ptr.2399.

Islam MS, and H Choi. 2008. Comparative effects of dietary ginger (*Zingiber officinale*) and garlic (*Allium sativum*) investigated in a type 2 diabetes model of rats. *Journal of Medicinal Food*, Mar; 11(1): 152–159. DOI: 10.1089/jmf.2007. 634.

Islam MS, and H Choi. 2008. Dietary red chilli (*Capsicum frutescens* L.) is insulinotropic rather than hypoglycemic in type 2 diabetes model of rats. *Phytotherapy Research*, Aug; 22(8): 1025–1029. DOI: 10.1002 /ptr.2417.

Iso H, Date C, Wakai K, Fukui M, Tamakoshi A, and the JACC Study Group. 2006. The relationship between green tea and total caffeine intake and risk for self-reported type 2 diabetes among Japanese adults. *Annals of Internal Medicine*, Apr; 144(8): 554–562. PMID: 16618952.

Jong-Anurakkun N, Bhandari MR, Hong G, and J Kawabata. 2008. α-Glucosidase inhibitor from Chinese aloes, *Fitoterapia*, 79(6): 456–457. DOI: 10.1016/j.fitote.2008.02.010.

Jung M, Park M, Lee HC, Kang YH, Kang ES, and SK Kim. 2006. Antidiabetic agents from medicinal plants. *Current Medicinal Chemistry*, 13(10): 1203–1218. PMID: 16719780.

Kaur R, Afzal M, Kazmi I, Ahamd I, Ahmed Z, Ali B, Ahmad S, and F Anwar. 2013. Polypharmacy (herbal and synthetic drug combination): a novel approach in the treatment of type-2 diabetes and its complications in rats. *Journal of Natural Medicine*, Jul; 67(3): 662–671. DOI: 10.1007/s11418-012-0720-5.

Kawakami M, Hirayama A, Tsuchiya K, Ohgawara H, Nakamura M, and K Umezawa. 2010. Promotion of β-cell differentiation by the alkaloid conophylline in porcine pancreatic endocrine cells. *Biomedicine and Pharmacotherapy*, Mar; 64(3): 226–231. DOI: 10.1016/j.biopha.2009.09.025.

Kim HY, and K Kim. 2007. Protective effect of ginseng on cytokine-induced apoptosis in pancreatic β-cells. *Journal of Agricultural and Food Chemistry*, Mar; 55(8): 2816–2823. DOI: 10.1021/jf062577r.

Kim S, Jwa H, Yanagawa Y, and T Park. 2012. Extract from *Dioscorea batatas* ameliorates insulin resistance in mice fed a high-fat diet. *Journal of Medical Food*, Jun; 15(6): 527–534. DOI: 10.1089 /jmf.2011.2008.

Kim S, Shin BC, Lee MS, Lee H, and E Ernst. 2011. Red ginseng for type 2 diabetes mellitus: a systematic review of randomized controlled trials. *Chinese Journal of Integrative Medicine*, Dec; 17(12): 937–944. DOI: 10.1007/s 11655-011-0937-2.

Kim WS, Lee YS, Cha SH, Jeong HW, Choe SS, Lee MR, Oh GT, Park HS, Lee KU, Lane MD, and JB Kim. 2009. Berberine improves lipid dysregulation in obesity by controlling central and peripheral AMPK activity. *American Journal of Physiology*, Apr; 296(4): E812–E819. DOI: 10.1152 /ajpendo.90710.2008.

Kodera T, Yamada S, Yamamoto Y, Hara A, Tanaka Y, Seno M, Umezawa K, Takei I, and I Kojima. 2009. Administration of conophylline and betacellulin-δ4 increases the β-cell mass in neonatal streptozotocin-treated rats. *Endocrine Journal*, 56(6): 799–806. DOI: 10.1507/endocrj.K09E-158.

Kjems LL, Holst JJ, Vølund A, and S Madsbad. 2003. The influence of GLP-1 on glucose-stimulated insulin secretion. Effects on β-cell sensitivity in Type 2 and nondiabetic subjects. *Diabetes*, Feb; 52(2): 380–386. https://doi.org/10.2337/diabetes.52.2.380.

Kojima I, and K Umezawa K. 2006. Conophylline: a novel differentiation inducer for pancreatic beta cells. *International Journal of Biochemistry and Cell Biology*, 8(5–6):923–930. DOI: 10.1016/j .biocel.2005.09.019.

Kok NN, Morgan LM, Williams CM, Roberfroid MB, Thissen JP, and NM Delzenne. 1998. Insulin, glucagon-like peptide 1, glucose-dependent insulinotropic polypeptide and insulin-like growth factor I as putative mediators of the hypolipidemic effect of oligofructose in rats. *Journal of Nutrition*, Jul; 128 (7): 1099–1103. PMID: 9649591.

Kwon DY, Hong SM, Lee JE, Sung SR, and S Park. 2007. Long-term consumption of fermented soybean-derived Chungkookjang attenuates hepatic insulin resistance in 90% pancreatectomized diabetic rats. *Hormone and Metabolic Research*, Oct; 39(10): 752–757. DOI: 10.1055/s-2007-990287.

Lee BH, Hsu WH, and TM Pan. 2011. Inhibitory effects of dioscorea polysaccharide on TNF-α-induced insulin resistance in mouse FL83B cells. *Journal of Agricultural and Food Chemistry*, May; 59(10): 5279–5285. DOI: 10.1021/jf200651c.

Lee HJ, Lee YH, Park SK Kang ES, Kim HJ, Lee YC, Choi CS, Park SE, Ahn CW, Cha BS, Lee KW, Kim KS, Lim SK, and HC Lee. 2009. Korean red ginseng (*Panax ginseng*) improves insulin sensitivity and attenuates the development of diabetes in Otsuka Long-Evans Tokushima fatty rats. *Metabolism*, Aug; 58(8): 1170–1177. DOI: 10.1016/j.metabol.2009.03.015.

Lee WK, Kao ST, Liu LM, and JT Cheng. 2007. Ginsenoside Rh2 is one of the active principles of *Panax ginseng* root to improve insulin sensitivity in fructose-rich chow-fed rats. *Hormone and Metabolic Research*, May; 39(5): 347–354. DOI: 10.1055/s-2007-976537.

Lee YS, Kim WS, Kim KH, Yoon MJ, Cho HJ, Shen Y, Ye JM, Lee CH, Oh WK, Kim CT, Hohnen-Behrens C, Gosby A, Kraegen EW, James DE, and JB Kim. 2006. Berberine, a natural plant product, activates AMP-activated protein kinase with beneficial metabolic effects in diabetic and insulin-resistant states. *Diabetes*, Aug; 55(8): 2256–2264. DOI: 10.2337/db06-0006.

Lekshmi PC, Arimboor R, Indulekha PS, and AN Menon. 2012. Turmeric (*Curcuma longa* L.) volatile oil inhibits key enzymes linked to type 2 diabetes. *International Journal of Food Sciences and Nutrition*, Mar; 63(7): 832–834. http://dx.doi.org/10.3109/09637486.2011.607156.

Li C, Cao L, and Q Zeng. 2004. *Astragalus* prevents diabetic rats from developing cardiomyopathy by down-regulating angiotensin II type2 receptors' expression. *Journal of Huazhong University of Science and Technology*, 24(4): 379–384. PMID: 15587404.

Li J, Liu T, Wang L, Xu T, Guo X, Wu L, Qin L, and W Sun. 2012. Antihyperglycemic and antihyperlipidemic action of cinnamaldehyde in C57BLKS/J db/db mice. *Journal of Traditional Chinese Medicine*, Sept; 32(3): 446–452. https://doi.org/10. 1016/S0254-6272(13)60053-9.

Liu M, Wu K, Mao X, Wu Y, and J Ouyang. 2010. Astragalus polysaccharide improves insulin sensitivity in KKAy mice: regulation of PKB/GLUT4 signaling in skeletal muscle. *Journal of Ethnopharmacology*, Jan; 127(1): 32–37. DOI: 10.1016/j.jep. 2009. 09.055.

Luo JZ, and L Luo. 2009. Ginseng on hyperglycemia: effects and mechanisms. *Evidence-Based Complementary and Alternative Medicine*, Jan: 6(4): 423-427. DOI: 10.1093/ecam/nem178.

Mae T, Kishida H, Nishiyama T, Tsukagawa M, Konishi E, Kuroda M, Mimaki Y, Sashida Y, Takahashi K, Kawada T, Nakagawa K, and M Kitahara. 2003. A licorice ethanolic extract with peroxisome prolif-erator-activated receptor-γ ligand-binding activity affects diabetes in KK-Ay mice, abdominal obesity in diet-induced obese C57BL mice and hypertension in spontaneously hypertensive rats. *Journal of Nutrition*, Nov; 133(11): 3369–3377. PMID: 14608046.

Mao XQ, Yu F, Wang N, Wu Y, Zou F, Wu K, Liu M, and JP Ouyang. 2009. Hypoglycemic effect of polysac-charide enriched extract of *Astragalus membranaceus* in diet induced insulin resistant C57BL/6J mice and its potential mechanism. *Phytomedicine*, May; 16(5): 416–425. DOI: 10.1016/j.phymed.2008.12.011.

Marles RJ, and NR Farnsworth. 1995. Antidiabetic plants and their active constituents. *Phytomedicine*, Oct; 2(2): 137–189. DOI: 10.1016/S0944-7113(11)80059-0.

Meng B, Li J, and H Cao. 2013. Antioxidant and antiinflammatory activities of curcumin on diabetes mellitus and its complications. *Current Pharmaceutical Design*, 19(11): 2101–2113. PMID: 23116316.

Meng F, Abedini A, Plesner A, Verchere CB, and DP Raleigh. 2010. The Flavanol (−)-epigallocatechin 3-gallate inhibits amyloid formation by islet amyloid polypeptide, disaggregates amyloid fibrils, and protects cultured cells against IAPP-induced toxicity. *Biochemistry*, Sept; 49(37): 8127–8133. DOI: 10.1021 /bi100939a.

Min KH, Kim HJ, Jeon YJ, and JS Han. 2011. *Ishige okamurae* ameliorates hyperglycemia and insulin resis-tance in C57BL/KsJ-db/db mice. *Diabetes Research and Clinical Practice*, Apr; 2011 Jul; 93(1): 70–76. DOI: 10.1016/j.diabres.2011.03.018.

Mohan V, and M Balasubramanyam. 2001. Fenugreek and insulin resistance. *The Journal of the Association of Physicians of India*, Nov; 49: 1055–1056. PMID: 11868854.

Noh JS, Kim HY, Park CH, Fujii H, and T Yokozawa. 2010. Hypolipidaemic and antioxidative effects of oli-gonol, a low-molecular-weight polyphenol derived from lychee fruit, on renal damage in type 2 diabetic mice. *British Journal of Nutrition*, Oct; 104(8): 1120–1128. DOI: 10.1017/S0007114510001819.

Noh JS, Park CH, and T Yokozawa. 2011. Treatment with oligonol, a low-molecular polyphenol derived from lychee fruit, attenuates diabetes-induced hepatic damage through regulation of oxidative stress and lipid metabolism. *British Journal of Nutrition*, Oct; 106(7): 1013–1022. DOI: 10.1017/S0007114511001322.

Ogata T, Li L, Yamada S, Yamamoto Y, Tanaka Y, Takei I, Umezawa K, and I Kojima. 2004. Promotion of β-cell differentiation by conophylline in fetal and neonatal rat pancreas. *Diabetes*, Oct; 53(10): 2596–2602. https://doi.org/10.2337/diabetes. 53.10.2596.

Ortsater H, N. Grankvist N, S. Wolfram S, N. Kuehn N, and A. Sjoholm. 2012. Diet supplementation with green tea extract epigallocatechin gallate prevents progression to glucose intolerance in db/db mice. *Nutrition and Metabolism*, 9(article 11).

Oubré AY, Carlson TJ, King SR, and GM Reaven. 1997. From plant to patient: an ethnomedical approach to the identification of new drugs for the treatment of NIDDM. *Diabetologia*, May; 40(5): 614–617. DOI: 10.1007/s001250050724.

Park S, Ahn IS, Kim JH, Lee MR, Kim JS, and HJ Kim. 2010. Glyceollins, one of the phytoalexins derived from soybeans under fungal stress, enhance insulin sensitivity and exert insulinotropic actions. *Journal of Agricultural and Food Chemistry*, Jan; 58(3): 1551–1557. DOI: 10.1021/jf903432b.

Patel DK, Prasad SK, Kumar R, and S Hemalatha. 2012. An overview on antidiabetic medicinal plants having insulin mimetic property. *Asian Pacific Journal of Tropical Biomedicine*, Apr; 2(4): 320–330. DOI: 10.1016/S2221-1691(12)60032-X.

Pavithran K. 1994. Fenugreek in diabetes mellitus. *The Journal of the Association of Physicians of India*, Jul; 42(7): 584.

Pérez YY, Jiménez-Ferrer E, Zamilpa A, Hernández-Valencia M, Alarcón-Aguilar FJ, Tortoriello J, Román-Ramos R. 2007. Effect of a polyphenol-rich extract from *Aloe vera* gel on experimentally induced insulin resistance in mice. *American Journal of Chinese Medicine*, 35(6): 1037–1046. DOI: 10.1142/S0192415 X07005491.

Pittler MH, Schmidt K, and E Erns. 2005. Adverse events of herbal food supplements for body weight reduction: systematic review. *Obesity Reviews*, Apr: 6(2): 93–111. PMID: 15051593.

Priya Rani M, Padmakumari KP, Sankarikutty B, Lijo Cherian O, Nisha M and KG Raghu. 2011. Inhibitory potential of ginger extracts against enzymes linked to type 2 diabetes, inflammation and induced oxidative stress. *International Journal of Food Sciences and Nutrition*, Sept; 62(2): 106–110. http://dx.doi.org/10.3109/09637486. 2010.515565.

Qin B, Dawson HD, Schoene NW, Polansky MM, and RA Anderson. 2012. Cinnamon polyphenols regulate multiple metabolic pathways involved in insulin signaling and intestinal lipoprotein metabolism of small intestinal enterocytes. *Nutrition*, Nov–Dec; 28(11–12): 1172–1179. DOI: 10.1016/j.nut.2012.03.020.

Qin B, Panickar KS, and RA Anderson. 2010. Cinnamon: potential role in the prevention of insulin resistance, metabolic syndrome, and type 2 diabetes. *Journal of Diabetes Science and Technology*, May; 4(3): 685–693. DOI: 10.1177/193229681000400324.

Ramadori G, Gautron L, Fujikawa T, Vianna CR, Elmquist JK, and R Coppari. 2009. Central administration of resveratrol improves diet-induced diabetes. *Endocrinology*, Dec; 150(12): 5326–5333. DOI: 10.1210/en.2009-0528.

Ramkumar KM, Lee AS, Krishnamurthi K, Devi SS, Chakrabarti T, Kang KP, Lee S, Kim W, Park SK, Lee NH, and P Rajaguru. 2009. *Gymnema montanum* H. Protects against alloxan-induced oxidative stress and apoptosis in pancreatic β-cells. *Cellular Physiology and Biochemistry*, Jul; 24(5–6): 429–440. DOI: 10.1159/000257480.

Rui YC. 1991. Advances in pharmacological studies of silymarin. *Memorias do Instituto Oswaldo Cruz*, 86(Suppl 2): 79–85.

Saito R, Yamada S, Yamamoto Y, Kodera T, Hara A, Tanaka Y, Kimura F, Takei I, Umezawa K, and I Kojima. 2012. Conophylline suppresses pancreatic stellate cells and improves islet fibrosis in Goto–Kakizaki rats. *Endocrinology*, Feb; 153(2): 621–630. DOI: 10.1210/en.2011-1767.

Sasidharan S, Sumathi V, Jegathambigai NR, and LY Latha. 2011. Antihyperglycaemic effects of ethanol extracts of *Carica papaya* and *Pandanus amaryfollius* leaf in streptozotocin-induced diabetic mice. *Natural Product Research*, Dec; 25(20): 1982–1987. DOI: 10.1080/14786419.2010.523703.

Saxena A, and NK Vikram. 2004. Role of selected Indian plants in management of type 2 diabetes: a review. *Journal of Alternative and Complementary Medicine*, July; 10(2): 369–378. https://doi.org/10.1089/107555304323062365.

Seymour EM, Tanone II, Urcuyo-Llanes DE, Lewis SK, Kirakosyan A, Kondoleon MG, Kaufman PB, and SF Bolling. 2011. Blueberry intake alters skeletal muscle and adipose tissue peroxisome proliferator-activated receptor activity and reduces insulin resistance in obese rats, *Journal of Medicinal Food*, Dec; 14(12): 1511–1518. https://doi.org/10.1089/jmf.2010.0292.

Shearer J, Farah A, De Paulis T, Bracy DP, Pencek RR, Graham TE, and DH Wasserman. 2003. Quinides of roasted coffee enhance insulin action in conscious rats. *Journal of Nutrition*, Nov; 133(11): 3529–3532. PMID: 14608069.

Singh J, Cumming E, Manoharan G, Kalasz H, and E Adeghate. 2011. Medicinal chemistry of the antidiabetic effects of *Momordica charantia*: active constituents and modes of actions. *Open Medicinal Chemistry Journal*, Sept; 5(Supp 2): 70–77. DOI: 10.2174/1874104501105010070.

Stull AJ, Cash KC, Johnson WD, Champagne CM, and WT Cefalu. 2010. Bioactives in blueberries improve insulin sensitivity in obese, insulin-resistant men and women. *Journal of Nutrition*, Oct; 140(10): 1764–1768. DOI: 10.3945/jn.110.125336.

Subash Babu P, Prabuseenivasan S, and S Ignacimuthu. 2007. Cinnamaldehyde—a potential antidiabetic agent. *Phytomedicine*, Jan; 14(1): 15–22. DOI: 10.1016/j.phymed.2006.11.005.

Subash-Babu P, Ignacimuthu S, Agastian P, and B Varghese. 2009. Partial regeneration of β-cells in the islets of Langerhans by Nymphayol a sterol isolated from *Nymphaea stellata* (Willd.) flowers. *Bioorganic and Medicinal Chemistry*, Feb; 17(7): 2864–2870. DOI: 10.1016/j.bmc.2009.02.021.

Takahashi T, and M Miyazawa. 2012. Potent alpha-glucosidase inhibitors from safflower (*Carthamus tinctorius* L.) seed. *Phytotherapy Research*, May; 26(5): 722–726. DOI: 10.1002/ptr.3622.

Thanopoulou AC, Karamanos BG, Angelico FV, Assaad-Khalil SH, Barbato AF, Del Ben MP, Djordjevic PB, Dimitrijevic-Sreckovic VS, Gallotti CA, Katsilambros NL, Migdalis IN, Mrabet MM, Petkova MK, Roussi DP, and MT Tenconi. 2003. Dietary fat intake as risk factor for the development of diabetes: multinational, multicenter study of the Mediterranean Group for the Study of Diabetes (MGSD). *Diabetes Care*, Feb; 26(2): 302–307. PMID: 12547853.

Thomsen C, Storm H, Holst JJ, and K Hermansen. 2003. Differential effects of saturated and monounsaturated fats on postprandial lipemia and glucagon-like peptide 1 responses in patients with type 2 diabetes. *American Journal of Clinical Nutrition*, Mar; 77(3): 605–611.

Ubillas RP, Mendez CD, Jolad SD, Luo J, King SR, Carlson TJ, and MD Fort. 2000. Antihyperglycemic acetylenic glucosides from *Bidens pilosa*. *Planta Medica*, 66(1): 82–83.

Uemura T, Hirai S, Mizoguchi N Goto T, Lee JY, Taketani K, Nakano Y, Shono J, Hoshino S, Tsuge N, Narukami T, Takahashi N, and T Kawada.2010. Diosgenin present in fenugreek improves glucose metabolism by promoting adipocyte differentiation and inhibiting inflammation in adipose tissues. *Molecular Nutrition and Food Research*, Nov; 54(11): 1596–1608. DOI: 10.1002/mnfr.200900609.

Urías-Silvas JE, Cani PD, Delmée E, Neyrinck A, López MG, and NM Delzenne. 2008. Physiological effects of dietary fructans extracted from *Agave tequilana* Gto. and *Dasylirion* spp. *British Journal of Nutrition*, Feb; 99(2): 254–261. DOI: 10.1017/S0007114507795338.

Valette G, Sauvaire Y, Baccou JC, and G Ribes. 1984. Hypocholesterolaemic effect of fenugreek seeds in dogs. *Atherosclerosis*, Jan: 50(1): 105–111. PMID: 6696779.

Van Dam RM, and FB Hu. 2005. Coffee consumption and risk of type 2 diabetes: a systematic review. *Journal of the American Medical Association*, July; 294(1): 97–104, DOI: 10.1001/jama.294.1.97.

Vetterli L, Brun T, Giovannoni L, Bosco D, and P Maechler. 2011. Resveratrol potentiates glucose-stimulated insulin secretion in INS-1E β-cells and human islets through a SIRT1-dependent mechanism. *Journal of Biological Chemistry*, Dec; 286(8): 6049–6060. DOI: 10.1074/jbc.M110.176842.

Vuksan V, Sievenpiper JL, Koo VYY, Francis T, Beljan-Zdravkovic U, Xu Z, and E Vidgen. 2000. American ginseng (*Panax quinquefolius* L.) reduces postprandial glycemia in nondiabetic subjects and subjects with type 2 diabetes mellitus. *Archives of Internal Medicine*, Apr: 160(7): 1009–1013. PMID: 10761967.

Vuksan V, Sung MK, Sievenpiper JL, Stavro PM, Jenkins AL, Di Buono M, Lee KS, Leiter LA, Nam KY, Arnason JT, Choi M, and A Naeem. 2008. Korean red ginseng (*Panax ginseng*) improves glucose and insulin regulation in well-controlled, type 2 diabetes: results of a randomized, double-blind, placebo-controlled study of efficacy and safety. *Nutrition, Metabolism and Cardiovascular Diseases*, Jan; 18(1): 46–56. DOI: 10.1016/j.numecd.2006.04.003.

Vuong T, Benhaddou-Andaloussi A, Brault A, Harbilas D, Martineau LC, Vallerand D, Ramassamy C, Matar C, and PS Haddad. 2009. Antiobesity and antidiabetic effects of biotransformed blueberry juice in KKA y mice. *International Journal of Obesity*, Jun; 33(10): 1166–1173. DOI:10.1038/ijo.2009.149.

Waltner-Law ME, Wang XL, Law BK, Hall RK, Nawano M, and DK Granner. 2002. Epigallocatechin gallate, a constituent of green tea, represses hepatic glucose production. *Journal of Biological Chemistry*, Sept; 277(38): 34933–34940. DOI: 10.1074/jbc.M204672200.

Wedick NM, Brennan AM, Sun Q, Hu FB, Mantzoros CS, and RM van Dam. 2011. Effects of caffeinated and decaffeinated coffee on biological risk factors for type 2 diabetes: a randomized controlled trial. *Nutrition Journal*, Sept; 10 (article 93). https://doi.org/10.1186/1475-2891-10-93.

Weidner C, de Groot JC, Prasad A, Freiwald A, Quedenau C, Kliem M, Witzke A, Kodelja V, Han CT, Giegold S, Baumann M, Klebl B, Siems K, Müller-Kuhrt L, Schürmann A, Schüler R, Pfeiffer AF, Schroeder FC, Büssow K, and S Sauer. 2012. Amorfrutins are potent antidiabetic dietary natural products. *Proceedings of the National Academy of Sciences USA*, May; 109(19): 72577–72562. DOI: 10.1073/pnas.1116971109.

Wickenberg J, Ingemansson SL, and J Hlebowicz. 2010. Effects of *Curcuma longa* (turmeric) on postprandial plasma glucose and insulin in healthy subjects. *Nutrition Journal*, 9(1): article 43. https://doi.org/10.1186/1475-2891-9-43.

Wolfram S, Raederstorff D, Preller M, Wang Y, Teixeira SR, Riegger C, and P Weber. 2006. Epigallocatechin gallate supplementation alleviates diabetes in rodents. *Journal of Nutrition*, Oct; 136(10): 2512–2518. PMID: 16988119.

Wu F, and X Chen. 2004. A review of pharmacological study on *Astragalus membranaceus* (Fisch.) Bge. *Journal of Chinese Medicinal Materials* (*Zhong Yao Cai*), Mar; 27(3): 232–234.

Wu Y, Ou-Yang JP, Wu K, Wang Y, Zhou YF, and CY Wen. 2005. Hypoglycemic effect of Astragalus polysaccharide and its effect on PTP1B. *Acta Pharmacologica Sinica*, Mar; 26(3): 345–352. DOI: 10.1111 /j.1745-7254.2005. 00062.x.

Wu Z, Luo JZ, and L Luo. 2007. American ginseng modulates pancreatic beta cell activities. *Chinese Medicine*, 2(article 11). DOI: 10.1186/1749-8546-2-11.

Xie JT, Wang CZ, Ni M, Wu JA, Mehendale SR, Aung HH, Foo A, and CS Yuan. 2007. American ginseng berry juice intake reduces blood glucose and body weight in ob/ob mice. *Journal of Food Science*, 72(8): S590–S594. DOI: 10.1111/j.1750-3841.2007.00481.x.

Yongchaiyudha S, Rungpitarangsi V, Bunyapraphatsara N, and O Chokechaijaroenporn. 1996. Antidiabetic activity of *Aloe vera* L. juice. I. Clinical trial in new cases of diabetes mellitus. *Phytomedicine*, Nov; 3(3): 241–243. https://doi.org/10.1016/S0944-7113(96)80060-2.

Yoo KM, Lee C, Lo YM, and B Moon. 2012. The hypoglycemic effects of American red ginseng (*Panax quinquefolius* L.) on a diabetic mouse model. *Journal of Food Science*, Jul; 77(7): H147–H152. DOI: 10.1111/j.1750-3841.2012.02748.x.

Yun SN, Moon SJ, Ko SK, Im BO, and SH Chung. 2004. Wild ginseng prevents the onset of high-fat diet induced hyperglycemia and obesity in ICR mice. *Archives of Pharmacal Research*, Jul; 27(7): 790–796. PMID: 15357009.

Zhang H, and Y Teng. 1986. Effect of li ren (semen litchi) anti-diabetes pills in 45 cases of diabetes mellitus. *Journal of Traditional Chinese Medicine*, Dec; 6(4): 277–278. PMID: 3600021.

Zhang Y, Cai J, Ruan H, Pi H, and J Wu. 2007. Antihyperglycemic activity of kinsenoside, a high yielding constituent from *Anoectochilus roxburghii* in streptozotocin diabetic rats. *Journal of Ethnopharmacology*, Nov; 114(2): 141–145. DOI: 10.1016/j.jep.2007.05.022.

Zhao M, Zhang ZF, Ding Y, Wang JB, and Y Li. 2012. Astragalus polysaccharide improves palmitate-induced insulin resistance by inhibiting PTP1B and NF-kappaB in C2C12 myotubes. *Molecules*, Jun; 17(6): 7083–7092. DOI: 10.3390/molecules17067083.

10 Selected Botanicals and Plant Products That Lower Blood Glucose (Continued)

10.1 LYCHEE—LOWERING BLOOD SUGAR BY INHIBITING GLUCONEOGENESIS

It will be shown in the following chapter that white mulberry leaf, either as an extract or as tea, decreases absorption of sugars and carbohydrates by inhibiting the action of the enzyme α-glucosidase in the digestive tract. This inhibition lowers the rate of glucose absorption through delayed carbohydrate digestion and extended digestion time. There are other consumables that lower blood glucose by other means. Prominent among these is lychee (*Litchi chinensis*). Lychee contains the (potentially liver toxic) compound methylene cyclopropyl-alanine, also known as hypoglycin A (HGA), that induces hypoglycemia by inhibiting gluconeogenesis.

It is this substance in lychee that was implicated in the mystery illness that plagued and indeed killed a number of children in the town of Muzaffarpur in Bihar, India, in 1995 (Vashishtha. 2016).

Gluconeogenesis is the formation of glucose from precursors other than carbohydrates, especially by the liver and kidneys, using amino acids from proteins, glycerol from fats, or lactate produced by muscle during anaerobic glycolysis. It occurs primarily in the liver and kidneys whenever the supply of carbohydrates is insufficient to meet the body energy needs. Gluconeogenesis is stimulated by cortisol and other glucocorticoids and by the thyroid hormone thyroxine.

Lychee features prominently in glycemic control also for its contribution to the possible slowing of cataract formation, even prevention: Aldose reductase is the principal enzyme of the polyol pathway that plays a vital role in the development of diabetic complications including cataracts. Many phytochemical compounds in lychee have been reported to be aldose reductase inhibitors (Veeresham, Rao, and Kaleab. 2013; Lee, Park, Park et al. 2009). The aldose reductase and the polyol pathway and its role in cataract formation are detailed below.

10.1.1 Nutrients, Antioxidants, and Other Constituents of Lychee

The lychee is the fruit of an evergreen tree about 50 to 60 ft tall with foliage that resembles that of the Lauraceae family. The fruits mature in 80 to 110 days depending on the climate, location, and cultivar. They vary in shape from round to oval, to that resembling a heart. The thin, tough inedible skin is green when immature, ripening to red or pink-red, and is smooth or covered with small, sharp protuberances. It turns brown and dries when left out after harvesting.

The fleshy, edible portion of the fruit is an aril, an extra seed covering, surrounding one dark brown inedible seed. Some cultivars produce a high percentage of fruits that have shriveled, aborted, seeds known as "chicken tongues." These fruits typically bring a higher price because they have more edible flesh (Menzel, Christopher and Geoff. 2005).

L. chinensis belongs to the Sapindaceae family and is also well known to the Indian traditional healing system, Ayurveda, for its traditional uses. The parts of the plant used are leaves, flowers, fruits, seed, pulp, and pericarp. All parts of the plant are rich sources of phytochemicals:

- Epicatechin, procyanidin A2, and procyanidin B2
- Leucocyanidin, cyanidin glycoside, malvidin glycoside, and saponins
- Isolariciresinol
- Kaempferol
- Rutin
- Stigmasterol

Nutrients: Fresh whole lychee contains a total 72 mg of vitamin C per 100 g of fruit, an amount representing 86% of the daily value. On an average, consuming nine peeled lychee fruits will meet an adult person's daily vitamin C requirement, but other than that, the lychee supplies little nutrient content. A 100-g serving of raw lychee fruit provides about 7% of the copper, 4% of the phosphorus, and 4% of the potassium daily requirements. Lychees are low in saturated fat and sodium.

Phytochemicals: Leaves: (–)-Epicatechin, procyanidin A2, and procyanidin B2 (Castellain, Gesser, Tonini et al. 2014).

Fruit: 5-Hydroxymethyl-2-furfurolaldehyde, benzyl alcohol, hydrobenzoin, and (+)-catechin (Zhou, Wang, Yang et al. 2012).

Seed: Leucocyanidin, cyanidin glycoside and malvidin glycoside, and saponins.

Pericarp: A methylene-linked flavan-3-ol dimer, bis(8-epicatechinyl)methane (1) was recently isolated from the pericarps of *L. chinensis* Sonn. (Sapindaceae), together with dehydrodiepicatechin A (2), proanthocyanidin A1 (3), proanthocyanidin A2 (4), (–)-epicatechin (5), 8-(2-pyrrolidinone-5-yl)-(–)-epicatechin (6), (–)-epicatechin 8-C-β-D-glucopyranoside (7), naringenin 7-O-(2,6-di-O-α-L-rhamnopyranosyl)-β-D-glucopyranoside (8), and rutin (9) (Kilari, and Putta. 2016). It was the first report of compound 2 as a natural product, and compounds 6–8 from this species.

Compounds 1, 2, and 6–8 were evaluated for antioxidant activity. The ferric reducing antioxidant powers (FRAP) of compounds 1 and 6 were comparable to that of L-ascorbic acid, and the scavenging activities of compounds 1, 2, 6, and 7 toward 1,1-diphenyl-2-picrylhydrazyl (DPPH) radicals and 2,2′-azinobis(3-ethylbenzthiazoline-6-sulfonic acid) radical cations were more potent than those of L-ascorbic acid; compound 8 was weak in FRAP and DPPH assays (Ma, Xie, Li et al. 2014).

The journal *Fitoterapia* published a study titled "Characterization and preparation of oligomeric procyanidins from *L. chinensis* pericarp." The purpose of the study was to prepare A-type oligomeric procyanidins from litchee pericarp (*L. chinensis Baila*). The variety of oligomeric procyanidins in the sample was characterized by LC-ESI-MS analysis.

There were (+)-catechin, (–)-epicatechin, 12 dimers, and 6 trimers of procyanidins in litchee pericarp extracts. A-type procyanidins were much more abundant than B-type procyanidins.

The main flavan-3-ol monomer and oligomeric procyanidins in litchee pericarp were (–)-epicatechin, A-type dimers (A1 and A2), and trimer [epicatechin-(4β-8, 2β-O-7)-epicatechin-(4β-8)-epicatechin].

Procyanidin A1 [epicatechin-(4β-8, 2β-O-7)-catechin] was identified by nuclear magnetic resonance (NMR) in litchee pericarp for the first time. (–)-Epicatechin and oligomeric procyanidins were prepared by the combination of AB-8 column chromatography and Toyopearl HW-40S column chromatography.

It should be noted that the concentration of active constituents in lychee is not uniform across cultivars. A report in the journal *Molecules* aimed to determine the varietal differences in phenolic profiles and antioxidant activity of litchee fruit pericarp (LFP) from nine commercially available cultivars. The total phenolic and flavonoid contents ranged from 9.39 to 30.16 mg gallic acid equivalents/g fresh weight (FW) and from 7.12 to 23.46 mg catechin equivalents/g FW, respectively.

The total anthocyanin contents ranged from 1.77 to 20.94 mg cyanidin-3-glucoside equivalents/100 g FW. Three anthocyanins, including cyanidin-3-rutinoside, cyanidin-3-glucoside, and malvidin-3-glucoside, were detected, and cyanidin-3-rutinoside was the predominant constituent that contributes from 68.8% to 100% of the total anthocyanins, The total procyanidin contents ranged from 4.35 to 11.82 mg epicatechin equivalents/g FW.

Procyanidin B2, epicatechin, A-type procyanidin trimer, and procyanidin A2 were detected in all nine litchee varieties.

The oxygen radical absorbance capacity (ORAC) activities and DPPH radical-scavenging activities ranged from 430.49 to 1752.30 μmol TE/100 g FW and from 4.70 to 11.82 mg/g (IC50), respectively.

These results indicate that there are significant differences in phytochemical profiles and anti-oxidant activity among the tested varieties. Knowing the phenolic profiles and antioxidant activity of LFP of different varieties helps its potential health-promoting application (Li, Liang, Zhang et al. 2012).

A detailed review of the medicinal uses, phytochemistry, and pharmacology of *L. chinensis* appears in Mohamed and Ibrahim (2015) (*Journal of Ethnopharmacology*, Nov; 174: 492–513) and also in Chang, Lin, Bartolome et al. (2013) (Evidence Based Complementary and Alternative Medicine, 2013: 378657).

10.1.2 Methylene Cyclopropyl-Alanine (a.k.a. Hypoglycin A) and Gluconeogenesis

Gluconeogenesis is a metabolic pathway that leads to the synthesis of glucose from pyruvate and other noncarbohydrate precursors. It occurs in all microorganisms, fungi, plants, and animals, and the reactions are essentially the same, leading to the synthesis of one glucose molecule from two pyruvate molecules. Therefore, it is in essence glycolysis in reverse, the latter going from glucose to pyruvate, and glycolysis and gluconeogenesis share seven enzymes in common. In higher animals, gluconeogenesis occurs in the liver, renal cortex, and the epithelial cells of the small intestine (enterocytes).

The liver is the major site of gluconeogenesis, accounting for about 90% of the synthesized glucose, followed by kidney cortex with about 10%.

It is generally agreed that the constituent of lychee that interferes with sugar absorption causing hypoglycemia is methylene cyclopropyl-alanine (a.k.a. hypoglycin A) found in all parts of the lychee plant. Methylene cyclopropyl-alanine inhibits gluconeogenesis.

Gluconeogenesis and glycolysis are reciprocally regulated: Gluconeogenesis and glycolysis are coordinated so that, within a cell, one pathway is relatively inactive while the other is highly active. However, the amounts and activities of the distinctive enzymes of each pathway are controlled so that both pathways are not highly active at the same time. The rate of glycolysis is also determined by the concentration of glucose and the rate of gluconeogenesis by the concentrations of lactate and other precursors of glucose (Berg, Tymoczko, and Stryer. 2002).

10.1.3 Inhibition of Aldose Reductase May Prevent Cataract Formation

In Chapter 5, reference was made to the role of aldose reductase and the polyol pathway in the formation of cataracts. That issue is elaborated here in connection with the inhibitory action of extracts from lychee.

The *Journal of Enzyme Inhibition and Medicinal Chemistry* reported pharmacological investigations of the rat lens using extracts of the fruits of *L. chinensis* (Sapindaceae) to inhibit the action of the enzyme aldose reductase. There is published support for the theory that the initiating mechanism in diabetic cataract formation is the generation of polyols from glucose by aldose reductase, which results in increased osmotic stress in the lens fibers, leading in turn to their swelling, rupture, and opacification.

The extracts and organic fractions of *L. chinensis* tested yielded a methanol extract and an ethyl acetate fraction found to be potent inhibitors of rat lens aldose reductase (RLAR) *in vitro*, their IC50 values being 3.6 and 0.3 μg/mL, respectively. The IC50 is the concentration of an inhibitor where the response (or binding) is reduced by half.

From the active ethyl acetate fraction, four minor compounds with diverse structural moieties were isolated and identified as d-mannitol (1), 2,5-dihydroxybenzoic acid (2), delphinidin 3-O-β-galactopyranoside-39,59-di-O-β-glucopyranoside (3), and delphinidin 3-O-β-galactopyranoside-39-O-β-glucopyranoside (4).

The investigators concluded that delphinidin 3-O-β-galactopyranoside-39-O-β-glucopyranoside was the most potent aldose reductase inhibitor (IC50 = 0.23 μg/mL) and may be useful in the prevention and/or treatment of diabetic complications (Lee, Park, Park, et al. 2009).

The *Saudi Journal of Ophthalmology* supplied the following information about some fruits that inhibit aldose reductase (Kaur, Gupta, Christopher et al. 2017):

- *Belamcanda chinensis* (blackberry): Tectoridin, tectorigenin
- *Myrciaria dubia* (Rumberry): Ellagic acid
- *Syzygium cumini* (jamun): Ellagic acid
- *L. chinensis* (lychee): Delphinidin 3-O-β-galactopyranoside-3′-O-β-glucopyranoside
- *Citrus limon* (lemon): Rutin
- *Citrus aurantium* (orange): Rutin
- *Psidium guajava* (guava): Quercetin derivatives
- *Malus pumila* (apple): Quercetin, epicatechin, procyanidin
- *Vitis vinifera* (grapes): Citronellol

The importance of inhibiting aldose reductase is that the enzyme catalyzes the reduction of glucose to sorbitol through the polyol pathway, a process linked to the development of diabetic cataract. Extensive research has focused on the central role of the aldose reductase pathway as the initiating factor in diabetic cataract formation.

The high concentration of sorbitol leads to osmotic changes resulting in hydropic lens fibers that degenerate and form sugar cataracts (Kinoshita. 1974; Kinoshita, Fukushi, Kador et al. 1979). Sorbitol is produced faster than it can be converted to fructose in the lens by the enzyme sorbitol dehydrogenase. In addition, the polar character of sorbitol prevents its intracellular removal through diffusion. The increased accumulation of sorbitol creates a hyperosmotic effect that results in an infusion of fluid to countervail the osmotic gradient. The intracellular accumulation of polyols leads to a collapse and liquefaction of lens fibers, which ultimately results in the formation of lens opacities (Kinoshita. 1974; Kinoshita. 1965).

According to a detailed report in the *Journal of Ophthalmology*, these findings were the basis of the "Osmotic Hypothesis" of sugar cataract formation, emphasizing that the intracellular increase of fluid in response to aldose reductase-mediated accumulation of polyols results in lens swelling associated with complex biochemical changes ultimately leading to cataract formation (Kinoshita. 1974; Kinoshita, Fukushi, Kador et al. 1979; Kador, and Kinoshita. 1984).

The osmotic stress in the lens caused by sorbitol accumulation (Srivastava, Ramana, and Bhatnagar. 2005) induces apoptosis in lens epithelial cells (Takamura, Sugimoto, Kubo et al. 2001), which is another factor that contributes to the development of cataracts (Li, Kuszak, Dunn et al. 1995). Impairments in the osmoregulation may make the lens susceptible to even small increases of aldose reductase-mediated osmotic stress, potentially leading to progressive cataract formation.

A study reported in the journal *Investigative Ophthalmology and Visual Science* aimed to determine whether aldose reductase is linked to the development of adult diabetic cataracts. Levels of aldose reductase in red blood cells of patients under 60 years of age with a short duration of diabetes were positively correlated with the prevalence of posterior subcapsular cataracts (Oishi, Morikubo, Takamura et al. 2006).

A negative correlation was shown between the amount of aldose reductase in erythrocytes and the density of lens epithelial cells known to be decreased in diabetic individuals, compared to those nondiabetic (Kumamoto, Takamura, Kubo et al. 2007).

The polyol pathway has been described as the primary mediator of diabetes-induced oxidative stress in the lens. Osmotic stress caused by the accumulation of sorbitol induces stress in the endoplasmic reticulum, the principal site of protein synthesis, ultimately leading to the generation of free radicals. Endoplasmic reticulum stress may also result from fluctuations of glucose levels initiating an unfolded protein response that generates reactive oxygen species (ROS) and causes oxidative stress damage to lens fibers (Chung, Ho, Lam et al. 2003; Mulhern, Madson, Danford et al. 2006).

In addition to increased levels of free radicals, diabetic lenses show an impaired antioxidant capacity, increasing their susceptibility to oxidative stress. The loss of antioxidants is exacerbated by glycation and inactivation of lens antioxidant enzymes like superoxide dismutases (Ookawara, Kawamura, Kitagawa et al. 1992; Pollreisz, and Schmidt-Erfurth. 2010).

Parenthetically, copper-zinc superoxide dismutase 1 (SOD1) is the most dominant superoxide dismutase isoenzyme in the lens (Behndig, Karlsson, Johansson et al. 2001), which is important for the degradation of superoxide radicals ($O2^-$) into hydrogen peroxide (H_2O_2) and oxygen (McCord, and Fridovich. 1969).

More detailed information is available in a thorough review by Devalaraja, Jain, and Yadav (2011) (*Food Research International*, Aug; 44(7): 1856–1865). For additional tables, go to: https://www.ncbi.nlm.nih.gov/pmc/articles/PMC3156450/.

You will see their table of the biological activities of lychee ("Litchi") in Table 10.1.

The references are Guo, Li, Pan et al. (2004); Huang, and Wu (2002); Sakurai, Nishioka, Fujii et al. (2008); Kong, Zhang, Liao et al. (2010); Lee, Park, Park et al. (2009); Cheung, Mitchell, and Wong (2010); and Obrosova, Chung, and Kador (2010).

10.1.4 Multiple Protective Functions of Oligonol from Lychee

Oligonol is a polyphenol extracted from lychee fruit known in particular to be an antioxidant. However, it has also been shown to have many other benefits. For instance:

- It improved the lipid profile in a population of obese women (Bahijri, Ajabnoor, Hegazyx et al. 2017).
- It alleviated diet-induced insulin resistance by suppressing mTOR (mammalian target of rapamycin)/SREBP-1 (sterol regulatory element-binding protein-1)–mediated lipogenesis in liver and restoring insulin signaling in skeletal muscle (Wei, Chang, Chen et al. 2016).
- It suppressed inflammatory cytokine production from human monocytes (Lee, Shin, Kang et al. 2016).
- Oligonol is antioxidative and it reduces high-fat diet (HFD)–induced dysregulated expression of genes for adipokines in adipocytes (Sakurai, Nishioka, Fujii et al. 2008).
- Oligonol from lychee reduces diabetes-induced renal damage through the advanced glycation end product (AGE)–related pathway in an animal model (Park, Yokozawa, and Noh. 2014).
- It reduces the effect of oliginol on cortisol and related cytokines in healthy young men (Lee, Shin, Min et al. 2010).
- Oligonol prevents the impairment of endothelial nitric oxide synthase (eNOS) activity that is otherwise induced by high glucose, and it does so by reversing altered eNOS phosphorylation status (Zhang, Yokoo, Nishioka et al. 2010).

For additional references, go to oligonol published papers (https://www.aminoup.co.jp/researcher /papers/oligonol/).

The British Journal of Nutrition reported a study that identified the effects of oligonol derived from lychee fruit on oxidative stress and lipid metabolism in a Type 2 diabetes animal model. Oligonol was orally administered at 10 or 20 mg/kg body weight per day for 8 weeks to db/db mice, and its effects were compared with those of vehicle in db/db as well as in m/m mice. Serum and

TABLE 10.1
Biological Activities of *Litchi*

	Anti-Adipocity	Antihyperlipidemia/Dyslipidemia	Antihyperglycemia	Anti-Inflammation	Antioxidant	Other(s)
Litchi	Decreased body weight gain, which correlates with adipocity (Guo, Li, Pan et al. 2004)	Decreased total cholesterol, triaglycerol, free fatty acid, leptin in type II diabetic rats (Guo, Li, Pan et al. 2004)	Decreased blood glucose in type II diabetic rats (Guo, Li, Pan et al. 2004)	Decreased TNFα, increased PGE2 production in type II diabetic rats (Huang, and Wu. 2002; Guo, Li, Pan et al. 2004).	Dose-dependent free radical scavenging activity, decreased SOD and ROS levels in mouse adipocytes (Sakurai, Nishioka, Fujii et al. 2008; Kong, Zhang, Liao et al., 2010)	Reduced glucose induced cataract shown through aldose reductase in vitro (Lee, Park, Park et al. 2009; Cheung, Mitchell, and Wong. 2010; Obrosova, Chung, and Kador. 2010)

Source: From Devalaraja, Jain, and Yadav. 2011. *Food Research International*, Aug; 44(7): 1856–1865. With permission.

hepatic biochemical factors, and protein and mRNA expression related to lipid metabolism, were measured.

In the oligonol group, there was significant reduction of ROS, lipid peroxidation, and the chylomicron triacylglyceride (TAG) and total cholesterol concentrations in both the serum and liver. Oligonol reduced oxidative stress through the inhibition of AGE formation and its receptor expression. The augmented expressions of NF-κBp65 and of inducible NOS in the db/db mice were downregulated to the levels of m/m mice in the group treated with oligonol at 20 mg/kg.

It was also found in the db/db mice that treatment with lychee extracts caused a reduction of hepatic lipids, which resulted from the downregulation of both (1) the activity of SREBP-1 and (2) its target gene, which produces lipogenic enzymes in the liver.

The investigators concluded that oligonol has protective effects against ROS-related inflammation and excess lipid deposition in the Type 2 diabetic liver (Noh, Park, and Yokozawa. 2011).

A report in the journal *Bioscience, Biotechnology, and Biochemistry* described the antioxidative effects of oligonol (Amino Up Chemical Co., Ltd., Sapporo, Japan) in adipocytes: The levels of ROS and the expression of adipokine genes decreased in HW mouse white adipocytes with treatment with oligonol compared to that in control cells. The transcriptional activity of nuclear factor-kappaB (NF-κB) and the activation of extracellular signal-regulated kinase (ERK) 1/2 were also downregulated by oligonol. In addition, when C57BL/6J mice were fed an HFD for 5 weeks, the levels of epididymal white adipose tissue (WAT) mass and lipid peroxidation in WAT both increased, but oligonol intake clearly inhibited such HFD-induced increases. Furthermore, dysregulated expression of genes for adipokines in WAT of mice fed solely an HFD was attenuated by oligonol intake.

These results suggest that oligonol has antioxidative effects, and that it attenuates HFD-induced dysregulated expression of genes for adipokines in adipocytes (Sakurai, Nishioka, Fujii et al. 2008).

The journal *Food Science and Nutrition* reported an investigation of the value of the antidiabetic properties of α-glucosidase and aldose reductase inhibition, and antioxidant activity of selected folk remedies. It was found that lychee extract exhibited the best dose-dependent inhibitory activity against α-glucosidase with an IC50 of 10.4 mg/mL.

Interestingly, the antioxidant activities of selected fruits and vegetables were found related to their beneficial health effects, insofar as there was positive correlation between total flavonoid content and aldose reductase inhibitory activity (Wu, Luo, and Xu. 2015). The journal *Food Chemistry* reported a study that found that two flavanone compounds isolated from lychee seeds exhibited strong α-glucosidase inhibitory activity (Ren, Xu, Pan et al. 2011).

Parenthetically, the results from the Wu, Luo, and Xu (2015) study identified the potential antidiabetic function of fruits other than lychee: For example, blueberry and plum also inhibited α-glucosidase, with IC50 values of 13.0 and 10.9 mg/mL, respectively.

Plum was the second most effective α-glucosidase inhibitor compared to the IC50 of the selected samples. Plum contained the highest amount of total flavonoids (15.2 mg CE/g). The result supported other findings (Kim, Jeong, and Lee. 2003) that plums were good source of dietary flavonoids, which can also be regarded as α-glucosidase inhibitors (Gao and Kawabata. 2005).

For α-glucosidase, the IC50 values of extracts from all the selected samples including blueberry, lemon peel, and wolfberry were better than (lower than) those of the prescription medication acarbose. Nevertheless, the investigators wisely counseled that eating the fruits instead of relying on medications "is not recommended" (Wu, Luo, and Xu. 2015).

10.1.4.1 Safety of Oligonol

The journal *Food and Chemical Toxicology* published a report titled "Evaluation of the safety and toxicity of the oligomerized polyphenol oligonol." The report states that oligonol is an optimized phenolic product containing catechin-type monomers and lower oligomers of proanthocyanidin that result from the conversion of polyphenol polymers into oligomers.

In a single dose of 2000 mg/kg of body weight toxicity study, administration of oligonol by gavage for 4 weeks was found to be safe, with no side effects such as abnormal behavior or alopecia. Body weight gain and food consumption were within normal range. Oligonol had no observed toxicity at the dose 1/25 of the LD_{50}, administered for 6 months. This suggests that oligonol is probably safe for humans at repeated doses lower than 200 mg/day. The highest dose used in this study is equal to 12 g daily for an adult man with 60 kg body weight. The LD_{50} was calculated to be 5.0 g/kg body weight.

Studies conducted on healthy volunteers consuming oligonol at doses of 100 mg/day and 200 mg/day for 92 days showed good bioavailability. The biochemical parameters relating to liver and kidney function, as well as hematological parameters, were within normal ranges.

The potential of oligonol to induce gene mutation (a reverse mutation test) was tested using *Salmonella typhimurium* TA98, TA100, TA104, TA1535, TA153, as well as *Escherichia coli* WP2uvrA. Oligonol was not mutagenic to the tested strains. The lack of toxicity supports the potential use of oligonol as a food or dietary supplement and for use as an additive in pharmaceutical and cosmetic applications (Fujii, Sun, Nishioka et al. 2007). For those not wishing to take a supplement, eating lychees will provide at least some levels of this promising compound.

10.1.5 Lychee and Glycemic Control

In a report titled "Biological and phytopharmacological descriptions of *Litchi chinensis*," published in the journal *Pharmacognosy Review*, the investigators warn that "Lychee may lower blood sugar levels. Caution is advised when taking insulin or drugs for diabetes: consumption by mouth should be monitored closely" (Kilari, and Putta. 2016). In that review, they detail the description of lychee, its traditional medicinal uses, and phytoconstituents, and investigate the pharmacological activities in its various parts.

A report in the *Journal of Clinical Biochemistry and Nutrition* described a study aimed to evaluate the glycemic index and peak incremental indices of healthy participants to those with Type 2 diabetes consuming six popular fruits in Taiwan: grapes, Asian pears, guavas, golden kiwifruit, lychees, and bananas. Glycemic index values were tested according to the standard glycemic index testing protocol. The glycemic index and peak incremental indices were calculated according to published formulas.

In Type 2 diabetes participants, the glycemic index values were as follows:

- Grapes, 49.0 ± 4.5
- Asian pears, 25.9 ± 2.9
- Guavas, 32.8 ± 5.2
- Golden kiwifruit, 47.0 ± 6.5
- Lychees, 60.0 ± 8.0
- Bananas, 41.3 ± 3.5

In healthy participants, the glycemic index values were as follows:
- Grapes 49.1 ± 7.3
- Asian pears, 18.0 ± 5.4
- Guavas, 31.1 ± 5.1
- Golden kiwifruit, 47.3 ± 12.1
- Lychees, 47.9 ± 6.8
- Bananas, 35.1 ± 5.6

There was no significant difference in glycemic index values between healthy and Type 2 diabetes participants. There was also no significant difference in peak incremental indices when comparing healthy participants to those with Type 2 diabetes. It was concluded that glycemic index and peak incremental indices in healthy participants can be approximately the same for Type 2 diabetes (Chen, Wu, Weng et al. 2011).

Section 10.1.8 will provide some caveats and limitations on the use of lychee nuts for the control of hyperglycemia.

10.1.6 Effect of Lychee Fruit Extract (Oligonol) on Peripheral Circulation

As noted in Chapter 3, Type 2 diabetes has an adverse impact on cardiovascular and heart action because it jeopardizes blood circulation. One of the ways that it does that is by jeopardizing endothelial blood vessel relaxation by the NO pathway.

The *Natural Medicine Journal* reported a pilot study where skin thermography showed the vasodilation effects of the polyphenol oligonol. The authors maintained that poor blood circulation often manifests as small but chronic temperature differences in the peripheral extremities and that the surface of the skin may be an indication of abnormal blood flow and, thus, more serious vascular or circulation disorders.

This is illustrated in their Figure 4. See Kitadate, Aoyagi, and Homma (2014) [*Natural Medicine Journal*, Jul; 6(7)], which can be accessed at https://www.naturalmedicinejournal.com/journal/2014 -07/effect-lychee-fruit-extract-oligonol-peripheral-circulation-pilot-study (accessed 2.9.18). Areas of skin showing a red or yellow color are warmer, while blue and green areas are colder. The results suggested that oligonol might act as a vasodilator and be an effective treatment for a variety of vasoconstriction symptoms such as cold hands and feet, shoulder discomfort, and diabetes-related vascular problems (Kitadate, Aoyagi, and Homma. 2014). The thermograph appears to represent symptoms of Raynaud's disease. The study makes no mention of that.

10.1.7 Antioxidant Activity of Lychee

Reporting in the journal *Molecules*, investigators identified polysaccharides with strong antioxidant activity in *L. chinensis* Sonn. Four different polysaccharide-enriched fractions were isolated from lychee pulp tissue and were partially purified by standard preparation and determination by gas chromatography and infrared spectrophotometry.

These four polysaccharide-enriched fractions exhibited a dose-dependent free radical scavenging activity as shown by their DPPH radical, superoxide anion and hydroxyl radical quenching, chelating ability, and reducing power. Among the different fractions, LFP-III showed the strongest scavenging activity against 2,2-diphenyl-2-picrylhydrazyl hydrate (DPPH) radical, superoxide and hydroxyl radicals, and chelating ability.

These findings suggested to the authors that lychee polysaccharides from pulp tissue have a potential as *functional foods* with enhanced antioxidant activity (Kong, Zhang, Liao et al. 2010).

Likewise, the journal *Food Chemistry* reported the phenolic profiles and antioxidant activity of 13 varieties of lychee pulp. The free, bound, and total phenolic contents were 66.17–226.03, 11.18–40.54, and 101.51–259.18 mg of gallic acid equivalents/100 g, respectively.

The free, bound, and total flavonoid contents were 16.68–110.33, 10.48–22.75, and 39.43–129.86 mg of catechin equivalents/100 g, respectively.

Free phenolics and flavonoids contributed on average 80.1% and 75% to their total contents, respectively. Six individual phenolics [gallic acid, chlorogenic acid, (+)-catechin, caffeic acid, (−)-epicatechin, and rutin] were detected in lychee pulp by high-performance liquid chromatography (HPLC). The contents of each compound in free and bound fractions were determined.

Significant varietal differences in antioxidant activity were also found by FRAP and DPPH scavenging capacity methods. Antioxidant activity was significantly correlated with phenolic and flavonoid contents. Phenolics and flavonoids exist mainly in the free form in lychee pulp.

There were significant varietal differences in phytochemical contents and antioxidant activity of lychee pulp (Zhang, Zeng, Deng et al. 2013).

A study of lychee pericarp methanol extracts, published in the journal *Food Chemistry*, reported finding a novel phenolic, 2-(2-hydroxyl-5-(methoxycarbonyl) phenoxy)benzoic acid compound, together with kaempferol, isolariciresinol, stigmasterol, butylated hydroxytoluene, 3,4-dihydroxyl benzoate, methyl shikimate, and ethyl shikimate.

Antioxidant activity of the compounds was determined by a DPPH radical scavenging assay, and the results showed that 2-(2-hydroxy-5-(methoxycarbonyl) phenoxy)benzoic acid, kaempferol, isolariciresinol, butylated hydroxytoluene, and 3,4-dihydroxy benzoate exhibited good antioxidant activities. An interesting finding was that butylated hydroxytoluene, generally understood to be a synthetic antioxidant used as a food preservative, was detected as a natural antioxidant in this analysis. The novel compound exhibited no inhibitory effects against tyrosinase and α-glucosidase activities (Jiang, Lin, Wen et al. 2013).

The journal *PLoS One* reported a study that evaluated the content of total proanthocyanidins in lychee (*L. chinensis* Sonn.) pulp of 32 cultivars as well as the total phenolics, and flavonoids, for antioxidant activity.

One cultivar, Hemaoli, showed the highest total proanthocyanidins and total phenolics, and DPPH or ABTS radical scavenging activities. ESI-MS and NMR analysis of the Hemaoli pulp crude extracts (HPCE) showed that procyanidins composed of (epi)catechin units with a degree of polymerization of 2–6 were dominant proanthocyanidins in HPCE.

After the HPCE was fractionated by a Sephadex LH-20 column, 32 procyanidins were identified by LC-ESI-Q-TOF-MS in lychee pulp for the first time. Quantification of individual procyanidin in HPCE indicated that epicatechin, procyanidin B2, procyanidin C1, and A-type procyanidin trimer were the main procyanidins.

The radical scavenging activities of different fractions of HPCE as well as six procyanidin standards were evaluated by both DPPH and ABTS assays. HPCE fractions showed similar antioxidant activities with those of ascorbic acid (Vc), and six individual procyanidins, the IC50 of which ranged from 1.88 ± 0.01 to 2.82 ± 0.10 μg/mL for the DPPH assay and from 1.52 ± 0.17 to 2.71 ± 0.15 μg/mL for the ABTS assay.

The investigators concluded that these results indicate that lychee cultivars rich in proanthocyanidins are good sources of dietary antioxidants and have the potential to contribute to human health (Lv, Luo, Zhao et al. 2015).

Likewise, the journal *Food Chemistry* reported finding that lychee pulp contains phenolic compounds that are strong antioxidants. In that study, the major contributors to the antioxidant activity of fresh lychee pulp were identified as well as their cellular antioxidant activity. Aqueous acetone extracts of lychee pulp were fractionated on polyamide resin, and those fractions with the largest antioxidant and radical scavenging activities were selected using cellular antioxidant activity and oxygen radical absorbance capacity assays.

Three compounds that were major contributors to the antioxidant activity in these fractions were obtained by reverse-phase preparative HPLC and identified as quercetin 3-O-rutinoside-7-O-α-L-rhamnosidase (quercetin 3-rut-7-rha), quercetin 3-O-rutinoside (rutin), and (−)-epicatechin, using NMR spectroscopy, HMBC, and ESI-MS spectrometry. The concentration of quercetin 3-rut-7-rha was 17.25 mg per 100 g of lychee pulp fresh weight.

The investigators concluded that this is the identification and definition of the cellular antioxidant activity of quercetin 3-rut-7-rha from lychee pulp (Su, Ti, Zhang et al. 2014).

10.1.8 Lychee: Cautions, Contraindications, and Interactions with Medications

Lychee may lower blood sugar levels and therefore caution is advised when taking insulin or other drugs for diabetes: consumption by mouth should be monitored closely, especially just before elective surgery.

Methylenecyclopropylglycine (MCPG) and HGA are naturally occurring amino acids found in some soapberry fruits. Lychee is the Chinese tropical fruit tree *L. chinensis*, of the soapberry family. Fatalities have been reported worldwide as a result of HGA ingestion, and exposure to MCPG has been implicated recently in the Asian outbreaks of hypoglycemic encephalopathy.

In response to an outbreak linked to soapberry ingestion, the authors of a study published in the *Journal of Agricultural and Food Chemistry* developed the first method to simultaneously quantify MCPG and HGA in soapberry fruits from 1 to 10,000 parts per million of both toxins in dried fruit aril. Further, this is the first report of HGA in litchi, longan, and mamoncillo arils. This method is presented to specifically address the laboratory needs of public health investigators in the hypoglycemic encephalitis outbreaks linked to soapberry fruit ingestion (Isenberg, Carter, Hayes et al. 2016).

Lychee may increase the risk of bleeding when taken with drugs including aspirin, anticoagulants such as warfarin or heparin, antiplatelet drugs such as clopidogrel, and nonsteroidal anti-inflammatory drugs such as ibuprofen or naproxen. It also interacts with anticancer agents, anti-inflammatory agents, antivirals, cardiovascular agents, cholesterol- or lipid-lowering agents, immune modulating agents, and pain relievers.

Lychee may also increase the risk of bleeding when taken with herbs and supplements that are believed to increase the risk of bleeding. Multiple cases of bleeding have been reported with the simultaneous use of *Ginkgo biloba*, and fewer cases with garlic and saw palmetto (Kilari, and Putta. 2016).

Given the serious adverse events that lychee nuts can cause (hypoglycemia, hypoglycemic encephalopathy, and bleeding if ingested while on medications and/or nutraceuticals that are anticoagulants), we *advise against* consuming lychee nuts on a regular basis, as a means to control blood sugar (or otherwise), or to exercise great caution in doing so. It is not as benign as it appears to be. Lychee is one example among many of fruits that can be toxic.

10.2 MILK THISTLE (*SILYBUM MARIANUM*)

Milk thistle (*S. marianum*, family Asteraceae) is a traditional medicine that has been well researched for the treatment of liver disease. The active complex of milk thistle is a lipophilic extract from the seeds of the plant, and is composed of three isomer flavonolignans (silybin, silydianin, and silychristin) collectively known as silymarin.

Silybin is the component with the greatest degree of biological activity and makes up 50% to 70% of silymarin. Silymarin is found in the entire plant, but is concentrated in the fruit and seeds.

Silymarin functions as an antioxidant by reducing free radical production and lipid peroxidation. It has antifibrotic activity and may act as a toxin blockade agent by inhibiting binding of toxins to the hepatocyte cell membrane receptors.

In animal models, silymarin has been shown to reduce liver injury caused by acetaminophen, carbon tetrachloride, radiation, iron overload, phenylhydrazine, alcohol, cold ischemia, and *Amanita phalloides*—commonly known as the "Death Cap mushroom," a deadly poisonous basidiomycete fungus, one of many in the genus *Amanita*.

Silymarin has been used to treat alcoholic liver disease, acute and chronic viral hepatitis, and toxin-induced liver diseases (Abenavoli, Capasso, Milic et al. 2010).

10.2.1 Composition of Milk Thistle

The thistles contain

- Silymarin at 1.5% to 3% of dry weight (to be elucidated later)
- Silyhermin and both Neosilyhermin A and B
- Protein and mucilage (taking up 25% to 30% of the herb by dry weight)
- Quercetin and the dihydro variant known as taxifolin
- Kaempferol, dihydrokaempferol, and the 7-glucoside and 3-sulfate of kaempferol
- Apigenin (and 7-O-glucoside, 4,7-diglucoside, and 7-O-glucuronide)
- Eriodyctiol, chrysoeriol, and naringin
- 5,7-Dihydroxychromone

- Vitamin E at 0.038%
- Sterols (cholesterol, campesterol, stigmasterol, and sitosterol) at 0.63%

The leaves further contain

- Luteolin and its 7-O-glucoside
- Triterpene acetate
- Fumaric acid (Abenavoli, Capasso, Milic et al. 2010)

When processed into an ethanolic extract and sold as milk thistle extract (the most common supplemental form), the composition tends to be

- 65% to 80% silymarin (concentrated from 1.5% to 3% of the plant) (Kroll, Shaw, and Oberlies. 2007)
- 20% to 35% fatty acids (approximately linoleic at 60%, oleic at 30%, and palmitic at 9% (Abenavoli, Capasso, Milic et al. 2010)

The silymarin component specifically includes

- Silybinin (diastereoisomeric blend of silybinin A and silybinin B; Kroll, Shaw, and Oberlies. 2007; Kim, Graf, Sparacino et al. 2003; Lee, and Liu. 2003), which comprises 50%–70% of silymarin (and, by extension, 39% to 56% of milk thistle extract)
- Isosilibin (isosilybin A and isosilybin B comprising about 5% of silymarin; Kroll, Shaw, and Oberlies. 2007; Kim, Graf, Sparacino et al. 2003; Lee, and Liu. 2003)
- Silychristine and isosilychristine at around 20% silymarin (Kim, Graf, Sparacino et al. 2003)
- Silydianin at around 10% silymarin (Kim, Graf, Sparacino et al. 2003)
- Taxifolin (quercetin conjugate known as dihydroquercetin) usually in nearly undetectable levels (Kim, Graf, Sparacino et al. 2003)

The term "flavonolignans" is used to refer to seven compounds with the prefix sily- or isosily- (Kroll, Shaw, and Oberlies. 2007). These compounds are shown at the website https://examine.com /supplements/milk-thistle/#ref4.

Milk thistle as an herb contains a variety of compounds, but most studies use an ethanolic extract with a high silymarin component; this silymarin component is mostly just seven flavonolignans that are seen as unique to milk thistle.

10.2.2 Pharmacology—Absorption

A phytosome is a complex of natural active ingredient and a phospholipid—mostly lecithin. It is claimed that a phytosome formulation increases absorption of conventional herbal extracts or isolated active principles, both topically and orally. Phytosomes are said to enhance the bioavailability of milk thistle supplements and are commercially available.

Enzymatic Interactions: Silymarin (mixture) appears to inhibit the enzyme xanthine oxidase, with an IC50 of 27.58 ± 3.48 mM and a K_i of 5.85 mM *in vitro via* mixed (noncompetitive and uncompetitive) inhibition (Sheu, Lai, and Chiang. 1998). When assessing the silibinin content (isomeric mixture), 50 μM of silybinin can reduce superoxide production by xanthine oxidase by 20% and still confer inhibition of the enyzme, this effect apparently having a potency comparable to that of allopurinol *in vitro*; yet, it conferred less inhibition than both quercetin and luteolin (all at the same concentrations) (Pauff, and Hille. 2009).

Silymarin (mixture) at 50 µM has been shown to accumulate daunomycin, the substrate of P-glycoprotein (P-Gp), in cells expressing P-Gp, with no effect on cells that do not express P-Gp. This study noted accumulation of 445% ± 12%, which was similar to phloretin and slightly less than Morin (from *Morus alba*) and Biochanin A (Zhang, and Morris. 2003). Silymarin did not appear to influence the protein content of P-Gp, did not interact with the ATPase activity of P-Gp, and inhibited vermapril-induced ATPase activity on P-Gp; the inhibition at 100 µM reaches 61.2% ± 20.7% *in vitro*, comparable to that of vinblastine (Zhang, and Morris. 2003).

A study reported in the *Journal of Pharmacology and Experimental Therapeutics* noted enhancement of doxorubicin cytotoxicity due to P-Gp inhibition, which has been noted in prostatic cells due to silybinin (Tyagi, Singh, Agarwal et al. 2002) and noted elsewhere with silybin (Maitrejean, Comte, Barron et al. 2000), and the lack of changes to P-Gp protein content was replicated over 24 h (Tyagi, Singh, Agarwal et al. 2002; Zhou, Lim, and Chowbay. 2004).

This inhibition of P-glycoprotein has been demonstrated *in vivo* to aid in the absorption of berberine when berberine is taken with 105 mg of milk thistle (60% flavonolignans) (see Chapter 11) (Di Pierro, Villanova, Agostini et al. 2012), but another study using 300 mg (80% silymarin) three times a day failed to find significant alterations to digoxin kinetics (Gurley, Barone, Williams et al. 2006) (see also https://examine. com/supplements/milk-thistle/).

10.2.3 MILK THISTLE AND HYPERGLYCEMIA

The *Review of Diabetic Studies* reports that apart from its use in liver and gallbladder disorders, milk thistle has recently gained attention because of its hypoglycemic and hypolipidemic properties. A substance from milk thistle has been shown to possess peroxisome proliferator-activated receptor γ (PPARγ) agonist properties.

PPARγ is the molecular target of thiazolidinediones, which are used clinically as insulin sensitizers to lower blood glucose levels in Type 2 diabetes patients. The thiazolidinedione type of PPARγ ligands is an agonist with a very high binding affinity. However, this ligand type demonstrates a range of undesirable side effects, thus necessitating the search for new effective PPARγ agonists.

Studies indicate that partial agonism of PPARγ induces promising activity patterns by retaining the positive effects attributed to the full agonists, with reduced side effects (Kazazis, Evangelopoulos, Kollas et al. 2014). PPAR agonists can help to improve blood glucose levels and levels of blood lipids (fats and cholesterol) and may also reduce risks of atherosclerosis, because PPARs regulate the expression of genes that affect (1) blood lipid metabolism, (2) the generation of adipocytes, and (3) the control of blood glucose.

A number of risk factors for cardiovascular disease tend to occur together, including insulin resistance, elevated blood glucose levels, Type 2 diabetes, blood lipid abnormalities, and inflammation. Therefore, there is a search to find therapeutic agents that might address all of these risk factors at once.

The currently available PPAR agonists aimed at control of diabetes are known as thiazolidinediones or "glitazones." These include pioglitazone (brand name Actos) and rosiglitazone (Avandia). These drugs increase the sensitivity of body tissues to the action of insulin. The thiazolidinediones exert this effect by binding to and activating PPARγ, and in addition, they may inhibit certain chemokines that attract inflammatory cells and thus promote atherosclerosis (No authors listed. June 15, 2006. PPAR agonists. *Diabetes Self Management*; https://www.diabetesselfmanagement.com/diabetes-resources/definitions/ppar-agonists/; accessed 8.27.17).

The *Journal of Diabetes Research* published a study showing that silymarin administration was associated with a significant reduction in fasting blood glucose (FBG) levels (mean difference, −26.86 mg/dL in four trials) (Fallahzadeh, Dormanesh, Sagheb et al. 2012; Velussi, Cernigoi, Ariella et al. 1997).

The aim of a study published in the journal *Phytotherapy Research* was to verify that the herbal medicine *S. marianum* seed extract (silymarin) confers antioxidant benefits on the glycemic profile in diabetic patients.

A 4-month clinical trial was conducted in Type 2 diabetes patients in two well-matched groups: The first group received a silymarin (200 mg) tablet three times a day plus conventional therapy. The second group received the same conventional therapy but a placebo tablet instead of silymarin.

The patients were visited monthly and glycosylated hemoglobin (HbA1c), FBG, insulin, total cholesterol, low-density lipoprotein (LDL) and high-density lipoprotein (HDL), triglyceride, SGOT, and SGPT levels were determined at the beginning and at the end of the study.

The results showed a significant decrease in HbA1c, FBG, total cholesterol, LDL, triglyceride, SGOT, and SGPT levels in the silymarin-treated patients compared with placebo, as well as with values for both groups compared to the beginning of the study, keeping in mind that some improvement would be expected even in the placebo group, given that conventional therapy was also being applied.

The investigators concluded that 4 months of silymarin treatment in Type 2 diabetes patients has a beneficial effect on the glycemic profile (Huseini, Larijani, Heshmat et al. 2006).

Similarly, compared with placebo, silymarin administration significantly reduced HbA1c levels, as reported in a publication titled "Silymarin in Type 2 diabetes mellitus: a systematic review and meta-analysis of randomized controlled trials," in the *Journal of Diabetes Research* (Voroneanu, Nistor, Dumea et al. 2016).

The *Journal of Medicinal Food* published a study titled "Silymarin as an adjunct to glibenclamide therapy improves long-term and postprandial glycemic control and body mass index in type 2 diabetes." Glibenclamide, also known as glyburide, is an antidiabetic drug in a class of medications known as sulfonylureas, closely related to sulfonamide antibiotics. The aim of the study was to determine whether the antioxidant flavonoid silymarin could improve long-term and postprandial glycemic control, and weight control, in Type 2 diabetic patients also being treated with glibneclamide.

Type 2 diabetes patients, previously maintained on 10 mg/day glibenclamide and diet control, but with poor glycemic control, were assigned to one of three groups: The first two groups were treated with either 200 mg/day silymarin, or placebo, as adjuncts to glibenclamide, and the third group was maintained on glibenclamide alone, with both groups being followed for 120 days.

Fasting and 4-h postprandial plasma glucose (PPG), glycated hemoglobin (HbA1c), and body mass index (BMI) were assessed at baseline and again after 120 days.

At 120 days, compared to placebo, silymarin treatment significantly reduced both fasting plasma glucose (FPG) and PPG excursions, and also significantly reduced HbA1c levels and BMI. No significant differences were observed for the placebo group, compared to the group getting glibenclamide alone.

The investigators concluded that the use of silymarin as an adjunct to glibenclamide improves the glycemic control targeted by glibenclamide, both in fasting levels and in postprandial levels (Hussain. 2007).

The Review of Diabetic Studies published an article titled "The therapeutic potential of Milk Thistle in diabetes" that cites a number of relevant clinical studies on milk thistle as an adjunct treatment in Type 2 diabetes, and its complications.

For instance, in patients with diabetes and alcoholic liver cirrhosis, a silymarin daily dose of 600 mg for 6 months produced a significant reduction in FBG and mean daily glucose levels from the second month of treatment onward, without any increase in episodes of hypoglycemia, compared to the pretreatment period.

Insulin requirement was also decreased by 20% by silymarin treatment. A significant decrease of 0.5% in HbA1c levels and a decrease in levels of malondialdehyde (MDA) were also noted after 6 months of treatment, with a patient satisfaction rate of 100% (Velussi, Cernigoi, Viezzoli et al. 1993).

In another study, diabetic patients with end-stage renal disease received a 350-mg intravenous dose of silibin over 24 h. In the treated patients, the cellular surface thiol status in peripheral blood lymphocytes was restored. The same phenomenon was observed at the intracellular level 48 h later, with subsequent improvement in T-cell activation and reduction of TNFα levels and inflammation.

The investigators attributed these effects to the activation of γ-glutamyl transferase in the lymphocyte's membrane and to functional improvement of intracellular γ-glutamyl-cysteine synthetase and/or glutathione synthetase that regulates glutathione synthesis (Dietzmann, Thiel, Ansorge et al. 2002).

Another study published in the journal *Phytotherapy Research* reported that Type 2 diabetes patients treated for 4 months with 200 mg silimarin, three times a day before meals, experienced a significant reduction in blood glucose levels (from 156 ± 46 mg/dL down to 133 ± 39 mg/dL), as compared to an increase observed in the placebo-treated group.

In the treatment period, HbA1c levels fell from 7.82% ± 2.01% to 6.78% ± 1.05%; likewise, total cholesterol, HDL cholesterol, LDL cholesterol, triglyceride, AST, and ALT levels were significantly improved. The authors concluded that silimarin reduces blood glucose levels by mechanisms that are independent of insulin production (Huseini, Larijani, Heshmat et al. 2006).

10.2.3.1 Combining Milk Thistle with *Berberis vulgaris*

Berberine (*B. vulgaris*) is an isoquinoline alkaloid used to improve the glucidic and lipidic profiles of patients with hypercholesterolemia, metabolic syndrome, and Type 2 diabetes. It is detailed in the next chapter. The limitation of berberine seems to be its poor oral bioavailability, which is affected by the presence, in enterocytes, of P-glycoprotein—an active adenosine triphosphate (ATP)–consuming efflux protein that extrudes berberine back into the intestinal lumen, thus limiting its absorption. According to some sources, silymarin, derived from *S. marianum*, could be considered a P-glycoprotein antagonist.

The aim of a study published in the journal *Clinical Pharmacology* was to determine the benefits in Type 2 diabetes of adding a P-glycoprotein antagonist (silymarin), to a product containing *Berberis aristata* extract. Patients with Type 2 diabetes with suboptimal glycemic control were treated with diet, hypoglycemic drugs, and, in cases of concomitant alterations of the lipid profile, hypolipidemic agents.

The patients received an add-on therapy consisting of either a standardized extract of *B. aristata* (titrated to 85% berberine) corresponding to 1000 mg/day of berberine, or Berberol, a fixed combination containing the same standardized extract of *B. aristata* plus a standardized extract of *S. marianum* (titrated as more than 60% in silymarin), for a total intake of 1000 mg/day of berberine and 210 mg/day of silymarin. It was found that both treatments similarly improved fasting glucose, total cholesterol, LDL cholesterol, triglyceride, and liver enzyme levels. However, HbA1c values were reduced to a greater extent by the fixed combination.

The investigators concluded that the combination of berberine plus silymarin proved to be more effective than berberine alone in reducing HbA1c, when administered at the same dose, and in the form of standardized extracts, to Type 2 diabetic patients (Di Pierro, Putignano, Villanova et al. 2013).

10.2.4 ANTIOXIDANT AND ANTI-INFLAMMATORY PROFILE OF *S. MARIANUM*

A clinical trial on the effects of silymarin supplementation on oxidative stress indices and also on hs-CRP on patients with Type 2 diabetes was reported in the journal *Phytomedicine*.

Type 2 diabetes patients 25 to 50 years old, and on stable medication, were recruited from the Iranian Diabetes Society and endocrinology clinics in East Azarbayjan (Tabriz, Iran). They were assigned to two groups: Patients in the silymarin treatment group received 140 mg, three times daily of dried extracts of *S. marianum*, and those in the placebo group received identical placebos for 45 days.

Data about height, weight, waist circumference, and BMI, as well as food consumption, were collected at baseline, and at the conclusion of the study. Fasting blood samples were obtained, and antioxidant indices and hs-CRP were assessed at baseline as well as at the end of the trial.

All patients completed the study and did not report any adverse effects or symptoms from the silymarin supplementation. Silymarin supplementation significantly increased superoxide dismutase (SOD) by 12.85%, glutathione peroxidase (GPX) activity by 30.32%, and total antioxidant capacity (TAC) by 8.43%, compared to patients given the placebo. These changes are statistically significant.

The hs-CRP values for the silymarin group were 26.83% lower than for the placebo group, and MDA concentration significantly decreased by 12.01% in the silymarin group compared to baseline. It was concluded that silymarin supplementation improves antioxidant indices (SOD, GPX, and TAC) and decreases hs-CRP levels in Type 2 diabetes patients (Ebrahimpour Koujan, Gargari, Mobasseri et al. 2014).

According to a report in the journal *Antioxidants* (Basel, Switzerland), silymarin contains flavonolignans (as noted earlier in this chapter, silybin is the major one). In many cases, the antioxidant properties of silymarin are considered the basis of its protective actions. The possible antioxidant mechanisms of silymarin are as follows:

1. Direct scavenging of free radicals and chelating free Fe^{++} and Cu^{++}, mainly effective in the gut
2. Preventing free radical formation by inhibiting specific ROS-producing enzymes, or improving the integrity of mitochondria in stress conditions
3. Maintaining an optimal redox balance in the cell by activating a range of antioxidant enzymes and nonenzymatic antioxidants, mainly via Nrf2 activation, probably the main driving force of the antioxidant action of silymarin
4. Decreasing inflammatory responses by inhibiting NF-κB pathways, which is emerging as a new mechanism for understanding the protective effects of sylimarinin in treating liver toxicity and various other liver diseases
5. Activating vitagenes, responsible for synthesis of protective molecules, including heat shock proteins, thioredoxin, and sirtuins
6. Affecting the microenvironment of the gut, including silymarin–bacteria interactions (Surai. 2015)

10.2.5 Safety of Milk Thistle

According to a report in the *Journal of Clinical Pharmacology*, consumption of 140, 280, 560, and 700 mg of silimarin every 8 h, for 7 days, in noncirrhotic patients with chronic hepatitis C did not produce any adverse reactions or abnormal findings from follow-up, which included physical examination, biochemical tests, and electrocardiogram. There were two reported events of nausea and headache, but these appeared to be unrelated to silymarin administration (Hawke, Schrieber, Soule et al. 2010).

In another study, patients with chronic hepatitis C received 600 and 1200 mg/day silimarin treatment for 12 weeks. The patients reported symptoms from the gastrointestinal tract; two patients reported headache/dizziness, and one reported pruritus (Gordon, Hobbs, Bowden et al. 2006).

Generally, silymarin is considered safe, even at doses as high as 13 g/day, with no interactions (at least at low concentrations, such as 10 μM) with chemotherapeutic agents like vincristine or L-asparaginase. Additional studies of the safety of this botanical in diverse patient populations can be found in Kazazis, Evangelopoulos, Kollas et al. (2014) [*The Review of Diabetic Studies*, Summer; 11(2): 167–174].

10.3   BERBERINE

Berberine is a naturally occurring yellow plant alkaloid extract with a long history of medicinal use in both Ayurvedic and Chinese medicine—it is also well known in Iranian medicine. It is found in the roots, rhizomes, stems, and bark of various plants including *Hydrastis canadensis* (goldenseal), *Coptis chinensis* (Coptis or goldenthread), *Berberis aquifolium* (Oregon grape), *B. vulgaris* (barberry), *B. aristata* (tree turmeric), and *Phellodendron amurense* (phellodendron), not to be confused with the unrelated household plant, philodendron (No authors listed. 2000).

Berberine extracts and decoctions have demonstrated significant antimicrobial activity against a variety of organisms including bacteria, viruses, fungi, protozoans, helminths, and chlamydia.

10.3.1   THE EFFECTS OF BERBERINE ON HYPERGLYCEMIA

According to a report in the *Journal of Ethnopharmacology*, berberine extracted from *Coptis* root and *P. amurense* has been frequently used in China for the adjunctive treatment of Type 2 diabetes, hyperlipidemia, and hypertension. This report reviews the efficacy and safety of berberine in the treatment of Type 2 diabetes, hyperlipidemia, and hypertension, based on meta-analysis of available clinical data.

The investigators searched the English databases PubMed, ScienceDirect, Cochrane library, EMBASE, and so on, as well as Chinese databases including the China biomedical literature database (CBM), the Chinese Technology Journal Full-text Database, the Chinese journal full text database (CNKI), and the Wanfang digital periodical full text database.

It was found that berberine, along with lifestyle intervention, significantly lowers the level of FPG, PPG, and HbA1c, compared to lifestyle intervention alone, or placebo. There was no statistically significant difference between berberine and prescription oral hypoglycemic agents.

Berberine plus lifestyle intervention was significantly better than lifestyle intervention alone for the treatment of hyperlipidemia; berberine with oral lipid-lowering drugs was significantly better than lipid-lowering drugs alone in reducing the levels of total cholesterol and LDL cholesterol, and in raising the level of HDL cholesterol (Lan, Zhao, Dong et al. 2015).

A study intended to determine how berberine controls blood sugar reported that it does so by activating the enzyme adenosine monophosphate kinase (AMPK). However, it was not clear how AMPK is activated by berberine. An animal model study published in the *American Journal of Physiology-Endocrinology and Metabolism* aimed to determine the mechanism of action for berberine *in vivo* and *in vitro*.

Berberine increased insulin sensitivity after 5 weeks of administration to dietary obese rats. Fasting insulin and homeostasis model assessment for insulin resistance (HOMA-IR) declined by 46%, and 48%, respectively.

In cell lines including 3T3-L1 adipocytes, L6 myotubes, C2C12 myotubes, and H4IIE hepatocytes, berberine increased glucose consumption, 2-deoxyglucose uptake, and, to a lesser degree, 3-O-methylglucose uptake independently of insulin.

The insulin-induced glucose uptake was enhanced by berberine in the absence of change in IRS-1 (Ser307/312), Akt, p70 S6, and ERK phosphorylation. AMPK phosphorylation was reportedly increased by berberine at 0.5 h, and the increase lasted for up to, and, in some instances, more than, 16 h.

Aerobic and anaerobic respiration were assessed to understand the action of berberine: The long-lasting phosphorylation of AMPK was found to be associated with persistent elevation in the AMP/ATP ratio and reduction in oxygen consumption. An increase in glycolysis was observed with an increase in lactic acid production.

Berberine showed no cytotoxicity, and it protected the plasma membrane in L6 myotubes in cell culture.

These results suggested to the investigators that berberine enhances glucose metabolism by stimulation of glycolysis, which is related to inhibition of glucose oxidation in mitochondria. Berberine-induced AMPK activation is likely a consequence of mitochondria inhibition that increases the AMP/ATP ratio (Yin, Gao, Liu et al. 2007).

Berberine reduces blood glucose by a number of mechanisms, for example, by reducing glucose release from glycolysis in the liver and by lowering fasting glucose, fasting insulin, and postprandial glucose. Interestingly, it lowers HbA1c by inducing the growth of new insulin receptors. Here are further reports:

A study published in *The Journal of Clinical Endocrinology and Metabolism* aimed to determine the efficacy and safety of berberine in the treatment of Type 2 diabetic patients with dyslipidemia. These patients were to receive either berberine (1.0 g daily), or placebo, for 3 months.

The berberine group saw FPG decline from 7.0 ± 0.8 down to 5.6 ± 0.9 and postload plasma glucose decline from 12.0 ± 2.7 down to 8.9 ± 2.8 mm/L; HbA1c declined from $7.5\% \pm 1.0\%$ down to $6.6\% \pm 0.7\%$; triglycerides declined from 2.51 ± 2.04 down to 1.61 ± 1.10 mm/L; total cholesterol declined from 5.31 ± 0.98 down to 4.35 ± 0.96 mm/L; and LDL cholesterol declined from 3.23 ± 0.81 down to 2.55 ± 0.77 mm/L. All parameters differed significantly from those of the placebo group.

The authors concluded that berberine is effective and safe in the treatment of Type 2 diabetes and dyslipidemia (Zhang, Li, Zou et al. 2008).

The journal *Metabolism* reported a study that aimed to determine the efficacy and safety of berberine in the treatment of Type 2 diabetic patients. One group of adult participants with newly diagnosed Type 2 diabetes was given berberine, whereas the other was given metformin (0.5 g t.i.d.), in a 3-month trial.

The hypoglycemic effect of berberine was found to be similar to that of metformin. Significant decreases observed in the berberine group were reductions in HbA1c from $9.5\% \pm 0.5\%$ down to $7.5\% \pm 0.4\%$, FBG from 10.6 ± 0.9 mmol/L down to 6.9 ± 0.5 mmol/L, postprandial blood glucose from 19.8 ± 1.7 down to 11.1 ± 0.9 mmol/L, and plasma triglycerides from 1.13 ± 0.13 mmol/L down to 0.89 ± 0.03 mmol/L.

In a second study, adult participants with poorly controlled Type 2 diabetes were given supplementary berberine in a 3-month trial.

Berberine lowered FBG and postprandial blood glucose from week 1 until the end of the trial. HbA1c decreased from $8.1\% \pm 0.2\%$ down to $7.3\% \pm 0.3\%$. Fasting plasma insulin and HOMA-IR were reduced by 28.1% and 44.7%, respectively. Total cholesterol and LDL cholesterol declined significantly as well.

It was also reported that 34.5% of the patients suffered from transient adverse gastrointestinal effects: These events included diarrhea (10.3%), constipation (6.9%), flatulence (19.0%), and abdominal pain (3.4%). The side effects were observed only in the first 4 weeks in most patients. In 24.1% of the patients, berberine dosage was lowered from 0.5 g t.i.d. to 0.3 g t.i.d., as a consequence of gastrointestinal adverse events.

However, no functional liver or kidney damage was observed in any patients. The investigators concluded that this pilot study found berberine to be a potent oral hypoglycemic agent with beneficial effects on lipid metabolism (Yin, Xing, and Ye. 2008).

A report in the journal *Metabolism* concluded that "Berberine lowers blood glucose in type 2 diabetes patients through increasing insulin receptor expression." In this study, the investigators found that berberine significantly lowered FBG, HbA1c, triglycerides, and insulin levels in patients with Type 2 diabetes. The FBG- and HbA1c-lowering efficacies of berberine were comparable to those of metformin and rosiglitazone.

In the berberine-treated patients, the percentages of peripheral blood lymphocytes that express the insulin receptor gene (InsR) were significantly elevated as a result of the therapy. Berberine also effectively lowered FBG in patients with chronic hepatitis B or C, comorbid with Type 2 diabetes or impaired fasting glucose. Liver function was improved greatly in these patients, as evidenced by meaningful reduction of the elevated liver enzymes.

The investigators confirmed the activity of berberine on the insulin receptor gene in humans and its relationship to the glucose-lowering effect, and concluded that berberine is, therefore, an ideal medicine for patients with Type 2 diabetes and that its mode of action differs from that of metformin and rosiglitazone (Zhang, Wei, Xue et al. 2010).

In addition, there are many excellent reviews that detail the benefits of berberine in treating hyperglycemia, including the following:

- Pang, Zhao, Zhou et al. (2015). Application of berberine on treating Type 2 diabetes mellitus. *International Journal of Endocrinology*, Feb; 2015 (Article ID 905749): 12 pages. http://dx.doi.org/10.1155/2015/905749.
- Dong, Wang, Zhao et al. (2012). Berberine in the treatment of Type 2 diabetes mellitus: a systemic review and meta-analysis. *Evidence-Based Complementary and Alternative Medicine*, Jul; 2012 (Article ID 591654): 12 pages. http://dx.doi.org/10.1155/2012/591654.

10.3.2 BERBERINE IN INSULIN RESISTANCE AND POLYCYSTIC OVARY SYNDROME

Polycystic ovary syndrome is a frequent reproductive and metabolic disorder associated with insulin resistance. A study published in the *European Journal of Endocrinology* aimed to compare the effects of berberine to those of metformin on the metabolic features of women with polycystic ovary syndrome.

Patients with polycystic ovary syndrome, and patients with insulin resistance, were assigned to 3 months of therapy in one of three groups: (A) berberine + the compound cyproterone acetate (CPA), (B) metformin + CPA, and (C) placebo + CPA. Compared to metformin, treatment with berberine (500 mg three times daily, for 3 months) resulted in a decrease in waist circumference and in waist-to-hip ratio, lower total cholesterol, lower triglycerides, and lower LDL cholesterol, as well as increases in HDL cholesterol and in sex hormone-binding globulin.

Similarly, compared to placebo, treatment with berberine resulted in decreased waste to-hip ratio, lower FPG, lower fasting insulin, lower HOMA-IR, lower area under the curve of insulin, lower total cholesterol, LDLC, and TG, as well as increase in HDLC and sex hormone-binding globulin (Wei, Zhao, Wang et al. 2012; An, Sun, Zhang et al. 2013).

Berberine activates adenosine monophosphate-activated protein kinase (AMPK) and inhibits protein-tyrosine phosphatase 1B. Activating AMPK reverses insulin resistance, thus promoting glycolysis (that is to say, increasing the metabolic consumption of glucose) and reducing oxidative stress. One result of activating AMPK is suppression of hepatic glucose output, so that insulin and IGF-1 levels are lower. Both berberine and metformin activate AMPK.

10.3.3 WHAT IS A SAFE AND EFFECTIVE DOSE OF BERBERINE?

One clinical source reported in the journal *Metabolism* that berberine 500 mg twice daily for 3 months is effective in treating diabetes (Yin, Xing, and Ye. 2008). Some studies show a benefit at three times daily. However, one should not take an entire day's dose of berberine all at once, because of poor intestinal uptake. As with most herbs, it is better to take berberine in multiple doses spread throughout the day.

10.3.3.1 Berberine May Be Hazardous in Pregnancy

According to the Natural Medicine database, berberine is rated LIKELY UNSAFE during pregnancy because it crosses the placenta and may harm the baby. In one study, newborn infants exposed to berberine had elevations of bilirubin to such an extent that kernicterus developed. Kernicterus is a very rare type of brain damage that occurs in newborns with severe jaundice. It is caused by a high level of bilirubin in the blood. If left untreated, the bilirubin can then become deposited in the brain, where it causes long-term damage.

A study on the effect of berberine, the major ingredient of the Chinese herb huanglian (*C. chinensis*), on the protein binding of bilirubin, using the peroxidase kinetic method, published in the journal *Biology of the Neonate*, reported it to pose some risk for kernicterus among jaundiced newborn Chinese infants. The molar displacing effect of berberine was found *in vitro* to be about 10-fold that of phenylbutazone, a known potent displacer of bilirubin, and about 100-fold that of papaverine, a berberine-type alkaloid.

The chronic intraperitoneal administration of berberine (10 and 20 µg/g) to adult rats (mixed breed of Wistar and Sprague-Dawley), once daily for 1 week, resulted in a significant decrease in mean bilirubin serum protein binding due to an *in vivo* displacement effect, and a persistent elevation in steady-state serum concentrations of unbound and total bilirubin, possibly due to inhibition of metabolism.

The use of the herb and other traditional Chinese medicines that contain a high proportion of berberine is best avoided in jaundiced neonates and pregnant women (Chan. 1993). Furthermore, limited data suggest that berberine may cause preterm contractions. Similarly, berberine is considered LIKELY UNSAFE in nursing women as it can be transferred to the baby in breast milk.

It is suggested that it may be best to limit the duration of berberine to only 8 weeks or so at a time, and then take a break to relieve the effect of the herb on the cytochrome P450 (CYP) system in the liver. Note: The "CYP" designation is pronounced like "sip". Hence, for example, CYP3A4 would be pronounced sip3A4.

Many animal model studies have reported interactions between berberine-containing products and some of the P450 cytochromes, but little is known about whether berberine alters CYP activities in humans, especially after repeated doses. The *European Journal of Clinical Pharmacology* reported a study on healthy men, on the effects of ingesting berberine (300 mg, t.i.d., p.o.) on the metabolism of the probe drugs midazolam, omeprazole, dextromethorphan, losartan, and caffeine for 2 weeks, to evaluate the effects of berberine on the activity of the P450 enzymes CYP3A4, CYP2C19, CYP2D6, CYP2C9, and CYP1A2, respectively.

It was found that, as a result of the continued administration of berberine:

1. The activity of CYP2D6 was inhibited, causing urinary excretion of dextromethorphan/dextrorphan to increase ninefold.
2. The activity of CYP2C9 was inhibited, causing the losartan/E-3174 ratio to double.
3. The activity of CYP3A4 was inhibited, as the C_{max}, $AUC_{0-\infty}$, and AUC_{0-12} of midazolam were increased 38%, 40%, and 37%, respectively.
4. Compared to the placebo group, in the berberine-treated subjects the T_{max} and $T_{1/2}$ of midazolam were prolonged from 3.03 ± 0.27 to 3.66 ± 0.37 h and 0.66 ± 0.08 to 0.99 ± 0.09 h, respectively. The oral clearance of midazolam was decreased 27%, and the phenotypic indices of 1-h midazolam/1′-hydroxymidazolam increased 59%.
5. There were no statistically significant differences in the pharmacokinetic parameters of the other probe drugs, between placebo and the berberine-treated group.

The authors concluded that repeated administration of berberine (300 mg, t.i.d., p.o.) inhibited the activity of the enzymes CYP2D6, 2C9, and CYP3A4. Drug–drug interactions should therefore be considered when berberine is administered (Guo, Chen, Tan et al. 2012).

10.4   THE ANTIHYPERGLYCEMIC EFFECT OF SELECTED MUSHROOMS

Large numbers of mushroom species are commonly consumed as food. While some mushrooms are quite poisonous, many have known medicinal value (Cargill. 2016). The description of the anti-glycemic and the anti-inflammatory activity of certain mushroom species is given here *pro forma* because their use is not likely to be implemented as adjunctive treatment for diabetes—although that was the case elsewhere over the years.

It is important to keep in mind that there is a vast array of botanicals that are antiglycemic, antihypertensive, anti-inflammatory, antilipidemic, antibacterial, and so on. Both geographic regional differences and changes in eating habits make many of these botanicals unlikely to appear in the daily diet of Westerners. This is especially true in modern diets with a large proportion of preprocessed foods that exclude these botanicals, and where, paradoxically, they might do the most good (Stamets, and Zwickey. 2014; Lindequist, Niedermeyer, and Jülich. 2005).

10.4.1 Mushrooms That Lower Blood Glucose

Effective and safe treatments of Type 2 diabetes patients were reported focusing on overcoming peripheral insulin resistance with edible mushrooms. According to a report in the *International Journal of Medicinal Mushrooms*, a polysaccharide fraction of maitake (*Grifola frondosa*; SX fraction, p.o.; a.k.a. Hen of the woods) showed antihyperglycemic action in patients with Type 2 diabetes (Konno, Aynehchi, Dolin et al. 2002).

Ganoderan A and B, glucans from reishi mushroom (*Ganoderma lucidum*; a.k.a. lingzhi) or mushroom fruiting bodies (Hikino, Konno, Mirin et al. 1985), and an acidic glucuronoxylomannan from the fruiting bodies of witch's butter (*Tremella aurantia Schwein*) (Kiho, Morimoto, Kobayashi et al. 2000) all exhibited antihyperglycemic effects in several test systems and ameliorated the symptoms of diabetes.

The *International Journal of Medicinal Mushrooms* reported a study that aimed to determine the efficacy and safety of ganopoly (polysaccharide fractions extracted from reishi [*G. lucidum*] by a patented technique) in patients older than 18 years, with confirmed Type 2 diabetes of more than 3 months duration who were not receiving insulin.

The patients exhibited normal vital signs appropriate for their age and disease state, normal electrocardiogram, and FPG level in sulfonylurea-naive patients, or an FPG less than 10 mmol/L before washout in sulfonylurea-treated patients.

The patients were assigned to either reishi orally at 1800 mg, three times daily for 12 weeks, or placebo. The patients underwent 4 weeks of dose adjustment, followed by 8 weeks of dose maintenance. HbA1c, plasma glucose, insulin, and C-peptide were monitored at predetermined intervals. Adverse events and hypoglycemic episodes were recorded. The reishi treatment significantly decreased the mean HbA1c from 8.4% at baseline to 7.6% 12 weeks later.

Significant changes in mean fasting and postprandial levels of plasma glucose were seen at the last visit, and these paralleled the changes in mean HbA1c: At baseline, the mean FPG and PPG values in patients who were about to be treated with reishi were 12.0 and 13.6 mmol/L, respectively.

At week 12, mean postprandial values had decreased from 13.6 to 11.8 mmol/L, whereas these values did not change (or actually increased slightly) in patients receiving placebo. The between-group difference in postprandial levels at week 12 was significant. Changes in fasting insulin, 2-h postprandial insulin, fasting C-peptide, and 2-h postprandial C-peptide were consistent, with the between-group differences in these end points being significant at the last visit. Overall, reishi was well tolerated (Gao, Lan, Dai et al. 2004).

There are numerous studies of mushroom extracts in treatment of hyperglycemia in animal models. For instance, tremellastin from yellow brain fungus (*Tremella mesenterica*) containing 40% to 45% acidic polysaccharide glucuronoxylomannan, and obtained by alcohol precipitation of culture broth, decreased blood glucose levels as well as triglyceride levels in rats after 15 days of treatment (p.o. 100 mg kg^{-1}; 500 mg kg^{-1}) (Wasser, Tan, and Elisashvili. 2002).

Oral preparations of the traditional Chinese drug cordyceps (caterpillar fungus) and of its fermented mycelia ameliorate diabetes in a diabetic animal model using streptozotocin (STZ)-induced rats (Hsu, and Lo. 2002). Additionally, polysaccharides from cultured mycelium of cordyceps have shown significant activity after intraperitoneal injection (Kiho, Ookubo, Usui et al. 1996).

10.4.2 ANTI-INFLAMMATORY MUSHROOMS

Ethanolic extracts and a proteoglycan from meshimakobu, a.k.a. *Phellinus linteus*, a medicinal mushroom used in Japan, Korea, and China for centuries, show anti-inflammatory effect in the collagen-induced arthritis model as well as in the croton oil-induced ear edema test in mice, and show an antinociceptive effect in the writhing test (Kim, Song, Kim et al. 2004; Kim, Kim, Hwang et al. 2003). The writhing test is a chemical method used to induce pain of peripheral origin by injection of an irritant like phenylquinone, acetic acid, or acetylsalicylic acid in mice (Gawade. 2012). Other compounds effective in the writhing test are the ganoderic acids A (8c), B (8a), G (8g), and H (8h), isolated from *G. lucidum.*

According to a report in the *International Journal of Medicinal Mushrooms*, a methanolic extract of *Pleurotus pulmonarius* (Fr.) Quél.—commonly known as the Indian oyster or Italian oyster mushroom—fruiting bodies (500 and 1000 mg kg^{-1}) reduced carrageenan-induced and formalin-induced paw edema in mice. The activity was comparable to the reference diclofenac (10 mg kg^{-1}). The effect seemed to be related to the significant antioxidant activity of the extract.

The IC50 value for hydroxyl-radical scavenging was 476 μg mL^{-1}, and for lipid peroxidation inhibition, it was 960 μg mL^{-1} (Jose, Ajith, and Jananrdhanan. 2002).

The edible maitake mushroom (*G. frondosa*) contains ergosterol, ergosta-4-6-8(14),22-tetraen-3-one (21), and 1-oleoyl-2-linoleoyl-3-palmitoylglycerol, which inhibit cyclooxygenases 1 and 2 activity (Zhang, Mills, and Nair. 2002). More detail is available from Lindequist, Niedermeyer, and Jülich (2005) [*Journal of Agricultural and Food Chemistry*, Dec; 50(26): 7581–7585].

10.4.3 A NOTE OF CAUTION

A review in the *International Journal of Medicinal Mushrooms* presented an overview of the reported efficacy and mechanism(s) of action of medicinal mushrooms for glucose control in diabetes, including the inhibition of glucose absorption, protection against beta-cell (β-cell) damage, increase of insulin release, enhancement of antioxidant defenses, attenuation of inflammation, modulation of carbohydrate metabolism pathway, and regulation of insulin-dependent and insulin-independent signaling pathways.

However, the authors caution that there is still insufficient evidence to draw definitive conclusions about the efficacy of individual medicinal mushrooms for diabetes. In addition, the wide variability, the lack of standards for production, and the lack of testing protocols to assess product quality are still problems in producing medicinal mushroom products. Well-designed randomized controlled trials with long-term consumption are needed to guarantee the bioactivity and safety of medicinal mushroom products for diabetic patients (Lo, and Wasser. 2011).

10.5 SAFFLOWER (*CARTHAMUS TINCTORIUS* L.) SEEDS, EXTRACT, AND OIL LOWER BLOOD GLUCOSE

Safflower (*C. tinctorius*) is a thistle-like annual plant. It is native to environments having seasonal rain and it is commercially cultivated for the vegetable oil extracted from the seeds. The journal *Food Chemistry* reported a study about the chemical composition and oxidative stability of safflower oil prepared from safflower seed, roasted at different temperatures (284°F to 356°F) to determine oxidative stability. It was compared to oil from unroasted safflower.

The color development and phosphorus content increased significantly as roasting temperature rose; however, the fatty acid compositions did not change with roasting temperature. The major fatty acid was linoleic acid (ca. 80%).

Four phospholipid classes, namely, phosphatidylethanolamines, phosphatidyinositols, phosphatidic acids, and phosphatidylcholines, were identified. The major phospholipid component of safflower seed oil is phosphatidyinositols. As the roasting temperature rose, the proportion of PI in the safflower oil increased significantly while the proportion of phosphatidylethanolamines decreased significantly. Tocopherol and tocotrienol homologs were identified, namely, α-, β-, and γ-tocopherols, and γ- and δ-tocotrienols, whereas no δ-tocopherol or α- and β-tocotrienols were detected.

A report on the "Chemical composition and oxidative stability of flax, safflower and poppy seed and seed oils" appeared in the journal *Bioresource Technology*. Three Turkish seed samples, flax, poppy, and safflower, were analyzed for their fatty acids, tocols (tocopherols and tocotrienols) and total phenolic composition, and oxidative stability of their oil. The major fatty acid in the flax oil was α-linolenic acid (ALA) (58.3% of total fatty acids), whereas poppy and safflower oils were rich in linoleic acid (74.5% and 70.5%, respectively). The amount of total tocols was 14.6 mg/100 g flax, 11.0 mg/100 g poppy, and 12.1 mg/100 g safflower seed.

Flax and poppy oil were rich in γ-tocopherol as 79.4 mg/100 g oil and 30.9 mg/100 g oil, respectively, while α-tocopherol (44.1 g/100 g oil) was dominant in safflower oil. Only α- and γ-tocotrienol were found in the oils.

The authors concluded that all of the seeds investigated provided a healthy profile (Bozan, and Temelli. 2008).

A number of reports suggest that safflower seed, or oil, may be helpful in the treatment of hyperglycemia. For instance, a study in the journal *Phytotherapy Research* reports that safflower seed contains a "potent α-glucosidase inhibitor." The active α-glucosidase inhibitor compounds were serotonin derivatives [e.g., *N*-p-coumaroyl serotonin (1) and *N*-feruloyl serotonin (2)]. These compounds showed a potent inhibitory activity in the IC50 values calculated as 47.2 μm (1) and 99.8 μm (2), while that of the reference drugs acarbose and 1-deoxynojirimycin were evaluated as 907.5 and 278.0 μm, respectively.

The IC50 represents how small, or large, the concentration of a molecule has to be, to inhibit a given enzyme by 50%. Thus, the lower the number, the more potent the agent is compared to those with a higher IC50. Hence, the data above indicate that the compounds in safflower are far more potent than the reference drugs. Regarding the structure of the serotonin derivative, the existence of the hydroxyl group at the 5-position in the serotonin moiety and the linkage of cinnamic acid and serotonin are essential for the inhibitory activities against α-glucosidase.

The authors conclude that these results support the potential application of safflower seed as "traditional medicine" for the treatment of diabetes. In particular, the serotonin compounds could be used as a lead compound for a new potential α-glucosidase inhibitor derived from the plant (Takahashi, and Miyazawa. 2012).

The aim of a study published in the journal *Clinical Nutrition* was to determine the effects of conjugated linoleic acid (CLA) and safflower oil on glycemia, blood lipids, and inflammation, because the metabolic effects of the quality of dietary intake in people with Type 2 diabetes are not known. The investigators tested the hypothesis that safflower oil will improve glycemic and inflammatory markers in a time-dependent way that follows accumulation of linoleic acid and CLA isomers in the serum of participants supplemented with dietary oils.

Postmenopausal obese women with Type 2 diabetes were given 8 g daily of CLA and safflower oil for 16 weeks each.

CLA did not alter measured metabolic parameters. Safflower oil decreased HbA1c (−0.64% ± 0.18%) and C-reactive protein (−13.6 ± 8.2 mg/L) and increased the Quantitative Insulin-Sensitivity Check Index (0.0077 ± 0.0035) with a minimum time to effect observed 16 weeks after treatment. Safflower oil increased HDL cholesterol (0.12 ± 0.05 mmol/L) with the minimum time to detect an effect of safflower oil at 12 weeks. The minimum time to detect an increase of c9t11-CLA, t10c12-CLA, and linoleic acid in serum of women supplemented with CLA or safflower oil, respectively, was 4 weeks.

The investigators concluded that 8 g of safflower oil daily improved glycemia, reduced inflammation, and improved blood lipids, indicating that small changes in dietary fat quality may augment diabetes treatments to improve risk factors for diabetes-related complications (Asp, Collene, Norris et al. 2011).

Effect of *C. tinctorius* (safflower) was also observed on FBG and insulin levels in alloxan-induced diabetic rabbits. Healthy male rabbits were assigned to one of five groups: (1) normal control, (2) diabetic control, (3) diabetic treated orally for 30 days with glibenclamide, (4) diabetic treated with *C. tinctorius* extract at a dose of 200 mg/kg, and (5) the same agent, at a dose of 300 mg/kg of body weight. Blood glucose levels and insulin levels were observed after the 15th and 30th day of treatment with standard reagent kits.

It was found that *C. tinctorius* has a significant antihyperglycemic effect at 200 and 300 mg/kg doses, compared to the diabetic control group (Qazi, Khan, Rizwani et al. 2014).

Safflower extract has also been shown to reduce arterial stiffness as evidenced by changes in augmentation index. A study published in the journal *Vascular Health and Risk Management* reported that safflower seed extract contains characteristic polyphenols and serotonin derivatives [*N*-(p-coumaroyl)serotonin and *N*-feruloylserotonin], which are reported to inhibit oxidation of LDL, inhibit formation of atherosclerotic plaques, and decrease arterial stiffness as assessed by pulse wave analysis in animal models.

The study also evaluated the effects of long-term supplementation with safflower seed extract on arterial stiffness in men between the ages of 35 and 65 and postmenopausal women 55 to 65 years old with high-normal blood pressure, or mild hypertension, who were not undergoing treatment.

The participants received safflower seed extract (70 mg/day as serotonin derivatives) or placebo for 12 weeks, and pulse wave measurements, that is, second derivative of photoplethysmogram (SDPTG), augmentation index, and brachial–ankle pulse wave velocity (baPWV), were conducted at baseline and at weeks 4, 8, and 12.

It was found that vascular age estimated by SDPTG aging index improved in the safflower seed extract–supplemented group when compared to the placebo group at 4 and 12 weeks.

A trend of augmentation index reduction was observed in the safflower seed extract–supplemented group, but reduction of baPWV was not observed.

The safflower seed extract–supplemented group also showed a trend toward a lower MDA-modified LDL autoantibody titer at 12 weeks from baseline. Taken together, these results suggest that long-term consumption of safflower seed extract could help reduce arterial stiffness (Suzuki, Tsubaki, Fujita et al. 2010).

See Chapter 2 for further information on plethysmography, blood vessel flexibility, and augmentation index, and also see Elgendi (2012) (Standard terminologies for photoplethysmogram signals. *Current Cardiology Reviews*, 8, 215–219).

10.6 FLAX (*LINUM USITATISSIMUM*) SEEDS, EXTRACT, AND OIL LOWER BLOOD GLUCOSE

Flaxseed is one of the richest plant sources of the ω-3 fatty acid ALA. According to a report in the *American Journal of Clinical Nutrition*, dietary recommendations based on a large body of evidence from epidemiologic and controlled clinical studies have been made for n-3 fatty acids (n-3 meaning the same as ω-3), including ALA, eicosapentaenoic acid (EPA), and docosahexaenoic acid (DHA), to prevent and treat cardiovascular disease.

The n-3 fatty acid recommendation to achieve nutritional adequacy, defined as the amount necessary to prevent deficiency symptoms, is 0.6%–1.2% of energy for ALA; up to 10% of this can be provided by EPA or DHA. To achieve recommended ALA intakes, food sources including flaxseed and flaxseed oil, walnuts and walnut oil, and canola oil are recommended.

The evidence base supports a dietary recommendation of approximately 500 mg/day of EPA and DHA for cardiovascular disease risk reduction/prevention. For treatment of existing cardiovascular disease, 1 g/day is recommended.

A dietary strategy for achieving the 500 mg/day recommendation is to consume two fish meals per week (preferably fatty fish from cold waters). Foods enriched with EPA and DHA, or fish oil supplements, are a suitable alternate to achieve the minimum recommended intakes and may be necessary to achieve the pharmacological-level intakes of 1 g/day (Gebauer, Psota, Harris et al. 2006).

10.6.1 Secoisolariciresinol Diglucoside, a "New Antidiabetic Agent"

The *Journal of Food Science and Technology* reported that flaxseed is an important functional food ingredient due to its rich contents of ALA (ω-3 fatty acid), lignans, and fiber, with potential health benefits such as a reduction of risk for cardiovascular disease, atherosclerosis, diabetes, cancer, arthritis, osteoporosis, autoimmune disorders, and neurological disorders.

Flax protein helps prevent and treat heart disease, and it supports the immune system. As a functional food ingredient, flax or flaxseed oil has been incorporated into baked foods, juices, milk and dairy products, muffins, dry pasta products, macaroni, and meat products.

Dietary fibers, lignans, and ω-3 fatty acids, present in flaxseed, have a protective effect against diabetes risk (Prasad, Mantha, Muir et al. 2000; Prasad. 2001; Adlercreutz. 2007). Flaxseed lignan secoisolariciresinol diglucoside has been shown to inhibit expression of the phosphoenolpyruvate carboxykinase gene, which codes for a key enzyme responsible for glucose synthesis in the liver (Prasad. 2002).

Supplementing diet in Type 2 diabetes with 10 g of flaxseed powder per day for 1 month reduced FBG by 19.7% and HbA1c by 15.6%.

A study published in the *Journal of Dietary Supplements* reported exploratory evidence that when flaxseed was incorporated in recipes, it resulted in a reduction in the glycemic index of the food items. These observations prompted the investigators to determine the efficacy of flaxseed supplementation in Type 2 diabetics.

Participants were assigned to an experimental group daily receiving 10 g of a flaxseed powder supplement per day for a period of 1 month. A control group received placebo "supplementation." During the study, diet and drug intake of the subjects remained unaltered. The efficacy of supplementation with flaxseed was evaluated through a battery of clinico-biochemical parameters.

It was found that supplementation with flaxseed reduced FBG by 19.7% and HbA1c by 15.6%. A favorable reduction in total cholesterol (14.3%), triglycerides (17.5%), LDL cholesterol (21.8%), and apolipoprotein B and an increase in HDL cholesterol (11.9%) were also observed.

Several small studies, including one published in the *British Journal of Nutrition*, using a fasting glucose tolerance approach, reported a reduction in postprandial blood glucose levels of women consuming flaxseed (Cunnane, Ganguli, Menard et al. 1993). In another study titled "Nutritional attributes of traditional flaxseed in healthy young adults," published in *The American Journal of Clinical Nutrition*, the objective was to determine the effect of consuming 50 g of flaxseed per day for 4 weeks on several indices of nutrition in young healthy adults.

It was found that during the flaxseed consumption trial period, α-linolenate was increased significantly in adipose tissue, and n-3 polyunsaturates were increased in plasma lipids. Plasma LDL cholesterol was reduced by up to 8%, and total urinary lignan excretion rose more than fivefold.

Muffins containing 25 g of flaxseed did not differ significantly from control muffins in their content of thiobarbituric acid–reactive substances, and α-linolenate in the muffins was not significantly reduced by baking. Antioxidant vitamins and lipid hydroperoxides in plasma were not significantly affected by flaxseed consumption.

Bowel movements, per week, increased by 30% while flaxseed was consumed. It was concluded that traditional flaxseed has modest beneficial effects without compromising antioxidant status (Cunnane, Hamadeh, Liede et al. 1995).

A report in the journal *Ethnomedicine* investigated the effect of supplementation of flaxseed powder in menopausal women with diabetes. Patients were provided 15 and 20 g/day of flaxseed powder for a period of 2 months. Postprandial blood glucose levels were found to have declined by 7.9% and 19.1%, respectively, indicating that there was a dose-dependent response (Kapoor, Sachdeva, and Kochhar. 2011).

Similar results were also reported in a study published in *The Indian Journal of Nutrition and Dietetics* conducted on diabetic participants who were supplemented with flaxseed powder in bread form for 90 days. The investigators found a significant reduction in blood glucose levels after supplementation (Nazni, Amrithaveni, and Poongodi. 2006).

It should be noted, however, that some investigators failed to replicate the beneficial effects of flaxseed: In a study published in the *Journal of Oleo Science*, it was reported that 10 g/day of flaxseed oil had no effect on fasting blood serum glucose, insulin levels, or HbA1c levels (Barre, Mizier-Barre, Griscti et al. 2008; Goyal, Sharma, Upadhyay et al. 2014).

10.7 ANTIHYPERGLYCEMIC EFFECTS OF BITTER MELON (*MOMORDICA CHARANTIA*)

According to a report in the *Asian Pacific Journal of Tropical Disease*, it has been estimated that up to one-third of patients with diabetes use some form of complementary and alternative medicine, and the plant that has received the most attention for its antidiabetic properties is bitter melon, *M. charantia*.

Bitter melon, a.k.a. bitter gourd, bitter squash, karela, or balsam pear, is a valuable tropical and subtropical vine of the family Cucurbitaceae, widely grown for its edible fruit in Asia, Africa, and the Caribbean. The plant is a climbing perennial with elongated fruit that resembles a warty gourd or cucumber.

The unripe fruit is white or green in color and has a bitter taste that becomes more pronounced as the fruit ripens. The fruit is commonly used for the treatment of diabetes and related conditions of the indigenous populations of Asia, South America, India, and East Africa (Joseph, and Jini. 2013).

Bitter melon is included here with a note of caution that invariably accompanies its description elsewhere. There are case reports concerning dangerously low blood sugar, atrial fibrillation, and even coma associated with bitter melon consumption. It is contraindicated in patients with impaired liver function.

The red arils that cover the seeds of bitter melon are poisonous to humans, and consuming this part of the fruit causes a reaction that includes vomiting, diarrhea, and possibly death, according to Memorial Sloan-Kettering Cancer Center (https://www.mskcc.org/cancer-care/integrative-medicine/herbs/bitter-melon; accessed 9.29.17).

It should be noted also that while research on the hypoglycemic effect of this botanical in animal models of Type 2 diabetes shows it to be uniformly effective, that is not the case in human clinical studies. As the studies cited below will show, there is considerable disagreement about its effectiveness in glycemic control in humans suffering from chronic hyperglycemia.

10.7.1 ACTIVE CONSTITUENTS AND MODE OF ACTION OF BITTER MELON

The main constituents that appear to be responsible for the antihyperglycemic (and possibly hypoglycemia-inducing) properties of *Momordica* are charantin, insulin-like peptide [plant (p)-insulin], cucurbutanoids, momordicin, and oleanolic acids (Harinantenaina, Tanaka, Takaoka et al. 2006). P-insulin is similar to bovine insulin and is composed of two polypeptide chains held together by disulfide bonds.

Bitter melon also has numerous other constituents including proteins (momordin), glycosides, saponins, and minerals. It is also rich in vitamins A and C and β-carotene, as well as the minerals iron, phosphorus, and potassium (No authors listed. 2007).

In an animal model study published in the journal *Phytotherapy Research*, a methanol extract of *M. charantia* was administered to diabetic rats to determine the long-term effect of the extract on the lipid profile and the oral glucose tolerance test. Treatment for 30 days showed a significant decrease in triglycerides and in LDL and a significant increase in HDL. A significant effect on oral glucose tolerance was also noted.

Chronic administration showed an improvement in the oral glucose tolerance curve. The effect was more pronounced when the test was done on animals fed the extract on the day of the test, compared to tests done on animals that were not fed the extract on the same day. The authors claim that bitter melon extract increases glucose utilization by the liver (Chaturvedi, George, Milinganyo et al. 2004).

Another animal model study published in the journal *Diabetes Research and Clinical Practice* aimed to determine the effects of 10 weeks of feeding *M. charantia* fruit extract on blood plasma and tissue lipid profiles in normal and STZ-induced Type 1 diabetic rats.

The results show that in STZ-induced diabetic rats that were untreated, there was as expected a significant increase in plasma nonesterified cholesterol, triglycerides, and phospholipids, accompanied by a decrease in HDL cholesterol. A moderate increase in plasma lipid hydroperoxide (LPO) (a measure of oxidative injury) and MDA and an about twofold increase in kidney LPO were also observed in these STZ-induced diabetic rats. The treatment of diabetic rats with *M. charantia* fruit extract over a 10-week period returned these levels to close to normal. In addition, the *charantia* fruit extract also exhibited an inhibitory effect on membrane LPO under *in vitro* conditions.

The investigators concluded that *M. charantia* fruit extract exhibits hypolipidemic as well as antihyperglycemic effects in the STZ-induced diabetic rat (Ahmed, Lakhani, Gillett et al. 2001).

Extracts of *M. charantia* have also been shown to enhance cellular uptake of glucose, to promote insulin release and potentiate its effect, and to increase the number of insulin-producing β-cells in the pancreas of diabetic animals (No authors listed. 2007).

A study published in *The Biochemistry Journal* reported that a 95% ethanolic extract of *M. charantia* lowered blood glucose in an animal model of diabetes by depressing production in the liver through depression of the key gluconeogenic enzymes, glucose-6-phosphatase and fructose-1,6-bisphosphatase, and also by enhancing glucose oxidation by the shunt pathway (through activation of its principal enzyme, G6PDH) (Shibib, Khan, and Rahman. 1993).

Another study in the *Biological and Pharmaceutical Bulletin* reported that the protein from Thai bitter gourd (*M. charantia*) fruit pulp was extracted and its glycemic effect was evaluated. Subcutaneous administration of the protein extract (5 and 10 mg/kg) significantly and markedly decreased plasma glucose concentrations in both normal and STZ-induced diabetic rats, in a dose-dependent manner. The onset of the protein extract–induced antihyperglycemia/hypoglycemia was observed at 4 h in diabetic rats and at 6 h in normal rats.

In perfused rat pancreas, the protein extract (10 μg/mL) raised insulin secretion but not glucagon secretion. The increase in insulin secretion was apparent within 5 min of administration and was persistent during the 30 min of administration. Furthermore, the protein extract enhanced glucose uptake into C2C12 myocytes and 3T3-L1 adipocytes. Time course experiments performed in rat adipocytes revealed that *M. charantia* protein extract significantly increased glucose uptake after 4 and 6 h of incubation.

The investigators concluded that the *M. charantia* protein extract, a slow-acting chemical, exerted both insulin secretagogue and insulinomimetic activities to lower blood glucose concentrations *in vivo* (Yibchok-anun, Adisakwattana, Yao et al. 2006).

In an animal model study published in the journal *Acta Biologica et Medica Germanica*, an aqueous extract from the unripe fruits of *M. charantia* was found to stimulate insulin release from β-cell–rich pancreatic islets isolated from obese hyperglycemic mice. The stimulation of insulin release was partially reversible, and it differed from that of D-glucose and other commonly employed insulin secretagogues in not being suppressed by L-epinephrine, and in even being potentiated by the removal of Ca^{2+}.

This anomaly was not associated with general effects on the metabolism of the β-cells, as indicated by an unaltered oxidation of D-glucose.

Studies of 45Ca fluxes suggest that the insulin-releasing action is the result of perturbations of membrane functions. In support for the idea of direct effects on membrane lipids, the action of the extract was found to mimic that of saponin in inhibiting the Ca^{2+}/H^+ exchange mediated by the ionophore A23187 in isolated chromaffin granules and in releasing Ca^{2+} from preloaded liposomes (Welihinda, Arvidson, Gylfe et al. 1982).

In a study published in the journal *Diabetes Research and Clinical Practice*, the investigators aimed to determine the effect of *M. charantia* fruit juice on the distribution and number of α-, β-, and δ-cells in the pancreas of STZ-induced diabetic rats using immunohistochemical methods.

It was found that there was a significant increase in the number of β-cells in *M. charantia*–treated animals, compared with untreated diabetic animals. However, their number was still significantly less than that observed in normal rats. There was also a significant increase in the number of δ-cells in STZ-diabetic rats compared to nondiabetic rats. The increase in the number of δ-cells was not affected by *M. charantia* treatment.

The number of α-cells did not change significantly in *M. charantia*–treated diabetic rats when compared with untreated diabetic rats. These results suggested to the investigators that oral administration of *M. charantia* fruit juice may help renewal of β-cells in STZ-diabetic rats or it may permit the recovery of partially destroyed β-cells (Ahmed, Adeghate, Sharma et al. 1998).

10.7.2 BITTER MELON LOWERS BLOOD GLUCOSE

A study published in the journal *Pharmacological Research* reported that alcohol-extracted charantin from *M. charantia* consists of mixed steroids, and in an animal model of diabetes, it improved glucose tolerance to a degree similar to that of the oral antihyperglycemic agent, tolbutamide (Sarkar, Pranava, and Marita. 1996).

A clinical study published in the *Upsala Journal of Medical Sciences* reported the result of the treatment of diabetic patients with an insulin-like compound obtained from vegetable source (vegetable insulin). The active hypoglycemic principle, purified protein extract, was obtained from fruits as well as from tissue cultures of the plant *M. charantia* L. As described earlier in this chapter, this extract was homologous to insulin obtained from animal pancreas. It showed a consistent antihyperglycemic effect in patients with diabetes.

The average fall in blood sugar level at the peak effect of vegetable insulin was statistically significant. The onset of action was within 30 to 60 min, with the peak effect 6 h after the administration of the dose of plant insulin (Baldwa, Bhandari, Pangaria et al. 1977). This effect is similar to that of long-acting (NPH) insulin, which has an onset at 1½ to 2 h with a peak effect from 4 to 12 h after administration. However, curiously, no administration dosages could be found in the Baldwa et al. report.

Oral bitter melon preparations have also been shown to be effective in clinical trials of Type 2 diabetes, one reported in the *Journal of Ethnopharmacology*. This study resulted in a statistically significant improvement in glucose tolerance in Type 2 diabetes patients. The patients, 38 years old on average, were given 100 mL of bitter melon juice 30 min before a glucose load.

Improved glucose tolerance was observed in 73% of the patients (Welihinda, Karunanayake, Sheriff et al. 1986).

An uncontrolled trial titled "Antidiabetic and adaptogenic properties of *M. charantia* extract. An experimental and clinical evaluation" was published in the journal *Phytotherapy Research*. It aimed to evaluate two bitter melon extracts. Five grams of dried fruit powder was administered three times daily to participants with unspecified type of diabetes. A second set of participants received an aqueous extract containing 100 g of fruit per 100 mL of water.

After 3 weeks, the participants in the fruit powder group experienced an average decline in blood sugar of 25%, while those in the aqueous extract group experienced an average 54% decline in blood sugar. HbA1c examined in a subset of participants decreased an average of 17% after the 3-week trial (which is astoundingly good, given the usual lag time of a month or more until a drop in blood sugar can be reflected in a drop in HbA1c levels). The antihyper-glycemic effects in diabetic patients were found to be highly significant at the end of the trial but were cumulative and gradual, unlike that produced by insulin (Srivastava, Venkatakrishna-Bhatt, Verma et al. 1993).

The aim of a study published in the *Journal of Ethnopharmacology* was to assess the efficacy and safety of three doses of bitter melon, compared with metformin, in a 4-week trial. Patients were assigned to four groups: three of them received bitter melon, at either 500, 1000, or 2000 mg/day, and a fourth group received metformin, 1000 mg/day.

It was found that there was a significant decline in fructosamine at week 4 for the metformin group as well as for the bitter melon 2000 mg/day group. Bitter melon at the lower doses of 500 and 1000 mg/day did not significantly decrease fructosamine levels.

The investigators concluded that in patients with Type 2 diabetes, bitter melon had a modest antihyperglycemic effect, and that it significantly reduced fructosamine levels from baseline among patients who received the highest dose (2000 mg/day). However, the antihyperglycemic effect of bitter melon was less than that of metformin at 1000 mg/day (Fuangchan, Sonthisombat, Seubnukarn et al. 2011).

Because previous data offered relatively inconclusive and inconsistent results about the benefits of bitter melon in patients with diabetes, a review published in the journal *Nutrition and Diabetes* aimed to determine whether it has a favorable effect in lowering plasma glucose in such patients.

The investigators searched PubMed, EMBASE, and the Cochrane Library from inception to July 2013, without any language restrictions, for randomized controlled trials evaluating bitter melon against no treatment in patients with Type 1 or Type 2 diabetes. Conventional search methods were employed.

The review revealed that compared with no treatment, bitter melon did not significantly lower A1C, or FPG, and it was concluded that bitter melon supplementation compared with no treatment did not show significant glycemic improvements on either A1c or FPG (Yin, Lee, Hirpara et al. 2014).

A comprehensive and thorough literature review aimed to assess the effects of *M. charantia* for Type 2 diabetes was published in *The Cochrane Database of Systematic Reviews*. The authors concluded that "… there is insufficient evidence on the effects of momordica charantia for Type 2 diabetes mellitus. Further studies are therefore required to address the issues of standardization and the quality control of preparations. For medical nutritional therapy, further observational trials evaluating the effects of momordica charantia are needed before randomized control trials (RCTs) are established to guide any recommendations in clinical practice" (Ooi, Yassin, and Hamid. 2012).

Finally, the summary of a review titled "Bitter melon (*M. charantia*): a review of efficacy and safety" published in the *American Journal of Health-System Pharmacy* states that:

…Bitter melon (*Momordica charantia*) is an alternative therapy that has primarily been used for lowering blood glucose levels in patients with diabetes mellitus. Components of bitter melon extract appear to have structural similarities to animal insulin…. Four clinical trials found bitter melon juice, fruit, and dried powder to have a moderate hypoglycemic effect. These studies were small and were not randomized or double-blind, however. Reported adverse effects of bitter melon include hypoglycemic coma and convulsions in children, reduced fertility in mice, a favism-like syndrome, increases in gamma-glutamyltransferase and alkaline phosphatase levels in animals, and headaches. Bitter melon may have additive effects when taken with other glucose-lowering agents. Adequately powered, randomized, placebo-controlled trials are needed to properly assess safety and efficacy before bitter melon can be routinely recommended. Bitter melon may have hypoglycemic effects, but data are not sufficient to recommend its use in the absence of careful supervision and monitoring.

From Basch, Gabardi, and Ulbricht (2003) [*American Journal of Health-System Pharmacy, Feb; 60(4): 356–359. With permission*].

10.7.3 Drug–Botanical Interactions, Side Effects, and Toxicity

Due to its ability to provoke outright hypoglycemia, even to the point of coma, bitter melon extracts could excessively potentiate the effects of insulin and oral hypoglycemic medications. Individuals should be advised to closely monitor blood sugar when adding this botanical to a treatment regimen, and to be certain to have foodstuffs at the ready (orange juice, sucking candies, etc.) in case hypoglycemic symptoms come on.

Oral consumption of bitter melon fruit is generally thought to be safe as demonstrated by long-term consumption of the fruit in Asian cultures. Subcutaneous injection of p-insulin extracted from bitter melon appears to be safe; however, intravenous injection of extracts is significantly more toxic and is not recommended.

Bitter melon seeds contain momorcharin, which has been shown to have antifertility effects in female mice. β-Momorcharin is a basic glycoprotein found in the seeds of *M. charantia* L. While it differs immunologically from α-momorcharin, also of the same source, nevertheless it has midterm abortifacient activity.

Intraperitoneal administration of β-momocharin in mice on days 4 and 6 of pregnancy led to an inhibition of pregnancy. *In vitro* study showed that the protein disturbed peri-implantation development by (a) blocking the hatching of embryos from the zona pellucida, (b) decreasing the incidence of successful attachment of the blastocyst, (c) reducing the trophoblast outgrowth, and (d) disrupting the development of the inner cell mass.

Therefore, bitter melon seed consumption is not recommended in women who are seeking to become pregnant (as well as for those who are already pregnant, as a sensible precaution) (Chan, Tam, and Yeung. 1984). This plant has "figured out" a fascinating mechanism for reducing the number of progeny (and hence the population size) of predators who would eat the seeds.

A note to the reader: Please see the chart in the Appendix for a summary of the therapeutic and other effects of the selected botanicals described in this chapter.

REFERENCES

Abenavoli L, Capasso R, Milic N, and F Capasso. 2010. Milk thistle in liver diseases: past, present, future. *Phytotherapy Research*, Oct; 24(10): 1423–1432. DOI: 10.1002/ptr.3207.

Adlercreutz H. 2007. Lignans and human health. *Critical Reviews in Clinical Laboratory Sciences*, 44(5–6): 483–525. DOI: 10.1080/10408360701612942.

Ahmed I, Adeghate E, Sharma AK, Pallot DJ, and J Singh. 1998. Effects of *Momordica charantia* fruit juice on islet morphology in the pancreas of the streptozotocin-diabetic rat. *Diabetes Research and Clinical Practice*, Jun; 40(3): 145–1451. PMID: 9716917.

Ahmed I, Lakhani M, Gillett M, John A, and H Raza. 2001. Hypotriglyceridemic and hypocholesterolemic effects of anti-diabetic *Momordica charantia* (karela) fruit extract in streptozotocin-induced diabetic rats. *Diabetes Research and Clinical Practice*, Mar; 51(3): 155–161. PMID: 11269887.

An Y, Sun Z, Zhang Y, Liu B, Guan Y, and M Lu. 2013. The use of berberine for women with polycystic ovary syndrome undergoing IVF treatment. *Clinical Endocrinology*, Aug; Mar; 80(3): 425–431. DOI: 10.1111/cen.12294.

Asp ML, Collene AL, Norris LE, Cole RM, Stout MB, Tang S-Y, Hsu JC, MA Belury. 2011. Time-dependent effects of safflower oil to improve glycemia, inflammation and blood lipids in obese, post-menopausal women with type 2 diabetes: a randomized, double-masked, crossover study. *Clinical Nutrition*, Aug; 30(4): 443–449. DOI: 10.1016/j.clnu.2011.01.001.

Bahijri SM, Ajabnoor GM, Hegazyx GA, Alsheikh L, Moumena MM, Bashanfar BM, and AH Alzahrani. 2017. Supplementation with Oligonol, prevents weight gain and improves lipid profile in overweight and obese Saudi females. *Current Nutrition and Food Science*, 13(4) (2017). DOI: 10.2174/1573401313666170609101408.

Baldwa VS, Bhandari CM, Pangaria A, and RK Goyal. 1977. Clinical trial in patients with diabetes mellitus of an insulin-like compound obtained from plant sources. *Upsala Journal of Medical Sciences*, 82(1): 39–41. DOI: 10.3109/03009737709179057.

Barre DE, Mizier-Barre KA, Griscti O, and K Hafez. 2008. High dose flaxseed oil supplementation may affect fasting blood serum glucose management in human type 2 diabetics. *Journal of Oleo Science*, 57(5): 269–273. PMID: 18391475.

Basch E, Gabardi S, and C Ulbricht. 2003. Bitter melon (*Momordica charantia*): a review of efficacy and safety. *American Journal of Health-System Pharmacy*, Feb; 60(4): 356–359. PMID: 12625217.

Behndig A, Karlsson K, Johansson BO, Brännström T, and SL Marklund. 2001. Superoxide dismutase isoenzymes in the normal and diseased human cornea. *Investigative Ophthalmology and Visual Science*, Sept; 42(10): 2293–2296. PMID: 11527942.

Berg JM, Tymoczko JL, and L Stryer. 2002. *Biochemistry*. 5th edition. New York: W H Freeman. Section 16.4.

Bozan B, and F Temelli. 2008. Chemical composition and oxidative stability of flax, safflower and poppy seed and seed oils. *Bioresource Technology*, Sep; 99(14): 6354–6359. DOI: 10.1016/j.biortech.2007.12.009.

Cargill M. 2016. A history of medicinal mushrooms. *Spirit of Change*; http://www.spiritofchange.org/Spring-2016/A-History-of-Medicinal-Mushrooms/; accessed 9.16.17.

Castellain RC, Gesser M, Tonini F, Schulte RV, Demessiano KZ, Wolff FR, Delle-Monache F, Netz DJ, Cechinel-Filho V, de Freitas RA, de Souza MM, and C Meyre-Silva. 2014. Chemical composition, antioxidant and antinociceptive properties of *Litchi chinensis* leaves. *The Journal of Pharmacy and Pharmacology*, Dec; 66(12): 1796–1807. Epub 2014 Sep 12. DOI: 10.1111/jphp.12309.

Chan E. 1993. Displacement of bilirubin from albumin by berberine. *Biology of the Neonate*, 63(4): 201–208. PMID: 8513024.

Chan WY, Tam PP, and HW Yeung. 1984. The termination of early pregnancy in the mouse by beta-momorcharin. *Contraception*, Jan; 29(1): 91–100. PMID: 6734206.

Chaturvedi P, George S, Milinganyo M, Tripathi Y. 2004. Effect of *Momordica charantia* on lipid profile and oral glucose tolerance in diabetic rats. *Phytotherapy Research*, 18: 954–956. DOI: 10.1002/ptr.1589.

Chen Y-Y, Wu P-C, Weng S-F, and J-F Liu. 2011. Glycemia and peak incremental indices of six popular fruits in Taiwan: healthy and Type 2 diabetes subjects compared. *Journal of Clinical Biochemistry and Nutrition*, Nov; 49(3): 195–199. DOI: 10.3164/jcbn.11-11.

Cheung N, Mitchell P, and TY Wong. 2010. Diabetic retinopathy. *Lancet*, Jul; 376(9735): 124–136. DOI: 10.1016/S0140-6736(09)62124-3.

Chung SSM, Ho ECM, Lam KSL, and SK Chung. 2003. Contribution of polyol pathway to diabetes-induced oxidative stress. *Journal of the American Society of Nephrology*, Aug; 14(3): S233–S236. PMID: 12874437.

Cunnane SC, Ganguli S, Menard C, Liede AC, Hamadeh MJ, Chen ZY, Wolever TM, and DJ Jenkins. 1993. High alpha-linolenic acid flaxseed (*Linum usitatissimum*): some nutritional properties in humans. *British Journal of Nutrition*, Mar; 69(2): 443–453. PMID: 8098222.

Cunnane SC, Hamadeh MJ, Liede AC, Thompson LU, Wolever TM, and DJ Jenkins. 1995. Nutritional attributes of traditional flaxseed in healthy young adults. *The American Journal of Clinical Nutrition*, Jan; 61(1): 62–68. PMID: 7825540.

Di Pierro F, Putignano P, Villanova N, Montesi L, Moscatiello S, and G Marchesini. 2013. Preliminary study about the possible glycemic clinical advantage in using a fixed combination of *Berberis aristata* and *Silybum marianum* standardized extracts versus only *Berberis aristata* in patients with type 2 diabetes. *Clinical Pharmacology*, Nov; 5: 167–174. DOI: 10.2147/CPAA.S54308. eCollection 2013.

Devalaraja S, Jain S, and H Yadav. 2011. Exotic fruits as therapeutic complements for diabetes, obesity and metabolic syndrome. *Food Research International*, Aug; 44(7): 1856–1865. DOI:10.1016/j.foodres.2011.04.008.

Di Pierro F, Villanova N, Agostini F, Marzocchi R, Soverini V, and G Marchesini. 2012. Pilot study on the additive effects of berberine and oral type 2 diabetes agents for patients with suboptimal glycemic control. *Diabetes, Metabolic Syndrome and Obesity*, 5: 213–217. DOI: 10.2147/DMSO.S33718.

Dietzmann J, Thiel U, Ansorge S, Neumann KH, and M Täger. 2002. Thiol-inducing and immunoregulatory effects of flavonoids in peripheral blood mononuclear cells from patients with end-stage diabetic nephropathy. *Free Radical Biology and Medicine*, Nov; 33(10): 1347–1354. DOI: 10.1002/14651858.CD007845.pub3.

Dong H, Wang N, Zhao L, and F Lu. 2012. Berberine in the treatment of Type 2 diabetes mellitus: a systemic review and meta-analysis. *Evidence-Based Complementary and Alternative Medicine*, Jul; 2012 (Article ID 591654): 12 pages. http://dx.doi.org/10.1155/2012/591654.

Ebrahimpour Koujan S, Gargari BP, Mobasseri M, Valizadeh H, and M Asghari-Jafarabadi. 2014. Effects of *Silybum marianum* (L.) Gaertn. (silymarin) extract supplementation on antioxidant status and hs-CRP in patients with type 2 diabetes mellitus: a randomized, triple-blind, placebo-controlled clinical trial. *Phytomedicine*, 2015 Feb; 22(2): 290–296. DOI: 10.1016/j.phymed.2014.12.010.

Elgendi M. 2012. Standard terminologies for photoplethysmogram signals. *Current Cardiology Reviews*, 8, 215–219. DOI: 10.2174/157340312803217184.

Fallahzadeh MK, Dormanesh B, Sagheb MM, Roozbeh J, Vessal G, Pakfetrat M, Daneshbod Y, Kamali-Sarvestani E, and KB Lankarani. 2012. Effect of addition of Silymarin to renin-angiotensin system inhibitors on proteinuria in Type 2 diabetic patients with overt nephropathy: a randomized, double-blind, placebo-controlled trial. *American Journal of Kidney Diseases*, Dec; 60(6): 896–903. DOI: http://dx. doi.org/10.1053/j.ajkd.2012.06.005.

Fuangchan A, Sonthisombat P, Seubnukarn T, Chanouan R, Chotchaisuwat P, Sirigulsatien V, Ingkaninan K, Plianbangchang P, and ST Haines. 2011. Hypoglycemic effect of bitter melon compared with metformin in newly diagnosed type 2 diabetes patients. *Journal of Ethnopharmacology*, Mar; 134(2): 422–428. DOI: 10.1016/j.jep.2010.12.045.

Fujii H, Sun B, Nishioka H, Hirose A, and OI Aruoma. 2007. Evaluation of the safety and toxicity of the oligomerized polyphenol Oligonol. *Food and Chemical Toxicology*, Mar; 45(3): 378–387. DOI: 10.1016/j.fct.2006.08.026.

Gao H, and J Kawabata. 2005. alpha-Glucosidase inhibition of 6-hydroxyflavones. Part 3: Synthesis and evaluation of 2,3,4-trihydroxybenzoyl-containing flavonoid analogs and 6-aminoflavones as alpha-glucosidase inhibitors. *Bioorganics and Medicinal Chemistry*, Mar; 13(5): 1661–1671. DOI: 10.1016/j.bmc.2004.12.010.

Gao Y, Lan J, Dai X, Ye J, and S Zhou. 2004. A phase I/II study of ling zhi mushroom *Ganoderma lucidum* (W.Curt.:Fr.)Lloyd (Aphyllophoromycetidae) extract in patients with type II diabetes mellitus. *International Journal of Medicinal Mushrooms*, 4; 6(1): 33–39. DOI: 10.1615/IntJMedMushr.v6.i1.30.

Gawade SP. 2012. Acetic acid induced painful endogenous infliction in writhing test on mice. *Journal of Pharmacology and Pharmacotherapeutics*, Oct–Dec; 3(4): 348. DOI: 10.4103/0976-500X.103699.

Gebauer SK, Psota TL, Harris WS, and PM Kris-Etherton. 2006. n-3 fatty acid dietary recommendations and food sources to achieve essentiality and cardiovascular benefits. *American Journal of Clinical Nutrition*, Jun; 83(6 Suppl): 1526S–1535S. PMID: 16841863.

Gordon A, Hobbs DA, Bowden DS, Bailey MJ, Mitchell J, Francis AJ, and SK Roberts. 2006. Effects of *Silybum marianum* on serum hepatitis C virus RNA, alanine aminotransferase levels and well-being in patients with chronic hepatitis C. *Journal of Gastroenterology and Hepatology*, Jan; 21(1 Pt 2): 2752–2780. DOI: 10.1111/j.1440-1746.2006.04138.x.

Goyal A, Sharma V, Upadhyay N, Gill S, and M Sihag. 2014. Flax and flaxseed oil: an ancient medicine & modern functional food. *Journal of Food Science and Technology*, Sep; 51(9): 1633–1653. DOI: 10.1007/s13197-013-1247-9.

Guo J, Li L, Pan J, Qiu G, Li A, Huang G, and L Xu. 2004. Pharmacological mechanism of Semen Litchi on antagonizing insulin resistance in rats with type 2 diabetes [article in Chinese]. *Journal of Chinese Medicine* (Zhong Yao Cai). Jun; 27(6): 435–438. PMID: 15524300.

Guo Y, Chen Y, Tan ZR, Klaassen CD, and HH Zhou. 2012. Repeated administration of berberine inhibits cytochromes P450 in humans. *European Journal of Clinical Pharmacology*, Feb; 68(2): 213–217. DOI: 10.1007/s00228-011-1108-2.

Gurley BJ, Barone GW, Williams DK, Carrier J, Breen P, Yates CR, Song PF, Hubbard MA, Tong Y, and S Cheboyina. 2006. Effect of milk thistle (*Silybum marianum*) and black cohosh (*Cimicifuga racemosa*) supplementation on digoxin pharmacokinetics in humans. *Drug Metabolism and Disposition*, Jan; 34(1): 69–74. DOI: 10.1124/dmd.105.006312.

Harinantenaina L, Tanaka M, Takaoka S, Oda M, Mogami O, Uchida M, and Y Asakawa. 2006. *Momordica charantia* constituents and antidiabetic screening of the isolated major compounds. *Chemical and Pharmaceutical Bulletin* (Tokyo), 54: 1017–1021.

Hawke RL, Schrieber SJ, Soule TA, Wen Z, Smith PC, Reddy KR, Wahed AS, Belle SH, Afdhal NH, Navarro VJ, Berman J, Liu QY, Doo E, and MW Fried, and SyNCH Trial Group. 2010. Silymarin ascending multiple oral dosing phase I study in noncirrhotic patients with chronic hepatitis C. *Journal of Clinical Pharmacology*, Apr; 50(4): 434–449. DOI: 10.1177/0091270009347475.

Hikino H, Konno C, Mirin Y, and T Hayashi. 1985. Isolation and hypoglycemic activity of ganoderans A and B, glycans of *Ganoderma lucidum* fruit bodies 1. *Planta Medica*, Aug; 51(4): 339–340. DOI: 10.1055/s-2007-969507.

Hsu TH, and HC Lo. 2002. Biological activity of Cordyceps (Fr.) Link species (ascomycetes) derived from a natural source and from fermented mycelia on diabetes in STZ-induced rats. *International Journal of Medicinal Mushrooms*, 4: 111–125.

Huang CJ, and MC Wu. 2002. Differential effects of foods traditionally regarded as 'heating' and 'cooling' on prostaglandin E(2) production by a macrophage cell line. *Journal of Biomedical Science*, Nov–Dec; 9(6 Pt 2): 596–606. DOI: 67288.

Huseini HF, Larijani B, Heshmat R, Fakhrzadeh H, Radjabipour B, Toliat T, and M Raza. 2006. The efficacy of *Silybum marianum* (L.) Gaertn. (silymarin) in the treatment of type II diabetes: a randomized, double-blind, placebo-controlled, clinical trial. *Phytotherapy Research*, Dec; 20(12): 1036–1039. DOI: 10.1002/ptr.1988.

Hussain S A-R. 2007. Silymarin as an adjunct to glibenclamide therapy improves long-term and postprandial glycemic control and body mass index in type 2 diabetes. *Journal of Medicinal Food*, Jul; 10(3): 543–547. https://doi.org/10.1089/jmf.2006. 089.

Isenberg SL, Carter MD, Hayes SR, Graham LA, Johnson D, Mathews TP, Harden LA, Takeoka GR, Thomas JD, Pirkle JL, and RC Johnson. 2016. Quantification of toxins in soapberry (Sapindaceae) arils: hypoglycin A and methylenecyclopropylglycine. *Journal of Agricultural and Food Chemistry*, Jul; 64 (27): 5607–5613. DOI: 10.1021/acs.jafc.6b02478.

Jiang G, Lin S, Wen L, Jiang Y, Zhao M, Chen F, Prasad KN, Duan X, and B Yang. 2013. Identification of a novel phenolic compound in litchi (*Litchi chinensis* Sonn.) pericarp and bioactivity evaluation. *Food Chemistry*, Jan 15; 136(2): 563–568. DOI: 10.1016/j.foodchem.2012.08.089.

Jose N, Ajith TA, and KK Jananrdhanan. 2002. Antioxidant, anti-inflammatory, and antitumor activities of culinary-medicinal mushroom *Pleurotus pulmonarius* (Fr.) Quél. (Agaricomycetidae). *International Journal of Medicinal Mushrooms*, 4: 329–335.

Joseph B, and D Jini. 2013. Antidiabetic effects of *Momordica charantia* (bitter melon) and its medicinal potency. *Asian Pacific Journal of Tropical Disease*, Apr; 3(2): 93–102. DOI: 10.1016/S2222-1808(13)60052-3.

Kador PF, and JH Kinoshita. 1984. Diabetic and galactosaemic cataracts. *Ciba Foundation Symposium*, 106: 110–131. PMID: 6439498.

Kapoor S, Sachdeva R, and A Kochhar. 2011. Efficacy of flaxseed supplementation on nutrient intake and other lifestyle pattern in menopausal diabetic females. *Ethnomedicine*, Dec; 5(3): 153–160.

Kaur A, Gupta V, Christopher AF, Malik MA, and P Bansala. 2017. Nutraceuticals in prevention of cataract—an evidence based approach. *Saudi Journal of Ophthalmology*, Jan–Mar; 31(1): 30–37. DOI: 10.1016/j.sjopt.2016.12.001.

Kazazis CE, Evangelopoulos AA, Kollas A, and NG Vallianou. 2014. The therapeutic potential of Milk Thistle in diabetes. *The Review of Diabetic Studies*, Summer; 11(2): 167–174. DOI: 10.1900/RDS.2014.11.167.

Kiho T, Morimoto H, Kobayashi T, Ysai S, Ukai S, Aizawa K, and T Inakuma. 2000. Effect of a polysaccharide (TAP) from the fruiting bodies of *Tremella aurantia* on glucose metabolism in mouse liver. *Bioscience, Biotechnology, and Biochemistry*, Feb; 64: 417–419. DOI: 10.1271/bbb.64.417.

Kiho TA, Yamane J, Hui S, Usui S, and S Ukai. 1996. Polysaccharides in fungi. XXXVI. Hypoglycemic activity of a polysaccharide (CS-F30) from the cultural mycelium of *Cordyceps sinensis* and its effect on glucose metabolism in mouse liver. *Biological and Pharmaceutical Bulletin*, 19: 294–296.

Kilari EK, and S Putta. 2016. Biological and phytopharmacological descriptions of *Litchi chinensis*. *Pharmacognosy Review*. Jan–Jun; 10(19): 60–65. DOI: 10.4103/0973-7847.176548.

Kim DO, Jeong SW, and CY Lee. 2003. Antioxidant capacity phenolic phytochemicals from various cultivars of plums. *Food Chemistry*, Jun; 81:321–326. https://doi.org/10.1016/S0308-8146(02)00423-5.

Kim GY, Kim SH, Hwang SY, Kim HY, Park YM, Park SK, Lee MK, Lee SH, Lee TH, and JD Lee. 2003. Oral administration of proteoglycan isolated from *Phellinus linteus* in the prevention and treatment of collagen-induced arthritis in mice. *Biological and Pharmaceutical Bulletin*, Jun; 26(6): 823–831. PMID: 12808294.

Kim NC, Graf TN, Sparacino CM, Wani MC, and ME Wall. 2003. Complete isolation and characterization of silybins and isosilybins from milk thistle (*Silybum marianum*). *Organic and Biomolecular Chemistry*, May 21; 1(10): 1684–1689. PMID: 12926355.

Kim SH, Song YS, Kim SK, Kim BC, Lim CJ, and EH Park. 2004. Anti-inflammatory and related pharmacological activities of the n-BuOH subfraction of mushroom *Phellinus linteus*. *Journal of Ethnopharmacology*, Jul; 93: 141–116. DOI: 10.1016/j.jep.2004.03.048.

Kinoshita JH, Fukushi S, Kador P, and LO Merola. 1979. Aldose reductase in diabetic complications of the eye. *Metabolism*, Apr; 28(4): 462–469. PMID: 45423.

Kinoshita JH. 1965. Cataracts in galactosemia. The Jonas S. Friedenwald memorial lecture. *Investigative Ophthalmology*, Oct; 4(5): 786–799. PMID: 5831988.

Kinoshita JH. 1974. Mechanisms initiating cataract formation. Proctor lecture. *Investigative Ophthalmology*, Oct; 13(10): 713–724. PMID: 4278188.

Kitadate K, Aoyagi K, and K Homma, 2014. Effect of Lychee Fruit extract (Oligonol) on peripheral circulation, a pilot study. Skin thermography demonstrates vasodilatation effects of polyphenol. *Natural Medicine Journal*, Jul; 6(7).

Kong F, Zhang M, Liao S, Yu S, Chi J, and Z Wei. 2010. Antioxidant activity of polysaccharide-enriched fractions extracted from pulp tissue of *Litchi chinensis* Sonn. *Molecules*, Mar 25; 15(4): 2152–2165. DOI: 10.3390/molecules15042152.

Konno S, Aynehchi S, Dolin DJ, Schwartz AM, Choudhury MS, and HN Tazakin. 2002. Anticancer and hypoglycemic effects of polysaccharides in edible and medicinal Maitake mushroom [*Grifola frondosa* (Dicks.:Fr.) S.F.Gray]. *International Journal of Medicinal Mushrooms*, 4: 185–195.

Kroll DJ, Shaw HS, and NH Oberlies. 2007. Milk thistle nomenclature: why it matters in cancer research and pharmacokinetic studies. *Integrative Cancer Therapies*, Jun; 6(2): 110–119. DOI: 10.1177/1534735407301825.

Kumamoto Y, Takamura Y, Kubo E, Tsuzuki S, and Y Akagi. 2007. Epithelial cell density in cataractous lenses of patients with diabetes: association with erythrocyte aldose reductase. *Experimental Eye Research*, Sept; 85(3): 393–399. DOI: 10.1016/j.exer.2007.06.007.

Lan J, Zhao Y, Dong F, Yan Z, Zheng W, Fan J, and G Sun. 2015. Meta-analysis of the effect and safety of berberine in the treatment of type 2 diabetes mellitus, hyperlipemia and hypertension. *Journal of Ethnopharmacology*, Feb; 161: 69–81. DOI: 10.1016/j.jep.2014.09.049.

Lee DY, and Y Liu. 2003. Molecular structure and stereochemistry of silybin A, silybin B, isosilybin A, and isosilybin B. Isolated from *Silybum marianum* (milk thistle). *Journal of Natural Products*, Sep; 66(9):1171–1174. DOI: 10.1021/np030163b.

Lee J-B, Shin Y-O, Min Y-K, and H-M Yang. 2010. The effect of Oligonol intake on cortisol and related cytokines in healthy young men. *Nutrition Research and Practice*, Jun; 4(3): 203–207. DOI: 10.4162/nrp.2010.4.3.203.

Lee N, Shin MS, Kang Y, Park K, Maeda T, Nishioka H, Hajime F, Kanga I, and I Kang, 2016. Oligonol, a lychee fruit-derived low-molecular form of polyphenol mixture, suppresses inflammatory cytokine production from human monocytes. *Human Immunology*, Jun; 77(6): 512–525. DOI: 10.1016/j.humimm.2016.04.011.

Lee S-J, Park WH, Park SD, and H-I Moon. 2009. Aldose reductase inhibitors from *Litchi chinensis* Sonn. *Journal of Enzyme Inhibition and Medicinal Chemistry*, Apr; 24(4): 957–959. http://dx.doi.org/10.1080/14756360802560867.

Li W, Liang H, Zhang MW, Zhang RF, Deng YY, Wei ZC, Zhang Y, and XJ Tang. 2012. Phenolic profiles and antioxidant activity of litchi (*Litchi chinensis* Sonn.) fruit pericarp from different commercially available cultivars. *Molecules*, Dec; 17(12): 14954–14967. DOI: 10.3390/molecules171214954.

Li W-C, Kuszak JR, Dunn K, Wang R-R, Ma W, Wang G-M, Spector A, Leib M, Cotliar AM, Weiss M, Espy J, Howard G, Farris RL, Auran J, Donn A, Hofeldt A, Mackay C, Merriam J, Mittl R, and TR Smith. 1995. Lens epithelial cell apoptosis appears to be a common cellular basis for non-congenital cataract development in humans and animals. *Journal of Cell Biology*, Jul; 130(1):169–181. PMCID: PMC2120521.

Lindequist U, Niedermeyer THJ, and W-D Jülich. 2005. The pharmacological potential of mushrooms. *Evidence Based Complementary and Alternative Medicine*, Sep; 2(3): 285–299. DOI: 10.1093/ecam/neh107; https://www.ncbi.nlm.nih.gov/pmc/articles/PMC1193547/.

Lo HC, and SP Wasser. 2011. Medicinal mushrooms for glycemic control in diabetes mellitus: history, current status, future perspectives, and unsolved problems (review). *International Journal of Medicinal Mushrooms*, 13(5): 401–426. PMID: 22324407.

Lv Q, Luo F, Zhao X, Liu Y, Hu G, Sun C, Li X, and K Chen. 2015. Identification of proanthocyanidins from Litchi (*Litchi chinensis* Sonn.) pulp by LC-ESI-Q-TOF-MS and their antioxidant activity. *PLoS One*, 10(3): e0120480. DOI: 10.1371/journal.pone. 0120480.

Ma Q, Xie H, Li S, Zhang R, Zhang M, and X Wei. 2014. Flavonoids from the pericarps of *Litchi chinensis*. *Journal of Agricultural and Food Chemistry*, Feb 5; 62(5): 1073–1078. DOI: 10.1021/jf405750p.

Maitrejean M, Comte G, Barron D, El Kirat K, Conseil G, and A Di Pietro. 2000. The flavanolignan silybin and its hemisynthetic derivatives, a novel series of potential modulators of P-glycoprotein. *Bioorganic and Medicinal Chemistry Letters*, Jan 17; 10(2): 157–160. PMID: 10673101.

McCord JM, and I Fridovich. 1969. Superoxide dismutase. An enzymic function for erythrocuprein (hemocuprein). *Journal of Biological Chemistry*. 1969; 244(22):6049–6055. PMID: 5389100.

Menzel C, Christopher M and K Geoff. 2005. *Litchi and Longan: Botany, Production and Uses*. Cambridge, MA: CABI Publishing USA. p. 26.

Mohamed GA, and SRM Ibrahim, 2015. *Litchi chinensis*: Medicinal uses, phytochemistry, and pharmacology. *Journal of Ethnopharmacology*, Sept; 174: 491–513. DOI: 10.1016/j.jep.2015.08.054.

Mulhern ML, Madson CJ, Danford A, Ikesugi K, Kador PF, and T Shinohara. 2006. The unfolded protein response in lens epithelial cells from galactosemic rat lenses. *Investigative Ophthalmology and Visual Science*, Sept; 47(9): 3951–3959. DOI: 10.1167/iovs.06-0193.

Nazni P, Amrithaveni M, and VT Poongodi. 2006. Impact of flaxseed based therapeutic food on selected type II diabetic patients. *The Indian Journal of Nutrition and Dietetics*, 43: 141–145.

No authors listed. 2000. Berberine. *Alternative Medicine Review*, Apr; 5(2): 175–177. PMID: 10767672.

No authors listed. 2007. *Momordica charantia*. *Alternative Medicine Review*, 12(4): 360–363. http://www.altmedrev.com/publications/12/4/360.pdf.

No authors listed. 2006. PPAR agonists. Diabetes Self Management; https://www.diabetesselfmanagement.com/diabetes-resources/definitions/ppar-agonists/; accessed 8.27.17

Noh JS, Park CH, and T Yokozawa. 2011. Treatment with oligonol, a low-molecular polyphenol derived from lychee fruit, attenuates diabetes-induced hepatic damage through regulation of oxidative stress and lipid metabolism. *The British Journal of Nutrition*, Oct; 106(7): 1013–1022. DOI: 10.1017/S0007114511001322.

Obrosova IG, Chung SS, and PF Kador. 2010. Diabetic cataracts: mechanisms and management. *Diabetes/Metabolism Research and Reviews*, Mar; 26(3): 172–180. DOI: 10.1002/dmrr.1075.

Oishi N, Morikubo S, Takamura Y, Kubo E, Tsuzuki S, Tanimoto T, and Y Akagi. 2006. Correlation between adult diabetic cataracts and red blood cell aldose reductase levels. *Investigative Ophthalmology and Visual Science*, May; 47(5): 2061–2064. DOI: 10.1167/iovs.05-1042.

Ooi CP, Yassin Z, and TA Hamid. 2012. *Momordica charantia* for type 2 diabetes mellitus. *The Cochrane Database of Systematic Reviews*, Aug; (8): CD007845.

Ookawara T, Kawamura N, Kitagawa Y, and N Taniguchi. 1992. Site-specific and random fragmentation of Cu,Zn-superoxide dismutase by glycation reaction. Implication of reactive oxygen species. *Journal of Biological Chemistry*. Sept; 267(26): 18505–18510. PMID: 1326527.

Pang B, Zhao L-H, Zhou Q, Zhao T-Y, Wang H, Gu C-J, and X-L Tong. 2015. Application of berberine on treating Type 2 diabetes mellitus. *International Journal of Endocrinology*, Feb; 2015 (Article ID 905749): 12 pages. http://dx.doi.org/10.1155/2015/905749.

Park CH, Yokozawa T, and JS Noh. 2014. Oligonol, a low-molecular-weight polyphenol derived from lychee fruit, attenuates diabetes-induced renal damage through the advanced glycation end product-related pathway in db/db mice. *The Journal of Nutrition*, Aug; 144(8): 1150–1157. DOI: 10.3945/jn.114.193961.

Pauff JM, and R Hille R. 2009. Inhibition studies of bovine xanthine oxidase by luteolin, silibinin, quercetin, and curcumin. *Journal of Natural Products*, Apr; 72(4): 725–731. DOI: 10.1021/np8007123.

Pollreisz A, and U Schmidt-Erfurth. 2010. Diabetic cataract—pathogenesis, epidemiology and treatment. *Journal of Ophthalmology*, Nov; 244(22): 6049–6055.608751. DOI: 10.1155/2010/608751.

Prasad K, Mantha SV, Muir AD, and ND Westcott. 2000. Protective effect of secoisolariciresinol diglucoside against streptozotocin-induced diabetes and its mechanism. *Molecular and Cellular Biochemistry*, Mar; 206(1–2): 141–149. PMID: 10839204.

Prasad K. 2001. Secoisolariciresinol diglucoside from flaxseed delays the development of type 2 diabetes in Zucker rat. *The Journal of Laboratory and Clinical Medicine*, Jul; 138(1): 32–39. DOI: 10.1067/mlc.2001.115717.

Prasad K. 2002. Suppression of phospoenolpyruvate carboxykinase gene expression by secoisolariciresinol diglucoside (SDG), a new antidiabetic agent. *International Journal of Angiology*, Mar; 11(2): 107–109. DOI: 10.1007/s00547-001-0071.

Qazi N, Khan RA, Rizwani GH, and ZA Feroz. 2014. Effect of *Carthamus tinctorius* (Safflower) on fasting blood glucose and insulin levels in alloxan induced diabetic rabbits. *Pakistan Journal of Pharmaceutical Sciences*, Mar; 27(2): 377–380. PMID: 24577929.

Ren S, Xu DD, Pan Z, Gao Y, Jiang ZG, and QP Gao. 2011. Two flavanone compounds from lychee (*Lychee chinensis* Sonn.) seeds, one previously unreported, and appraisal of their α-glycosidase activities. *Food Chemistry*, 127:1760–1763.

Sakurai T, Nishioka H, Fujii H, Nakano N, Kizaki T, Radak Z, Izawa T, Haga S, and H Ohno. 2008. Antioxidative effects of a new lychee fruit-derived polyphenol mixture, oligonol, converted into a low-molecular form in adipocytes. *Bioscience, Biotechnology, and Biochemistry*, Feb; 72(2): 463–476. DOI: 10.1271/bbb.70567.

Sarkar S, Pranava M, and R Marita. 1996. Demonstration of the hypoglycemic action of *Momordica charantia* in a validated animal model of diabetes. *Pharmacological Research*, Jan; 33(1): 1–4. PMID: 8817639.

Sheu SY, Lai CH, and HC Chiang. 1998. Inhibition of xanthine oxidase by purpurogallin and silymarin group. *Anticancer Research*, Jan–Feb; 18(1A): 263–267. PMID: 9568088.

Shibib BA, Khan LA, and R Rahman. 1993. Hypoglycaemic activity of *Coccinia indica* and *Momordica charantia* in diabetic rats: depression of the hepatic gluconeogenic enzymes glucose-6-phosphatase and fructose-1,6-bisphosphatase and elevation of both liver and red-cell shunt enzyme glucose-6-phosphate dehydrogenase. *The Biochemistry Journal*, May 15; 292 (Pt 1): 267–270. PMCID: PMC1134299.

Srivastava SK, Ramana KV, and A Bhatnagar. 2005. Role of aldose reductase and oxidative damage in diabetes and the consequent potential for therapeutic options. *Endocrine Reviews*, May; 26(3): 380–392. DOI: 10.1210/er.2004-0028.

Srivastava Y, Venkatakrishna-Bhatt H, Verma Y, Venkaiah K, and BH Raval. 1993. Antidiabetic and adaptogenic properties of *Momordica charantia* extract. An experimental and clinical evaluation. *Phytotherapy Research*, July/August; 7(4): 285–289. DOI: 10.1002/ptr.2650070405.

Stamets P, and H Zwickey. 2014. Medicinal mushrooms: ancient remedies meet Modern science. *Integrative Medicine*, (Encinitas). Feb; 13(1): 46–47. PMCID: PMC4684114.

Su D, Ti H, Zhang R, Zhang M, Wei Z, Deng Y, and J Guo. 2014. Structural elucidation and cellular antioxidant activity evaluation of major antioxidant phenolics in lychee pulp. *Food Chemistry*, Sep; 158: 385–391. DOI: 10.1016/j.foodchem.2014.02.134.

Surai PF. 2015. Silymarin as a natural antioxidant: an overview of the current evidence and perspectives. *Antioxidants* (Basel), Mar; 4(1): 204–247. DOI: 10.3390/antiox4010204.

Suzuki K, Tsubaki S, Fujita M, Koyama N, Takahashi M, and K Takazawa. 2010. Effects of safflower seed extract on arterial stiffness. *Vascular Health and Risk Management*, Nov; 6: 1007–1014. DOI: 10.2147 /VHRM.S13998.

Takahashi T, and M Miyazawa. 2012. Potent α-glucosidase inhibitors from safflower (*Carthamus tinctorius* L.) seed. *Phytotherapy Research*, May; 26(5): 722–726. DOI: 10.1002/ptr.3622.

Takamura Y, Sugimoto Y, Kubo E, Takahashi Y, and Akagi. 2001. Immunohistochemical study of apoptosis of lens epithelial cells in human and diabetic rat cataracts. *Japanese Journal of Ophthalmology*, Nov–Dec; 45(6): 559–563. PMID: 11754895.

Tyagi AK, Singh RP, Agarwal C, Chan DC, and R Agarwal. 2002. Silibinin strongly synergizes human prostate carcinoma DU145 cells to doxorubicin-induced growth Inhibition, G2-M arrest, and apoptosis. *Clinical Cancer Research*, Nov; 8(11): 3512–3519. PMID: 12429642.

Vashishtha VM. 2016. Outbreaks of hypoglycemic encephalopathy in Muzaffarpur, India: Are these caused by toxins in litchi fruit? The counterpoint. *Indian Pediatrics*, May 8; 53(5): 399–402. PMID: 27254049.

Veeresham C, Rao AR, and A Kaleab. 2013. Aldose reductase inhibitors of plant origin. *Phytotherapy Research*, Mar; 28(3): 1–17. DOI: 10.1002/ptr.5000.

Velussi M, Cernigoi AM, Ariella DM, Dapas F, Caffau C, and M Zilli. 1997. Long-term (12 months) treatment with an anti-oxidant drug (silymarin) is effective on hyperinsulinemia, exogenous insulin need and malondialdehyde levels in cirrhotic diabetic patients. *Journal of Hepatology*, Apr; 26(4): 871–879, 1997. DOI: http://dx.doi.org/10.1016/S0168-8278(97)80255-3.

Velussi M, Cernigoi AM, Viezzoli L, Dapas F, Caffau C, and M Zilli. 1993. Silymarin reduces hyperinsulinemia, malondialdehyde levels, and daily insulin need in cirrhotic diabetic patients. *Current Therapeutic Research*, 53(5): 533–545.

Voroneanu L, Nistor I, Dumea R, Apetrii M, and A Covic. 2016. Silymarin in Type 2 diabetes mellitus: a systematic review and meta-analysis of randomized controlled trials. *Journal of Diabetes Research*, 2016: 5147468. DOI: 10.1155/2016/5147468.

Wasser SP, Tan KK, and VI Elisashvili. 2002. Hypoglycemic, interferonogenous, and immunomodulatory activity of Tremellastin from the submerged culture of *Tremella mesenterica* Retz.:Fr. (Heterobasidiomycetes). *International Journal of Medicinal Mushrooms*, 4(3): 215–227. DOI: 10.1615 /IntJMedMushr.v4.i3.40.

Wei CC, Chang S-J, Chen YA, and SJ Chang. 2016. Flavanol-rich lychee fruit extract alleviates diet-induced insulin resistance via suppressing mTOR/SREBP-1 mediated lipogenesis in liver and restoring insulin signaling in skeletal muscle. *Molecular Nutrition and Food Research*, Oct; 60(10): 2288–2296. DOI: 10.1002/mnfr. 201501064.

Wei W, Zhao H, Wang A, Sui M, and Y Guan. 2012. A clinical study on the short-term effect of berberine in comparison to metformin on the metabolic characteristics of women with polycystic ovary syndrome. *European Journal of Endocrinology*, Jan; 166(1): 99–105. DOI: 10.1530/EJE-11-0616.

Welihinda J, Arvidson G, Gylfe E, Hellman B, and E Karlsson. 1982. The insulin releasing activity of the tropical plant *Momordica charantia*. *Acta Biologica et Medica Germanica*, Jan; 41(12): 1229–1240. PMID: 6765165.

Welihinda J, Karunanayake EH, Sheriff MH, and KS Jayasinghe. 1986. Effect of *Momordica charantia* on the glucose tolerance in maturity onset diabetes. *Journal of Ethnopharmacology*, Sept; 17(3): 277–282. PMID: 3807390.

Wu T, Luo J, and B Xu. 2015. In vitro antidiabetic effects of selected fruits and vegetables against glycosidase and aldose reductase. *Food Science and Nutrition*, Nov; 3(6): 495–505. DOI: 10.1002/fsn3.243.

Yibchok-anun S, Adisakwattana S, Yao CY, Sangvanich P, Roengsumran S, and WH Hsu. 2006. Slow acting protein extract from fruit pulp of *Momordica charantia* with insulin secretagogue and insulinomimetic activities. *Biological and Pharmaceutical Bulletin*, Jun; 29(6): 1126–1131. PMID: 16755004.

Yin J, Gao Z, Liu D, Liu Z, and J Ye. 2007. Berberine improves glucose metabolism through induction of glycolysis. *American Journal of Physiology-Endocrinology and Metabolism*, Jan; 294(1): E148–E156. DOI: 10.1152/ajpendo.00211.2007.

Yin J, Xing H, and J Ye. 2008. Efficacy of berberine in patients with Type 2 diabetes. *Metabolism*, May; 57(5): 712–717. DOI: 10.1016/j.metabol. 2008.01.013.

Yin RV, Lee NC, Hirpara H, and OJ Phung. 2014. The effect of bitter melon (*Momordica charantia*) in patients with diabetes mellitus: a systematic review and meta-analysis. *Nutrition and Diabetes*, Dec; 4(12): e145. DOI: 10.1038/nutd. 2014.42.

Zhang H, Wei J, Xue R, Wu JD, Zhao W, Wang ZZ, Wang SK, Zhou ZX, Song DQ, Wang YM, Pan HN, Kong WJ, and JD Jiang. 2010. Berberine lowers blood glucose in type 2 diabetes mellitus patients through increasing insulin receptor expression. *Metabolism*, Feb; 59(2): 285–292. DOI: 10.1016/j .metabol.2009.07.029.

Zhang R, Zeng Q, Deng Y, Zhang M, Wei Z, Zhang Y, and X Tang. 2013. Phenolic profiles and antioxidant activity of litchi pulp of different cultivars cultivated in Southern China. *Food Chemistry*, Feb 15; 136(3–4): 1169–1176. DOI: 10.1016/j.foodchem.2012.09.085.

Zhang S, and ME Morris. 2003. Effects of the flavonoids biochanin A, morin, phloretin, and silymarin on P-glycoprotein-mediated transport. *Journal of Pharmacology and Experimental Therapeutics*, Mar; 304(3): 1258–1267. DOI: 10.1124/jpet.102.044412.

Zhang X-H, Yokoo H, Nishioka H, Fujii H, Matsuda N, Hayashi T, and Y Hattori. 2010. Beneficial effect of the oligomerized polyphenol oligonol on high glucose- induced changes in eNOS phosphorylation and dephosphorylation in endothelial cells. *British Journal of Pharmacology*, Feb; 159: 928–938. DOI: 10.1111/j.1476-5381.2009. 00594.x.

Zhang Y, Li X, Zou D, Liu W, Yang J, Zhu N, Huo L, Wang M, Hong J, Wu P, Ren G, and G Ning. 2008. Treatment of Type 2 Diabetes and dyslipidemia with the natural plant alkaloid berberine. *The Journal of Clinical Endocrinology and Metabolism*, Jul; 93(7): 2559–2565, https://doi.org/10.1210/jc.2007-2404.

Zhang Y, Mills G, and MG Nair. 2002. Cyclooxygenase inhibitory and antioxidant compounds from the mycelia of the edible mushroom *Grifola frondosa*. *Journal of Agricultural and Food Chemistry*, Dec; 50(26): 7581–7585. PMID: 12475274.

Zhou S, Lim LY, and B Chowbay. 2004. Herbal modulation of P-glycoprotein. *Drug Metabolism Reviews*, Feb; 36(1): 57–104. DOI: 10.1081/DMR-120028427.

Zhou Y, Wang H, Yang R, Huang H, Sun Y, Shen Y, Lei H, and H Gao. 2012. Effects of *Litchi chinensis* fruit isolates on prostaglandin E(2) and nitric oxide production in J774 murine macrophage cells. *BMC Complementary and Alternative Medicine*, Mar 1; 12:12. DOI: 10.1186/1472-6882-12-12.

11 Selected Functional Foods That Combat the Effects of Hyperglycemia and Chronic Inflammation

One quarter of what you eat keeps you alive. The rest keeps your doctor alive.

Anonymous

11.1 HYPERGLYCEMIA AND CHRONIC SYSTEMIC INFLAMMATION

There is a wealth of evidence that supports the theory that the etiology of most cardiovascular diseases is linked to chronic systemic inflammation. A report in the *Central European Journal of Immunology* tells us that this is particularly the case in atherosclerosis. In fact, the title of the report is "Atherosclerosis: a chronic inflammatory disease mediated by mast cells" (Conti, and Shaik-Dasthagirisae. 2015).

There is also substantial evidence that chronic hyperglycemia, as in Type 2 diabetes, is linked to chronic systemic inflammation. A report in the *Journal of Clinical Investigation* concludes that "...the available evidence strongly suggests that Type 2 diabetes is an inflammatory disease and that inflammation is a primary cause of obesity-linked insulin resistance, hyperglycemia, and hyperlipidemia rather than merely a consequence" (Wellen, and Hotamisligil. 2005).

White blood cell (WBC) count is a clinical marker of inflammation. It has been known for some time that it is elevated in Type 2 diabetes, but the first large-scale study of this phenomenon was conducted on a Chinese population and reported in the *International Journal of Environmental Research and Public Health*: The investigators aimed to determine the relationship between white blood cell count and glucose metabolism.

Nearly 10,000 participants—average age, 59—were recruited, and they were classified into groups: those with normal glucose tolerance, those with isolated impaired fasting glucose, and those with impaired glucose tolerance and Type 2 diabetes. It was found that in the Type 2 diabetes group, white blood cell count increased as glucose metabolism disorders worsened. White blood cell count also correlated positively with waist–hip ratio, body mass index (BMI), smoking, triglycerides, glycosylated hemoglobin (HbA1c), and 2-h postprandial glucose. In addition, high-density lipoprotein (HDL) and female gender were factors inversely correlated with white blood cell count.

The white blood cell count, while elevated in Type 2 diabetes, does not increase as the duration of the disease increases. The investigators concluded that elevated white blood cell count is independently associated with worsening of glucose metabolism in the middle-aged and elderly in their population (Jiang, Yan, Li et al. 2014).

And so the question is: Does inflammation cause insulin resistance, the main feature of Type 2 diabetes, or is it the other way around?

A study reported in *Nature Reviews. Immunology* (London) concluded that inflammation *participates* in the pathogenesis of Type 2 diabetes. The preliminary results from clinical trials with salicylates, and interleukin-1 antagonists, support this notion and have opened the door for immune-modulatory strategies for the treatment of Type 2 diabetes that simultaneously lower blood glucose levels and potentially reduce the severity and prevalence of the associated complications of this disease—meaning inflammation (Donath, and Shoelson. 2001).

A report published in the *World Journal of Diabetes* concluded that low-grade inflammation in Type 2 diabetes has given an impetus to the field of immuno-metabolism linking inflammation to insulin resistance and β-cell dysfunction. Many cellular factors point to a causal link between metabolic stress and inflammation including factors that trigger inflammatory signaling cascades. Therefore, Type 2 diabetes can be considered an inflammatory disorder triggered by disordered metabolism. Cellular mechanisms like activation of Toll-like receptors, endoplasmic reticulum stress, and inflammasome activation are related to the excess of glucose, linking pathogenesis and progression of Type 2 diabetes with inflammation (Hameed, Masoodi, Mir et al. 2015).

And so, logic dictates the conclusion that treatment, conventional or "integrative," will work best when it simultaneously addresses both insulin resistance and chronic systemic inflammation.

One approach of integrative treatment is the selection of treatment substances that, in combination, target hyperglycemia and chronic systemic inflammation: selected "functional foods" are a ready source. In fact, in many respects, they may be superior to currently available prescription medications tailored to aim at only one specific target, *via* one specific pathway.

11.2   FUNCTIONAL FOODS

The term *functional foods* was chosen here rather than *supplements*, or *nutraceuticals*, to distance this category from the common definition of those terms. First, *supplement* implies solitary substances that take up the slack for inadequate supply in the diet—as noted in the next two chapters. Second, nutraceutical implies stepping through a loophole in US Federal medicine claims–limitations statutes. Foods proposed here, especially those in this section, are not intended to replace pharmaceutical prescription medications. Furthermore, chronic inflammation, albeit described in detail by medicine, is not presently recognized as a *pro forma* routinely treatable clinical disorder.

Two types of functional foods were chosen for inclusion in the selection: First, foods that help normalize blood glucose levels, and second, foods that help reduce the effects of chronic inflammation. In most cases, the latter are foods that in one way or another supply antioxidants.

In the first type, namely, foods that normalize blood glucose levels, there is no known deficiency of the active constituents of the functional food. For instance, although there is no known deficiency of gingerols in the body, ginger, as reported in the *Iranian Journal of Pharmaceutical Research*, helps improve fasting blood sugar, hemoglobin A1c, and lowers levels of malondialdehyde (MDA) in Type 2 diabetic patients. (Khandouzi, Shidfar, Rajab et al. 2015) Malondialdehyde is a conventional marker of lipid peroxidation (Gaweł, Wardas, Niedworok et al. 2004).

In the second type, a functional food may supply a constituent that makes up a known deficiency. For example, iodine deficiency is reaching epidemic proportions in the United States. Its consequences are not simply thyroid malfunction, given that iodine deficiency is strongly implicated in Type 2 diabetes as well as in the chronic inflammation that leads to early formation of atherosclerosis (Joffe, and Distiller. 2014).

11.3   THE TWO-PRONGED APPROACH TO ANTIOXIDATION

In addition to detailing the antihyperglycemic properties of the functional foods cited, this chapter will also describe their role in reducing free radicals by one or both of two pathways: One pathway is to "neutralize" free radicals with exogenous antioxidants. By analogy, the common practice is to protect ourselves from the damage caused by the heat of a fire; alternatively, we can put out the fire.

Benjamin Franklin put it wisely... *"An ounce of prevention is worth a pound of cure."* So, in this chapter, the focus is on the alternative, eliminating the formation of free radicals at their source. This is done by *quenching* inflammation—chronic or acute.

11.4 INFLAMMATION CAUSES OXIDATIVE STRESS

Inflammation is the natural reaction of the body to infection by bacteria, viruses, fungi, and so on, as well as to toxins, and/or to physical, chemical, or traumatic injury. In a sense, inflammation is a complex process that aims to protect against injury while the body is figuring out how to heal. It usually but not invariably causes pain. Where there is infection, inflammation is the way that the body responds and that is not to be confused with the infection, rather it is the response of the body to the cause of the infection.

Inflammatory conditions can range from minor nuisance to those leading to fatality, as in *sepsis.* Some sources even hold that chronic inflammation can set the stage for cancer (Salzano, Checconi. Hanschmann et al. 2014).

In many instances, chronic systemic—read whole body—inflammation is not confined to a particular tissue, but may involve the lining of blood vessels, the lining of joints, the digestive tract, and many other internal organs and systems including the brain. This inflammatory process is the source of oxidative stress and may not cause pain, as some internal organs do not register and relay pain. When there is no pain, one may simply remain unaware of the serious damage that the systemic inflammation may be causing. In many cases, it leads to debilitating and even life-threatening diseases.

One set of clinical investigators made that point clear in the title of their publication, "Inflammation as a cardiovascular risk factor," in their report published in *Circulation*, the journal of the American Heart Association (AHA), in 2004.

Their report emphasizes that inflammation occurs in blood vessels in response to injury, including that caused by lipid peroxidation and infection. Various risk factors, including hypertension, diabetes, and smoking, are exaggerated by the harmful effects of oxidized low-density lipoprotein (LDL) cholesterol, initiating a chronic inflammatory reaction that may result in unstable arterial vessel plaque prone to rupture and thrombosis.

Epidemiological and clinical studies have shown strong and consistent relationships between markers of inflammation and risk of future cardiovascular events (Willerson, and Ridker. 2004).

A report published in *Diabetes*, the journal of the American Diabetes Association, is titled, "Inflammatory cytokines and the risk to develop Type 2 diabetes." Cytokines are protein molecules that affect the function of other cells, in this case, immune system cells in inflammation. The report tells us that a subclinical inflammatory reaction has been shown to precede the onset of Type 2 diabetes. In other words, Type 2 diabetes may result from activation of the immune system consonant with chronic inflammation (Spranger, Kroke, Möhlig et al. 2003).

However, note the term "subclinical." This means that it goes largely undetected. Many conditions that are clinical disorders seem to also harbor chronic inflammation. An article published in *Circulation*, titled "Chronic subclinical inflammation as part of the insulin resistance syndrome. The Insulin Resistance Atherosclerosis Study (IRAS)" (Festa, D'Agostino, Howard et al. 2000) likewise confirms the link between chronic systemic inflammation and Type 2 diabetes.

11.5 C-REACTIVE PROTEIN—A STANDARD MARKER OF INFLAMMATION

One way to assess the severity of inflammation is by observing C-reactive protein (CRP), principal among the biomarkers of inflammation. It is a protein made by the liver and released into the blood within a few hours after tissue injury, after the start of an infection, or other cause of inflammation. CRP is most commonly thought of in connection with detection of heart "events" (Ridker. 2003).

However, many conventional routine "blood panel" tests include CRP, and it is a good idea to keep track of that value and, if it is elevated without an obvious cause, it might be wise to ask for further testing to detect the cause of the possible chronic inflammation.

11.6 CRP AND CHRONIC HYPERGLYCEMIA

In one recent study, CRP appeared to be a better predictor of cardiovascular and heart disease than LDL cholesterol level (Datta, Iqbal, and Prasad. 2011). Another recent study published in *Diabetes* notes that elevated CRP levels helped to identify women at high risk of developing Type 2 diabetes (Hu, Meigs, Li et al. 2004). The authors raised the possibility that low-grade systemic inflammation may be an important factor causing Type 2 diabetes.

The American Heart Association notes that the CRP test is most helpful for primary prevention of cardiovascular and heart disease for patients who are at intermediate risk based on their other risk factors, that is, those patients who have a 10% to 20% risk for cardiovascular and heart disease. The test may not be as helpful for people who already have cardiovascular and heart disease or diabetes, or who are at low risk for cardiovascular and heart disease.

Already having Type 2 diabetes is considered a cardiovascular and heart disease risk-equivalent: Research has shown that people with diabetes are as likely to have a heart attack as those without diabetes who have a history of a heart attack.

A study appearing in the journal *Inflammation*, conducted on a Tunisian population, concluded that elevated CRP levels are independently associated with Type 2 diabetes: A significant difference in mean values of body mass index (BMI), plasma lipids, fasting plasma glucose (FPG), insulin, and homeostatic model assessment of insulin resistance (HOMA-IR) was observed between participants with and without Type 2 diabetes. CRP level was significantly higher in participants with Type 2 diabetes than in those without it, and this result persisted even after adjustment for age, gender, BMI, smoking, and alcohol consumption.

CRP was significantly associated with fasting plasma glucose (FPG), insulin, and HOMA-IR. Participants with elevated CRP levels (greater than 5 mg/L) had an increased risk of Type 2 diabetes (odds ratio [OR], 2.02) than those whose CRP levels were less than or equal to 5 mg/L. Even after adjustment for potentially confounding factors, the risk of Type 2 diabetes was still higher in participants with elevated CRP levels (OR, 1.91) (Belfki, Ben Ali, Bougatef et al. 2012).

Investigators reported in the journal *Diabetes Research and Clinical Practice* that compared with normal control participants, serum high-sensitivity CRP (hs-CRP) was significantly increased in groups with impaired glucose tolerance, or with Type 2 diabetes. hs-CRP was negatively correlated with HDL cholesterol, insulin sensitivity index, and adiponectin levels and positively correlated with systolic blood pressure, FPG, BMI, waist-to-hip ratio, postprandial 2-h plasma glucose, fasting serum insulin, and postprandial serum insulin.

Adiponectin was a significantly independent determinant for serum hs-CRP. Thyroglobulin, insulin sensitivity index, hs-CRP, fasting serum insulin, 2-h plasma glucose, and waist-to-hip ratio were significantly independent determinants for serum adiponectin concentration (Yuan, Zhou, Tang et al. 2006). Adiponectin is a protein involved in regulating glucose levels as well as fatty acid breakdown.

A report published in the *Journal of Endocrinological Investigation* concluded that men with Type 2 diabetes, but without cardiovascular and heart disease, had CRP levels similar to nondiabetic patients with cardiovascular and heart disease; whereas the CRP levels of men with both Type 2 diabetes and cardiovascular and heart disease were higher than in nondiabetic men with cardiovascular and heart disease.

Because of positive correlation between serum hs-CRP and HbA1c, the following pathologies may be thought to jointly contribute to the cardiovascular risk in men with Type 2 diabetes: elevated fasting insulin and HOMA-IR, inflammation, insulin resistance, and hyperglycemia

(Bahceci, Tuzcu, Ogun et al. 2005). As reported in the journal *Diabetologia*, it was also found that elevated serum ferritin levels predict new-onset Type 2 diabetes (Forouhi, Harding, Allison et al. 2007). Ferritin is a blood protein that transports iron. Elevated levels can indicate a number of possible medical conditions, but absent those, it is most likely an indication of inflammation.

11.6.1 STATIN THERAPY AND CRP LEVEL IN TYPE 2 DIABETES—THE CONTROVERSY

Investigators reported in the *Current Health Sciences Journal* that CRP, also found within macrophages of atherosclerotic plaques, is causally or mechanistically related to atherothrombosis and that inflammation plays an important role in the pathogenesis of Type 2 diabetes. The lowering of elevated CRP levels by statins may reduce the risk of cardiovascular events independently of the effect of statins on lipid levels.

Because increased levels of CRP have been associated with arterial-wall inflammation, statins can prevent ischemia by both inhibiting deposition of lipids and decreasing inflammation. The authors concluded that inflammation underlies diabetes and may even predict it (Ionică, Moța, Cătălina et al. 2009).

However, a number of studies including the following published in the *Revista da Associacao Medica Brasileira* (*Journal of the Brazilian Medical Association*) contend that statins may be associated with a higher incidence of new cases of diabetes. The investigators reviewed articles published up to June 2015 in the Scielo and PubMed databases, which assessed or described the association between use of statins and risk of diabetes. They found that statins are associated with a small increase in incidence of diabetes in patients predisposed to glycemic alteration.

However, they concluded that since the benefit of cardiovascular risk reduction prevails even in this group, there is no evidence that this finding should change the recommendation of starting statin therapy (Bernardi, Rocha, and Faria-Neto. 2015).

11.7   SELECTED FUNCTIONAL FOODS THAT FIGHT INFLAMMATION AND SUPPORT GLYCEMIC CONTROL

The following is a partial listing and description of functional foods that science reveals may help to reduce chronic systemic inflammation as well as hyperglycemia. These foods, readily available in most homes or nearby health food stores, have been scientifically shown to be helpful in controlling blood glucose and in reducing chronic systemic inflammation as well.

The list is not comprehensive because that is not the aim of this book. However, even this brief list may raise awareness that there are self-help products at home and nearby, and this may encourage further exploration. One helpful source is the US Department of Health and Human Services, National Center for Complementary and Integrative Health, Dietary and Herbal Supplements website: https://nccih.nih.gov/health/supplements. There are also others.

11.8   GINGER (*ZINGIBER OFFICINALE* ROSCOE)

Ginger (*Z. officinale* Roscoe) is a flowering perennial plant whose rhizome (meaning the root) is widely used as a spice or as folk medicine. It contains pungent phenolic substances known as gingerols. 6-Gingerol is the major pharmacologically active component of ginger known to be anti-inflammatory and antioxidant. Due to its efficacy and regulation of multiple targets, as well as its safety for human use, 6-gingerol has received considerable interest as a potential therapeutic agent for the prevention and/or treatment of various medical conditions.

Gingerols are reportedly counter-inflammatory due to the analgesic and anti-inflammatory effects of 6-gingerol (the pungent constituent of ginger) (Young, Luo, Cheng et al. 2005; Semwal, Semwal, Combrinck et al. 2015). In fact, investigators reported in the journal *Planta Medica* that ginger dry extract, conformed into solution and plasters for topical application, likewise showed anti-inflammatory action (Minghetti, Sosa, Cilurzo et al. 2007).

The original discovery in the early 1970s, that ginger can inhibit formation of prostaglandins that mediate inflammation, has been repeatedly confirmed. This discovery identified ginger as an herbal medicinal that shares pharmacological properties with nonsteroidal anti-inflammatory drugs (NSAIDs). The pharmacological property of ginger distinguishes it from NSAIDs though it may have a better therapeutic profile and fewer side effects than NSAIDs (Grzanna, Lindmark, and Frondoza. 2005).

In fact, a report in *Food and Function*, in 2013, affirms the gastro-protective effects of ginger (Haniadka, Saldanha, Sunita et al. 2013). Ginger has been shown to be effective in preventing gastric ulcers induced by NSAIDs such as indomethacin and aspirin and by *Helicobacter pylori*–induced gastric ulcerations (in laboratory animals). Various studies have also shown ginger to possess anti-emetic effects. However, there are conflicting reports in connection with the prevention of chemotherapy-induced nausea and vomiting as well as motion sickness.

Ginger has been shown to possess free radical scavenging antioxidants and promotes inhibition of lipid peroxidation. These properties might have contributed to the observed gastro-protective effects (Haniadka, Saldanha, Sunita et al. 2013).

Gingerol easily undergoes dehydration reactions to form the corresponding shogaols that impart the characteristic taste to dried ginger. Both gingerols and shogaols are anti-inflammatory, antioxidant, antimicrobial, and antiallergic. Shogaols appear to be more potent than the gingerols.

The numerous reports that ginger counters inflammation led to the following study appearing in the *Advanced Pharmaceutical Bulletin*, in 2013. It aimed to evaluate the effects of ginger on pro-inflammatory cytokines (substances such as interferon and interleukin that are secreted by immune system cells) and the acute phase protein hs-CRP in Type 2 diabetes. As stated above, the notation "hs" stands for "high sensitivity."

Patients were assigned to ginger or placebo comparison groups, and they received two tablets per day of either for 2 months. The concentrations of cytokines and hs-CRP were analyzed in blood samples before and after the intervention. It was found that supplementation of ginger significantly reduced the levels of both cytokines and hs-CRP in the ginger group in comparison to the control group (Mahluji, Ostadrahimi, Mobasseri et al. 2013).

A study published in the *Journal of Traditional and Complementary Medicine*, in 2015, aimed to test the effects of ginger powder supplementation on nitric oxide (NO) and CRP-reactive protein in elderly patients with osteoarthritis of the knee. The study was designed to determine the effect of ginger powder supplementation on some inflammatory markers (NO and hs-CRP) in these patients. This was a clinical trial with a follow-up period of 3 months, conducted on outpatients with moderately painful knee osteoarthritis given 500 mg of ginger powder, compared to a control group given placebo for 3 months.

Before the intervention, there was no significant difference in inflammatory markers (i.e., NO and hs-CRP) between the two groups. However, for the group receiving ginger, after 3 months of supplementation, serum concentration of NO and hs-CRP decreased in the ginger group, and after 12 weeks, the concentration of these markers declined even further. Ginger powder supplementation at a dose of 1 g/day can reduce inflammatory markers in patients with knee osteoarthritis, and it was recommended as a suitable supplement for these patients (Naderi, Mozaffari-Khosravi, Dehghan et al. 2015).

11.8.1 GINGER AND CHRONIC HYPERGLYCEMIA

A study reported in the *Iranian Journal of Pharmaceutical Research* in 2015 aimed to investigate the effects of ginger on fasting blood sugar, hemoglobin A1c, and malondialdehyde (MDA) in Type 2 diabetes patients. Diabetic patients assigned to the ginger group received 2 g/day of ginger powder supplement; a comparison group received lactose as placebo for 12 weeks. The serum concentrations of fasting blood sugar, HbA1c, and MDA were analyzed before and after the intervention.

Ginger supplementation significantly reduced the levels of fasting blood sugar, HbA1c, and MDA in the ginger treatment group in comparison to baseline as well as to the control group. Elevated MDA, as previously noted, is a marker of lipid peroxidation and oxidative stress. It seems that in Type 2 diabetes patients, oral administration of ginger powder supplement can improve fasting blood sugar and HbA1c and can lower MDA levels (Khandouzi, Shidfar, Rajab et al. 2015).

Insulin resistance is also a prime feature of metabolic syndrome. A study published in the journal *Complementary Therapies in Medicine* aimed to identify the effect of ginger on insulin resistance. Participants affected by diabetes were assigned to ginger and comparison groups. The ginger group received three 1-g capsules containing ginger powder, whereas the comparison (control) group received three 1-g placebo capsules daily for 8 weeks.

Mean fasting blood sugar declined by 10.5% in the ginger group, whereas the placebo comparison group showed a mean increase of 21%. The change in mean HbA1c showed the same trend as the fasting blood sugar. The investigators concluded that daily consumption of 3 g of ginger powder for 8 weeks helps patients with Type 2 diabetes by reducing fasting blood sugar, and HbA1c, as well as by improving insulin resistance indices (*via* the quantitative insulin sensitivity check index [QUICKI]) (Mozaffari-Khosravi, Talaei, Jalali et al. 2014).

The *Journal of Complementary and Integrative Medicine* published a study on the effect of ginger supplementation on glycemic indices in Iranian patients with Type 2 diabetes. They found that after 3 months, the differences between the ginger and placebo groups were statistically significant: serum glucose declined (−19.41 ± 18.83 vs. 1.63 ± 4.28 mg/dL), HbA1c percentage declined (−0.77% ± 0.88% vs. 0.02% ± 0.16%), insulin declined (−1.46 ± 1.7 vs. 0.09 ± 0.34 µIU/mL), insulin resistance declined (−16.38 ± 19.2 vs. 0.68 ± 2.7), high-sensitive CRP declined (−2.78 ± 4.07 vs. 0.2 ± 0.77 mg/L), paraoxonase-1 (PON-1) rose (22.04 ± 24.53 vs. 1.71 ± 2.72 U/L), total antioxidant capacity (TAC) rose (0.78 ± 0.71 vs. −0.04 ± 0.29 µIU/mL), and MDA declined (−0.85 ± 1.08 vs. 0.06 ± 0.08 µmol/L).

Paraoxonase 1 (PON1 is an enzyme that can protect against lipid oxidation.

This report concluded that the 3 months supplementation with ginger improved glycemic indices, TAC, and PON-1 activity in patients with Type 2 diabetes (Shidfar, Rajab, Rahideh et al. 2015).

Similarly, a clinical study with conventional protocols, published in the *International Journal of Food Science and Nutrition*, reported that ginger supplementation significantly lowered the levels of insulin (11.0 ± 2.3 vs. 12.1 ± 3.3), LDL cholesterol (67.8 ± 27.2 vs. 89.2 ± 24.9), TG (127.7 ± 43.7 vs. 128.2 ± 37.7), and the HOMA index (3.9 ± 1.09 vs. 4.5 ± 1.8), and increased the QUICKI (0.313 ± 0.012 vs. 0.308 ± 0.012) in comparison to a control group. The quantitative insulin sensitivity check index (QUICKI) is determined by the inverse of the sum of the logarithms of the fasting insulin and fasting glucose: 1/(log(fasting insulin µU/mL) + log(fasting glucose mg/dL)).

This index correlates well with glucose clamp studies (r_{xy} = 0.78) and is useful for measuring insulin sensitivity, which is the inverse of insulin resistance. It has the advantage that it can be obtained from a fasting blood sample, and it is the preferred method for certain types of clinical research.

In summary, ginger supplementation improved insulin sensitivity, as well as some fractions of the lipid profile, in Type 2 diabetes patients (Mahluji, Attari, Mobasseri et al. 2013).

11.8.2   How Safe Is Consumption of Ginger?

Ginger is said by the U.S. Food and Drug Administration to be a food additive that is "generally recognized as safe." Observational human studies provided no evidence that it causes fetal malformation when used as a treatment for early pregnancy nausea. According to a report in the *American Journal of Obstetrics & Gynecology*, administration of ginger beginning at the first trimester of pregnancy showed no increase in the rates of major malformations above the baseline rate of 1% to 3%.

The Motherisk Program aimed also to establish the safety of ginger in treatment of nausea and vomiting of pregnancy (NVP). The primary objective of the study was to examine the safety, and the secondary objective was to examine the effectiveness of ginger for NVP. The women taking ginger were compared to a group of women who were exposed to nonteratogenic drugs that were not antiemetic medications. Teratogenic means causing fetal deformity. The women were followed up to ascertain the outcome of the pregnancy and the health of their infants. They were also asked on a scale of 0 to 10 how effective the ginger was for their symptoms of NVP.

There was no significant difference between the ginger group and the comparison group other than that there were more infants weighing less than 2500 g (5.5 lb) in the comparison group. These results suggested that ginger has a mild effect in the treatment of nausea and vomiting in pregnancy (NVP) and that it does not appear to increase the rates of major malformations above the baseline rate of 1% to 3% (Portnoi, Chng, Karimi-Tabesh et al. 2003a). Overall, clinical studies indicate that ginger consumption appears to be quite safe with very limited side effects (Bode, and Dong. 2011). It should be noted, however, that a study appearing in *Archives of Pharmacal Research*, in 2008, reported some cytotoxic components extracted from the dried rhizomes of *Z. officinale* Roscoe (Portnoi, Chng, Karimi-Tabesh et al. 2003b).

11.9   GREEN TEA

Green tea is made from *Camellia sinensis* leaves that have not undergone the same withering and oxidation when processing it into oolong tea and black tea. It is loaded with polyphenols like flavonoids and catechins, which are antioxidants. Black tea is the tea most commonly consumed in the Western world. It is fully fermented before drying and is more oxidized than oolong, green, and white teas. It is generally stronger in flavor than the less oxidized teas.

Researchers from the College of Medicine, National Taiwan University, Taipei, reported in the *Journal of Agricultural and Food Chemistry* on "Factors affecting the levels of tea polyphenols and caffeine in tea leaves." They report that a laboratory procedure was developed for the simultaneous determination of caffeine and six catechins in tea samples: When 31 commercial teas extracted by boiling water, or 75% ethanol, were analyzed by this technique, the levels of (−)-epigallocatechin-3-gallate (EGCG) and total catechins in teas were in the following order of concentration: green tea (old leaves) was found to have greater concentrations than green tea (young leaves), and oolong tea was found to have greater concentrations than black tea and Pu-erh tea.

Note: (−)-epigallocatechin 3-gallate is a catechin and the most concentrated in tea. Catechin is a natural phenol and antioxidant. It is a plant secondary metabolite that belongs to the group of flavan-3-ols, part of the chemical family of flavonoids.

The contents of caffeine and catechins also have been measured in fresh tea leaves from the Tea Experiment Station in Wen-Shan or Taitung. The old tea leaves were found to contain less caffeine but more EGCG and total catechins than young ones.

To compare caffeine and catechins in the same strain of tea but manufactured by different fermentation processes, the level of caffeine in different manufactured teas was in the following order of concentration: black tea was found to be greater than oolong tea… greater than green tea… greater than fresh tea leaf.

The levels of EGCG and total catechins were in the following order of concentration: green tea greater than oolong tea… greater than fresh tea leaf… greater than black tea. In addition, six commercial tea extracts were used to test the biological functions including hydroxyl radical scavenging, nitric oxide (NO) suppression, and apoptotic effects. The Pu-erh tea extracts protected plasmid DNA from damage as well as the comparison control (which was a known protector of DNA) at a concentration of 100 μg/mL (Lin, Tsai, Tsay et al. 2003).

11.9.1 Tea Reduces Inflammation

Green tea has been shown to combat inflammation. An unusual property of green tea is described in an article in the journal *Food & Function*, in 2013, explaining that effect. Flavanols from tea were shown to have an unusual affinity for cell nuclei and have been reported to accumulate in the cell nucleus in considerable concentrations.

The nature of this phenomenon, which could provide novel approaches to understanding the well-known beneficial health effects of tea phenols, is investigated in this study, and it was found that selected polyphenols displayed affinity for all of the selected cell nuclear structures. Theaflavin-digallate was shown to display the highest affinity for DNA reported for any naturally occurring molecule reported so far. This finding may have implications for understanding the role of tea phenolics as "life span essentials" (Mikutis, Karaköse, Jaiswal et al. 2013a).

Writing in the journal *Current Medicinal Chemistry*, investigators concluded that catechins, the major polyphenolic compounds in green tea, exert vascular protective antioxidative, antihypertensive, anti-inflammatory, antiproliferative, antithrombotic, and lipid-lowering effects. They report that tea catechins are free radical scavengers; reduce intestinal lipid absorption, thereby improving blood lipid profile; activate endothelial NO; prevent the vascular inflammation that plays a critical role in the progression of atherosclerotic lesions; and suppress platelet adhesion, thereby inhibiting formation of blood clots (Mikutis, Karaköse, Jaiswal et al. 2013b).

In 2007, the journal *Cardiovascular and Hematological Disorders—Drug Targets* confirmed that EGCG in green tea polyphenols is a free radical scavenger and the major, and the most active, component in green tea. It protects against cellular damage by inhibiting DNA damage and oxidation of LDL. EGCG can also reduce the inflammatory response associated with local tissue by lowering lipid peroxidation and oxidative stress and by inhibiting the overproduction of pro-inflammatory cytokines and mediators and reducing the formation of reactive oxygen species (ROS).

EGCG effectively prevents cellular damage by lowering inflammation, reducing lipid peroxidation, and reducing NO-generated radicals leading to oxidative stress (Tipoe, Leung, Hung et al. 2007).

11.9.2 (Mostly Green) Tea and Type 2 Diabetes

Many studies have shown the beneficial effects of green tea in decreasing blood pressure, LDL cholesterol, oxidative stress, and a marker of chronic inflammation—not only on cardiovascular diseases but also on obesity and Type 2 diabetes (Nantz, Rowe, Bukowski et al. 2009; Iso, Date, Wakai et al. 2006; Wu, Lu, Chang et al. 2003).

In a retrospective cohort study performed in Japan, a 33% reduction of the risk of developing Type 2 diabetes was found in participants who consumed six or more cups of green tea daily, compared to those consuming less than one cup per week (Wu, Lu, Chang et al. 2003). It was also reported in the journal *Metabolism* that Taiwanese participants who had habitually consumed tea for more than 10 years showed lower body fat composition and smaller waist circumference. Evidence from epidemiological studies suggests the possibility of green tea being a novel strategy for treatment or prevention of obesity and diabetes (Mackenzie, Leary, and Brooks. 2007; see also Kim, and Kim. 2013).

EGCG, the most abundant form of catechin in green tea, has been known to be the main attributable factor of beneficial effects of green tea (Higdon, and Frei. 2003). EGCG inhibits adipocyte proliferation and differentiation in 3T3-L1 cells (Furuyashiki, Nagayasu, Aoki et al. 2004), increases fat oxidation (Klaus, Pultz, Thone-Reineke et al. 2005), and increases expression of GLUT-4 in adipose tissue (in an animal model) (Wu, Juan, Hwang et al. 2004).

In human studies, clear increases in energy expenditure were documented (Rumpler, Seale, Clevidence et al. 2001). Also, some of the studies suggested the protective function of EGCG for cytokine-induced β-cell destruction mediated by inhibition of nuclear factor κB (NF-κB) activation (Han. 2003).

Recently, investigators showed that green tea polyphenols had an antiobesity effect by upregulating adiponectin levels (in rats). They suggested that the involved mechanisms were the inhibition of Erk activation, alleviation of peroxisome proliferator-activated receptor γ (PPARγ) phosphorylation, and increases in PPARγ expression (Tian, Ye, Zhang et al. 2013).

Another study showed the ambivalent role of gallated catechin in green tea, including EGCG, in glucose tolerance. Gallated catechin reduces blood glucose levels mainly through its activities in the alimentary tract, while increasing the glucose level when in the circulation, by blocking normal glucose uptake into the tissues. The investigators suggested the development of nonabsorbable derivatives of gallated catechin with only positive luminal effect as a prevention strategy for Type 2 diabetes and obesity (Park, Jin, Baek et al. 2009).

In this study, reported in the *Diabetes and Metabolism Journal*, the investigators demonstrated the possibility that green tea extract may be antiobesic and/or antidiabetic when co-administered with another dietary supplement, poly-γ-glutamic acid (γ-PGA), in db/db mice, potentially through the action of intestinal green tea extract. γ-PGA is a main constituent of the viscous material in Korean chungkookjang and Japanese natto. The study reported the results of nuclear magnetic resonance spectroscopy that γ-PGA can interact with EGCG, and this possible complex formation may delay the absorption of GCs to systemic circulation from the intestine, resulting in decreased blood glucose level.

The protective effects of green tea extract + γ-PGA regimen on body weight gain and development of glucose intolerance were much better than treatment with either green tea extract or γ-PGA alone. Therefore, they suggested that green tea extract + γ-PGA treatment may be a promising preventive and therapeutic tool for obesity and Type 2 diabetes.

The investigators proposed that future studies are warranted to confirm these benefits in patients with diabetes, or healthy persons as well, so as to define the precise molecular mechanisms of action of green tea supplementation (Bae, Park, Na et al. 2013).

The aim of a study published in the journal *PLoS ONE* was to determine the effects of green tea extract on insulin resistance in Type 2 diabetes patients. The participants in the therapeutic group were given 500 mg of green tea extract, three times a day, while the control group received cellulose with the same dose and frequency to complete the 16-week study.

Within-group comparisons showed that green tea extract caused a significant decrease in triglyceride and homeostasis model assessment of insulin resistance (HOMA-IR) index after 16 weeks. Green tea extract also significantly increased the levels of HDL cholesterol, which is beneficial. The HOMA-IR index decreased from 5.4 ± 3.9 to 3.5 ± 2.0 in the treatment group only. Adiponectin, apolipoprotein A1, and apolipoprotein B100 rose significantly in both groups, but only glucagon-like peptide 1 increased in the therapeutic group.

The authors concluded that green tea extract significantly improved insulin resistance and increased glucagon-like peptide 1 (Liu, Huang, Huang et al. 2014).

Glucose control and insulin sensitivity play a significant role in metabolic syndrome, a source of chronic systemic inflammation. Low-grade inflammation is characteristic of the metabolic syndrome (Devaraj, Singh, and Jialal. 2009).

A report in the *Journal of the American College of Nutrition* concluded that "green tea may be beneficial for people with decreased insulin sensitivity and increased oxidative stress, such as those with the metabolic syndrome or type 2 diabetes" (Hininger-Favier, Benaraba, Coves et al. 2009. *Journal of the American College of Nutrition*, Aug; 28(4): 355–561). A more recent study in the same journal reported the outcome of a meta-analysis of the effect of green tea on human insulin sensitivity. The authors concluded that green tea significantly decreased fasting glucose and HbA1c concentrations (Liu, Zhou, Wang et al. 2013). Insulin insensitivity is a component of metabolic syndrome, in turn a major contributor to oxidative stress and chronic inflammation. That makes tea a valuable functional food in combating oxidative stress–related chronic inflammation.

A study published in the *Journal of Agricultural and Food Chemistry* showed that teas differ in their capacity to enhance insulin activity although they all do it to a greater or lesser extent. Tea, as normally consumed, was shown to increase insulin activity more than 15-fold *in vitro* in an experimental fat-cell assay. Black, green, and oolong teas were all shown to increase insulin activity (Anderson, and Polansky. 2002).

Nevertheless, it needs to be mentioned that a limited number of clinical trials using green tea, green tea extracts, or its main ingredient catechin have shown disappointing results in controlling hyperglycemia in Type 2 diabetes patients or protection from the condition in healthy people. A report in the journal *Obesity* showed that plasma glucose levels and A1c did not improve after 12 weeks of supplementation with catechin in patients with Type 2 diabetes (Nagao, Meguro, Hase et al. 2009; see also Mackenzie, Leary, and Brooks. 2007; Ryu, Lee, Lee et al. 2006). However, they showed that the addition of catechin decreased A1c level and increased serum insulin levels compared to the placebo group in a subgroup of patients who have been treated with insulin therapy.

11.9.3 Tea Reduces Inflammation and Protects Blood Vessels by Promoting Endothelium NO Formation

Epidemiological studies indicate that tea has beneficial cardiovascular effects. Are different types of tea superior in their cardiovascular benefits? In this study published in *Basic Research in Cardiology*, investigators compared green and black tea NO production and vasodilation. They chose a highly fermented black tea and determined concentrations of individual tea compounds in both green and black tea of the same type (Assam). The fermented black tea was almost devoid of catechins.

Both types of tea triggered the endothelium NO enzyme, eNOS, and blood vessel relaxation to the same extent in animal models, bovine aortic endothelial cells, and rat aortic rings. However, in green tea, only EGCG resulted in pronounced NO production and NO-dependent vasorelaxation in aortic rings. It is thought that during tea processing to produce black tea, the catechins are converted to theaflavins and thearubigins. Individual black tea theaflavins showed a higher potency than EGCG in NO production and vasorelaxation. The thearubigins in black tea are highly efficient stimulators of vasodilation and NO production.

These results show that highly fermented black tea is equally potent as green tea in promoting beneficial endothelial effects. Theaflavins and thearubigins predominantly counterbalance the lack of catechins in black tea. The findings may underline the contribution of black tea consumption in prevention of cardiovascular diseases (Lorenz, Urban, Engelhardt et al. 2009).

11.9.4 It Is Best to Leave Out the Milk

One of the more powerful compounds in green tea is the polyphenolic bioflavonoid antioxidant EGCG. The aim of a study published in the *European Journal of Clinical Nutrition* was to assess the antioxidant capacity of green and black tea as well as the effect of adding milk to the beverage. Conventional antioxidant capacity assessment methods were used on two groups each of which consumed 300 mL of either black or green tea, after overnight fast: The human plasma antioxidant capacity (TRAP) was measured before and 30, 50, and 80 min after consuming tea.

Note: In measurement for cooking, a cup is 250 mL (236 mL, or 8 oz in the United States).

When the experiment was repeated on a separate day, 100 mL of whole milk was added to the tea (ratio 1:4). Both teas inhibited dose-dependent antioxidant capacity, but the green tea was sixfold more potent than black tea until milk was added. The addition of milk totally inhibited antioxidant capacity (Serafini, Ghiselli, and Ferro-Luzzi. 1996).

Besides leaving out milk if one wants the full antioxidant effect, brewing loose tea is probably the best way to consume it in the long run—matcha green tea can also be mixed into cold water without losing its properties. According to a study published in the *International Journal of Food Science and Nutrition*, tea bag materials—acting as a sort of filter—may prevent some extraction of flavonoids into the tea beverage (Langley-Evans. 2000).

11.9.5   GREEN TEA VERSUS BLACK TEA. BREWING "LOOSE" TEA VERSUS TEA BAGS—THE CASE FOR LOWER OXALATE LEVELS

For individuals with kidney stones disease, green tea brewed from loose tea leaves may be preferable to tea in other conventional forms including black tea and oolong tea made from both loose leaf tea and from tea bags. Thirty-two commercially available teas consisting of green, oolong, and black teas purchased in local markets in New Zealand were examined for the soluble oxalate content of the infusate made from each of the teas.

The mean soluble oxalate content of black tea in tea bags and loose tea leaves was 4.68 and 5.11 mg/g tea, respectively, while green teas and oolong tea had lower oxalate content, ranging from 0.23 to 1.15 mg/g tea.

A regular tea drinker consuming six cups of tea/day would have an intake of between 26.46 and 98.58 mg soluble oxalate/day from loose black tea and between 17.88 and 93.66 mg soluble oxalate/day from black tea in tea bags. The oxalate intake from the regular daily consumption of black teas is modest when compared to the amounts of soluble oxalate that can be found in common foods. However, oxalate in black teas has the potential to bind to a significant proportion of calcium in the milk, which is commonly consumed with the black teas (Charrier, Savage, and Vanhanen. 2002).

Some tea bags are treated with epichlorohydrin to prevent them from disintegrating or tearing. Epichlorohydrin is mainly used in the production of epoxy resins, and when it comes in contact with water, it breaks down to 3-MCPD, a known carcinogen that has also been linked to infertility and suppressed immune function. According to the *Institute of Food Science and Technology* (UK) Issues Statement on 3-MCPD, 25 March 2003, its presence in foodstuffs should be reduced to undetectable level (http://www.food navigator.com/Science/IFST-issues-statement-on-3-MCPD).

11.9.6   IS IT SAFE TO DRINK A LOT OF TEA?

Some people will say that they drink a lot of tea every day, just as they will say that they drink a lot of coffee. Just how much is "a lot"? The following study in the journal *Clinical Cancer Research* addressed the question, "What is a lot?" in connection with tea as part of a cancer treatment project because green tea and green tea polyphenols were shown to possess cancer preventive activities in preclinical model systems.

In preparation for future green tea intervention trials, the investigators conducted a clinical study to determine the safety and the way that green tea polyphenols move through the body (pharmacokinetics) after 4 weeks of daily oral consumption of EGCG or Polyphenon E (a defined, decaffeinated green tea polyphenol mixture).

Adverse events reported during the 4-week treatment period included excess gas, upset stomach, nausea, heartburn, stomach ache, abdominal pain, dizziness, headache, and muscle pain. All of the reported events were rated as "mild events." For most events, the incidence reported in the polyphenol-treated groups was not more than that reported in a comparison placebo group. No significant changes were observed in blood counts, and blood chemistry profiles, after repeated consumption of green tea polyphenol products.

The investigators concluded that it is safe for healthy individuals to take green tea polyphenol products in amounts equivalent to the EGCG content in 8 to 16 cups of green tea once a day, or in divided doses twice a day for 4 weeks (Chow, Cai, Hakim et al. 2003).

The journal *Drug Safety* reported that regulatory agencies in France and Spain suspended market authorization of a weight-loss product containing green tea extract because of concerns about possible liver damage. Adverse event case reports involving green tea products were cited. In response, the US Pharmacopeia Dietary Supplement Information Expert Committee (DSI EC) systematically reviewed the safety information for green tea products in order to reevaluate the current safety class to which these products are assigned.

Clinical pharmacokinetics and animal toxicological information indicated that consumption of green tea concentrated extracts, on an empty stomach, are more likely to lead to adverse effects than consumption in the fed state. However, based on this safety review, the DSI EC determined that when dietary supplement products containing green tea extracts are used and formulated appropriately, the committee is unaware of significant safety issues that would prohibit monograph development, provided a caution statement is included in the labeling section (Sarma, Barrett, Chavez et al. 2008).

11.10 BEETS (BEETROOT—*BETA VULGARIS*) ARE ANTI-INFLAMMATORY AND ANTIGLYCEMIC

Beets (red beetroot) are rich in nitrates that metabolize to nitrite that, in turn, delivers NO essential to blood vessel function and, therefore, cardiovascular health (Hobbs, Kaffa, George et al. 2012; Lundberg, Weitzberg, and Gladwin. 2008). In fact, NO also helps maintain healthy blood glucose levels, and it protects blood vessels often impaired in diabetes.

Because inorganic nitrate and nitrite yield NO in the body, some of its properties, for example, regulation of glucose metabolism, vascular homeostasis, and insulin signaling pathway, have recently led to proposing that they may be potential therapeutic agents in Type 2 diabetes. In a review published in the journal *Nutrition and Metabolism (London)*, the investigators examined experimental and clinical studies on the effect of nitrate/nitrite administration on various clinical aspects of Type 2 diabetes.

For the most part, the studies they sampled showed that an altered metabolism of nitrate/nitrite resulting in an impaired NO pathway occurs in diabetes, which could contribute to its complications. Some important beneficial properties, including regulation of glucose homeostasis and insulin signaling, improvement of insulin resistance and vascular function, along with blood pressure–lowering, lipid-lowering, and anti-inflammatory and antioxidative effects were reported to occur after administration of inorganic nitrate/nitrite.

The investigators pointed to some well-known mechanisms that could explain the impairment of the NO pathway in Type 2 diabetes. The list includes chronic hyperglycemia, increased oxidative stress, and activation of nuclear factor κB (NF-κB), as well as accumulation of advanced glycation end products AGE), which are documented disruptive factors in the nitrate/nitrite/NO pathway (Oelze, Schuhmacher, and Daiber. 2010).

Furthermore, in diabetes, increased plasma levels of asymmetric dimethylarginine (ADMA), an endogenous competitive inhibitor of NO synthase, is also a known hyperglycemia-induced impairment factor of the NO pathway (Lin, Ito, Asagami et al. 2002). In addition, decreased NOS activity and decreased production of NO from L-arginine, as well as increased arginase activity (which leads to decreased L-arginine bioavailability and thus decreased NO synthesis), are other disrupted pathways in NO homeostasis in diabetic conditions (Romero, Caldwell, and Caldwell. 2006). Since activation of NOS is regulated also by insulin, and the Akt signaling pathway, impaired insulin secretion and insulin resistance due to diabetes could affect NO synthesis (Vincent, Montagnani, and Quon. 2003).

Some investigators have concluded that dietary nitrate/nitrite could be a compensatory means of supporting a jeopardized nitrate/nitrite/NO pathway and related disorders in diabetes (Bahadoran, Ghasemi, Mirmiran et al. 2015).

The evidence that a diet rich in nitrate or its supplementation (e.g., from beets or beet products) is beneficial in Type 2 diabetes is consonant with the evidence that endothelial dysfunction is an early and, ultimately, a cardinal feature of that disorder. As noted in a previous chapter, endothelial dysfunction is considered a major contributing factor in coronary artery disease. Many studies shed light on the role of diabetes in impairing endothelial function—among them are the following:

In a review published in the journal *Endocrine and Metabolic Disorders*, titled "Endothelial dysfunction in diabetes mellitus: Molecular mechanisms and clinical implications," the investigators concluded that endothelial dysfunction, attributed to Type 2 diabetes, contributes to the pathogenesis and clinical expression of atherosclerosis in diabetes (Tabit, Chung, Hamburg et al. 2010). This goes to a point made previously in this book, namely, that early signs of cardiovascular risk tend to be focused primarily on poor lipid profiles, and that focus at the time of diagnosis may draw attention away from detecting early signs of diabetes.

The journal *Diabetologia* reported a study that aimed to determine the effects of endothelium-dependent and -independent vasodilators on forearm blood flow in patients with Type 2 diabetes, and in a control participant group, by means of venous occlusion plethysmography.

Increasing amounts of acetylcholine and glyceryl trinitrate (vasodilators) were infused through a brachial artery cannula in doses of 60, 120, 180 and 240 mmol/min, and 3, 6, and 9 nmol/min, respectively.

NG monomethyl-L-arginine, an inhibitor of *endothelium derived relaxing factor*, was infused to inhibit basal and stimulated release of NO. Forearm blood flow responses to each dose of acetylcholine were significantly greater in the control participants than in the diabetes patients.

NG monomethyl-L-arginine forearm blood flow declined in both control participants and in diabetic patients, from maximal stimulated values when responses were compared with the natural decline to acetylcholine. However, it had no effect on basal blood flow responses. Forearm blood flow responses to each dose of glyceryl trinitrate were significantly greater in the control participants than in the diabetic patients. The investigators concluded that these data provide evidence for endothelial and smooth muscle dysfunction in diabetes (McVeigh, Brennan, Johnston et al. 1992).

A footnote to history: The investigators of this particular study used the term *endothelium-derived relaxing factor*—EDRF—because before 1992, when that study was conducted, it was not known that EDRF was, in fact, NO. S. Moncada (Glaxo-Wellcome, UK Ltd) was the first to publish the identity of EDRF as NO in the journal *Biochemical Pharmacology* in 1989 (Moncada, Palmer, and Higgs. 1989).

In a review published in the journal *Biochimica et Biophysica Acta*, the authors report that patients with diabetes invariably show an impairment of endothelium-dependent vasodilation. They therefore propose that understanding and treating endothelial dysfunction should be a major focus in the prevention of vascular complications associated with all forms of diabetes (Sena, Pereira, and Seiça. 2013).

11.10.1 THE CASE FOR BEETS IN SUPPLEMENT FORM VERSUS WHOLE BEETS

In the following study published in the journal *Nutrition Research*, it was reported that in healthy older adults, plasma nitrate and nitrite are increased by a high-nitrate supplement but not necessarily by high-nitrate foods. The investigators examined the effect of a 3-day control diet versus high-nitrate diet, with and without a high-nitrate supplement (beetroot juice), on plasma nitrate and nitrite, and blood pressure.

It was found that a high-nitrate supplement consumed at breakfast elevated plasma nitrate and nitrite levels throughout the day (Miller, Marsh, Dove et al. 2012).

There are many beetroot supplements commercially available, including the products shown on the HumanN® website, https://www.humann.com/products/?gclid=CIy8gs3DqM8CFYwkhgodQVc Bmw. The science supporting these products is impressive.

The aims of the following study published in the *Journal of Nutritional Science* were to assess the phytochemical constituents of red beetroot juice and to measure the postprandial glucose and insulin responses elicited by either 225 mL beetroot juice (BEET), a control beverage matched for macronutrient content (MCON), or a glucose beverage in healthy adults.

Beetroot juice is a particularly rich source of betalain degradation compounds: The orange/yellow pigment neobetanin was found to be in particularly high quantities (providing 1.3 g in 225 mL). Healthy individuals were recruited and consumed the test meals in a controlled single-blind crossover design.

Results revealed a significant lowering of the postprandial insulin response in the early phase (0 to 60 min) and a significantly lower glucose response in the 0- to 30-min phase in the BEET treatment compared with MCON.

The investigators concluded that the betalains, polyphenols, and dietary nitrate found in the beetroot juice may each have contributed to the observed differences in the postprandial insulin concentration data (Wootton-Beard, Brandt, Fell et al. 2014).

11.10.2 Antioxidant and Anti-Inflammatory Properties of Beets

As noted above, the antioxidative and anti-inflammatory effects of beets are mediated also by high concentrations of betalains that give them the intense red color, as well as other phenolics. Betalain is a recently discovered class of antioxidants whose metabolites inhibit lipid peroxidation of membranes (Kanner, Harel, and Granit. 2001; Reddy, Alexander-Lindo, and Nair. 2005; Georgiev, Weber, Kneschke et al. 2010; Zielinska-Przyjemska, Olejni, Dobrowolska-Zachwieja et al. 2009).

The journal *Nutrients* published a report that concluded that betalains in beetroot extracts have emerged as potent anti-inflammatory agents (Clifford, Howatson, West et al. 2015). At least part of their anti-inflammatory effects seems to be their inhibition of pro-inflammatory signaling cascades, the most prominent of these being the NF-κB cascade that activates and transcribes most gene targets that regulate and amplify the inflammatory response (i.e., cytokines, chemokines, and apoptotic and phagocytic cells) (Baker, Hayden, and Ghosh. 2001). Consequently, NF-κB activity plays a central role in the inflammatory processes that manifest in chronic disease (Baker, Hayden, and Ghosh. 2001).

In a recent study published in the journal *Mediators of Inflammation*, NF-κB DNA-binding activity was shown to be dose-dependently attenuated in nephrotoxic rats administered a beetroot extract for 28 days (250 mg or 500 mg·kg·bm^{-1}). Kidney homogenates from the beetroot-treated rats had lower concentrations of immune cell-generated inflammatory mediators (tumor necrosis factor-alpha [TNF-α], interleukin-6 [IL-6], and myeloperoxidase) and reduced signs of oxidative damage (via lower levels of MDA), which could be directly related to the blunting of the NF-κB pathway.

The investigators concluded that these effects were likely mediated, at least in part, by the betalains present in beetroot (El Gamal, AlSaid, Raish et al. 2014). In another study published in the journal *Food and Chemical Toxicology*, it was reported that betanin treatment (25 and 100 mg/kg/day for 5 days) significantly inhibits NF-κB DNA-binding activity in rats with induced acute renal damage (Tan, Wang, Bai et al. 2015).

Betalains were also shown to suppress cyclooxygenase-2 (COX-2) expression *in vitro*. COX-2 is an important precursor molecule for pro-inflammatory arachidonic acid metabolites (prostaglandins) (Vidal, López-Nicolás, Gandía-Herrero et al. 2014). According to a report in the journal *Arteriosclerosis, Thrombosis and Vascular Biology*, as well as suppressing COX-2 synthesis, betanidin, extracted from beetroot, significantly inhibited (dose-dependently) lipoxygenase, a catalytic enzyme vital for the synthesis of pro-inflammatory leukotriene molecules (Ricciotti, and FitzGerald. 2011).

There are also studies on the anti-inflammatory effects of beetroot supplements *in vivo*. For instance, one study published in the journal *New Medicine* showed that therapeutic administration of betalain-rich oral capsules made from beetroot extracts alleviated inflammation and pain in osteoarthritis patients. The beet extract, a novel and proprietary food-based extract, *ProLain*, prepared from red beetroots, was obtained from FutureCeuticals, Inc. USA, where it was produced using a patent-pending technology that does not require use of organic solvents and that significantly reduces the amounts of sugar in the final material.

After 10 days of supplementation with 100, 70, or 35 mg/day of the beet extract, the pro-inflammatory cytokines TNF-α and IL-6 in these osteoarthritis patients had decreased from baseline by a range of 8.3% to 35% and 22% to 28%, respectively. The activity of the chemokines GRO-α (growth-regulated oncogene-alpha) and RANTES (regulated upon activation normal T cell growth) was also markedly inhibited by the beetroot treatment. This attenuation of the inflammatory response coincided with a significant reduction in self-reported pain on the McGill Pain Questionnaire (Pietrzkowski, Nemzer, Spórna et al. 2010).

11.10.3 BEETS PROMOTE NO SYNTHESIS WITH THE HELP OF ORAL BACTERIA

Beets supply the basics for endothelial NO synthesis, but antibacterial mouthwash might actually inhibit NO formation. In the following study titled "Concurrent beet juice and carbohydrate ingestion: influence on glucose tolerance in obese and nonobese adults," published in the *Journal of Nutrition and Metabolism*, the authors preface their report by stating that "Insulin resistance and obesity are characterized by low nitric oxide (NO) bioavailability. Insulin sensitivity is improved with stimulation of NO generating pathways. Consumption of dietary nitrate (NO_3^-) increases NO formation, via NO_3^- reduction to nitrite (NO_2^-) by oral bacteria."

The aim of their study was to determine whether "acute" dietary nitrate (beet juice) ingestion could improve insulin sensitivity in obese, albeit not in nonobese adults. Nonobese participants (BMI: 26.3 ± 0.8 kg/m^2) and obese participants (BMI: 34.0 ± 0.8 kg/m^2) consumed beet juice supplemented with 25 g of glucose (carbohydrate load: 75 g), with and without prior use of antibacterial mouthwash to inhibit NO_3^- reduction to NO_2^-.

Blood glucose concentrations after beet juice and glucose ingestion were greater in obese participants than in nonobese participants after the first 60 min and then after 90 min. Insulin sensitivity, as shown by the Matsuda Index (where higher values reflect greater insulin sensitivity), was lower in the obese than in the nonobese participants.

Antibacterial mouthwash rinsing decreased insulin sensitivity in the obese participants (5.7 ± 0.7 vs. 4.9 ± 0.6), but not in nonobese adult participants (8.1 ± 1.0 vs. 8.9 ± 0.9).

The investigators concluded that insulin sensitivity was improved in the obese but not in the nonobese participants, following co-ingestion of beet juice and glucose, when oral bacteria nitrate reduction was not inhibited. The investigators concluded also that obese adults may benefit from healthy nitrate-rich foods in their meals (Beals, Binns, Davis et al. 2017).

Parallel findings were reported in a study published in the journal *Free Radical Biology and Medicine*. The aim of the study was to determine whether suppression of the oral microflora affects systemic nitrite levels and hence blood pressure in healthy individuals.

The investigators measured blood pressure (clinic, home, and 24-h ambulatory) in healthy volunteers during an initial 7-day control period, followed by a 7-day treatment period with a *chlorhexidine*-based antiseptic mouthwash. Oral nitrate–reducing capacity and nitrite levels were measured after each study period.

It was found that antiseptic mouthwash treatment reduced oral nitrite production by 90% and plasma nitrite levels by 25%, compared to the control period.

Systolic and diastolic blood pressure rose by an average of 2 to 3.5 mmHg, and increases correlated significantly with a decrease in circulating nitrite concentrations. The blood pressure effect appeared within 1 day of disruption of the oral microflora and was sustained during the 7-day mouthwash intervention.

These results suggested that the recycling of endogenous nitrate by oral bacteria plays an important role in determination of plasma nitrite levels and thereby in the physiological control of blood pressure (Kapil, Haydar, Pearl et al. 2013). Similar results were reported more recently in a review titled "Oral microbiome and nitric oxide: the missing link in the management of blood pressure," published in the journal *Current Hypertension Reports*. The authors report that "The presence or absence of select and specific bacteria may determine steady-state blood pressure levels. Eradication of oral bacteria through antiseptic mouthwash or overuse of antibiotics causes blood pressure to increase. Allowing recolonization of nitrate- and nitrite-reducing bacteria can normalize blood pressure" (Bryan, Tribble, and Angelov. 2017).

11.10.4 BEET FIBER ALSO IMPROVES HYPERGLYCEMIA

The object of the following study published in the *European Journal of Clinical Nutrition* was to determine the effects of sugar beet fiber, in formula diet, on blood glucose, serum insulin, and serum hydroxyproline in human participants.

Two formula test meals, one experimental with 7 g of sugar beet fiber, namely, 5.1 g total dietary fiber, and one control without it, were consumed by the participants in a clinic, in the morning after a 12-h fast. The participants were healthy male volunteers, 25 years old, on average, with age ranging from 21 to 42 years. Both test meals held similar amounts of nutrients and supplied total energy of 1778 kJ (425 kcal). The total test time from the start of the meal was 155 min. Blood samples were drawn before and after the test meals.

It was found that the formula with sugar beet fiber significantly reduced the postprandial blood glucose response, the serum insulin response, and the serum hydroxyproline response, compared with the outcome of the formula without fiber.

The investigators concluded that sugar beet fiber, in a formula, could reduce hyperglycemia in enteral nutrition and be useful in therapeutic liquid and formula diets. In addition, sugar beet fiber fares well in heating and preparation in the process of canning, and it can diminish the glycemic responses in relatively small amounts (Thorsdottir, Andersson, and Einarsson. 1998).

11.10.5 CAVEAT

Persons forming kidney stones should be aware that the oxalate content of raw beets is quite high, at about 81.1 ± 23.8 mg per 100 g of beets (Urology/Kidney-Stones/Oxalate-Content-of-Foods.htm; accessed 11/6/17), and that raw beets have about 9 g of sugar per cup (136 g). One 8-oz glass of beet juice holds about 25 g of carbohydrates (https://www.webmd.com/food-recipes/features/truth-about-beetroot-juice; accessed 11/5/17), of which about 13 g is sugar.

However, the bioavailability of oxalates varies with the foods in which they are contained: the bioavailability of oxalates in beets is relatively poor—six times less so than spinach, for instance. Cooking the beets could cut levels by about 25%.

For the rare person with a condition like idiopathic calcium nephrolithiasis (a type of kidney stone), who needs a low-oxalate diet, other high-nitrate vegetable choices might be preferable (Michael Greger, MD; https://nutritionfacts.org/questions/oxalic-acid-in-beets/; accessed 11/5/17).

Although there are presently no anticipated adverse health outcomes associated with other constituents of beetroot, consumers should be aware that some supplements, that is, juices, could have a relatively high sugar content, which might have to be taken into consideration by some individuals suffering from diabetes (Tesoriere, Butera, Arpa et al. 2003; Clifford, Howatson, West et al. 2015).

11.11 CHILI PEPPERS

Sometimes they are green, sometimes they are red; they are rarely hot; they are never chilly; they are not even *pepper*. However, they are antioxidant and anti-inflammatory and they have been said to help glycemic control. They are chili pepper, the fruit of plants from the genus *Capsicum*, members of the *nightshade* family.

Chili is cited here to introduce a cautionary note that what is generally "good for the goose," as they say, is not invariably "good for the gander." While chili is antioxidant and anti-inflammatory, as shown below, and it is known to enhance cardiovascular health, it may in fact be harmful to consume it in the face of Type 2 diabetes.

Chili peppers originated in the Americas and many cultivars spread across the world are used as spices in foods and for medicine. The substances that give chili peppers their intense taste or sensation, when they are applied topically, are capsaicin (8-methyl-*N*-vanillyl-6-nonenamide) and several related compounds collectively called capsaicinoids.

Capsaicinoids bind to pain receptors in the mouth and throat that are responsible for sensing heat. Once activated by them, these receptors signal the brain that the person has consumed something hot. The brain responds to the burning sensation by raising the heart rate, increasing perspiration, and releasing endorphins.

The sensation of heat from consuming chili peppers was historically measured in *Scoville heat units* (SHU), based on the dilution of an amount of chili extract added to sugar syrup before its heat becomes undetectable to a panel of tasters: The more it has to be diluted to be undetectable, the more powerful the variety and therefore the higher the SHU rating.

Capsaicin is a potent inhibitor of *substance P*, a neuropeptide associated with inflammatory processes and more. A neuropeptide is a peptide (fragment of a protein) that acts as a neurotransmitter, conveying information within the nervous system. The hotter the chili pepper, the more capsaicin it contains.

11.11.1   *Capsicum baccatum* Is Anti-Inflammatory and It Has Been Said to Help Lower Blood Glucose

There is some controversy over the effectiveness of chili specifically in connection with glycemic control, although many animal models support it. For instance, such a study published in the journal *Phytotherapy Research* concluded that after 4 weeks of feeding of experimental diets, the serum insulin concentration was significantly reduced in a high red chili group, compared with a diabetic control and a low red chili group.

Blood HbA1c, liver weight, liver glycogen, and serum lipids were not influenced by the feeding of red chili–containing diets, but the data of this study suggested that 2% dietary red chili is insulinotropic, meaning stimulating or affecting the production and activity of insulin, rather than hypoglycemic, at least in this experimental condition (Islam, and Choi. 2008).

The objective of another study, published in *The American Journal of Clinical Nutrition*, was to determine the metabolic effects of a chili-containing meal after the consumption of a bland diet and a chili-blend (30 g/day; 55% cayenne chili) supplemented diet.

Participants 46 years old, on average, with a BMI of $26.3 \pm 4.6 \text{ kg/m}^2$, participated in an intervention study with two 4-week dietary periods.

The investigators evaluated the postprandial effects of a bland meal after a bland diet, a chili meal after a bland diet, and a chili meal after a chili-containing diet, and serum insulin, C-peptide, and glucose concentrations and energy expenditure were measured at fasting and up to 120 min postprandially.

General failure to detect differences ("significant heterogeneity") between the various meal pre- and post-combinations prevailed. The participants with a BMI greater than or equal to 26.3, the median BMI, also showed "heterogeneity" in C-peptide, iAUC C-peptide, and net AUC energy expenditure. AUC here means "area under the glucose curve."

However, the C-peptide/insulin quotient (an indicator of hepatic insulin clearance) was highest after the chili meal after a chili-containing diet. Therefore, the investigators concluded that regular consumption of chili may attenuate postprandial hyperinsulinemia (Ahuja, Robertson, Geraghty et al. 2006).

The anti-inflammatory effectiveness of *capsicum* is more strongly supported than its antiglycemic properties: A study appearing in *The Journal of Pharmacy and Pharmacology* aimed to evaluate the effects of the *C. baccatum* cultivar juice in an animal model of acute inflammation induced by two types of abdominal inflammatory substances.

The investigators reported that this is the first demonstration of the anti-inflammatory effect of *C. baccatum* juice and that the data suggest that this effect may be induced by capsaicin. Moreover, the anti-inflammatory effect induced by red pepper may be by inhibition of pro-inflammatory cytokine production at the inflammatory site (Spiller, Alves, Vieira et al. 2008).

Likewise, a study published in the journal *Food Chemistry* was conducted to determine the antioxidant vitamin content of paprika during ripening, processing, and storage. The most biologically effective antioxidant vitamins, such as ascorbic acid, tocopherols, and carotenoids, were separated, identified, and evaluated in different samples.

The rate of synthesis of the three antioxidants increased after onset of the ripening. As ripening progressed, antioxidant vitamins tended to increase proportionally except that ascorbic acid reached a maximum level at the color break II stage and then declined. During drying and storage, there was a dramatic decrease in the concentration of tocopherol and ascorbic acid as a result of active antioxidation activity, while carotenoid content decreased at a lower rate (Daood, Vinkler, Markus et al. 1996).

The close link between chronic inflammation and diabetes would support the inclusion of chili in this context. In fact, a report published in the journal *Phytotherapy Research* attributes the effect of chili more to the promotion of insulin secretion than to the reduction of glucose absorption.

This animal-model study aimed to determine whether a low or a high, but tolerable, dietary dose of red chili can ameliorate the diabetes related complications in a high-fat diet–fed streptozotocin (STZ)-induced rat model of Type 2 diabetes model. Sprague–Dawley rats were fed a high-fat diet for 2 weeks and then randomly assigned to four groups: normal control, diabetic control, red chili low (0.5%), and red chili high (2.0%) groups.

Diabetes was induced by an intraperitoneal injection of STZ (40 mg/kg BW) in all groups except the normal control group.

After 4 weeks of feeding experimental diets, the fasting blood glucose concentrations in both red chili–fed groups were not significantly different. The serum insulin concentration was significantly increased in the high red chili group compared to the diabetic control and the low chili groups. Blood HbA1c, liver weight, liver glycogen, and serum lipids were not influenced by the feeding of red chili–containing diets.

The results of this study suggested to the investigators that 2% dietary red chili may be insulinotropic rather than hypoglycemic, at least in this experimental condition (Islam, and Choi. 2008).

A note of caution concerning chili appeared in a review titled "Herbal therapies for Type 2 diabetes mellitus: chemistry, biology, and potential application of selected plants and compounds" published in the journal *Evidence Based Complementary and Alternative Medicine* (Chang, Lin, Bartolome et al. 2013).

Chili pepper extract, as previously noted, may exert an insulinotropic rather than a hypoglycemic action, implying its action on β-cells. As noted in a report in the journal *Biochemical and Biophysical Research Communications*, capsaicin activates AMPK in 3T3-L1 preadipocytes (Hwang, Park, Shin et al. 2005).

It has been suggested that the chili pepper and its active ingredients prevent Type 2 diabetes by regulating insulin resistance and probably β-cell function. However, there is a discrepancy in the use of capsaicin to treat Type 2 diabetes: Capsaicin might actually cause Type 2 diabetes by impairing insulin secretion. In fact, the authors of a study titled "Capsaicin-sensitive sensory fibers in the islets of Langerhans contribute to defective insulin secretion in Zucker diabetic rat, an animal model for some aspects of human type 2 diabetes," published in *The European Journal of Neuroscience*, concluded that the activity of islet-innervating capsaicin-sensitive fibers may have a role in the development of reduced insulin secretion in human Type 2 diabetes.

The investigators report that the system that regulates insulin secretion from β-cells has a capsaicin-sensitive inhibitory component. As calcitonin gene-related peptide (CGRP)–expressing primary sensory fibers innervate the islets, and a major proportion of the CGRP-containing primary sensory neurons are sensitive to capsaicin, the islet-innervating sensory fibers may represent the capsaicin-sensitive inhibitory component.

They therefore examined the expression of the capsaicin receptor, transient receptor potential vanilloid receptor type 1 (TRPV1), in CGRP-expressing fibers in the pancreatic islets and the effect of selective elimination of capsaicin-sensitive primary afferents on the decline of glucose homeostasis and insulin secretion in Zucker diabetic fatty (ZDF) rats, the model commonly used to study human Type 2 diabetes mellitus.

It was found that CGRP-expressing fibers in the pancreatic islets also express TRPV1. Furthermore, it was also found that systemic capsaicin application, before the development of hyperglycemia, prevented the increase of fasting, nonfasting, and mean 24-h plasma glucose levels, and the deterioration of glucose tolerance assessed on the fifth week following the injection.

These effects were accompanied by enhanced insulin secretion and a virtually complete loss of CGRP- and TRPV1-coexpressing islet-innervating fibers. These data were taken to indicate that CGRP-containing fibers in the islets are capsaicin sensitive and that elimination of these fibers contributes to the prevention of the deterioration of glucose homeostasis through increased insulin secretion in ZDF rats.

Based on these data, the investigators proposed that the activity of islet-innervating capsaicin-sensitive fibers may have a role in the development of reduced insulin secretion in human Type 2 diabetes (Gram, Ahrén, Nagy et al. 2007).

Taken as a whole, research on the effects of capsaicin in diabetes leads to the conclusion that the active substances in some functional foods as well as in supplements that benefit glycemic control do not do so simply because they are antioxidant and anti-inflammatory. Rather, some of them appear to be specific to insulin secretion and glucose absorption.

11.11.2 Types and Concentration of Carotenoids in Different Chili Fruits

The types and levels of carotenoids differ between different chili pepper fruits, and they are also influenced by environmental conditions. Yellow-orange colors of chili pepper fruits are mainly due to the accumulation of α- and β-carotene, zeaxanthin, lutein, and β-cryptoxanthin. Carotenoids such as capsanthin, capsorubin, and capsanthin-5,6-epoxide confer the red colors (del Rocío, Gómez-García, and Ochoa-Alejo. 2013).

11.11.3 Safety of Consumption of Chili

Capsicum and paprika are generally recognized to be safe as food by the U.S. Food and Drug Administration (No authors listed. 2007). A report in the *International Journal of Emergency Medicine* concerned a previously healthy young man who reported severe chest pain after using cayenne pepper pills for slimming: He sustained an extensive inferior myocardial infarction. Electrocardiography combined with a bedside echocardiogram confirmed the diagnosis. The patient denied using illicit substances, and he had no risk factors for coronary artery disease.

His medication history revealed that he had recently started taking cayenne pepper pills for slimming. A subsequent coronary angiogram revealed normal coronary arteries, suggesting that the mechanism was vasospasm. The authors postulated that the patient developed acute coronary vasospasm, and a myocardial infarction, in the presence of stimulating compounds. This case highlights the unlikely but nevertheless possible danger of capsaicin—even when used by otherwise healthy individuals (Sogut, Kaya, Gokdemir et al. 2012).

Although chili is a powerful antioxidant, and it is anti-inflammatory, and although chili-containing meals increase energy expenditure and fat oxidation (Janssens, Hursel, Martens et al. 2013), the preliminary evidence that it might actually damage β-cells and impair insulin secretion makes us conclude that its supplementation in Type 2 diabetes cannot be recommended.

11.12 CINNAMON

Cinnamon belonging to the Lauracea family is a popular spice used in flavoring baked goods. It is now known that it has beneficial antioxidant and anti-inflammatory properties and it is considered by many as an adjunct in complementary and alternative medicine (Kawatra, and Rajagopalan. 2015).

Cinnamon is exported mainly from Indonesia, China, Vietnam, and Sri Lanka as quills that are made by peeling the bark and then rolling it into pipes.

There are four types of cinnamon:

- True cinnamon, or Ceylon cinnamon (*Cinnamomum zeylanicum*)
- Indonesian cinnamon (*Cinnamomum burmanni*)
- Vietnamese cinnamon (*Cinnamomum loureiroi*)
- Cassia cinnamon or Chinese cinnamon (*Cinnamomum aromaticum*)

Cinnamomum cassia, a.k.a. Chinese cassia, is the most common type of cinnamon used as spice in the United States. Due to a blood anticoagulant constituent, coumarin, that could damage the liver, European health agencies have warned against consuming high amounts of cassia. However, a report appearing in the journal *Food and Chemical Toxicology* states that ordinary consumption is considered safe (Lake. 1999).

The author of an article in *Critical Reviews in Food Science and Nutrition* is from the *Central Food Technological Research Institute*, Mysore, India. He reports that there are several hundred different species of *Cinnamomum* distributed in Asia and Australia. *C. zeylanicum*, a common source of cinnamon bark and leaf oils, is native to Sri Lanka, although most oil now comes from cultivated areas.

C. zeylanicum is a spice widely applied in flavoring, perfumery, beverages, and medicines. Volatile oils from different parts of cinnamon such as leaves, bark, fruits, root bark, flowers, and buds have been isolated by conventional laboratory methods. The chemical compositions of more than 80 compounds have been identified from different parts of cinnamon. The leaf oil has a major component called eugenol.

Cinnamaldehyde and camphor have been reported to be the major components of volatile oils from stem bark and root bark, respectively, whereas trans-cinnamyl acetate was found to be the major compound in fruits, flowers, and fruit stalks. These volatile oils were found to exhibit antioxidant, anti-inflammatory, antimicrobial, and antidiabetic activities. *C. zeylanicum* bark and fruits were found to contain proanthocyandins (Jayaprakasha, and Rao. 2011).

11.12.1 CINNAMON IS ANTIOXIDANT AND ANTI-INFLAMMATORY

The antioxidant property of cinnamon is largely due to the eugenol component that inhibits lipid peroxidation: The ORAC value of cinnamon is very high (131,420) among the highest for common foods. ORAC stands for oxygen radical absorbance capacity and it is a measure of antioxidant activity of a food (see Cao, Alessio, and Cutler. 1993. Oxygen-radical absorbance capacity assay for antioxidants. *Free Radical Biology and Medicine*, Mar; 14(3): 303–311). A significant relationship was found between antioxidant capacity and total phenolic content, indicating that phenolic compounds are the major contributors to the antioxidant properties of these plants (Dudonne, Vitrac, Vouitiere et al. 2009; Mathew, and Abraham. 2006; Su, Yin, Charles et al. 2007).

Sri Lankan cinnamon (*C. zeylanicum*) was found to be one of the most potent anti-inflammatory foods among 115 foods tested by the authors of a study published in the journal *Food and Function* in 2015. Because knowledge of the exact nature of the anti-inflammatory compounds and their distribution in the two major cinnamon species used for human consumption is limited, the aim of this investigation was to determine the anti-inflammatory activity of *C. zeylanicum* and *C. cassia* and define their main compounds.

When extracts were tested in macrophages, most of the anti-inflammatory activity measured by downregulation of NO was observed in the extracts. The most abundant compounds in these extracts were E-cinnamaldehyde and o-methoxycinnamaldehyde. The highest concentration of E-cinnamaldehyde was found in the extract of *C. zeylanicum* or *C. cassia*. When these and other constituents were tested for their anti-inflammatory activity in macrophages, the most potent compounds were E-cinnamaldehyde and o-methoxycinnamaldehyde.

The authors concluded that these could be useful in the treatment of age-related inflammatory conditions (Gunawardena, Karunaweera, Lee et al. 2015).

According to a report published in the journal *BMC Complementary and Alternative Medicine*, the beneficial health effects of "true" cinnamon (*C. zeylanicum*) were (a) antimicrobial; (b) lowering of blood glucose, blood pressure, and serum cholesterol; (c) antioxidant and free radical scavenging properties; and (d) anti-inflammatory activity (Ranasinghe, Pigera, Premakumara et al. 2013).

11.12.2 Equivocal Data on Glycemic Control by Cinnamon in Chronic Hyperglycemia

Cinnamon has often been cited in connection with glycemic control. Glycemic control is complex and rests on many factors, a good number of them being medical issues involving also those in metabolic syndrome. The following studies reporting glycemic control with cinnamon are essentially generalizations that do not take into account individual medical considerations. This is, therefore, a reminder that information about the potential palliative value of any functional food, or beverage, in connection with a medical disorder, is not suggested as an alternative to competent conventional medical treatment. Besides, although reports of the efficacy of cinnamon in glycemic control are, by and large, positive, there are also conflicting reports in the medical literature.

The authors of the report in the *Annals of Family Medicine* tell us that cinnamon has been studied in clinical trials for its glycemic-lowering effects but that the studies have been small and show conflicting results. Therefore, they undertook systematic meta-analyses evaluating the effects of cinnamon on glycemia and lipid levels.

They searched Embase and Cochrane Central Register of Controlled Trials(CENTRAL) through February 2012. The trials evaluated cinnamon in patients with Type 2 diabetes and reported at least one of the following: glycated hemoglobin (A1c), fasting plasma glucose, total cholesterol, low-density lipoprotein cholesterol (LDL-C), high-density lipoprotein cholesterol (HDL-C), or triglycerides.

They report that cinnamon doses of 120 mg/day to 6 grams/day for four to eighteen weeks significantly reduced levels of fasting plasma glucose, total cholesterol, LDL-C, and triglycerides. Cinnamon also raised levels of HDLcholesterol. No significant effect on HbA1c levels was observed. It was further concluded however that the high degree of heterogeneity of the data may limit the ability to apply these results to patient care, because the preferred dose and duration of therapy are often unclear (Allen, Schwartzman, Baker et al. 2013).

Another meta-analysis reported in the *Journal of Medical Foods* reported that cinnamon intake, either as whole cinnamon or as cinnamon extract, results in a significant lowering in fasting blood sugar, while intake of cinnamon extract only lowered fasting blood sugar in people with Type 2 diabetes or prediabetes (Davis, and Yokoyama. 2011).

Another report of the review of several clinical trials of the effectiveness of cinnamon in Type 2 diabetes was published in the journal *Pharmacotherapy*. It concluded that cinnamon has a possible modest effect in lowering plasma glucose levels in patients with poorly controlled Type 2 diabetes. They stated that "… clinicians are strongly urged to refrain from recommending cinnamon supplementation in place of the proven standard of care, which includes lifestyle modifications, oral antidiabetic agents, and insulin therapy" (Pham, Kourlas, Pham et al. 2007. *Pharmacotherapy*, Apr; 27(4): 595–599).

Entering "cinnamon and Type 2 diabetes" into PubMed results in more than 100 citations. There is considerable scientific interest in that topic. It may be due in large measure to the fact that current interventions in glycemic control in Type 2 diabetes seem to leave much to be desired. The problem is that Type 2 diabetes is a health hazard of epidemic proportions. It would be good to be able to say authoritatively that cinnamon is a successful functional food and an effective adjunct to conventional medicine.

It is difficult to know why there is inconsistency in the outcome of studies of the effectiveness of cinnamon in glycemic control. There are many possibilities: varieties differ in type and concentration of effective constituents. The same variety has different concentration of constituents depending on the geographic regions in the world where it is cultivated. There are no data that would shed light on this debacle. For that reason, and because apparently valid clinical studies support the role of cinnamon in glycemic control, both sides of the picture are presented here.

Investigators from the Netherlands reported in the *Journal of Nutrition* that they found that the blood lipid profile of fasting subjects did not change after cinnamon supplementation. They therefore concluded that cinnamon (*C. cassia*) supplementation of 1.5 g/day does not improve whole-body insulin sensitivity or oral glucose tolerance, nor did it affect blood lipid profile in postmenopausal patients with Type 2 diabetes. They concluded that "… more research on the proposed health benefits of cinnamon supplementation is warranted before health claims should be made" (Vanschoonbeek, Thomassen, Senden et al. 2006. *Journal of Nutrition*, Apr; 136(4): 977–980). Another study also from a diabetes clinic in the Netherlands appearing in the journal *Nederlands Tijdschrift voor Geneeskunde* concluded that no evidence supports recommendation of cinnamon for improvement of glycemic control (Kleefstra, Logtenberg, Houweling et al. 2007).

11.12.3 SAFETY OF CONSUMING CINNAMON

Finally, as noted above, *cassia* cinnamon contains relatively high levels of coumarins that can be toxic in high doses. A daily intake of more than 0.1 mg/kg body weight (BW) can lead to conspicuous effect on the blood coagulation profile, if one is also on anticoagulant drugs such as warfarin (coumarin can also be highly toxic to the liver and its addition into food products is prohibited). However, due to the lack of awareness regarding the standard limits of cinnamon in these products, it is probably advisable for anyone with liver disorders to avoid cinnamon.

11.13 EDIBLE SEAWEED, A SEA VEGETABLE

Edible seaweed is included in this limited list of functional foods because it contains iodine, essential to healthy metabolic function, and diet is usually the sole source. Health authorities report that there is a significant worldwide iodine deficiency (Li, and Eastman. 2012). In the developed world, iodine deficiency has increased more than fourfold over the past 40 years: Nearly 74% of normal, "healthy" adults may no longer be consuming enough iodine (http://www.lifeextension.com/magazine/2011/10/the-silent-epidemic-of-iodine-deficiency/Page-01).

In 1922, David Cowie, chairman of the Pediatrics Department at the University of Michigan, proposed that the United States adopt salt iodinization to eliminate simple goiter (Markel. 1987).

In the United States, salt is iodized usually with potassium iodide at 100 parts per million (76 mg of iodine per kilogram of salt). However, approximately 70% of ingested salt now comes from processed food that is typically not iodinized. Iodine deficiency is still one of the most important public health issues globally, and an estimated 2.2 billion people live in iodine-deficient areas: The oceans are the main repositories of iodine; very little is found in the soil in most of the inhabited world.

Although the International Council for the Control of Iodine Deficiency Disorders Global Network estimates that the proportion of US households with access to iodized salt now exceeds 90%, data regarding actual usage is limited and the contribution of iodinized salt to the overall iodine sufficiency of the US population is uncertain. This is particularly the case as there is a trend in reducing table salt intake consistent with the rising concerns about "sodium" in diet and hypertension and cardiovascular and heart disease. In fact, *The Harvard Health Letter* (June 21, 2011) seemingly supported that trend in an article titled "Cut salt—it won't affect your iodine intake" (No authors listed. 2011). Actually, iodinized salt provides only a small fraction of ideal daily iodine intake.

While iodine deficiency has many implications for serious medical disorders, and poor cognitive function, the concern here is dietary deficiency that sets the stage for chronic inflammation and adverse impact on glycemic control, as noted in a previous chapter.

"Sea vegetables" are described here as a dietary source of iodine where it is suspected that the typical diet supplies insufficient amounts it. It is not intended to propose self-treatment for any thyroid condition related to iodine. Thyroid disease can be a serious medical problem and it needs to be addressed by competent medical means. In fact, even subclinical hypothyroidism may be a mild form of thyroid failure that needs to be treated medically (McDermott, and Ridgway. 2011). The Barnes self-test for at-home evaluation of possible iodine deficiency is described in Chapter 5.

11.13.1   KELP IS ON THE WAY

There are different varieties of edible seaweed/sea vegetables that are dietary sources of iodine. The better known varieties are as follows:

- Kelps, large seaweeds (algae) belonging to the brown algae Phaeophyceae in the order Laminariales. They typically have a long, tough stalk with a broad frond divided into strips. Some kinds grow to a very large size and form underwater "forests" that support a large population of animals. The Japanese version is kombu or haidai (*Laminaria japonica*)
- Nori or purple laver (*Porphyra* spp.)
- Wakame, quandai-cai (*Undaria pinnatifida*)
- Dulse (*Palmaria palmata*)

Seaweed, such as kelp, nori, kombu, and wakame, is one of the best food sources of iodine, but it is highly variable in its iodine content. It is used extensively as food in coastal cuisines around the world, and a rich source of iodine, an essential component of the thyroid hormones thyroxine (T4) and triiodothyronine (T3).

Iodine in food and iodized salt is present in chemical forms including sodium and potassium salts, inorganic iodine (I2), iodate, and iodide, the reduced form of iodine. Iodine rarely occurs as the element, but rather as a salt; for this reason, it is referred to as iodide and not iodine. Iodide is quickly and almost completely absorbed in the stomach and duodenum. It is reduced in the gastrointestinal tract and absorbed as iodide. When iodide enters the circulation, the thyroid gland concentrates it in appropriate amounts for hormone synthesis, and most of the remaining amount is excreted in urine.

11.13.2 IODINE CONTENT OF DIFFERENT VARIETIES

A report in the *Journal of Food and Drug Analysis* lists the following Asian seaweed iodine concentrations:

- Nori—29.3 to 45.8 mg/kg
- Wakame—93.9 to 185.1 mg/kg
- Kombu—241 to 4921 mg/kg (Yeh, Hung, and Lin. 2014)

The iodine concentration in samples of kelp from British Columbia, Canada, was reported in the journal *Thyroid* to range between 1259 and 1513 µg/g. The authors of that report also caution that iodine is water soluble in cooking and may vaporize in humid storage conditions, making average iodine content of prepared foods difficult to estimate. Also, it is possible that some Asian seaweed dishes may exceed the tolerable upper iodine intake level of 1100 µg/day (Teas, Pino, Critchley et al. 2004). Iodine can be effectively consumed also in commercially available kelp supplements that list the iodine content per capsule or pill.

11.13.3 SEA VEGETABLES HOLD POTENT ANTIOXIDANTS

The journal *Marine Drugs* published a review titled "Looking beyond the terrestrial: The potential of seaweed derived bioactives to treat non-communicable diseases" (Collins, Fitzgerald, Stanton et al. 2016). The review details the antioxidant and antidiabetic properties of consumable substances in seaweed. In particular, interest in using naturally obtained antioxidants for diabetic treatment has increased due to the inadequacy of synthetic antioxidants such as butylated hydroxyanisol(BHA), butylated hydroxytoluene (BHT) and tert-butylhydroquinone(TBHQ) that are available commercially (Chakraborty, Praveen, Vijayan et al. 2013).

Seaweeds are generally considered to be a rich source of antioxidant compounds. Pigments, such as fucoxanthin and astaxanthin, and polyphenolic compounds, such as phenolic acid, flavonoid, and tannins, have all exhibited antioxidant abilities proving useful even in Type 1 diabetes (Kang, Jin, Lee et al. 2010).

Polyphenolic compounds can act as reactive oxygen species (ROS) scavengers but there exist fundamental differences between the polyphenols produced by land plants and those produced by their marine counterpoints. Edible seaweeds are a good source of polyphenols, and it has been suggested that they have antidiabetic activity.

The brown seaweed *Tubinaria ornata* (Phaeophyceae), tropical brown algae of the order Fucales native to coral reef ecosystems of the South Pacific, has shown superoxide scavenging activity, which may be effective in reducing the level of O_2 that is elevated during oxidative stress in the body. The presence of phenolic compounds suggests that they are responsible for that action (Vijayabaskar, and Shiyamala. 2012).

Methanol extracts from *E. cava* edible marine brown algae species, found in the ocean off Japan and Korea, containing high levels of polyphenol and strong ROS scavenging ability, significantly reduce blood glucose levels and increase insulin concentration when fed to Type 1 diabetic rats. Blood alanine transaminase (ALT) levels were dramatically reduced to near-normal levels. Increased levels of alanine transaminase (ALT) in serum are often associated with health problems such as diabetes and liver damage. The antidiabetic effect appears to be at least partly mediated by the activation of both the AMP-activated protein kinase/acetyl-CoA carboxylase (ACC) and the Pl-3 kinase/Akt signal pathways (Kang, Ko, Shin et al. 2011).

Numerous other seaweeds have also been found to contain high amounts of phenolic compounds and exhibit strong antioxidant activity, including *Sargassum swartzii* (formerly *Sargassum wightii*), a species distributed throughout the temperate and tropical oceans of the world, where they generally inhabit shallow water and coral reefs, and the genus is widely known for its planktonic (free-floating) species (Meenakshi, Umayaparvathi, Arumugam et al. 2011); *Fucus serratus* (Phaeophyceae), a seaweed of the North Atlantic Ocean, known as "toothed wrack" or "serrated wrack," and *Fucus vesiculosus*, known by the common name "bladder wrack" or "bladderwrack," is a seaweed found on the coasts of the North Sea, the western Baltic Sea, the Atlantic Ocean, and the Pacific Ocean (O'Sullivan, O'Callaghan, O'Grady et al. 2011).

11.13.4   ANTI-INFLAMMATORY AND ANTIDIABETIC PROPERTIES OF SEAWEEDS

Seaweeds contain many constituents that are beneficial in the treatment of diabetes. In a review published by the journal *Marine Drugs* (Collins, Fitzgerald, Stanton et al. 2016), the investigators cite dietary fibers, unsaturated fatty acids, and polyphenolic compounds, bioactive compounds that are potentially useful in preventing or managing Type 2 diabetes by targeting various pharmacologically relevant routes including inhibition of enzymes such as α-glucosidase, α-amylase, lipase, aldose reductase, protein tyrosine phosphatase 1B(PTP1B) and dipeptidyl-peptidase-4(DPP-4).

Other mechanisms of action identified were anti-inflammatory, induction of hepatic antioxidant enzyme activities, stimulation of glucose transport and incretin hormone release, as well as β-cell cytoprotection (Sharifuddin, Chin, Lim et al. 2015).

The journal *Nutrition Research and Practice* published a clinical study aimed to determine the physiological effects of seaweed supplementation on blood glucose levels, lipid profile, and antioxidant enzyme activities in subjects with Type 2 diabetes. Patients were assigned to either a control group or a seaweed (wakame) supplementation group.

Pills with equal parts of dry powdered sea tangle (*Laminaria japonica*) and sea mustard (wakame) were provided to the seaweed supplementation group, three times a day for 4 weeks. Total daily consumption of seaweed was 48 g.

It was found that total dietary fiber intake was 2.5 times higher in participants receiving seaweed supplementation than in the control group. Accordingly, fasting blood glucose levels and 2-h postprandial blood glucose measurements were significantly lower in those ingesting seaweed. Furthermore, the serum concentrations of triglycerides were significantly lower and HDL cholesterol was significantly higher in the seaweed supplement group. However, the concentrations of total cholesterol and LDL cholesterol were not affected by seaweed supplementation.

The level of thiobarbituric acid reactive substances (TBARS) in erythrocytes was significantly lower with seaweed supplementation, compared to that in controls. Catalase and glutathione peroxidase activity with seaweed supplementation were significantly higher than that in the controls, but superoxide dismutase activity was not affected.

The investigators concluded that seaweed influences glycemic control, lowers blood lipids, and increases antioxidant enzyme activities (Kim, Kim, Choi et al. 2008).

Plants that have high polyphenol content can inhibit the activity of carbohydrate hydrolyzing enzymes such as α-amylase and α-glucosidase, thus lowering postprandial levels of glucose (Oboh, Ademiluyi, Akinyemi et al. 2012). Seaweeds are known to inhibit starch digestive enzymes and are currently an underexplored source of enzyme inhibitors for use in the treatment of diabetes (Heo, Hwang, Choi et al. 2009; Lee, Park, Heo et al. 2010).

A study investigating the α-amylase and α-glucosidase inhibitory effects of 15 Irish seaweeds found that cold water and ethanol extracts of *Ascophyllum nodosum* had a strong α-amylase inhibitory effect, while extracts of *F. vesiculosus* exhibited potent inhibition of α-glucosidase. The recorded effects of the extracts were associated with phenolic content and antioxidant activity (Lordan, Smyth, Soler-Vila et al. 2013).

Ascophyllum nodosum is a large common brown alga (*Phaeophyceae*), family *Fucaceae*, seaweed of the North Atlantic Ocean, also known as *feamainn bhuí*, rockweed, Norwegian kelp, knotted kelp, or knotted wrack. It is common also in east Greenland and the northeastern coast of North America.

The phenol-rich extracts of *A. nodosum* collected from UK waters have also been shown to inhibit α-amylase activity to some extent. In a study conducted with samples of *A. nodosum*, *P. palmata* and *Alaria esculenta* (Phaeophyceae), the *A. nodosum* extracts were found to be the most active of the three seaweeds. The same extracts were also able to inhibit the activity of α-glucosidase at low levels.

Following fractionation of the *Ascophyllum* extracts, it was found that the inhibitory activity was concentrated in the phlorotannin-rich fraction. It has been suggested that seaweeds accumulate phlorotannins to deter being eaten by predatory species such as molluscs and they have been shown to potently inhibit the digestive glycosidases of marine snails (Nwosu, Morris, Lund et al. 2011).

Two bromophenols (2,4,6-tribromophenol and 2,4-dibromophenol) isolated and purified from the red seaweed *Grateloupia elliptica* (Rhodophyta) were found to have high α-glucosidase inhibitory activity. *Grateloupia elliptica* is native to Jeju Island, Korea. Parenthetically, *Gelliptica* (Red Korean Seaweed) appears also to inhibit 5-*alpha*-reductase and thus it may help slow hair loss (Kang, Kim, Han et al. 2012).

According to a report in the journal *Food and Chemical Toxicology*, dieckol, a phlorotannin found in some seaweed species, isolated from *E. cava*, showed pronounced α-amylase and α-glucosidase inhibition, displaying higher activity than that of acarbose. Postprandial blood glucose levels in streptozotocin (STZ)-induced diabetic mice were also seen to be significantly suppressed (Lee, Park, Heo et al. 2010).

11.13.4.1 Antiobesity Effect of Fucoxanthin in Seaweed

Fucoxanthin is a marine carotenoid found in macroalgae and microalgae such as *Undaria pinnatifida* (wakame), *Laminaria japonica* (ma-kombu), *Phaeodactylum tricornutum*, and *Cylindrotheca closterium* (Kim, Jung, Kwon et al. 2012). Fucoxanthin has a unique molecular structure including an unusual allenic bond, a 5,6-monoepoxide, and nine conjugated double bounds. However, the unique structure and chirality of fucoxanthin are unstable: It is easily affected by heating, aerial exposure, and illumination (Zhao, Kim, Pan et al. 2014).

It is said that it was because of its unstable structure and the allenic bond that fucoxanthin has high antioxidant activity (Sangeetha, Bhaskar, and Baskaran. 2009). Moreover, fucoxanthin also showed antiobesity, antidiabetes, anti-inflammatory, and hepatoprotective activities as well as cardiovascular and cerebrovascular protective effects. Researchers found that fucoxanthin supplementation could play a beneficial role in antiobesity through various pathways.

Fucoxanthin has been shown to significantly reduce plasma and hepatic triglyceride concentrations, cholesterol, and cholesterol-regulating enzyme activities such as 3-hydroxy-3-methylglutaryl coenzyme A reductase and acyl coenzyme A (Woo, Jeon, Kim et al. 2010; Jeon, Kim, Woo et al. 2010).

A study in the journal *Nutrition Research and Practice* reported that, in rats with a high-fat diet, fucoxanthin supplementation could decrease the mRNA expression of hepatic acetyl-CoA carboxylase ACC, fatty acid synthase, glucose-6-phosphate dehydrogenase (G6PDH), hydroxy-3-methylglutaryl coenzyme A(HMG-CoA), acyl-CoA cholesterol acyltransferase (ACAT), and SREBP-1C. And the mRNA expression of lecithin-cholesterol acyltransferase (LCAT), CPT1, and CYP7A1 was significantly higher in the HF + Fxn group (Ha, and Kim. 2013).

In another study reported in the journal *Molecular Medicine Reports*, it was shown that dietary administration of high-fat diet resulted in expression of monocyte chemoattractant protein-1 (MCP-1) mRNA in mice. However, the increased expression of MCP-1 mRNA was normalized by fucoxanthin-rich wakame lipids. The results suggested that a wakame lipid diet could ameliorate high-fat diet–induced lipid metabolism disorders in mice (Maeda, Hosokawa, Sashima et al. 2009).

In a study published in the journal *Chemico-Biological Interactions*, it was also reported that fucoxanthin supplementation improves plasma and hepatic lipid metabolism, and blood glucose concentration, in high-fat diet–fed C57BL/6N mice: the activities of two key cholesterol regulating enzymes, acyl coenzyme A:cholesterol acyltransferase and 3-hydroxy-3-methylglutaryl coenzyme

A reductase, were significantly inhibited by fucoxanthin in mice. Relative mRNA expressions of acyl-coA oxidase 1, palmitoyl (ACOX1), and peroxisome proliferator-activated receptor α (PPARα) and γ (PPARγ) were also altered in a beneficial direction by fucoxanthin in the liver (Woo, Jeon, Kim et al. 2010).

Fucoxanthin might alter plasma leptin level elevated by the accumulation of fat in adipocytes. A study in the journal *Food and Chemical Toxicology* reported finding beneficial effects of *Undaria pinnatifida* ethanol extract (UEFx) in C57BL/6J mice. They found that fucoxanthin could significantly decrease plasma leptin levels associated with a significant decrement of the epididymal adipose tissue weight (Park, Lee, Park et al. 2011).

11.13.4.2 Antidiabetic Effect of Fucoxanthin

Diabetes mellitus often covaries with obesity because excessive energy intake and accumulation of lipids can elevate insulin resistance (Campfield, and Smith. 1999). Saturated fat intake can elevate the HbA1c level (Harding, Sargeant, Welch et al. 2001). The HbA1c level is a risk indicator of hyperglycemia and diabetic complications (Goldstein, Little, Lorenz et al. 1995). A study published in the journal *Chemico-Biological Interactions* aimed to determine the effects of fucoxanthin isolated from marine plant extracts on lipid metabolism, and blood glucose concentration in high-fat diet–fed C57BL/6N mice.

The mice were assigned to high-fat control (HFC; 20% fat, w/w), low-fucoxanthin (low-Fxn; HFC + 0.05% Fxn, w/w) and high-fucoxanthin (high-Fxn; HFC + 0.2% Fxn, w/w) groups.

It was found that fucoxanthin supplementation significantly lowered the concentration of plasma triglycerides with a concomitant increase of fecal lipids in comparison to the high-fat control group. The hepatic lipid contents were significantly lowered in the fucoxanthin-supplemented groups, which seemed to be due to the reduced activity of the hepatic lipogenic enzymes, glucose-6-phosphate dehydrogenase, enzymes that modify malic acid, fatty acid synthase, and phosphatidate phosphohydrolase and the enhanced activity of β-oxidation. Plasma HDL cholesterol concentrations and its percentage were markedly elevated by fucoxanthin supplementation. Activities of two key cholesterol regulating enzymes, 3-hydroxy-3-methylglutaryl coenzyme A reductase and acyl coenzyme A:cholesterol acyltransferase, were significantly suppressed by fucoxanthin regardless of the dosage. Relative mRNA expressions of acyl-coA oxidase 1, palmitoyl (ACOX1), and peroxisome proliferator activated receptors alpha (PPARalpha) and gamma (PPARgamma) were significantly altered in the liver by fucoxanthin supplementation.

Fucoxanthin also lowered blood glucose and HbA1c levels along with plasma resistin and insulin concentrations. These results suggest that fucoxanthin supplementation plays a beneficial role in regulating plasma and hepatic lipid metabolism and also for blood glucose–lowering action in high-fat diet–fed mice (Woo, Jeon, Kim et al. 2010).

The adipokine tumor necrosis factor-α (TNFα) is involved in the development of Type 2 diabetes. TNF-α is elevated in obesity and positively associated with insulin resistance (Hotamisligil, Shargill, and Spiegelman. 1993; Hotamisligil, Arner, Caro et al. 1995). A study published in the *Journal of Agricultural and Food Chemistry* showed that 0.2% fucoxanthin improved insulin resistance and markedly decreased blood glucose and plasma insulin concentrations in KK-Ay mice by downregulating TNF-α mRNA (Maeda, Hosokawa, Sashima et al. 2007).

In another study published in the journal *Molecular Medicine Reports*, it was found that a fucoxanthin-rich wakame lipid diet could ameliorate insulin resistance by promoting expression of glucose transporter 4 (GLUT4) mRNA in skeletal muscle tissues (Maeda, Hosokawa, Sashima et al. 2009).

A report published in the journal *Food and Chemical Toxicology* found that blood glucose level was positively associated with hepatic gluconeogenic enzyme activities, but negatively associated with hepatic glucokinase activity, and that fucoxanthin could decrease insulin resistance by elevating the ratio of hepatic glucokinase/glucose-6-phosphatase and glycogen content (Park, Lee, Park et al. 2011).

11.13.4.3   Anti-Inflammatory Effect of Fucoxanthin

A study published in the *European Journal of Pharmacology* aimed to determine the anti-inflammatory effect of fucoxanthin in lipopolysaccharide-stimulated murine macrophage RAW 264.7 cells. It was found that fucoxanthin could reduce the levels of pro-inflammatory mediators including NO, PGE2, IL-1β, TNF-α, and IL-6 by suppressing NF-κB activation and the MAPK phosphorylation.

In addition, fucoxanthin reduced the levels of iNOS and COX-2 proteins in a dose-dependent manner (Kim, Heo, Yoon et al. 2010).

11.13.5   Fucoxanthin as a Dietary Supplement

Fucoxantin is widely available as a dietary supplement, its link to weight loss and glycemic control is solid, but it is based primarily on reports of its effects in animal models. There is, however, an excellent review titled "Anti-obesity activity of the marine carotenoid Fucoxanthin" in the journal *Marine Drugs* (2015. Apr; 13(4): 2196–2214).

The authors conclude that

> fucoxanthin has many bioactivities potentially promoting human health. In particular, its potential anti-obesity effect was primarily detected by murine studies, which displayed an induction of uncoupling protein-1 in abdominal white adipose tissue mitochondria, leading to the oxidation of fatty acids and heat production.
>
> Even if further studies are necessary in order to authenticate these results in humans too, all the promising scientific findings might allow its future development as a marine nutraceutical and an interesting functional food.
>
> However, it is well recognized that basal metabolism, appetite and food intake are affected by many other factors including age, sex, body composition, physical activity levels, environmental factors (such as temperature), and also individual differences. These factors are likely to influence the balance of homeostatic controls and make it difficult to generalize; nevertheless, research and knowledge advancement in this area brings hope that potential novel strategies for weight control could be on the horizon. (From Gammone, and D'Orazio. 2015. *Marine Drugs*, Apr; 13(4): 2196–2214. With permission.)

11.13.6   Health Risk of Excessive Iodine Intake

High intakes of iodine can cause some of the same symptoms as iodine deficiency—including goiter, elevated TSH levels, and hypothyroidism—because excess iodine in susceptible individuals inhibits thyroid hormone synthesis and thereby increases TSH stimulation, which can produce goiter. Iodine-induced hyperthyroidism can also result from high iodine intakes, usually when iodine is administered to treat iodine deficiency.

Studies have also shown that excessive iodine intakes can cause thyroiditis and thyroid papillary cancer. Cases of acute iodine poisoning are rare and are usually caused by doses of many grams. Acute poisoning symptoms include burning of the mouth, throat, and stomach; fever; abdominal pain; nausea; vomiting; diarrhea; weak pulse; and coma. Some people, such as those with autoimmune thyroid disease and iodine deficiency, may experience adverse effects with iodine intakes considered safe for the general population.

The Food and Nutrition Board set iodine upper intake levels (ULs) from food and supplements. They make the following recommendations:

Men
- 14 to 18 years old: 900 µg
- 19 years or older: 1100 µg

Women
- 14 to 18 years old: 900 µg (includes pregnancy and lactation)
- 19 years or older: 1100 µg (includes pregnancy and lactation)

(Based on the Iodine Fact Sheets for Health Professionals. National Institutes of Health (NIH), Office of Dietary Supplements. https://ods.od.nih.gov/factsheets/Iodine-HealthProfessional/; accessed 2.23.18.)

In most people, iodine intakes from foods and supplements are unlikely to exceed the UL. Long-term intakes above the UL raise the risk of adverse health effects. The ULs do not apply to individuals receiving iodine for medical treatment under the care of a physician. (See No authors listed. 2001. Institute of Medicine, Food and Nutrition Board. Dietary reference intakes: vitamin A, vitamin K, arsenic, boron, chromium, copper, iodine, iron, manganese, molybdenum, nickel, silicon, vanadium, and zinc. Washington, DC: National Academy Press.)

11.13.7 INTERACTION WITH MEDICATIONS

Iodine supplements have the potential to interact with several types of medications including, of course, medications for an overactive thyroid. Selected examples are provided below. Individuals taking these medications on a regular basis should discuss their iodine intakes with their health care providers. There are many other conditions where medications may interact adversely with iodine supplementation. Medical consultation is strongly advised.

- Anti-thyroid medications: Anti-thyroid medications, such as methimazole (Tapazole), are used to treat hyperthyroidism. Taking high doses of iodine with anti-thyroid medications can have an additive effect and could cause medical problems.
- Angiotensin-converting enzyme (ACE) inhibitors: Angiotensin-converting enzyme ACE inhibitors, such as benazepril (Lotensin), lisinopril (Prinivil and Zestril), and fosinopril (Monopril), are used primarily to treat high blood pressure. Taking potassium iodide with ACE inhibitors can increase the risk of hyperkalemia (elevated blood levels of potassium).
- Potassium-sparing diuretics: Taking potassium iodide with potassium-sparing diuretics, such as spironolactone (Aldactone) and amiloride (Midamor), can increase the risk of hyperkalemia.

(See: Natural Medicines Comprehensive Database. Iodine; see also: https://ods.od.nih.gov/factsheets/Iodine-HealthProfessional/; see also: Does Iodine interact with any other medications. *Web*MD, http://answers.webmd.com/answers/1183554/does-iodine-interact-with-any-other; accessed 8.28.17.)

11.14 MUSHROOMS: SHITAKE AND OTHER FUNGI WITH ANTIDIABETIC PROPERTIES

Mushrooms are a widely consumed, low-calorie, low-cholesterol, and low-sodium health-promoting food. Some of the health-promoting properties have been attributed to the polysaccharides produced by different varieties of mushrooms. A comprehensive review of the medicinal property of mushrooms appears in a report titled "Mushroom polysaccharides: Chemistry and antiobesity, antidiabetes, anticancer, and antibiotic properties in cells, rodents, and humans," published in the journal *Foods* (Friedman. 2016).

More than 2000 species of edible and/or medicinal mushrooms have been identified to date. Their health-promoting properties are related to the bioactive compounds they produce including polysaccharides. Although β-glucans (homopolysaccharides) are believed to be the major bioactive polysaccharides of mushrooms, other types of mushroom polysaccharides (heteropolysaccharides) also possess biological properties. The mechanisms of bioactive action involve the gut microbiota; that is, the polysaccharides act as prebiotics in the digestive system.

11.14.1 ANTIDIABETIC AND ANTIOXIDANT ACTIVITY OF SELECTED MUSHROOMS

An evaluation of the effect of the culinary *Pleurotus ostreatus* (a.k.a. oyster mushroom) and *Pleurotus cystidiosus* mushrooms (a.k.a. maple oyster mushroom) (consumed as freeze-dried powders at a dose of 50 mg/kg BW) in healthy human volunteers and Type 2 diabetic patients showed (a) a reduction in fasting and postprandial serum glucose levels of healthy volunteers and (b) a reduction in postprandial serum glucose levels and increased serum insulin levels of Type 2 diabetic patients (Jayasuriya, Wanigatunge, Fernando et al. 2015).

The hypoglycemic activity seems to be associated with increased glucokinase activity and promotion of insulin secretion by the pancreas, thus increasing the utilization of glucose by peripheral tissues, inhibiting glycogen synthase kinase activity, and promoting glycogen synthesis (Friedman. 2016).

A study published in the *International Journal of Medicinal Mushrooms* aimed to assess the antidiabetic effects in different types of mushrooms of *in vitro* α-glycosidase and aldose reductase (AR) inhibitory assays, and antioxidant activity assay.

Ganoderma lucidum (a.k.a. lingzhi; a.k.a. reishi mushroom) extract exhibited the best dose-dependent inhibitory activity against α-glycosidase, with IC50 at 4.88 mg/mL, and also exhibited aldose reductase inhibitory potential with an IC50 value of 9.87 mg/mL.

Tremella fuciformis (a.k.a. snow fungus) demonstrated the highest aldose reductase inhibitory activity (IC50 = 8.39 mg/mL).

The antioxidant activity of selected mushrooms was evaluated based on the total phenolic content, total flavonoids content, and DPPH (2,2-diphenyl-1-picryl-hydrazyl-hydrate) free radical scavenging activity. It was found that *G. lucidum* (reishi mushroom) contained the highest total phenolic content (39.3 mg GAE/g sample extract), total flavonoids content (15.1 mg CE/g sample extract), and the strongest DPPH free radical scavenging activity (IC50 = 3.66 mg/mL) among the mushroom samples (Wu, and Xu. 2015).

According to a report in the *International Journal of Medicinal Mushrooms*, management of Type 2 diabetes by delaying or preventing glucose absorption, using natural products, is gaining significant attention. The reported investigation aimed to evaluate the antidiabetic activity of aqueous extracts of selected culinary–medicinal mushrooms, namely, *Pleurotus ostreatus* (oyster mushroom), *Calocybe indica* (abbreviated "*C. indica*") also known as milky mushroom), and *Volvariella volvacea* (straw mushroom), using *in vitro* models (α-amylase inhibition assay, glucose uptake by yeast cells, and glucose adsorption capacity). The most active extract was subsequently examined *in vivo* using the oral starch tolerance test in mice.

All prepared extracts showed dose-dependent inhibition of α-amylase and an increase in glucose transport across yeast cells. *C. indica* extract was the most active α-amylase inhibitor (half-maximal inhibitory concentration, 18.07 ± 0.75 mg/mL) and exhibited maximum glucose uptake by yeast cells (77.53% ± 0.97% at 35 mg/mL). All extracts demonstrated weak glucose adsorption ability. The positive *in vitro* tests for *C. indica* paved the way for *in vivo* studies.

C. indica extract (200 and 400 mg/kg) significantly reduced postprandial blood glucose peaks in mice challenged with starch. The extract (400 mg/kg) and acarbose normalized blood glucose levels at 180 min, when they were statistically similar to values in normal mice.

The investigators concluded that the antidiabetic effect of *C. indica* is mediated by inhibition of starch metabolism (α-amylase inhibition), increased glucose uptake by peripheral cells (promotion of glucose uptake by yeast cells), and mild entrapment (adsorption) of glucose (Singh, Bedi, and Shri. 2017).

Pleurotus sajor-caju (PSC) is an edible oyster mushroom featuring high nutritional values and pharmacological properties. The objective of an animal model study published in the journal *BioMed Research International* was to investigate the hypoglycemic and antidiabetic effects of single and repeated oral administration of PSC aqueous extract in normal and diabetic rats.

A single dose of 500, 750, or 1000 mg/kg of the PSC extract was given to an experimental group of patients to determine the effects on blood glucose and oral glucose tolerance test (OGTT). The effective dose (750 mg/kg) of the PSC extract was administered daily for 21 days to diabetic rats to examine its antidiabetic effects in terms of blood glucose control, body weight, urine sugar, HbA1c, and several serum profiles.

It was found that the 750-mg/kg dose showed the most significant blood glucose reduction (23.5%) in normal rats, 6 h after administration in the blood glucose study group. In the oral glucose tolerance (OGTT) study, the same dose produced a maximum blood glucose fall of 41.3% in normal rats and 36.5% in diabetic rats, 3 h after glucose administration.

In a 21-day study, treated diabetic rats showed significant improvement in fasting blood glucose, body weight, and urine sugar levels as compared to control untreated diabetic rats (Ng, Zain, Zakaria et al. 2015).

However, there are studies of mushroom effects in glycemic control and related disorders that do not yield encouraging results. For instance, a study published in the journal *Scientific Reports* aimed to evaluate the efficacy and safety of *G. lucidum* (lingzhi mushroom) for the treatment of hyperglycemia and other cardiovascular risk components of metabolic syndrome. Participants with Type 2 diabetes mellitus and metabolic syndrome were assigned to one of three intervention groups: (a) *G. lucidum*, (b) *G. lucidum* with *Cordyceps sinensis* (a rare combination of a caterpillar and a fungus native to Nepal and Tibet), or (c) placebo. The dosage was 3 g/day of *G. lucidum*, with or without *C. sinensis*, for 16 weeks. The primary outcome measure was blood HbA1c and FPG; a number of secondary outcome measures were also tested.

The combined intervention had no effect on any of the primary or secondary outcome measures over the course of the 16-week trial, and no overall increased risk of adverse events with either active treatment. Evidence from this randomized clinical trial does not support the use of *G. lucidum* for treatment of cardiovascular risk factors in people with diabetes or metabolic syndrome (Klupp, Kiat, Bensoussan et al. 2016).

11.15 TURMERIC

Turmeric (*Curcuma longa*) is a rhizomatous herbaceous perennial plant of the ginger family, zingiberaceae. A spice that comes from the turmeric plant contains curcumin commonly used in Asian cuisine. Turmeric is the main spice in curry. It has a warm, bitter taste and is frequently used to flavor or color curry powders, mustards, butters, and cheeses.

11.15.1 CURCUMIN IS ANTIOXIDANT AND ANTI-INFLAMMATORY

According to a report published in the journal *Advances in Experimental Medicine and Biology*, the anti-inflammatory effect of curcumin (diferuloylmethane) is probably its ability to inhibit important enzymes that mediate inflammatory processes (Menon, and Sudheer. 2007).

There are a considerable number of experimental studies of the effects of curcumin on inflammatory conditions that would affect us, such as oxidative stress, atherosclerosis, diabetes, and more. Most of these studies show encouraging positive outcome of curcumin treatment. However, due to the nature of the experimental procedures, they are often performed on animal models. The beneficial effects of curcumin are then, of necessity, extrapolated from those studies but, in all fairness, the extrapolation is not unreasonable.

A study published in the *Medical Science Monitor* aimed to determine the protective effect of curcumin against oxidative stress in chemically stressed rats. The subjects were made diabetic and then fed either only the AIN-93 (standard rodent formulation) diet or the AIN-93 diet containing 0.002%, 0.01%, or 0.5% curcumin for 8 weeks. Then, the levels of oxidative stress, and antioxidant enzymes, were determined in various tissues.

Hyperglycemia resulted in increased lipid peroxidation and protein components in red blood cells and other tissues, and it altered antioxidant enzyme activities. Curcumin reduced oxidative stress in the diabetic rats by inhibiting the increase in TBARS and protein components and reversing altered antioxidant enzyme activities without altering the hyperglycemic state in most of the tissues. Thiobarbituric acid reactive substances (TBARS) are formed as a by-product of lipid peroxidation (i.e., as degradation products of fats), which can be detected by the TBARS assay using thiobarbituric acid as a reagent.

The authors concluded that curcumin appears to be beneficial in preventing diabetes-induced oxidative stress in rats despite unaltered diabetic (hyperglycemic) status (Suryanarayana, Satyanarayana, Balakrishna et al. 2007).

According to a report in the journal *Trends in Pharmacological Sciences*, appearing in 2009, curcumin mediates its anti-inflammatory effects through the downregulation of inflammatory transcription factors (such as NF-κB), enzymes (such as cyclooxygenase 2 (COX2) and 5 lipoxygenase), and cytokines (such as tumor necrosis factor, interleukin 1, and interleukin 6) (Aggarwal, and Sung. 2009).

A study on human volunteers, published in the *Indian Journal of Physiology and Pharmacology*, in 1992, aimed to assess the effects of curcumin administration on the serum levels of cholesterol and lipid peroxides in healthy volunteers given 500 mg of curcumin per day, for 7 days. A significant decrease (33%) in the serum lipid peroxides, increase in HDL cholesterol (29%), and decrease in total serum cholesterol (11.63%) were noted (Soni, and Kuttan. 1992).

11.15.2 TURMERIC, CURCUMIN, AND GLYCEMIC CONTROL

The journal *Evidence Based Complementary and Alternative Medicine* published a comprehensive review of the research on the effects of curcumin on diabetes (Zhang, Fu, Gao et al. 2013). Curcumin is thought to be the main active ingredient derived from the root of turmeric and it has been cited as a potential therapeutic agent in experimental diabetes and for the treatment of the complications of diabetes patients including metabolic syndrome (Pérez-Torres, Ruiz-Ramírez, Baños et al. 2013), primarily because it is effective in reducing glycemia and hyperlipidemia in rodent models, and it is relatively inexpensive and safe (Goel, Kunnumakkara, and Aggarwal. 2008).

In fact, the ability of curcumin to control blood glucose levels was reported in the journal *Diabetes Care* in a clinical study of prediabetes. The aim of the study was to determine whether curcumin could delay development of Type 2 diabetes in a prediabetic population. Participants meeting criteria of prediabetes were assigned to receive either curcumin or placebo capsules for 9 months.

After 9 months of treatment, 16.4% of the participants in the placebo group were diagnosed with Type 2 diabetes, whereas none were diagnosed with Type 2 diabetes in the curcumin-treated group.

The curcumin-treated group showed a better overall function of β-cells, with higher HOMA-β (61.58 vs. 48.72), and lower C-peptide (1.7 vs. 2.17). The curcumin-treated group showed a lower level of HOMA-IR (3.22 vs. 4.04) and higher adiponectin (22.46 vs. 18.45) when compared to the placebo group.

The investigators concluded that a 9-month curcumin intervention in a prediabetic population significantly lowered the number of prediabetic individuals who eventually developed diabetes. In addition, the curcumin treatment appeared to improve overall function of β-cells, with very minor adverse effects. Therefore, this study demonstrated that the curcumin intervention in a prediabetic population may be beneficial (Chuengsamarn, Rattanamongkolgul, Luechapudiporn et al. 2012).

The *Evidence Based Complementary and Alternative Medicine* review cites extensive animal model (mostly rats) studies on the effects of curcumin on hyperglycemia and related cardiovascular and metabolic disorders. Some of these are summarized here and specific reference citations can be obtained in the original text (see Zhang, Fu, Gao et al. 2013. Volume 2013, Article ID 636053. DOI: 10.1155/2013/636053).

In alloxan-induced diabetic rats, STZ-induced rat-models, and STZ-nicotinamide-induced rat models, oral administration of various dosages of curcumin (80 mg/kg·BW for 21 days and 45 days; 60 mg/kg·BW for 14 days; 90 mg/kg·BW for 15 days; 150 mg/kg·BW for 49 days; 300 mg/kg·BW for 56 days; 100 mg/kg·BW for 4 weeks, 7 weeks, and 8 weeks) prevented body weight loss, reduced glucose levels, reduced hemoglobin (Hb) and HbA1c in blood, and improved insulin sensitivity.

Oral administration of turmeric aqueous extract (300 mg/kg·BW) or curcumin (30 mg/kg·BW) for 56 days resulted in a significant reduction in blood glucose in STZ-induced diabetes model in rats. In high-fat diet–induced insulin resistance and Type 2 diabetes models in rats, oral administration of curcumin (80 mg/kg·BW) for 15 and 60 days, respectively, showed an antihyperglycemic effect and improved insulin sensitivity. Dietary curcumin (0.5% in diet) was also effective in ameliorating the increased levels of fasting blood glucose, urine sugar, and urine volume in STZ-induced diabetic rats.

However, several researchers claimed that curcumin has no significant effect on blood glucose. One study reported in the journal *Bioscience, Biotechnology, and Biochemistry* found that the intragastric administration of curcumin (200 mg/kg·BW) for 14 days had no effect on serum concentration of glucose, insulin, and triacylglycerols in STZ- and high-fat diet–induced diabetic Sprague–Dawley rats (Nishizono, Hayami, Ikeda et al. 2000). In a similar vein, a study published in *The Journal of Cardiovascular Pharmacology* found that oral administration of curcumin from 4 weeks to 24 weeks (200 mg/kg·BW) had no significant effect on blood glucose and pressure in STZ diabetic rats. The investigators concluded that "… variations reported in antioxidant enzymes and vascular reactivity are due to the duration of diabetes or time after diabetes induction in STZ model and this cannot be completely reversed by chronic treatment with curcumin" (Majithiya, and Balaraman. 2005).

Nevertheless, there are a number of clinical studies that support curcumin as an adjunctive treatment in Type 2 diabetes. For instance, the *Indian Journal of Clinical Biochemistry* reported a study that aimed to determine the effect of turmeric as an adjunct to antidiabetic therapy.

Diabetic patients on metformin therapy were assigned to one of two groups: Group I received standard metformin treatment, while group II was on standard metformin therapy with turmeric (2 g) supplements for 4 weeks. Biochemical parameters were assessed at the time of recruitment for study and after 4 weeks of treatment.

It was found that turmeric supplementation in metformin-treated Type 2 diabetes patients significantly decreased fasting glucose (95 ± 11.4 mg/dL) and HbA1c levels (7.4% ± 0.9%). The turmeric-administered group showed reduction in lipid peroxidation, MDA (0.51 ± 0.11 μmol/L) and enhanced total antioxidant status (511 ± 70 μmol/L). Turmeric also exhibited beneficial effects on dyslipidemia LDL cholesterol (113.2 ± 15.3 mg/dL), non-HDL cholesterol (138.3 ± 12.1 mg/dL), LDL/HDL ratio (3.01 ± 0.61), and reduced inflammatory marker, hs-CRP (3.4 ± 2.0 mg/dL).

The investigators concluded that turmeric supplementation as an adjuvant in Type 2 diabetes patients on metformin treatment had an additional beneficial effect on blood glucose, oxidative stress, and inflammation (Maithili Karpaga Selvi, Sridhar, Swaminathan et al. 2015).

Finally, an animal model study published in the journal *Plant Foods for Human Nutrition* is noteworthy for its focus on the possible beneficial effects of turmeric on the polyol pathway relevant to cataract formation. The aim of the study was to determine the effect of turmeric and its active principle, curcumin, on diabetes mellitus in a rat model. Alloxan was used to induce diabetes and the turmeric or curcumin that was administered to diabetic rats significantly reduced blood sugar and glycosylated hemoglobin levels.

Turmeric and curcumin supplementation also reduced the oxidative stress in the diabetic rats observed as lower levels of TBARS (thiobarbituric acid reactive substances), which may have been due to the decreased influx of glucose into the polyol pathway leading to an increased NADPH/NADP ratio and elevated activity of the potent antioxdiant enzyme GPx. Moreover, the activity of sorbitol dehydrogenase, which catalyzes the conversion of sorbitol to fructose, was lowered significantly on treatment with turmeric or curcumin.

The authors concluded that curcumin was more effective in attenuating diabetes-related changes than turmeric (Arun, and Nalini. 2002).

11.15.3 How Safe Is It to Consume Curcumin?

A study on dosage safety of curcumin was reported in the journal *BMC Complementary & Alternative Medicine* in 2006. It detailed a dose-escalation study to determine the maximum tolerable dose and safety of a single oral dose of curcumin in healthy volunteers. They were given increasing doses of curcumin ranging from 500 to 12,000 mg, and safety was assessed for 72 h after administration. Seven of the participants who completed the trial experienced minimal toxicity that did not appear to be dose related: diarrhea, headache, rash, and yellow stool (Lao, Ruffin, Normolle et al. 2006).

In another study with human participants, curcumin at doses ranging from 0.45 to 3.6 g/day for 1 to 4 months was associated with nausea and diarrhea and caused an increase in serum alkaline phosphatase and lactate dehydrogenase contents (Sharma, Euden, Platton et al. 2004).

However, in one study, patients with advanced pancreatic cancer receiving curcumin (8 g/day) in combination with gemcitabine reported intractable abdominal pain after a few days to 2 weeks of curcumin intake. Thus, more studies are required to evaluate the long-term toxicity associated with curcumin before it can be recommended for human use at clinical high dosages (Epelbaum, Schaffer, Vizel et al. 2010).

A note to the reader: Please see the chart in the Appendix for a summary of the therapeutic and other effects of the selected functional foods described in this chapter.

REFERENCES

Aggarwal BB, and B Sung. 2009. Pharmacological basis for the role of curcumin in chronic diseases: an age-old spice with modern targets. *Trends in Pharmacological Sciences*, Feb; 30(2):85–94. DOI: 10.1016/j.tips.2008.11.002.

Ahuja KDK, Robertson IK, Geraghty DP, and MJ Ball. 2006. Effects of chili consumption on postprandial glucose, insulin, and energy metabolism. *The American Journal of Clinical Nutrition*, Jul; 84(1): 63–69.

Allen RW, Schwartzman E, Baker WL, Coleman CL, and OJ Phung. 2013. Cinnamon use in type 2 diabetes: an updated systematic review and meta-analysis. *Annals of Family Medicine*, Sep-Oct; 11(5):452–459. DOI: 10.1370/afm.1517.

Anderson RA, and MM Polansky. 2002. Tea enhances insulin activity. *Journal of Agricultural & Food Chemistry*, Nov 20; 50(24):7182–7186. PMID: 12428980.

Arun N, and N Nalini. 2002. Efficacy of turmeric on blood sugar and polyol pathway in diabetic albino rats. *Plant Foods for Human Nutrition*, Winter; 57(1): 41–52. PMID: 11855620.

Bae KC, Park JH, Na AY, Kim SJ, Ahn S, Kim SP, Oh BC, Cho HC, Kim YW, and DK Song. 2013. Effect of green tea extract/poly-gamma-glutamic acid complex in obese type 2 diabetic mice. *Diabetes and Metabolism Journal*, Jun; 37: 196–206. DOI: 10. 4093/dmj.2013.37.3.196.

Bahadoran Z, Ghasemi A, Mirmiran P, Azizi F, and F Hadaegh. 2015. Beneficial effects of inorganic nitrate/nitrite in type 2 diabetes and its complications. *Nutrition and Metabolism (Lond)*, May; 12: 16. DOI: 10.1186/s12986-015-0013-6.

Bahceci M, Tuzcu A, Ogun C, Canoruc N, Iltimur K, and C Aslan. 2005. Is serum C-reactive protein concentration correlated with HbA1c and insulin resistance in Type 2 diabetic men with or without coronary heart disease? *Journal of Endocrinological Investigation*, Feb; 28(2): 145–150. PMID: 15887860.

Baker RG, Hayden MS, and S Ghosh. 2001. NF-κB, inflammation, and metabolic disease. *Cell Metabolism*, Jan; 13(1): 11–22. DOI: 10.1016/j.cmet.2010.12.008.

Beals JW, Binns SE, Davis JL, Giordano GR, Klochak AL, Paris HL, Schweder MM, Peltonen GL, Scalzo RL, and C Bell. 2017. Concurrent beet juice and carbohydrate ingestion: influence on glucose tolerance in obese and nonobese adults. *Journal of Nutrition and Metabolism*, Jan; 2017: 6436783. DOI: 10.1155/2017/6436783.

Belfki H, Ben Ali S, Bougatef S, Ben Ahmed D, Haddad N, Jmal A, Abdennebi M, and H Ben Romdhane. 2012. Association between C-reactive protein and type 2 diabetes in a Tunisian population. *Inflammation*, Apr; 35(2): 684–689. DOI: 10.1007/s10753-011-9361-1.

Bernardi A, Rocha VZ, and JR Faria-Neto. 2015. Use of statins and the incidence of type 2 diabetes mellitus. *Revista da Associacao Medica Brasileira* (1992). Aug; 61(4): 375–380. DOI: 10.1590/1806 -9282.61.04.375.

Bode AM, and Z Dong. 2011. The amazing and mighty ginger. In Benzie, IFF, and S Wachtel-Galor, editors. *Herbal Medicine: Biomolecular and Clinical Aspects*. 2nd edition. Boca Raton (FL): CRC Press/Taylor & Francis.

Bryan NS, Tribble G, and N Angelov. 2017. Oral microbiome and nitric oxide: the missing link in the management of blood Pressure. *Current Hypertension Reports*, Apr; 19(4): 33. DOI: 10.1007/s11906-017-0725-2.

Campfield LA, and FJ Smith. 1999. The pathogenesis of obesity. *Bailliere's Best Practice and Research. Clinical Endocrinology and Metabolism*, Apr; 13(1):13–30. DOI: 10.1053/beem.1999.0004.

Cao G, Alessio HM, and RG Cutler. 1993. Oxygen-radical absorbance capacity assay for antioxidants. *Free Radical Biology and Medicine*, Mar; 14(3): 303–311. PMID: 8458588.

Chakraborty K, Praveen NK, Vijayan KK, and GS Rao. 2013. Evaluation of phenolic contents and antioxidant activities of brown seaweeds belonging to *Turbinaria* spp. (Phaeophyta, Sargassaceae) collected from Gulf of Mannar. *Asian Pacific Journal of Tropical Biomedicine*, Jan; 3(1): 8–16. DOI: 10.1016/S2221 -1691(13)60016-7.

Chang CLT, Lin Y, Bartolome AP, Chen, Y-C, Chiu S-C, and W-C Yang. 2013. Herbal therapies for Type 2 diabetes mellitus: chemistry, biology, and potential application of selected plants and compounds. *Evidence Based Complementary and Alternative Medicine*, 2013: 378657. DOI: 10.1155/2013/378657.

Charrier MJ, Savage GP, and L Vanhanen. 2002. Oxalate content and calcium binding capacity of tea and herbal teas. *Asia Pacific Journal of Clinical Nutrition*, 11(4): 298–301. PMID: 12495262.

Chow HH, Cai Y, Hakim IA, Crowell JA, Shahi F, Brooks CA, Dorr RT, Hara Y, and DS Alberts DS. 2003. Pharmacokinetics and safety of green tea polyphenols after multiple-dose administration of epigallocatechin gallate and polyphenon E in healthy individuals. *Clinical Cancer Research*, Aug; 9(9): 3312–3319. PMID: 12960117.

Chuengsamarn S, Rattanamongkolgul S, Luechapudiporn R, Phisalaphong C, and S Jirawatnotai. 2012. Curcumin extract for prevention of type 2 diabetes. *Diabetes Care*, Nov; 35(11): 2121–2127. DOI: 10.2337/dc12-0116.

Clifford T, Howatson G, West DJ, and EJ Stevenson. 2015. The potential benefits of red beetroot supplementation in health and disease. *Nutrients*, Apr; 7(4): 2801–2822. DOI: 10.3390/nu7042801.

Collins KG, Fitzgerald GF, Stanton C, and RP Ross. 2016. Looking beyond the terrestrial: the potential of seaweed derived bioactives to treat non-communicable diseases. *Marine Drugs*, Mar; 14(3): 60. DOI:10.3390/md14030060.

Conti P, and Y Shaik-Dasthagirisae. 2015. Atherosclerosis: a chronic inflammatory disease mediated by mast cells. *Central European Journal of Immunology*, Oct; 40(3): 380–386. DOI: 10.5114/ceji.2015.54603.

Daood HG, Vinkler, M, Márkus F, Hebshi EA, and PA Biacs. 1996. Antioxidant vitamin content of spice red pepper (paprika) as affected by technological and varietal factors. *Food Chemistry*, Apr; 55(4): 365–372. DOI: 10.1016/0308-8146(95)00136-0.

Datta S, Iqbal Z, and KR Prasad. 2011. Comparison between serum hsCRP and LDL cholesterol for search of a better predictor for ischemic heart disease. *Indian Journal of Clinical Biochemistry*, Apr; 26(2): 210–213. DOI: 10.1007/s12291-010-0100-4.

Davis PA, and W Yokoyama. 2011. Cinnamon intake lowers fasting blood glucose: meta-analysis. *Journal of Medical Foods*, Sep; 14(9): 884–889. DOI: 10.1089/jmf.2010.0180.

del Rocío Gómez-García M, and N Ochoa-Alejo. 2013. Biochemistry and molecular biology of carotenoid biosynthesis in chili peppers (Capsicum spp.). *International Journal of Molecular Sciences*, Sep; 14(9): 19025–19053. DOI: 10.3390/ijms1409 19025.

Devaraj S, Singh U, and I Jialal. 2009. Human C-reactive protein and the metabolic syndrome. *Current Opinion in Lipidology*, Jun; 20(3): 182–189. DOI: 10.1097/MOL.0b013e32832ac03e.

Donath MY, and SE Shoelson. 2001. Type 2 diabetes as an inflammatory disease. *Nature Reviews. Immunology (London)*. Feb; 11(2): 98–107. DOI: 10.1038/nri2925.

Dudonne S, Vitrac X, Vouitiere P, Woillez M, and JM Mérillon. 2009. Comparative study of antioxidant properties and total phenolic content of 30 plant extracts of industrial interest using DPPH, ABTS, FRAP, SOD, and ORAC assays. *Journal of Agricultural & Food Chemistry*, 57:1768–1774. DOI: 10.1021 /jf803011r.

El Gamal AA, AlSaid MS, Raish M, Al-Sohaibani M, Al-Massarani SM, Ahmad A, Hefnawy M, Al-Yahya M, Basoudan OAA, and S Rafatullah. 2014. Beetroot (*Beta vulgaris* L.) extract ameliorates gentamicin-induced nephrotoxicity associated oxidative stress, inflammation, and apoptosis in rodent model. *Mediators of Inflammation*, 2014: 983–952. DOI: 10.1155/2014/983952.

Epelbaum R, Schaffer M, Vizel B, Badmaev V, and G Bar-Sela. 2010. Curcumin and gemcitabine in patients with advanced pancreatic cancer. *Nutrition and Cancer*, 62 (8): 1137–1141. DOI: 10.1080/01635581.2010.513802.

Festa A, D'Agostino R, Howard G, Mykkänen L, Tracy RP, and SM Haffner. 2000. Chronic subclinical inflammation as part of the insulin resistance syndrome. The Insulin Resistance Atherosclerosis Study (IRAS). *Circulation*, https://doi.org/10.1161/01. CIR.102.1.42

Friedman M. 2016. Mushroom polysaccharides: chemistry and antiobesity, antidiabetes, anticancer, and antibiotic properties in cells, rodents, and humans. *Foods*, Dec; 5(4): 80. DOI: 10.3390/foods5040080.

Forouhi NG, Harding AH, Allison M, Sandhu MS, Welch A, Luben R, Bingham S, Khaw KT, NJ Wareham. 2007. Elevated serum ferritin levels predict new-onset type 2 diabetes: results from the EPIC-Norfolk prospective study. *Diabetologia*, May; 50(5): 949-56. DOI: 10.1007/s00125-007-0604-5.

Furuyashiki T, Nagayasu H, Aoki Y, Bessho H, Hashimoto T, Kanazawa K, and H Ashida. 2004. Tea catechin suppresses adipocyte differentiation accompanied by down-regulation of PPARgamma2 and C/EBPalpha in 3T3-L1 cells. *Bioscience, Biotechnology and Biochemistry*, 68(11): 2353–2359. DOI: 10.1271/bbb.68.2353.

Gammone MA, and N D'Orazio. 2015. Anti-obesity activity of the marine carotenoid Fucoxanthin. *Marine Drugs*, Apr; 13(4): 2196–2214. DOI: 10.3390/md13042196.

Gaweł S, Wardas M, Niedworok E, and P Wardas. 2004. Malondialdehyde (MDA) as a lipid peroxidation marker. *Wiadomorsci Lekarskie*, 57(9–10): 453–455. PMID: 15765761.

Georgiev VG, Weber J, Kneschke EM, Denev PN, Bley T, and AI Pavlov. 2010. Antioxidant activity and phenolic content of betalain extracts from intact plants and hairy root cultures of the red beetroot *Beta vulgaris* cv. Detroit dark red. *Plant Foods for Human Nutrition*, Jun; 65(2): 105–111. DOI: 10.1007/s11130-010-0156-6.

Goel A, Kunnumakkara AB, and BB Aggarwal. 2008. Curcumin as "Curecumin": from kitchen to clinic. *Biochemical Pharmacology*, Feb; 75(4): 787–809. DOI: 10.1016/j.bcp.2007.08.016.

Goldstein DE, Little RR, Lorenz RA, Malone JI, Nathan D, and CM Peterson. 1995. Tests of glycemia in diabetes. *Diabetes Care*, Jun; 18(6): 896–909. DOI: 10.2337/diacare.18.6.896.

Gram DX, Ahrén B, Nagy I, Olsen UB, Brand CL, Sundler F, Tabanera R, Svendsen O, Carr RD, Santha P, Wierup N, and AJ Hansen. 2007. Capsaicin-sensitive sensory fibers in the islets of Langerhans contribute to defective insulin secretion in Zucker diabetic rat, an animal model for some aspects of human type 2 diabetes. *The European Journal of Neuroscience*, Jan; 25(1): 213–223. DOI: 10.1111/j.1460-9568.2006.05261.x.

Grzanna R, Lindmark L, and CG Frondoza. 2005. Ginger—an herbal medicinal product with broad anti-inflammatory actions. *Journal of Medicinal Foods*, Summer; 8(2):125–132. DOI: 10.1089/jmf.2005.8.125.

Gunawardena D, Karunaweera N, Lee S, van Der Kooy F, Harman DG, Raju R, Bennett L, Gyengesi E, Sucher NJ, and G Münch. 2015. Anti-inflammatory activity of cinnamon (*C. zeylanicum* and *C. cassia*) extracts—identification of E-cinnamaldehyde and o-methoxy cinnamaldehyde as the most potent bioactive compounds. *Food and Function*, Mar; 6(3): 910–919. DOI: 10.1039/c4fo00680a.

Ha AW, and WK Kim. 2013. The effect of fucoxanthin rich power on the lipid metabolism in rats with a high fat diet. *Nutrition Research and Practice*, Aug; 7(4): 287–293. DOI: 10.4162/nrp.2013.7.4.287.

Hameed I, Masoodi SR, Mir SA, Nabi M, Ghazanfar K, and BA Ganai. 2015. Type 2 diabetes mellitus: from a metabolic disorder to an inflammatory condition. *World Journal of Diabetes*, May 15; 6(4): 598–612. DOI: 10.4239/wjd.v6.i4.598.

Han MK. 2003. Epigallocatechin gallate, a constituent of green tea, suppresses cytokine-induced pancreatic beta-cell damage. *Experimental and Molecular Medicine*, Apr; 35: 136–139. DOI: 10.1038/emm.2003.19.

Haniadka R, Saldanha E, Sunita V, Palatty PL, Fayadd R, and MS Baliga. 2013. A review of the gastroprotective effects of ginger (*Zingiber officinale* Roscoe). *Food and Function*, 4(6): 845–855. DOI: 10.1039/C3FO30337C.

Harding AH, Sargeant LA, Welch A, Oakes S, Luben RN, Bingham S, Day NE, Khaw KT, NJ Wareham and EPIC-Norfolk Study. 2001. Fat consumption and HbA(1c) levels: the EPIC-Norfolk study. *Diabetes Care*, Nov; 24(11): 1911–1916. DOI: 10. 2337/diacare.24.11.1911.

Heo SJ, Hwang JY, Choi JI, Han JS, Kim HJ, and Y Jeon. 2009. Diphlorethohydroxycarmalol isolated from *Ishige okamurae*, a brown algae, a potent alpha-glucosidase and alpha-amylase inhibitor, alleviates postprandial hyperglycemia in diabetic mice. *European Journal of Pharmacology*, Aug; 615(1–3): 252–256. DOI: 10.1016/j.ejphar.2009.05.017.

Higdon JV, and B Frei. 2003. Tea catechins and polyphenols: health effects, metabolism, and antioxidant functions. *Critical Reviews in Food Science and Nutrition*, 43(1): 89–143. DOI: 10.1080/10408690390826464.

Hininger-Favier I, Benaraba R, Coves S, Anderson RA, and AM Roussel. 2009. Green tea extract decreases oxidative stress and improves insulin sensitivity in an animal model of insulin resistance, the fructose-fed rat. *Journal of the American College of Nutrition*, Aug; 28(4): 355–561. PMID: 20368373.

Hobbs DA, Kaffa NW. George TW, Methven L, and JA Lovegrove. 2012. Blood pressure-lowering effects of beetroot juice and novel beetroot-enriched bread products in normotensive male subjects. *British Journal of Nutrition*, Dec; 108(11): 2066–2074. DOI: 10.1017/S0007114512000190.

Hotamisligil GS, Arner P, Caro JF, Atkinson RL, and BM Spiegelman. 1995. Increased adipose tissue expression of tumor necrosis factor-alpha in human obesity and insulin resistance. *Journal of Clinical Investigation*, May; 95(5): 2409–2415. DOI: 10.1172/jci117936.

Hotamisligil GS, Shargill NS, and BM Spiegelman. 1993. Adipose expression of tumor necrosis factor-alpha: direct role in obesity-linked insulin resistance. *Science*, Jan: 259(5091): 87–91. DOI: 10.1126/science.7678183.

Hu FB, Meigs JB, Li TY, Rifai N, and JE Manson. 2004. Inflammatory markers and risk of developing Type 2 diabetes in women. *Diabetes*, Mar; 53(3): 693–700. https://doi.org/10.2337/diabetes.53.3.693.

Hwang JT, Park IJ, Shin JI, Lee YK, Lee SK, Baik HW, Ha J, and OJ Park. 2005. Genistein, EGCG, and capsaicin inhibit adipocyte differentiation process via activating AMP-activated protein kinase. *Biochemical and Biophysical Research Communications*, Dec; 338(2): 694–699. DOI: 10.1016/j.bbrc.2005.09.195.

Ionică FE, Moța M, Cătălina Pisoschi C, Florica Popescu F, and E Gofiță. 2009. Statins therapy, C-reactive protein (CRP levels and type 2 diabetes). *Current Health Sciences Journal*, 2009, Apr–Jun (Quarterly); 35(2): 87–91.

Islam MS, and H Choi. 2008. Dietary red chili (*Capsicum frutescens* L.) is insulinotropic rather than hypoglycemic in type 2 diabetes model of rats. *Phytotherapy Research*, Aug; 22(8): 1025–1029. DOI: 10.1002/ptr.2417.

Iso H, Date C, Wakai K, Fukui M, Tamakoshi A and the JACC Study Group. 2006. The relationship between green tea and total caffeine intake and risk for self-reported type 2 diabetes among Japanese adults. *Annals of Internal Medicine*, Apr; 144: 554–562. PMID: 16618952.

Janssens PLHR, Hursel R, Martens EAP, and MS Westerterp-Plantenga. 2013. Acute effects of capsaicin on energy expenditure and fat oxidation in negative energy Balance. *PLoS ONE*. Jul: 8(7): e67786. DOI: 10.1371/journal.pone.0067786.

Jayaprakasha GK, and LJ Rao. 2011. Chemistry, biogenesis, and biological activities of *Cinnamomum zeylanicum*. *Critical Review in Food Science and Nutrition*, Jul; 51(6): 547–562. DOI: 10.1080/10408391003699550.

Jayasuriya WJABN, Wanigatunge CA, Fernando GH, Abeytunga DTU, and TS Suresh. 2015. Hypoglycaemic activity of culinary *Pleurotus ostreatus* and *P. cystidiosus* mushrooms in healthy volunteers and Type 2 diabetic patients on diet control and the possible mechanisms of action. *Phytotherapy Research*, Feb; 29(2): 303–309. DOI: 10.1002/ptr.5255.

Jeon SM, Kim HJ, Woo MN, Lee MK, Shin YC, Park YB, and MS Choi MS. 2010. Fucoxanthin-rich seaweed extract suppresses body weight gain and improves lipid metabolism in high-fat-fed C57BL/6J mice. *Biotechnology Journal*, Sep; 5(9): 961–969. DOI: 10.1002/biot.201000215.

Jiang H, Yan W-H, Li C-J, Wang A-P, Dou J-T, and Y-M Mu. 2014. Elevated white blood cell count is associated with higher risk of glucose metabolism disorders in middle-aged and elderly Chinese people. *International Journal of Environmental Research and Public Health*, May; 11(5): 5497–5509. DOI: 10.3390/ijerph11 0505497.

Joffe BI, and LA Distiller. 2014. Diabetes mellitus and hypothyroidism: Strange bedfellows or mutual companions? *World Journal of Diabetes*, Dec; 5(6): 901–904. DOI: 10.4239/wjd.v5.i6.901.

Kang C, Jin YB, Lee H, Cha M, Sohn ET, Moon J, Park C, Chun S, Jung ES, Hong JS, Kim SB, Kim JS, and E Kim. 2010. Brown alga *Ecklonia cava* attenuates type 1 diabetes by activating AMPK and Akt signaling pathways. *Food and Chemical Toxicology*, Feb; 48(2): 509–516. DOI: 10.1016/j.fct.2009.11.004.

Kang J-I, Kim S-C, Han S-C, Hong H-J, Jeon Y-J, Kim B, Koh Y-S, Yoo E-S, and H-K Kang. 2012. Hair-loss preventing effect of *Grateloupia elliptica*. *Biomolecules and Therapeutics* (Seoul), Jan; 20(1): 118–124. DOI: 10.4062/biomolther.2012.20.1.118.

Kang SI, Ko HC, Shin HS, Kim HM, Hong YS, Lee NH, and SJ Kim. 2011. Fucoxanthin exerts differing effects on 3T3-L1 cells according to differentiation stage and inhibits glucose uptake in mature adipocytes. *Biochemical and Biophysical Research Communications*, Jun 17; 409(4): 769–774. DOI: 10.1016/j.bbrc.2011.05.086.

Kanner J, Harel S, and R Granit. 2001. Betalains—a new class of dietary cationized antioxidants. *Journal of Agricultural and Food Chemistry*, Nov; 49(11): 5178–5185. DOI: 10.1021/jf010456f.

Kapil V, Haydar SMA, Pearl V, Lundberg JO, Weitzberg E, and A Ahluwalia. 2013. Physiological role for nitrate-reducing oral bacteria in blood pressure control. *Free Radical Biology and Medicine*, Feb; 55: 93–100. DOI: 10.1016/j.freeradbiomed.2012.11.013.

Kawatra P, and R Rajagopalan. 2015. Cinnamon: mystic powers of a minute ingredient. *Pharmacognosy Research*, Jun; 7(Suppl 1): S1–S6. DOI: 10.4103/0974-8490.157990.

Khandouzi N, Shidfar F, Rajab A, Rahideh T, Hosseini, and MM Taherif. 2015. The effects of ginger on fasting blood sugar, hemoglobin A1c, apolipoprotein B, apolipoprotein A-I and malondialdehyde in Type 2 diabetic patients. *Iranian Journal of Pharmaceutical Research*, Winter; 14(1): 131–140. PMCID: PMC4277626.

Kim HM, and J Kim. 2013. The effects of green tea on obesity and Type 2 diabetes. *Diabetes and Metabolism Journal*, Jun; 37(3): 173–175. DOI: 10.4093/dmj.2013.37.3.173.

Kim KN, Heo SJ, Yoon WJ, Kang SM, Ahn G, Yi TH, and YJ Jeon. 2010. Fucoxanthin inhibits the inflammatory response by suppressing the activation of NF-κB and MAPKs in lipopolysaccharide-induced RAW 264.7 macrophages. *European Journal of Pharmacology*, Dec; 649(1–3): 369–375. DOI: 10.1016/j.ejphar.2010.09.032.

Kim MS, Kim JY, Choi WH, and SS Lee. 2008. Effects of seaweed supplementation on blood glucose concentration, lipid profile, and antioxidant enzyme activities in patients with type 2 diabetes mellitus. *Nutrition Research and Practice*, Summer; 2(2): 62–67. DOI: 10.4162/nrp.2008.2.2.62.

Kim SM, Jung YJ, Kwon ON, Cha KH, Um BH, Chung D, and CH Pan. 2012. A potential commercial source of fucoxanthin extracted from the microalga *Phaeodactylum tricornutum*. *Applied Biochemistry and Biotechnology*, Apr; 166(7): 1843–1855. DOI: 10.1007/s12010-012-9602-2.

Klaus S, Pultz S, Thone-Reineke C, and S Wolfram. 2005. Epigallocatechin gallate attenuates diet-induced obesity in mice by decreasing energy absorption and increasing fat oxidation. *International Journal of Obesity (Lond)*, Jun; 29: 615–623. DOI: 10.1038/sj.ijo.0802926.

Kleefstra N, Logtenberg, SJ, Houweling ST, Verhoeven S, and HJ Bilo. 2007. Cinnamon: not suitable for the treatment of diabetes mellitus [article in Dutch]. *Nederlands Tijdschrift voor Geneeskunde*, Dec; 151(51): 2833–2837.

Klupp NL, Kiat H, Bensoussan A, Steiner GZ, and DH Chang. 2016. Double-blind, randomised, placebo-controlled trial of *Ganoderma lucidum* for the treatment of cardiovascular risk factors of metabolic syndrome. *Scientific Reports*, Aug; 6: 29540. DOI: 10.1038/srep29540.

Lake BG. 1999. Coumarin metabolism, toxicity and carcinogenicity: relevance for human risk assessment. *Food and Chemical Toxicology*, Apr; 37(4): 423–453. PMID: 10418958.

Langley-Evans SC. 2000. Antioxidant potential of green and black tea determined using the ferric reducing power (FRAP) assay. *International Journal of Food Science and Nutrition*, May; 51(3): 181–188. PMID: 10945114.

Lao CD, Ruffin MT, Normolle D, Heath DD, Murray SI, Bailey JM, Boggs ME, Crowell J, Rock CL, and DE Brenner. 2006. Dose escalation of a curcuminoid formulation. *BMC Complementary and Alternative Medicine*, 6:10. DOI: 10.1186/1472-6882-6-10.

Lee SH, Park MH, Heo SJ, Kang SM, Ko SC, Han JS, and YJ Jeon. 2010. Dieckol isolated from *Ecklonia cava* inhibits alpha-glucosidase and alpha-amylase in vitro and alleviates postprandial hyperglycemia in streptozotocin-induced diabetic mice. *Food and Chemical Toxicology*, Oct; 48(10): 2633–2637. DOI: 10.1016/j.fct.2010.06.032.

Li M, and CG Eastman. 2012. The changing epidemiology of iodine deficiency. *Nature Reviews Endocrinology*, advance online publication 3 April 2012. DOI: 10.1038/nrendo.2012.43.

Lin KY, Ito A, Asagami T, Tsao PS, Adimoolam S, Kimoto M, Tsao PS, Adimoolam S, Kimoto M, Tsuji H, Reaven GM, and JP Cooke. 2002. Impaired nitric oxide synthase pathway in diabetes mellitus: role of asymmetric dimethylarginine and dimethylarginine dimethylaminohydrolase. *Circulation*, Aug; 106(8): 987–992.

Lin YS, Tsai YJ, Tsay JS, and KS Lin. 2003. Factors affecting the levels of tea polyphenols and caffeine in tea leaves. *Journal of Agricultural and Food Chemistry*, Mar 26; 51(7): 1864–1873. DOI: 10.1021/jf021066b.

Liu C-Y, Huang C-J, Huang L-H, Chen I-J, Chiu J-P, and C-H Hsu. 2014. Effects of green tea extract on insulin resistance and glucagon-like peptide 1 in patients with Type 2 diabetes and lipid abnormalities: a randomized, double-blinded, and placebo-controlled trial. *PLoS ONE*, 9(3): e91163. https://doi.org/10.1371/journal.pone.0091163.

Liu K, Zhou R, Wang B, Chen K, Shi LY, Zhu JD, and MT Mi. 2013. Effect of green tea on glucose control and insulin sensitivity: a meta-analysis of 17 randomized controlled trials. *American Journal of Clinical Nutrition*, Aug; 98(2): 340–348. DOI: 10.3945/ajcn.112.052746.

Lordan S, Smyth TJ, Soler-Vila A, Stanton C, and RP Ross. 2013. The α-amylase and α-glucosidase inhibitory effects of Irish seaweed extracts. *Food Chemistry*, Dec; 141(3): 2170–2176. DOI: 10.1016/j.foodchem.2013.04.123.

Lorenz M, Urban J, Engelhardt U, Baumann G, Stangl K, and V Stangl. 2009. Green and black tea are equally potent stimuli of NO production and vasodilation: new insights into tea ingredients involved. *Basic Research in Cardiology*, Jan; 104(1): 100–110. DOI: 10.1007/s00395-008-0759-3.

Lundberg JO, Weitzberg E, and MT Gladwin. 2008. The nitrate–nitrite–nitric oxide pathway in physiology and therapeutics. *Nature Reviews. Drug Discovery*, Feb; 7(2):156–167. DOI: 10.1038/nrd2466.

Mackenzie T, Leary L, and WB Brooks. 2007. The effect of an extract of green and black tea on glucose control in adults with type 2 diabetes mellitus: double-blind randomized study. *Metabolism*, Oct; 56: 1340–1344. DOI: 10.1016/j.metabol.2007.05.018.

Maeda H, Hosokawa M, Sashima T, and K Miyashita. 2007. Dietary combination of fucoxanthin and fish oil attenuates the weight gain of white adipose tissue and decreases blood glucose in obese/diabetic KK-Ay mice. *Journal of Agricultural and Food Chemistry*, Sep; 55(19): 7701–7706. DOI: 10.1021/jf071569n.

Maeda H, Hosokawa M, Sashima T, Murakami-Funayama K, and K Miyashita. 2009. Anti-obesity and anti-diabetic effects of fucoxanthin on diet-induced obesity conditions in a murine model. *Molecular Medicine Reports*, Nov–Dec; 2(6): 897–902. DOI: 10.3892/mmr_00000189.

Mahluji S, Attari VE, Mobasseri M, Payahoo L, Ostadrahimi A, and SE Golzari. 2013. Effects of ginger (*Zingiber officinale*) on plasma glucose level, HbA1c and insulin sensitivity in type 2 diabetic patients. *International Journal of Food Science and Nutrition*, Sep; 64(6): 682–686. DOI: 10.3109/09637486.2013.775223.

Mahluji S, Ostadrahimi A, Mobasseri M, Attari VE, and L Payahoo. 2013. Anti-inflammatory effects of *Zingiber officinale* in Type 2 diabetic patients. *Advanced Pharmaceutical Bulletin*, Dec; 3(2): 273–276. DOI: 10.5681/apb.2013.044.

Maithili Karpaga Selvi N, Sridhar MG, Swaminathan, and R Sripradha. 2015. Efficacy of turmeric as adjuvant therapy in Type 2 diabetic patients. *Indian Journal of Clinical Biochemistry*, Apr; 30(2): 180–186. DOI: 10.1007/s12291-014-0436-2.

Majithiya JB, and R Balaraman. 2005. Time-dependent changes in antioxidant enzymes and vascular reactivity of aorta in streptozotocin-induced diabetic rats treated with curcumin. *The Journal of Cardiovascular Pharmacology*, Nov; 46(5): 697–705. PMID: 16220078.

Markel H. 1987. "When it rains it pours": endemic goiter, iodized salt, and David Murray Cowie, MD. *American Journal of Public Health*, Feb; 77(2): 219–229. PMCID: PMC1646845.

Mathew S, and E Abraham. 2006. Studies on the antioxidant activities of cinnamon (*Cinnamomum verum*) bark extracts, through various in vitro models. *Food Chemistry*, Mar; 94(4): 520–528.

McDermott MT, and EC Ridgway. 2011. Subclinical hypothyroidism is mild thyroid failure and should be treated. *The Journal of Clinical Endocrinology and Metabolism*, Oct; 86(10) DOI: 10.1210/jcem.86.10.7959.

McVeigh GE, Brennan GM, Johnston GD, McDermott BJ, McGrath LT, Henry WE, Andrews JW, and JR Hayes. 1992. Impaired endothelium-dependent and independent vasodilation in patients with Type 2 (non-insulin-dependent) diabetes mellitus. *Diabetologia*, Aug; 35(6): 771–776.

Meenakshi S, Umayaparvathi S, Arumugam M, and T Balasubramanian. 2011. *In vitro* antioxidant properties and FTIR analysis of two seaweeds of Gulf of Mannar. *Asian Pacific Journal of Tropical Biomedicine*, Sept; 1(1): S66–S70. DOI: 10.1016/S2221-1691(11)60126-3.

Menon VP, and AR Sudheer. 2007. Antioxidant and anti-inflammatory properties of curcumin. *Advances in Experimental Medicine and Biology*, 595: 105–125. DOI: 10.1007/978-0-387-46401-5_3.

Mikutis G, Karaköse H, Jaiswal R, LeGresley A, Islam T, Fernandez-Lahore M, and N Kuhnert. 2013a. Phenolic promiscuity in the cell nucleus—epigallocatechingallate (EGCG) and theaflavin-3,3′-digallate from green and black tea bind to model cell nuclear structures including histone proteins, double stranded DNA and telomeric quadruplex DNA. *Food and Function*, Feb; 4(2): 328–337. DOI: 10.1039/c2fo30159h.

Mikutis G, Karaköse H, R Jaiswal et al. 2013b. Green tea catechins and cardiovascular health: an update. *Current Medicinal Chemistry*, 15(18): 1840–1850.

Miller GD, Marsh AP, Dove, RW, Beavers D, Presley T, Helms C, Bechtold E, King SB, and D Kim-Shapiro. 2012. Plasma nitrate and nitrite are increased by a high-nitrate supplement but not by high-nitrate foods in older adults. *Nutrition Research*, Mar; 32(3): 160–168. DOI: 10.1016/j.nutres.2012.02.002.

Minghetti P, Sosa S, Cilurzo F, Casiraghi A, Alberti E, Tubaro A, Loggia RD, and I Montanari. 2007. Evaluation of the topical anti-inflammatory activity of ginger dry extracts from solutions and plasters. *Planta Medica*, Dec; 73(15): 1525–1530. DOI: 10.1055/s-2007-993741.

Moncada S, Palmer RM, and EA Higgs. 1989. Biosynthesis of nitric oxide from L-arginine. A pathway for the regulation of cell function and communication. *Biochemical Pharmacology*, Jun 1; 38(11): 1709–1715.

Mozaffari-Khosravi H, Talaei B, Jalali, BA, Najarzadeh A, and MR Mozayan. 2014. The effect of ginger powder supplementation on insulin resistance and glycemic indices in patients with type 2 diabetes: a randomized, double-blind, placebo-controlled trial. *Complementary Therapies in Medicine*, Feb; 22(1): 9–16. DOI: 10.1016/j.ctim.2013. 12.017.

Naderi Z, Mozaffari-Khosravi H, Dehghan A, Nadjarzadeh A, and HF Huseini. 2015. Effect of ginger powder supplementation on nitric oxide and C-reactive protein in elderly knee osteoarthritis patients: a 12-week double-blind randomized placebo-controlled clinical trial. *Journal of Traditional and Complementary Medicine*. DOI: 10.1016/j.jtcme.2014.12.007.

Nagao T, Meguro S, Hase T, Otsuka K, Komikado M, Tokimitsu I, Yamamoto T, and K Yamamoto. 2009. A catechin-rich beverage improves obesity and blood glucose control in patients with type 2 diabetes. *Obesity* (Silver Spring), Feb; 17: 310–317. DOI: 10.1038/oby.2008.505.

Nantz MP, Rowe CA, Bukowski JF, and SS Percival. 2009. Standardized capsule of *Camellia sinensis* lowers cardiovascular risk factors in a randomized, double-blind, placebo-controlled study. *Nutrition*, Feb; 25(2): 147–154. DOI: 10.1016/j.nut. 2008.07.018.

Ng SH, Zain MSM, Zakaria F, Ishak WRW, and WANW Ahmad. 2015. Hypoglycemic and antidiabetic effect of *Pleurotus sajor-caju* aqueous extract in normal and streptozotocin-induced diabetic rats. *BioMed Research International*, 2015: 214918. DOI: 10.1155/2015/214918.

Nishizono S, Hayami T, Ikeda I, and K Imaizumi. 2000. Protection against the diabetogenic effect of feeding tert-butylhydroquinone to rats prior to the administration of streptozotocin. *Bioscience, Biotechnology, and Biochemistry*, Jun; 64(6): 1153–1158. DOI: 10.1271/bbb.64.1153.

No authors listed. 2001. Dietary reference intakes: vitamin A, vitamin K, arsenic, boron, chromium, copper, iodine, iron, manganese, molybdenum, nickel, silicon, vanadium, and zinc. *Institute of Medicine*, Food and Nutrition Board Washington, D.C.: National Academy Press.

No authors listed. 2007. Final report on the safety assessment of capsicum annuum extract, capsicum annuum fruit extract, capsicum annuum resin, capsicum annuum fruit powder, capsicum frutescens fruit, capsicum frutescens fruit extract, capsicum frutescens resin, and capsaicin. *International Journal of Toxicology*, 26 Suppl 1:3–106.

No authors listed. 2011. Cut salt—it won't affect your iodine intake. Iodized salt provided only a small fraction of daily iodine intake. *The Harvard Health Letter*, Jun;21(10):1.bPMID: 21695856.

Nwosu F, Morris J, Lund VA, Stewart D, Ross HA, and GJ McDougall. 2011. Anti-proliferative and potential anti-diabetic effects of phenolic-rich extracts from edible marine algae. *Food Chemistry*, Jun; 126(3): 1006–1012. DOI: 10.1016/j.foodchem.2010.11.111.

O'Sullivan AM, O'Callaghan YC, O'Grady MN, Queguineur B, Hanniffy D, Troy DJ, Kerry JP, and NM O'Brien. 2011. *In vitro* and cellular antioxidant activities of seaweed extracts prepared from five brown seaweeds harvested in spring from the west coast of Ireland. *Food Chemistry*, Jun; 126(3): 1064–1070. DOI: 10.1016/j.foodchem.2010.11.127.

Oboh G, Ademiluyi AO, Akinyemi AJ, Henle T, Saliu JA, and U Schwarzenbolz. 2012. Inhibitory effect of polyphenol-rich extracts of jute leaf (*Corchorus olitorius*) on key enzyme linked to type 2 diabetes (α-amylase and α-glucosidase) and hypertension (*angiotensin I converting*) in vitro. *Journal of Functional Foods*, Apr; 4(2): 450–458. DOI: 10.1016/j.jff.2012.02.003.

Oelze M, Schuhmacher S, and A Daiber. 2010. Organic nitrates and nitrate resistance in diabetes: the role of vascular dysfunction and oxidative stress with emphasis on antioxidant properties of pentaerithrityl tetranitrate. *Experimental Diabetes Research*, 2010: Article ID 213176, 13 pages. http://dx.doi.org /10.1155/2010/213176.

Park HJ, Lee MK, Park YB, Shin YC, and MS Choi. 2011. Beneficial effects of *Undaria pinnatifida* ethanol extract on diet-induced-insulin resistance in C57BL/6J mice. *Food and Chemical Toxicology*, Apr; 49(4): 727–733. DOI: 10.1016/j.fct.2010.11.032.

Park JH, Jin JY, Baek WK, Park SH, Sung HY, Kim YK, Lee J, and DK Song. 2009. Ambivalent role of gal-lated catechins in glucose tolerance in humans: a novel insight into non-absorbable gallated catechin-derived inhibitors of glucose absorption. *Journal of Physiology and Pharmacology*, Dec; 60: 101–109. PMID: 20065503.

Pérez-Torres I, Ruiz-Ramírez A, Baños G, and M El-Hafidi. 2013. *Hibiscus sabdariffa* Linnaeus (Malvaceae), curcumin and resveratrol as alternative medicinal agents against metabolic syndrome. *Cardiovascular and Hematological Agents in Medicinal Chemistry*, Mar; 11(1): 25–37. PMID: 22721439.

Pham AQ, Kourlas H, and DQ Pham. 2007. Cinnamon supplementation in patients with type 2 diabetes mel-litus. *Pharmacotherapy*, Apr; 27(4): 595–599. DOI: 10.1592/phco.27.4.595.

Pietrzkowski Z, Nemzer B, Spórna A, Stalica P, Tresher W, Keller R, Jiminez R, Michalowski T, and S Wybraniec. 2010. Influence of betalin-rich extracts on reduction of discomfort associated with osteoar-thritis. *New Medicine*, 1: 12–17.

Portnoi G, Chng L, and AL Karimi-Tabesh. 2003b. Cytotoxic components from the dried rhizomes of *Zingiber officinale* Roscoe. *Archives of Pharmacal Research*, Apr; 31(4): 415–418.

Portnoi G, Chng LA, Karimi-Tabesh L, Koren G, Tan MP, and A Einarson. 2003a. Prospective comparative study of the safety and effectiveness of ginger for the treatment of nausea and vomiting in pregnancy. *American Journal of Obstetrics and Gynecology*, Nov; 189(5):1374–1377. PMID: 14634571.

Ranasinghe P, Pigera S, Premakumara GAS, Galappaththy P, Constantine GR, and P Katulanda. 2013. Medicinal properties of 'true' cinnamon (*Cinnamomum zeylanicum*): a systematic review. *BMC Complementary and Alternative Medicine*, 13: 275. DOI: 10.1186/1472-6882-13-275.

Reddy MK, Alexander-Lindo RK, and MG Nair. 2005. Relative inhibition of lipid peroxidation, cyclooxygen-ase enzymes, and human tumor cell proliferation by natural food colors. *Journal of Agricultural and Food Chemistry*, Oct; 53(23): 9268–9273. DOI: 10.1021/jf051399j.

Ricciotti E, and GA FitzGerald. 2011. Prostaglandins and inflammation. *Arteriosclerosis, Thrombosis and Vascular Biology*, May; 31(5): 986–1000. DOI: 10.1161/ATVBAHA.110.207449.

Ridker PM. 2003. Clinical application of C-reactive protein for cardiovascular disease detection and preven-tion. *Circulation*, Jan; 107(3): http://dx.doi.org/10.1161/01.CIR.0000053730.47739.3C.

Romero DHP MJ, Caldwell RB, and RW Caldwell. 2006. Does elevated arginase activity contribute to diabetes-induced endothelial dysfunction? *The Journal of Federation of American Societies for Experimental Biology*, 20 (Meeting Abstract Supplement): A1125.

Rumpler W, Seale J, Clevidence B, Judd J, Wiley E, Yamamoto S, Komatsu T, Sawaki T, Ishikura Y, and K Hosoda. 2001. Oolong tea increases metabolic rate and fat oxidation in men. *Journal of Nutrition*, Nov; 131: 2848–2852. PMID: 11694607.

Ryu OH, Lee J, Lee KW, Kim HY, Seo JA, Kim SG, Kim NH, Baik SH, Choi DS, and KM Choi. 2006. Effects of green tea consumption on inflammation, insulin resistance and pulse wave velocity in type 2 diabetes patients. *Diabetes Research and Clinical Practice*, Mar; 71: 356–358. DOI: 10.1016/j.diabres.2005.08.001.

Salzano S, Checconi P, Hanschmann E-M, Lillig CH, Bowler LD, Chan P, Vaudry D, Mengozzi M, Coppo L, Sacre S, Atkuri KR, Sahaf B, Herzenberg LA, Herzenberg LA, Mullen L, and P Ghezzi. 2014. Linkage of inflammation and oxidative stress via release of glutathionylated peroxiredoxin-2, which acts as a danger signal. *Proceedings of the National Academy of Sciences USA*, Aug; 111(33): 12157–12162. DOI: 10.1073/pnas.1401712111.

Sangeetha RK, Bhaskar N, and V Baskaran. 2009. Comparative effects of beta-carotene and fucoxanthin on retinol deficiency induced oxidative stress in rats. *Molecular and Cellular Biochemistry*, Nov; 331(1–2): 59–67. DOI: 10.1007/s11010-009-0145-y.

Sarma DN, Barrett ML, Chavez ML, Gardiner P, Ko R, Mahady GB, Marles RJ, Pellicore LS, Giancaspro GI, and T Low Dog. 2008. Safety of green tea extracts: a systematic review by the US Pharmacopeia. *Drug Safety*, 31(6): 469–484. PMID: 18484782.

Semwal RB, Semwal DK, Combrinck S, and AM Viljoen. 2015. Gingerols and shogaols: impor-tant nutraceutical principles from ginger. *Phytochemistry*, Sep; 117: 554–568. DOI: 10.1016/j.phytochem.2015.07.012.

Sena CM, Pereira AM, and R Seiça. 2013. Endothelial dysfunction—a major mediator of diabetic vas-cular disease. *Biochimica et Biophysica Acta*, Dec; 1832(12): 2216–2231. DOI: 10.1016/j.bbadis.2013.08.006.

Serafini M, Ghiselli A, and A Ferro-Luzzi. 1996. In vivo antioxidant effect of green and black tea in man. *European Journal of Clinical Nutrition*, 50(1): 28–32. PMID: 8617188.

Sharifuddin Y, Chin YX, Lim PE, and SM Phang. 2015. Potential bioactive compounds from seaweed for diabetes management. *Marine Drugs*, Aug 21; 13(8): 5447–5491. DOI: 10.3390/md13085447.

Sharma RA, Euden SA, Platton SL, Cooke DN, Shafayat A, Hewitt HR, Marczylo TH, Morgan B, Hemingway D, Plummer SM, Pirmohamed M, Gescher AJ, and WP Steward. 2004. Phase I clinical trial of oral curcumin: biomarkers of systemic activity and compliance. *Clinical Cancer Research*, Oct 15; 10(20): 6847–6854. DOI: 10.1158/1078-0432.CCR-04-0744.

Shidfar F, Rajab A, Rahideh T, Khandouzi N, Hosseini S, and S Shidfar. 2015. The effect of ginger (*Zingiber officinale*) on glycemic markers in patients with type 2 diabetes. *Journal of Complementary and Integrative Medicine*, Jun; 12(2): 165–170. DOI: 10.1515/jcim-2014-0021.

Singh V, Bedi GK, and R Shri. 2017. In vitro and in vivo antidiabetic valuation of selected culinary–medicinal mushrooms (Agaricomycetes). *International Journal of Medicinal Mushrooms*, 19(1): 17–25. DOI: 10.1615/IntJMedMushrooms.v19.i1.20.

Sogut O, Kaya H, Gokdemir MT, and Y Sezen. 2012. Acute myocardial infarction and coronary vasospasm associated with the ingestion of cayenne pepper pills in a 25-year-old male. *International Journal of Emergency Medicine*, 5:5. DOI: 10.1186/1865-1380-5-5.

Soni KB, and R Kuttan. 1992. Effect of oral curcumin administration on serum peroxides and cholesterol levels in human volunteers. *Indian Journal of Physiology and Pharmacology*, Oct; 36(4): 273–275. PMID: 1291482.

Spiller F, Alves MK, Vieira SM, Carvalho TA, Leite CE, Lunardelli A, Poloni JA, Cunha FQ, and JR de Oliveira. 2008. Anti-inflammatory effects of red pepper (*Capsicum baccatum*) on carrageenan- and antigen-induced inflammation. *The Journal of Pharmacy and Pharmacology*, Apr; 60(4): 473–478. DOI: 10.1211/jpp.60.4.0010.

Spranger J, Kroke A, Möhlig M, Hoffmann K, Bergmann MM, Ristow M, Boeing H, and AF Pfeiffer. 2003. Inflammatory cytokines and the risk to develop Type 2 diabetes. *Diabetes*, Mar; 52(3): 812–817. PMID: 12606524.

Su L, Yin J-J, Charles D, Zhou K, Moore J, and L Yu. 2007. Total phenolic contents, chelating capacities, and radical-scavenging properties of black peppercorn, nutmeg, rosehip, cinnamon and oregano leaf. *Food Chemistry*, 100(3): 990–997. DOI: 10.1016/j.foodchem.2005.10.058.

Suryanarayana P, Satyanarayana A, Balakrishna N, Kumar PU, and GB Reddy. 2007. Effect of turmeric and curcumin on oxidative stress and antioxidant enzymes in streptozotocin-induced diabetic rat. *Medical Science Monitor,* Dec; 13(12): BR286–BR292. PMID: 18049430.

Tabit CE, Chung WB, Hamburg NM, and JA Vita. 2010. Endothelial dysfunction in diabetes mellitus: molecular mechanisms and clinical implications. *Reviews in Endocrine and Metabolic Disorders*, Mar; 11(1): 61–74. DOI: 10.1007/s11154-010-9134-4.

Tan D, Wang Y, Bai B, Yang X, and J Han. 2015. Betanin attenuates oxidative stress and inflammatory reaction in kidney of paraquat-treated rat. *Food and Chemical Toxicology*, Apr; 78: 141–146. DOI: 10.1016/j.fct.2015.01.018.

Teas J, Pino S, Critchley A, and LE Braverman. 2004. Variability of iodine content in common commercially available edible seaweeds. *Thyroid*, 14(10): 836–847. DOI: 10.1089/thy.2004.14.836.

Tesoriere L, Butera D, D'Arpa D, Di Gaudio F, Allegra M, Gentile C, and MA Livrea. 2003. Increased resistance to oxidation of betalain-enriched human low density lipoproteins. *Free Radical Research*, Jun; 37(6): 689–696.

Thorsdottir I, Andersson H, and S Einarsson. 1998. Sugar beet fiber in formula diet reduces postprandial blood glucose, serum insulin and serum hydroxyproline. *European Journal of Clinical Nutrition*, Feb; 52(2): 155–156.

Tian C, Ye X, Zhang R, Long J, Ren W, Ding S, Liao D, Jin X, Wu H, Xu S, and C Ying. 2013. Green tea polyphenols reduced fat deposits in high fat-fed rats via erk1/2-PPARgamma-adiponectin pathway. *PLoS ONE*, 8: e53796.

Tipoe GL, Leung TM, Hung MW, and ML Fung. 2007. Green tea polyphenols as an anti-oxidant and anti-inflammatory agent for cardiovascular protection. *Cardiovascular and Hematological Disorders—Drug Targets*, Jun; 7(2): 135–144. PMID: 17584048.

Vanschoonbeek K, Thomassen BJ, Senden JM, Wodzig WK, and LJ van Loon. 2006. Cinnamon supplementation does not improve glycemic control in postmenopausal type 2 diabetes patients. *Journal of Nutrition*, Apr; 136(4): 977–980. PMID: 16549460.

Vidal PJ, López-Nicolás JM, Gandía-Herrero F, and F García-Carmona. 2014. Inactivation of lipoxygenase and cyclooxygenase by natural betalains and semi-synthetic analogues. *Food Chemistry*, Jul; 154: 246–254. DOI: 0.1016/j.foodchem.2014.01.014.

Vijayabaskar P, and V Shiyamala. 2012. Antioxidant properties of seaweed polyphenol from *Turbinaria ornata* (Turner) J. Agardh, 1848. *Asian Pacific Journal of Tropical Biomedicine*, Jan; 2: S90–S98. DOI: 10.1016/S2221-1691(12)60136-1.

Vincent MA, Montagnani M, and MJ Quon. 2003. Molecular and physiologic actions of insulin related to production of nitric oxide in vascular endothelium. *Current Diabetes Reports*, 2003 Aug; 3(4): 279–288.

Wellen KE, and GS Hotamisligil. 2005. Inflammation, stress, and diabetes. *Journal of Clinical Investigation*, May 2; 115(5): 1111–1119. DOI: 10.1172/JCI200525102.

Willerson JT, and PM Ridker. 2004. Inflammation as a cardiovascular risk factor. *Circulation*, Jun; 109(21 suppl 1): II2–10. DOI: 10.1161/01.CIR.0000129535.04194.38.

Woo MN, Jeon SM, Kim HJ, Lee MK, Shin SK, Shin YC, Park YB, and MS Choi. 2010. Fucoxanthin supplementation improves plasma and hepatic lipid metabolism and blood glucose concentration in high-fat fed C57BL/6N mice. *Chemico-Biological Interactions*, Aug; 186(3): 316–322. DOI: 10.1016/j.cbi.2010.05.006.

Wootton-Beard PC, Brandt K, Fell D, Warner S, and L Ryan. 2014. Effects of a beetroot juice with high neobetanin content on the early-phase insulin response in healthy volunteers. *Journal of Nutritional Science*, Apr3: e9. DOI: 10.1017/jns.2014.7.

Wu CH, Lu FH, Chang CS, Chang TC, Wang RH, and CJ Chang. 2003. Relationship among habitual tea consumption, percent body fat, and body fat distribution. *Obesity Research*, Sept; 11: 1088–1095. DOI: 10.1038/oby.2003.149.

Wu LY, Juan CC, Hwang LS, Hsu YP, Ho PH, and LT Ho. 2004. Green tea supplementation ameliorates insulin resistance and increases glucose transporter IV content in a fructose-fed rat model. *European Journal of Nutrition*, Apr; 43: 116–124. DOI: 10.1007/s00394-004-0450-x.

Wu T, and B Xu. 2015. Antidiabetic and antioxidant activities of eight medicinal mushroom species from China. *International Journal of Medicinal Mushrooms*, 17(2): 129–140. PMID: 25746618.

Yeh TS, Hung NH, and TC Lin. 2014. Analysis of iodine content in seaweed by GC-ECD and estimation of iodine intake. *Journal of Food and Drug Analysis*, Jun; 22(2): 189–196. DOI: http://dx.doi.org/10.1016/j.jfda.2014.01.014.

Young HY, Luo YL, Cheng HY, Hsieh WC, Liao JC, and WH Peng. 2005. Analgesic and anti-inflammatory activities of [6]-gingerol. *Journal of Ethnopharmacology*, Jan; 96(1–2): 207–210. DOI: 10.1016/j.jep.2004.09.009.

Yuan G, Zhou L, Tang J, Yang Y, Gu W, Li F, Hong J, Gu Y, Li X, Ning G, and M Chen. 2006. Serum CRP levels are equally elevated in newly diagnosed type 2 diabetes and impaired glucose tolerance and related to adiponectin levels and insulin sensitivity. *Diabetes Research and Clinical Practice*, Jun; 72(3): 244–250. DOI: 10.1016/j.diabres.2005.10.025.

Zhang D-w, Fu M, Gao S-H, and J-L Liu. 2013. Curcumin and diabetes: a systematic review. *Evidence Based Complementary and Alternative Medicine*, 2013: 636053. DOI: 10.1155/2013/636053.

Zhang H, Tang Y, Zhang Y, Zhang S, Qu J, Wang X, Kong R, Han C, and Z Liu. 2015. Fucoxanthin: a promising medicinal and nutritional ingredient. *Evidence Based Complementary and Alternative Medicine*, May; 2015: 723515. DOI: 10.1155/2015/723515.

Zhao D, Kim SM, Pan CH, and D Chung. 2014. Effects of heating, aerial exposure and illumination on stability of fucoxanthin in canola oil. *Food Chemistry*, Feb; 145: 505–513. DOI: 10.1016/j.foodchem.2013.08.045.

Zielinska-Przyjemska M, Olejni AA, Dobrowolska-Zachwieja A, and W Grajek. 2009. In vitro effects of beetroot juice and chips on oxidative metabolism and apoptosis in neutrophils from obese individuals. *Phytotherapy Research*, Jan; 23(1): 49–55. DOI: 10.1002/ptr.2535.

12 Functional Foods Continued
*White Mulberry (*Morus Alba*) Leaf Extract and Tea*

The Lord hath created medicines out of the earth; and he that is wise will not abhor them.

Ecclesiasticus 38:4

12.1 INTRODUCTION

The white mulberry (*Morus alba*) is a short-lived, fast-growing medium-sized tree, ranging between 30 and 60 feet in height. It is native to northern China where it was widely cultivated to feed the "worms" that are used in the production of silk. The "silkworm" is actually the larva of the domesticated silk moth, *Bombyx mori* (see Section 5.14.1). The tree is generally known as the Chinese mulberry (*Sang Ye*—桑), although it is now widely cultivated in North America, Mexico, Argentina, Australia, and Central Asia.

12.2 THE COMPLEX OF ACTIVE AGENTS IN MULBERRY LEAF

The *Chinese Journal of Natural Medicine* reports that flavonoids are a significant constituent of mulberry and they possess numerous biological properties, including the following:

- Antioxidant
- Antimicrobial
- Cytotoxic
- Antihypertensive
- Antidiabetic (α-glucosidase inhibition)
- Antihyperlipidemic
- Antiobesity
- Appetite suppressant
- Cardioprotective
- Hepatoprotective
- Renal protective

Many of these properties are detailed below.

The journal *Archives of Pharmacal Research* reports that nine flavonoids have been isolated from the leaves of *M. alba* (*Moraceae*) on the basis of spectroscopic and chemical studies. The structures of compounds were determined to be the following:

- Kaempferol-3-O-β-D-glucopyranoside (astragalin)
- Kaempferol-3-O-(6″-O-acetyl)-β-D-glucopyranoside
- Quercetin-3-O-(6″-O-acetyl)-β-D-glucopyranoside
- Quercetin-3-O-β-D-glucopyranoside
- Kaempferol-3-O-α-L-rhamnopyranosyl-(1→6)-β-D-glucopyranoside

- Quercetin-3-O-α-L-rhamnopyranosyl-(1→6)-β-D-glucopyranoside (rutin)
- Quercetin-3-O-β-D-glucopyranosyl-(1→6)-β-D-glucopyranoside
- Quercetin-3,7-di-O-β-D-glucopyranoside
- Quercetin

Compounds 7 and 9 exhibited significant radical scavenging effect on 1,1-diphenyl-2-picrylhydrazyl radical (Kim, Gao, Lee et al. 1999).

The journal *European Food Research and Technology* reported on the total phenolic content, phenolic acids, radical scavenging activity, and antiproliferative properties of different parts of mulberry (*M. alba* L.). "Antiproliferative" means to prevent or retard the spread of cells, especially malignant cells, into surrounding tissues.

The highest phenolic content was found in methanol extracts of mulberry root, followed by leaves, branches, and fruit (Chon, Kim, Park et al. 2009). The root bark of the mulberry contains stilbenoids (resveratrol is a stilbenoid) that have antimicrobial, cytotoxic, anti-inflammatory, and lipid-lowering properties (Chan, Lye, and Wong. 2016). These exert both anti-inflammatory and anticancer activity (Eo, Park, Park et al. 2014). In addition, a prenylated flavonoid isolated from the root bark of *M. alba* showed potent antiviral activity against herpes simplex type 1 virus (HSV-1).

Moralbanone, along with seven known compounds, kuwanon S, mulberroside C, cyclomorusin, eudraflavone B hydroperoxide, oxydihydromorusin, leachianone G, and α-acetyl-amyrin were isolated from the root bark of *M. alba* L. Leachianone G showed potent antiviral activity, whereas mulberroside C showed weak activity against HSV-1. Their structure was determined by spectroscopic methods (Du, He, Jiang et al. 2003).

Mulberry fruits are rich in anthocyanins and they have pharmacological properties, including antioxidant, antidiabetic, antiatherosclerotic, antiobesity, and hepatoprotective (which means to protect the liver).

There are various other compounds in mulberry extract that are now being investigated, and cyanidin 3-glucoside is the most abundant of those active compounds. It can increase antioxidant enzyme activities and regulate lipid metabolism to treat liver disease resulting from alcohol consumption, high-fat diet, lipopolysaccharides, and carbon tetrachloride exposure. It has also been shown to promote cancer cell self-destruction (apoptosis) (Huang, Ou, and Wang. 2013).

One study published in the journal *Molecule* reported developing laboratory procedures to identify polyhydroxylated alkaloids with potent glucosidase inhibitor activity in mulberry leaf. Numerous such compounds were identified including 1-deoxynojirimycin (DNJ) (see below).

12.3 ANTIOXIDANT AND ANTI-INFLAMMATORY PROPERTY OF WHITE MULBERRY LEAF OR EXTRACT FLAVONOIDS

A study in the journal *Food Chemistry* reports the flavonoid contents of 19 varieties of mulberry, determined by standard laboratory (spectrophotometric) procedures. Rutin equivalent varied from 11.7 to 26.6 mg/g in spring leaves and 9.84 to 29.6 mg/g in autumn leaves. Fresh leaves gave more extract than those air dried or oven dried. High-performance liquid chromatography showed that the mulberry leaves contain at least four flavonoids, two of which are rutin and quercetin.

The percentage of superoxide ion scavenged by extracts of mulberry leaves, branches, and bark were 46.6%, 55.5%, 67.5%, and 85.5%, respectively, at a concentration of 5 μg/mL. The scavenging effects of most mulberry extracts were greater than those of rutin (52.0%) (Jia, Tang, and Wu. 1999).

The antioxidant property of extracts from teas prepared from the medicinal plants *M. alba*, *Camellia sinensis* L., and *Cudrania tricuspidata* and their volatile components were reported in the *Journal of Agricultural and Food Chemistry*. All extracts exhibited antioxidant activity with a clear dose-related response in the aldehyde/carboxylic acid and the malonaldehyde/gas chromatography (MA/GC) assays.

The antioxidant activity of extracts at the level of 500 µg/mL ranged from 77.02% ± 0.51% (stems of *Burea* plant) to 52.57% ± 0.92% (fermented tea of *Camellia* and stems of mulberry tea) in the aldehydes/carboxylic acid assay. Their antioxidant activity at a concentration of 160 µg/mL ranged from 76.17% ± 0.27% (roots of Burea plant) to 59.32% ± 0.27% (stems of mulberry tea) in the mass spectrometry–gas chromatography (MA/GC) assay.

Among the positively identified compounds, there were 11 terpenes and terpenoids; 15 alkyl compounds; 26 nitrogen-containing heterocyclic compounds; 9 oxygen-containing heterocyclic compounds; 18 aromatic compounds; 7 lactones; 6 acids; and 3 miscellaneous compounds, eugenol, 2,5-dihydroxyl acetophenone, and isoeugenol. These exhibited antioxidant activity comparable to that of butylated hydroxytoluene in both assays. The plant components vanillin and 2-acetylpyrrole showed potent antioxidant activity in the aldehydes/carboxylic acid assay but only moderate activity in the mass spectrometry–gas chromatography assay.

The investigators concluded that the consumption of antioxidant-rich beverages prepared from mulberry plants may be beneficial to human health (Nam, Jang, and Shibamoto. 2012).

In a study published in the *International Journal of Molecular Sciences*, it was reported that leaves of three indigenous varieties of mulberry, namely, *M. alba* L., *Morus nigra* L., and *Morus rubra* L., were investigated for their antioxidant potential. The stem bark extract had the most potent inhibitory activity against lipid peroxidation with IC50 = 145.31 µg/mL. In addition, the reducing capacity on ferrous ion was in the following order: stem barks > root bark > leaves > fruits. The content of phenolics, flavonoids, flavonols and proanthocyanidins of stem barks was found to be higher than other extractives.

The investigators concluded that because of the high correlation between phenolic contents and antioxidant potentials of the extracts, the plant extracts could serve as an effective free radical inhibitor, or scavenger, which may make them good candidates for pharmaceutical plant-based products (Khan, Abdur Rahman, Islam et al. 2013).

12.3.1 CYTOTOXICITY OF *M. ALBA* (VARIETY *BARAMATIWALI*)

The *Journal of Medicinal Plants* reported a study of the antioxidant and cytotoxic properties of *M. alba* var. *Baramatiwali*. In the study, the leaves of mulberry, *M. alba* L. were extracted by using 80% methanol in the laboratory. The extract was found to be high in antioxidant activity of the phenolic compound (44.66 µg of GAE/mg of fresh weight).

The cytotoxicity of the extract was tested on MCF-7 (breast cancer cell line), HT-29 (colorectal cancer cell line), and WRL-68 (normal liver cell line), and the results showed cytotoxicity activity on IC50 values of 78.87, 77.50, and 78.29 µg/mL, respectively (Khyade. 2016). The IC50 is the concentration of an inhibitor where the response (or binding) is reduced by half.

12.4   CAUTION

Due to the lack of standardization of the tea brewing process, and the unavailability of information about the concentration of the active constituent (1-DNJ, see below) in any *M. alba* plant product, be it tea or extract in any form, it is not safe to consume any of these without supervision by a competent healthcare provider and without regularly monitoring blood sugar levels with a glucometer, as well as blood pressure with a conventional blood pressure device. It is easy to exceed safe concentrations in tea or extracts, and that may rapidly result in dangerous hypoglycemia and a precipitous decline in blood pressure.

12.5   1-DEOXYNOJIRIMYCIN

DNJ, also called *duvoglustat* or *moranolin*, is an α-glucosidase inhibitor. α-Glucosidase is an enzyme that breaks down starches and disaccharides to glucose. α-Glucosidase inhibitors are in common use in oral antidiabetic prescription medications (e.g., acarbose) used primarily to treat Type 2 diabetes, because they prevent the digestion of carbohydrates such as starch and table sugar that can be absorbed through the intestine.

12.5.1 Leaf DNJ Concentration

Based on laboratory analytical data, it was shown that the average content of DNJ in 29 mulberry leaf samples is 1.53 mg/g, while the total contents of DNJ in those leaf samples ranged from 0.20 to 3.88 mg/g. The content reached the highest levels with harvest in early August. The authors hold that these data may provide an important reference for the quality of mulberry leaves used as herbal medicine for the treatment of diabetes (Ji, Li, Su et al. 2016).

Interestingly, as reported in the journal *Molecule*, DNJ was found to be concentrated 2.7-fold by silkworms feeding on mulberry leaves. Although DNJ in mulberry leaves is a potent inhibitor of mammalian digestive glucosidases, it does not inhibit silkworm midgut glycosidases. Fortuitously, the silkworm has enzymes specially adapted to enable it to feed on mulberry leaves (Asano, Yamashita, Yasuda et al. 2001).

More than 100 polyhydroxylated alkaloids have been isolated from plants and microorganisms. As noted in a previous chapter, these alkaloids can be potent and highly selective glucosidase inhibitors and are arousing great interest as potential therapeutic agents. However, only three of the natural products so far have been widely studied for therapeutic potential, due largely to the limited commercial availability of the other compounds (Alison, Watson, Fleet et al. 2001).

It has been shown that mulberry tea with high DNJ content can be made from the shoots of varieties such as *Burirum 60* (found in Thailand), which contains 300 mg/100 g of dry weight. Tea-making conditions can be optimized for highest DNJ extraction in a research setting using *response surface methodology*, a sequence of designed experiments to obtain an optimal response.

In a recent study, approximately 95% of total DNJ in high-DNJ content dry tea was extracted when temperature was maintained at 98°C (208°F) for 400 s (ca. 6.6 min). One cup (normal serving of 230 mL) of DNJ-enriched mulberry tea contained enough DNJ (6.5 mg) to effectively suppress postprandial blood glucose (Vichasilp, Nakagawa, Sookwong et al. 2012).

The *Journal of Agricultural and Food Chemistry* published a report about mulberry leaf–derived DNJ to help prevent diabetes. However, they found that DNJ contents in commercial mulberry products are typically as low as about 0.1%, that is, 100 mg/100 g of dry product—too low for bioavailability.

The investigators aimed first to produce food-grade mulberry powder containing a maximally high DNJ content and, second, to determine, through clinical trials, the optimal dose of the DNJ-enriched powder for the suppression of postprandial blood glucose. To that end, they determined DNJ concentrations in mulberry leaves from different cultivars, different harvest seasons, and different leaf locations (using hydrophilic interaction chromatography with evaporative light scattering detection).

They found that young mulberry leaves taken from the top part of the branches in summer contained the highest amount of DNJ. After optimization of the harvesting and drying processes for young mulberry leaves (*M. alba* L. var. *Shin ichinose*), DNJ-enriched powder of 1.5% was produced.

Healthy volunteers received 0, 0.4, 0.8, and 1.2 g of DNJ-enriched powder (corresponding to 0, 6, 12, and 18 mg of DNJ, respectively), followed by 50 g of sucrose. Plasma glucose and insulin were determined before and 30 to 180 min after the DNJ/sucrose administration. The single oral administration of 0.8 and 1.2 g of DNJ-enriched powder significantly suppressed the elevation of postprandial blood glucose and secretion of insulin, indicating the effective dose.

The results of this study suggest that the newly developed DNJ-enriched powder can be used as a dietary supplement for preventing the effects of diabetes (Kimura, Nakagawa, Kubota et al. 2007).

The journal *LWT—Food Science and Technology* reported on the value of mulberry DNJ to suppress postprandial blood glucose. They pointed out that mulberry leaf dry teas are now commercially available as "functional foods" in many countries including the United States, but that these products may not provide the effective dose of 6 mg DNJ/60 kg human weight, due to their low DNJ content (about 100 mg/100 g of dry weight) (60 kg = 132 lb). Therefore, development of tea with higher DNJ content is desirable.

To accomplish this end, the investigators examined DNJ content and α-glucosidase inhibitory activity in 35 Thai mulberry varieties. They found that DNJ content in young leaves varied among mulberry varieties from 30 to 170 mg/100 g of dry leaves weight. Varieties having the highest DNJ content were *Kam*, *Burirum 60*, and *Burirum 51*. Leaf "position" affected DNJ content—content is greater in shoots than in young leaves, and these are greater than in mature leaves.

DNJ concentration and α-glucosidase inhibitory activity were highly correlated, confirming that the α-glucosidase inhibitory activity of mulberry leaves is mainly due to DNJ. Consequently, high DNJ content mulberry tea was produced from shoots of varieties such as *Burirum 60*, which contains 300 mg/100 g of dry weight.

As previously noted, approximately 95% of total DNJ in high–DNJ content dry tea was extracted when temperature was maintained at 98°C (208.4°F) for 400 s (6.67 min); these conditions could be applicable for preparation of commercial products with high DNJ content. One cup of DNJ-enriched mulberry tea (230 mL, or 7.77 fluid oz), a normal serving, contained enough DNJ (6.5 mg) to effectively suppress postprandial blood glucose (Vichasilp, Nakagawa, Sookwong et al. 2012). High DNJ concentration can also be accomplished by extraction from *Bacillus* and *Streptomyces* species (Onose, Ikeda, Nakagawa et al. 2013).

A detailed chemical analysis of DNJ can be found in Gao, Zheng, Wang et al. (2016) (*Molecules*, 21, 1600).

12.6   DNJ LOWERS POSTPRANDIAL BLOOD GLUCOSE

The authors of a study published in *Diabetes Care*, a journal of the American Diabetes Association, report evaluating the effect of enriched DNJ on postprandial hyperglycemia in participants with impaired glucose metabolism. The test was a conventional experimental control procedure to assess the effects of a single ingestion of mulberry leaf extract (3, 6, or 9 mg DNJ), or a placebo substance, on blood glucose and insulin concentrations 2 h after a carbohydrate (200 g of boiled white rice) challenge, in participants with fasting plasma glucose (FPG) ranging from 100 to 140 mg/dL.

A second study was likewise a conventional controlled trial to assess the efficacy of a 12-week extract supplementation (6 mg DNJ, t.i.d.) for long-term glycemic control in participants with the same fasting blood glucose levels range.

In the first part of the study, it was found that consumption of the mulberry leaf extract tea led to a lower post-challenge acute glycemia in a dose-dependent manner. In the second part of the study, the serum 1,5-anhydroglucitol concentration, a sensitive indicator of postprandial glycemic control, rose and was significantly higher than that in the placebo control group over the 12-week treatment period.

The investigators concluded that long-term consumption of mulberry leaf extract with enriched DNJ content can result in improved postprandial glycemic control in individuals with impaired glucose metabolism [Asai, Nakagawa, Higuchi et al. 2011; note: these trials were registered with UMIN (Japan) Clinical Trials Registry].

Blood glucose response and sucrose absorption with DNJ in Type 2 diabetes and normoglycemia were tested in a study reported in the journal *Nutritional Science and Vitaminology* (Tokyo). It was shown that mulberry leaf

- Lowers blood glucose in normal rats (Miyahara, Miyazawa, Satoh et al. 2004)
- Lowers blood glucose in rats with diabetes induced by streptozotocin (Chen, Nakashima, Kimura et al. 1995) or alloxan (Ye, Shen, Qiao et al. 2002)

- Reduces fasting blood glucose and A1c concentrations in individuals with Type 2 diabetes (Murata, Yatsunami, Mizukami et al. 2003)
- Reduces fasting blood glucose, serum lipids, and lipid peroxidation indicators in individuals with Type 2 diabetes, relative to treatment with glybenclamide (an antidiabetic drug in a class of medications known as sulfonylureas closely related to sulfonamide antibiotics) (Andallu, Suryakantham, Lakshmi Srikanthi et al. 2001)

The study cited in that journal aimed to determine how consumption of mulberry extract and 75 g of sucrose influenced the blood glucose response and sucrose absorption in both Type 2 diabetic and nondiabetic individuals. Participants in this clinical trial included healthy control participants ranging in age from 24 to 61 years and participants with Type 2 diabetes otherwise healthy, ranging in age from 59 to 75 years.

In the morning, participants were randomly given mulberry extract (1 g) or an inert placebo, plus 75 g of sucrose in 500 mL of hot water. The test was repeated in 1 week with the opposite treatment. Hourly breath samples for H_2 measurements were obtained for 8 h (Strocchi, Corazza, Ellis et al. 1993). Blood glucose was assessed by means of an AccuCheck glucometer (Roche Diagnostics, Indianapolis, Indiana) before and at intervals over 120 min after sucrose ingestion in control participants and additionally at 180 and 240 min in the Type 2 diabetic participants. A lunch low in producing levels of H_2 was provided after completion of glucose measurements.

On the test day, participants kept track of the severity of abdominal and other symptoms rated from 0 (none) to 4 (severe). Sucrose malabsorption was estimated from breath H_2 concentrations (Zhong, Furne, and Levitt. 2006).

Compared to placebo, the simultaneous ingestion of mulberry extract with 75 g of sucrose significantly reduced the increase in blood glucose observed over the initial 120 min of testing in the control and Type 2 diabetic participants. Blood glucose decline at the tail end of the study were smaller in the mulberry extract group. Thus, peak-to-trough fluctuations in blood glucose were markedly reduced by mulberry consumption.

Similar results were reported in a study published in the journal *Diabetes Care*: Changes in blood glucose concentration from the fasting concentration of healthy control participants were compared to those in participants with Type 2 diabetes after consuming 75 g of sucrose with 1.0 g of mulberry leaf extract, or placebo. The blood glucose concentrations in the mulberry group were significantly lower than those in the placebo group over the first 120 min of the study (Mudra, Ercan-Fang, Zhong et al. 2007).

The mulberry-induced reduction in blood glucose presumably reflects the ability of mulberry to inhibit intestinal absorption of sucrose. The increased H_2 observed with mulberry indicates that this supplement induced sucrose malabsorption.

The *Journal of Medical Food* published a study using conventional experimental control procedures to assess the efficacy of 4 weeks of mulberry leaf aqueous extract supplementation (5g/day) for postprandial glycemic control in participants with impaired fasting glucose tolerance.

Postprandial responses in the glucose, insulin, and C-peptide levels were measured after a carbohydrate load at baseline and after 4 weeks of mulberry leaf aqueous extract supplementation. The postprandial glycemic response was reduced in the mulberry leaf aqueous extract group after the treatment period, particularly 30 and 60min after loading. In addition, 4 weeks of mulberry leaf aqueous extract supplementation improved postprandial glycemic control in individuals with impaired fasting glucose tolerance (Kim, Ok, Kim et al. 2015).

The journal *Evidence Based Complementary and Alternative Medicine* reported a study aimed at determining the antihyperglycemic effect of a standardized extract of white mulberry (*M. alba*) leaves compared to acarbose. The study evaluated the α-glucosidase inhibitory effect and acute single oral toxicity, as well as blood glucose reduction, in both animals and patients with impaired glucose tolerance.

The extract was found to inhibit α-glucosidase at a fourfold higher level than the positive control, acarbose, in a concentration-dependent manner. Blood glucose concentration was decreased by the extract *in vivo*.

Clinical signs and weight changes in the animals were observed when evaluating the acute toxicity of the extract by a single-time administration with clinical observations conducted more than once each day, for 14 days.

The inhibitory effects of rice coated with the extract on postprandial glucose were evaluated in a group of impaired glucose tolerance patients and in a group of normoglycemic persons. The extract had a clear inhibitory effect on postprandial hyperglycemia in both groups. Overall, it was reported to show excellent potential for improving postprandial hyperglycemia (Hwang, Li, Lim et al. 2016).

Some individuals prefer an herbal over a pharmaceutical preparation, and these people might find mulberry extract more acceptable and better tolerated than medications. In addition, mulberry extract contains compounds such as fagomine, which induces insulin secretion (Taniguchi, Asano, Tomino et al. 1998), as well as antioxidants that putatively reduce lipid peroxidation (Enkhmaa, Shiwaku, Katsube et al. 2005; Varadacharylul. 2004).

12.6.1 "SUGAR-COATING" GLYCEMIC CONTROL

This curious study, reported in the journal *Nutrition and Metabolism*, aimed to determine the effective ratio of extract of white mulberry leaves to sucrose to formulate a confection that could suppress the elevation of postprandial blood glucose and insulin.

The formulations were tested on healthy men and women. They included dessert items such as mizu-yokan (a traditional Japanese jelly dessert), to which was added 30 g of sucrose and either 1.5 or 3.0 g of mulberry leaf extract; daifuku-mochi (a small round glutinous rice cake stuffed with sweet filling), to which was added 9.0 g of starch in addition to 30 g of sucrose and either 1.5 or 3.0 g of extract; and chiffon cake, to which was added 24 g of sucrose, starch, and either 3.0 or 6.0 g of extract.

When consuming 30 g of sucrose, with 1.2 or 3.0 g of extract, the elevations of postprandial blood glucose and insulin were effectively suppressed. The extract-containing confection, with a ratio of extract to sucrose of 1:10, was the most effective in suppressing the increases of both postprandial blood glucose and insulin. The extract does this by inhibiting the intestinal absorption of sucrose (Nakamura, Nakamura, and Oku. 2009).

12.7 COMPARING DNJ TO GLYBURIDE

A clinical study published in the *International Journal of Clinical Chemistry* (*Clinica Chimica Acta*) reported comparing treatment with mulberry leaf extract to treatment with glibenclamide, the generic version of the antidiabetic drug glyburide (a sulfonylurea).

Mulberry leaf extract lowered fasting blood sugar by 27% (from 153 to 111 mg/dL), while fasting blood sugar in those taking glyburide decreased by only 8% (from 154 to 142 mg/dL). In other words, in this study, the mulberry leaf extract (with its various components, including DNJ) was three times more effective than a conventional antidiabetic medication in lowering fasting blood sugars in diabetic patients.

Moreover, the patients treated with mulberry leaf extract saw their blood levels of hemoglobin A1c fall by 10%, on average, whereas the patients treated with glyburide had no such decrease (Andallu, Suryakantham, Lakshmi Srikanthi et al. 2001). Thus, the extract was superior to a gold-standard medication not only in terms of reducing fasting blood sugars but also in lowering glycosylated hemoglobin (HbA1c) levels as well.

Additional benefits were noted in participants taking mulberry leaf: There was a 12% decrease in total cholesterol; a 16% decrease in triglycerides; and high-density lipoprotein (HDL) levels rose by 18%, compared to 3% in the glyburide group. In the glyburide group, no meaningful improvements in these lipid factors were noted.

In a similar study, patients with mulberry treatment significantly improved their glycemic control as compared to those on glyburide treatment. The results from the analysis of blood plasma and urine samples, from pre- and posttreatment, showed that the mulberry therapy significantly decreased the concentration of serum total cholesterol by 12%, triglycerides by 16%, low-density lipoprotein (LDL) cholesterol by 23%, and very-low-density lipoprotein (VLDL) cholesterol by 17%, while increasing HDL cholesterol by 18%.

In contrast, the patients treated with glyburide showed only marginal improvement in glycemic control, and the changes in the lipid profiles were not statistically significant except for triglycerides, down 10%. In this particular study, neither the extract nor the glyburide produced any apparent effect on HbA1c in diabetic patients. However, the fasting blood glucose concentrations of diabetic patients were significantly reduced by the mulberry therapy (Andallu, Suryakantham, Lakshmi Srikanthi, et al. 2017).

12.8 THE PROPRIETARY FORMULATION REDUCOSE AND POSTPRANDIAL BLOOD GLUCOSE LEVEL

A study, reported in the journal *PLoS ONE*, aimed to determine whether Reducose®, a proprietary mulberry leaf extract, can reduce blood glucose responses after dietary carbohydrate intake. Conventional experimental control conditions were imposed to study the glycemic and insulinemic response to Reducose, in comparison to three "test products," at the Functional Food Centre, Oxford Brooks University, UK.

Participants ranged in age between 19 and 59, and had body mass index (BMI) greater than or equal to 20 kg/m^2, and equal to or less than 30 kg/m^2. For purposes of comparison, in both men and women, standard BMI ranges are as follows:

- Underweight: BMI is less than 18.5.
- Normal weight: BMI is 18.5 to 24.9.
- Overweight: BMI is 25 to 29.9.
- Obese: BMI is 30 or more.

The objective was to determine the effect of three doses of the proprietary mulberry product, Reducose, versus a placebo preparation, on blood glucose and insulin responses when co-administered with 50 g of maltodextrin to normoglycemic healthy adults.

It was found that Reducose significantly reduced the expected increase in both total blood glucose and insulin, after ingestion of maltodextrin over 120 min. The pattern followed a classical dose–response curve. There were no statistically significant differences between any of the treatment groups, including the placebo group, in the odds of experiencing gastrointestinal symptoms (Lown, Fuller, Lightowler et al. 2017).

This absence of gastrointestinal side effects, from what is basically a mulberry leaf extract, is of great clinical importance, given that one of the main reasons that acarbose, an FDA (Food and Drug Administration)-approved prescription α-glucosidase inhibitor, did not gain much traction among diabetologists in the United States is that many patients who tried it reported a great deal of very unpleasant gassiness—which reduced compliance.

12.9 THE HAZARDS OF FREQUENT HYPOGLYCEMIA

Patients with Type 2 diabetes who are not treated with insulin are strongly urged by their physicians to lower their blood sugar level with a variety of medications, usually in combination. The *Indian Journal of Endocrinology and Metabolism* cautions us to beware of the complications of the hypoglycemia that can result from these medications.

Hypoglycemia is an important complication of glucose-lowering therapy in patients with diabetes, because intensive glycemic control invariably raises the risk of hypoglycemia. A sixfold increase in deaths due to diabetes has been attributed to patients experiencing severe hypoglycemia in comparison to those not experiencing that. Repeated episodes of hypoglycemia can lead to impairment of the counter-regulatory system, with the potential for development of "hypoglycemia unawareness."

The short- and long-term complications of diabetes-related hypoglycemia are reported to include myocardial infarction, neurocognitive dysfunction, retinal cell death and loss of vision, and injuries from falls, in addition to health-related quality of life issues pertaining to sleep, driving, employment, and recreational activities involving exercise and travel.

There is an urgent need to examine the clinical spectrum and burden of hypoglycemia so that adequate control measures can be implemented against this neglected life-threatening complication. Early recognition of hypoglycemia risk factors, self-monitoring of blood glucose, selection of appropriate treatment regimens with minimal or no risk of hypoglycemia, and appropriate educational programs for healthcare professionals and patients with diabetes are the major ways forward to maintain good glycemic control, minimize the risk of hypoglycemia, and thereby prevent long-term complications (Kalra, Mukherjee, Venkataraman et al. 2013).

12.10 EFFECT OF *M. ALBA* EXTRACT ON BLOOD PRESSURE

An animal-model study published in the journal *Molecular Nutrition and Food Research* aimed to investigate the mechanisms and effects of *M. alba* extract on arterial blood flow in mice. It was reported that the extract causes endothelial vasorelaxation through a nitric oxide (NO)-dependent pathway due to an increase in activity of endothelial NO synthase (eNOS). As expected, *in vivo* administration of *M. alba* extract reduced blood pressure levels in wild-type mice, whereas it failed to reduce blood pressure in eNOS-deficient mice.

The investigators concluded that *M. alba* extract exerts antihypertensive action in an experimental model of arterial hypertension, and that it does so through its enhancement of eNOS signaling; *M. alba* extract could act as a food supplement for the regulation of the cardiovascular system, mainly in clinical conditions characterized by eNOS dysfunction, such as arterial hypertension (Carrizzo, Ambrosio, Damato et al. 2016). Moreover, given that the erectile tissues in men and women become less efficient with age (or as a result of diabetes) as eNOS activity declines in those tissues, *M. alba* should theoretically be beneficial in treating sexual dysfunctions that are "vascular" in nature.

The aim of another animal-model study published in the *International Journal of Pharmacology* was to determine the scientific basis for the medicinal use of *M. alba* in hypertension. It was found that a crude extract induced a dose-dependent (10 to 100 mg kg^{-1}) fall in arterial blood pressure in anaesthetized rats. In isolated guinea pig atria, it caused inhibition of atrial force and rate of spontaneous contractions, similar to that exhibited by verapamil. When tested in rat aortic ring preparations, *M. alba* relaxed high K$^+$ (80 mM) and phenylephrine (1 μM)-induced contractions, and shifted the Ca^{++} dose–response curves to the right, like that caused by verapamil, at a concentration range of 0.1 to 10 mg/mL.

These data indicate that the blood pressure-lowering action of *M. alba* is due to blockade of a Ca^{++} channel pathway, which provides evidence for the pharmacological basis to justify its effectiveness in hypertension (Khan, Khan, Rehman et al. 2014).

12.11 EFFECTS OF MULBERRY LEAF EXTRACT ON PLASMA LIPIDS

The blood pressure-lowering effect of DNJ was also observed in a clinical study reported in the *Journal of Clinical Biochemistry and Nutrition*. It had been previously shown by these investigators that Mulberry leaves, rich in DNJ, inhibit α-glucosidase, thereby suppressing elevation of postprandial blood glucose in humans.

The objective of this study was to evaluate the effects of a DNJ-rich mulberry leaf extract on the human plasma lipid profile. A conventional control study was conducted in participants with initial serum triglyceride levels greater than or equal to 200 mg/dL. The participants were given capsules containing 12 mg of DNJ-rich mulberry leaf extract, three times daily, before meals, for weeks.

A modest decrease in serum triglyceride levels and beneficial changes in the lipoprotein profile were observed after this 12-week administration of the DNJ-rich mulberry leaf extract. No significant changes in hematological or biochemical parameters (other than those beneficial ones referred to above) were observed during the study period; no adverse events associated with DNJ-rich mulberry leaf extract occurred (Kojima, Kimura, Nakagawa et al. 2010).

The *Journal of Agricultural and Food Chemistry* reported an animal-model study based on high-cholesterol–fed New Zealand white rabbits, as well as an *in vitro* experiment on aortic vascular smooth muscle cells to investigate the impact of mulberry leaf extract on the development of atherosclerosis.

Both the *in vivo* and the *in vitro* studies showed a decreased presence of the fatty material that forms arterial atheroma burden. In the *in vivo* model, the mulberry leaf extract significantly reduced the elevated levels of serum cholesterol, triglycerides, and LDL. It also improved liver function as evidenced by decreases from the baseline elevations of liver function tests. Both mulberry leaf extract and mulberry leaf polyphenol extract improved endothelial function, inhibited proliferation and migration of aortic vascular smooth muscle cells, and reduced the extent of atheromas in the blood vessel walls.

The investigators concluded that in addition to exerting lipid-lowering effects, mulberry leaf extract and mulberry leaf polyphenol extract can effectively inhibit proliferation and migration of aortic vascular smooth muscle cells, improve vascular endothelial function, and reduce atheroma burden, thereby preventing atherosclerosis (Chan, Yang, Lin et al. 2013).

It should be noted that this study showed improved vascular endothelial function. These complimentary functions are typically controlled by NO. Blood vessel function is jeopardized when the endothelium can no longer synthesize NO and, at the same time, cannot relax in response to NO. These two developments are typically the result of atherosclerosis damaging the endothelium, and that damage manifests itself as cardiovascular and heart disease, and also of course as male erectile dysfunction.

Atherogenesis is considered to result from the uptake of oxidized LDL (ox-LDL) by macrophages. In a study published in the *Journal of Agricultural and Food Chemistry*, the aim was to determine the antiatherogenic effect of mulberry leaf extracts and the polyphenolic content of the plant, which includes quercetin, naringenin, and gallocatechin gallate.

Both the mulberry leaf extracts and polyphenolic extracts inhibited the oxidation and lipid peroxidation of LDL, although the polyphenolic extracts were shown to be more potent. Whereas 1.0 mg/mL mulberry leaf extracts reduced ox-LDL–generated reactive oxygen species (ROS) by 30%, it took only 0.5 mg/mL of the polyphenolic extracts to decrease the ROS by 46%. The polyphenolic extracts were also shown to be more potent in increasing the activity of superoxide dismutase-1 as well as that of glutathione peroxidase in macrophages.

At that same dose of 0.5 mg/mL, the polyphenolic extracts exhibited 1.5-fold greater potency than mulberry leaf extracts in decreasing the formation of foam cells. Both mulberry leaf extracts, and polyphenolic extracts, reduced the expression of the glitazone receptor, or NR1C3 (PPARγ), CD36, and SR-A, implicating the molecular regulation on ox-LDL uptake. These results suggested that polyphenolic extracts potentially could be developed as an antiatherogenic agent and deserve further investigation (Yang, Huang, Chan et al. 2011).

The journal *High Blood Pressure and Cardiovascular Prevention* reported a clinical study aimed to determine the effects of three nutraceutical combinations plus white mulberry extract on glicolipid metabolism in patients with hypercholesterolemia not treated with statin medications.

After 2 weeks of placebo treatment, patients were assigned to treatment:

- First, combination A [policosanol, red yeast rice (monakolin K 3 mg), berberine 500 mg, astaxanthine, folic acid, and coenzyme Q10] for 4 weeks
- Followed by 4 weeks of combination B [red yeast rice (monakolin K 3.3 mg), berberine 531.25 mg, and leaf extract of *M. alba*] for 4 weeks
- Then, an additional 4 weeks of combination A

Combination B reduced LDL cholesterol below 130 mg/dL in 56% of the patients, whereas with combination A, it was reduced below that cutoff in only 22% of them.

Both combination treatments reduced plasma levels of triglycerides, along with total and LDL cholesterol, and both increased HDL cholesterol. Total and LDL cholesterol reduction was more pronounced in patients taking combination B. Combination B also reduced glycated hemoglobin, fasting glucose, and insulin plasma levels, as well as HOMA index. HOMA stands for homeostatic model assessment, and it is a method for assessing pancreatic β-cell function and insulin resistance from fasting glucose and insulin concentrations.

The investigators concluded that an increased content of berberine and monacolin K and the addition of *M. alba* extract improve the effect on plasma cholesterol and on glucose metabolism of the nutraceutical combinations (Trimarco, Izzo, Stabile et al. 2015).

Lowering elevated triglycerides: The *Journal of Clinical Biochemistry and Nutrition* reported a study of patients with elevated triglycerides, averaging 312 mg/dL, treated with mulberry leaf extract. A level of 312 mg/dL is more than double the upper limit of the normal range. The patients were instructed to consume 12 mg of DNJ-rich mulberry leaf extract before meals, three times daily.

After 12 weeks, average triglyceride levels had fallen to 252 mg/dL. This is lower, but at a level still considered dangerous. In 20% of the patients, triglyceride levels dropped to under 150 mg/dL—a reduction of more than 50%. There was also a significant decline in small or VLDL cholesterol particles, which are especially dangerous because they are readily oxidized and are strongly associated with atherosclerosis (Kojima, Kimura, Nakagawa et al. 2010).

The purpose of a study reported in the journal *Phytotherapy Research* was to evaluate the lipid-lowering effect of mulberry leaf in nondiabetic patients with mild dyslipidemia. Patients who met the criteria guideline for dyslipidemia and did not benefit from a 4-week diet therapy were enrolled and assigned to receive three 280-mg mulberry leaf tablet three times a day before meals, for a period of 12 weeks.

Routine blood analyses including lipid parameters and liver function tests were performed every 4 weeks. At 4 and 8 weeks of mulberry leaf tablet therapy, triglycerides were significantly decreased from baseline by 10.2% and 12.5%, respectively.

At the end of the study, total cholesterol, triglyceride, and LDL were significantly lower by 4.9% and 5.6%, respectively, from baseline whereas HDL was significantly increased by 19.7%. Even though some patients experienced side effects such as mild diarrhea (26%), dizziness (8.7%), or constipation and bloating (4.3%), mulberry leaf tablet therapy is believed to be a safe way to reduce cholesterol levels and enhance HDL in patients with mild dyslipidemia (Aramwit, Petcharat, and Supasyndh. 2011).

12.11.1 Effects of Mulberry Leaf Extract on Systemic Inflammation in Dyslipidemia

Dyslipidemia is an elevation of plasma cholesterol, triglycerides, or both, or a low level of HDL, all or any of which contributes to the development of atherosclerosis. C-reactive protein (CRP) is a marker of the inflammation in blood vessels that can be caused by dyslipidemia (among other factors). The journal *BioMed Research International* reported a study that aimed to determine the antioxidant property of mulberry leaf powder, using the antioxidant scavenging DPPH assay to gauge the effect of mulberry leaf powder on the lipid profile as well as on CRP level.

Patients received three tablets of 280-mg mulberry leaf powder three times a day before meals for 12 weeks. After those 12 weeks of mulberry leaf consumption, levels of serum triglycerides and LDL were significantly lower, and in more than half of all the patients, the CRP levels decreased every month as well. The mean serum 8-isoprostane level, a marker of oxidative stress, was significantly lower after mulberry treatment for the 12 weeks.

The investigators concluded that mulberry leaf powder is an antioxidant and shows promise in controlling serum triglycerides, LDL, and CRP levels in mild dyslipidemia patients, without causing severe adverse reactions (Aramwit, Supasyndh, Siritienthong et al. 2013).

According to the journal *Revista Brasileira de Farmacognosia* (*Brazilian Journal of Pharmacognosy*), *M. alba* L. leaves are used in Brazilian herbal medicines to combat fever, to protect the liver, and to lower blood pressure and cholesterol levels. An aqueous extract of leaves of *M. alba* at a dose of 150 mg/kg/day for 14 days, given by mouth to rats that had been made hyperlipidemic by a diet enriched with cholesterol (1% by weight), significantly reduced the levels of plasma triglycerides by 55.01% (Zeni, and Dall'Molin. 2010).

12.12 1-DNJ ENHANCES INSULIN SENSITIVITY

It has also been shown that mulberry leaf extract enhances insulin sensitivity by boosting the number of cellular transporter protein molecules "GLUT4" that transport sugar out of the bloodstream and into cells. GLUT4 is the insulin-regulated glucose transporter protein highly expressed in adipose tissues and striated muscle. It was shown in an animal model that mulberry leaf extract can increase glucose uptake in cells by as much as 54% (Naowaboot, Pannangpetch, Kukongviriyapan et al. 2012).

12.13 *M. ALBA* INHIBITS PLATELET AGGREGATION

Simply put—very simply, in fact—platelets are the corks of blood vessels. While they do so in a very complex fashion, their primary function is to repair damage to blood vessels in order to stem blood loss. In order to do that, they must be able to clump together, that is, to aggregate to form a clot (called a thrombus). Aggregation involves a process of cell adhesion necessary to stem blood flow (hemostasis) in the event of an injury. Aggregation involves platelet-to-platelet adhesion and is necessary for effective hemostasis after the initial adhesion of platelets to the site of injury (Kim, Ji, Rhee et al. 2014).

The *Journal of Atherosclerosis and Thrombosis* reported a study that aimed to determine the effects of morusinol, a flavonoid derived from *M. alba* root bark, on platelet aggregation and thromboxane B(2) formation *in vitro* and on thrombus formation *in vivo*. The antiplatelet potential of morusinol was assessed by *in vitro* rabbit platelet aggregation and *in vivo* by an induced thrombosis model. Morusinol significantly inhibited induced platelet aggregation and thromboxane B(2) formation in cultured platelets, and did so in a concentration-dependent manner.

The investigators concluded that morusinol may significantly inhibit arterial thrombosis *in vivo* due to its antiplatelet activity. Thus, morusinol may exert beneficial effects on thrombotic problems such as transient ischemic attacks, stroke, deep venous thrombosis, pulmonary embolism, angina, and myocardial infarction, via its down-modulation of platelet activation (Lee, Yang, Yoo et al. 2012).

12.14 REDUCOSE® (PHYNOVA GROUP LIMITED), A PATENTED COMMERCIAL STANDARDIZED WATER-SOLUBLE EXTRACT OF *M. ALBA* LEAVES

The *International Journal of Toxicology* reports that *M. alba* leaves and their constituents, particularly iminosugars (or azasugars), have gained interest for their ability to maintain normal blood glucose concentrations. Reducose (Phynova Group Limited) is a patented commercial water-soluble extract of *M. alba* leaves standardized to 5% DNJ, an iminosugar with α-glucosidase inhibition properties.

There is a long history of the consumption of *M. alba* leaves in certain regions, suggesting that the leaves and their extracts have a relatively good safety profile. However, there are no known safety assessments on an extract containing higher amounts of DNJ than would occur naturally.

A 28-day repeated dose oral toxicity study in rats, conducted according to Organisation for Economic Co-operation and Development guidelines, was carried out to assess the safety of Reducose. Male and female Hsd.Han Wistar rats were administered Reducose *via* gavage—typically through a tube leading down the throat to the stomach—at doses of 0, 1000, 2000, and 4000 mg/kg body weight/day.

No treatment-related mortality or adverse effects per clinical observations, body weight/weight gain, food consumption, ophthalmoscopy, clinical pathology, gross pathology, organ weights, or histopathology were observed, and no target organs were identified. The no-observed-adverse-effect level was determined to be 4000 mg/kg body weight/day for both male and female rats, the highest dose tested (Marx, Glávits, Endres et al. 2016).

12.15 COMMERCIALLY AVAILABLE FORMULATION PRODUCTS

White mulberry leaf products are widely sold on the consumer market. They are sold as packages of loose tea leaves, in tea bags, as "extract" in capsule form, and as proprietary formulations. How much DNJ is in a product? Products sold in capsule form may specify "500 mg" of "extract" per capsule, but it is not certain what it is that there is 500 mg of. It is probably 500 mg of powdered leaf, as there is little evidence for most of these products that it is actually an "extract." What's more, the SUPPLEMENT FACTS generally read "(Morus Alba) standardized to 1.2% alkaloids." If that means 1.2% 1-DNJ, then a 500-mg capsule holds about 5 mg of 1-DNJ. The recommendation of one to two capsules per day may benefit someone with normal blood glucose levels by lowering it marginally, but the data from experiments reported above would suggest that this is likely to be a dose too small to have an impact on anyone with chronic hyperglycemia.

Fortunately, there are extraction forms that yield determinable quantities of DNJ. These were described in an earlier section, but in particular, the *Brazilian Journal of Microbiology* reported fermentation with the microorganism *Ganoderma lucidum* can improve DNJ extraction from mulberry leaf.

The optimum extraction yield was analyzed by response surface methodology (RSM). The extracted DNJ was determined using a reverse-phase high-performance liquid chromatograph equipped with a fluorescence detector. The results of RSM showed that the optimal condition for mulberry fermentation was at pH 6.97, with potassium nitrate content at 0.81%, and an inoculum volume of 2 mL. The extraction efficiency reached 0.548% maximum, which is a 2.74-fold increase of the levels of DNJ in mulberry leaf (Jiang, Wang, Jin et al. 2014).

From this study, it can be inferred that the concentration of DNJ in unfermented leaf extract should be far less than the 0.55% obtained from the fermented extract. How much is extracted in brewing is yet another question. However, a study published in *Advances in Medical Sciences* provides one answer. The aim of the study was to determine the effect of mulberry leaf extract supplementation on human starch digestion and absorption.

Healthy participants, 19 to 27 years old, were given a 13C starch breath test performed twice in a crossover and single-blind design. The 13C starch breath test is a test of pancreatic function. The participants were initially to ingest cornflakes that are naturally abundant in the 13C isotope of carbon (50 g of cornflakes + 100 mL of low fat milk), taken either with the mulberry leaf extract (36 mg of the active component DNJ), or the placebo, and each subject received the opposite preparation 1 week later. It was found that the cumulative percentage dose recovery of the 13C isotope in the exhaled breath was lower for the mulberry leaf extract test than for the placebo test. A significant decrease was detectable from minute 120 after the ingestion.

The investigators concluded that a single 36-mg dose of DNJ in mulberry leaf extract taken with a test meal decreases starch digestion and absorption (Józefczuk, Malikowska, Glapa et al. 2017).

Yet another study found DNJ effective at an even lower dosage than the 36 mg in the study cited above. The *Journal of Diabetes Investigation* reported a study that aimed to determine the effects of a single ingestion of mulberry leaf extract (3, 6, or 9 mg DNJ) or placebo on blood glucose and insulin concentrations 2 h after a carbohydrate (200 g boiled white rice) challenge in participants with FPG in the range of 100–140 mg/dL. The second part of the study was to assess the efficacy of 12-week extract supplementation (6 mg DNJ, t.i.d.) for long-term glycemic control in participants with FPG in the range of 110–140 mg/dL.

It was found in the first part of the study that ingestion of the mulberry leaf extract led to attenuated post-challenge acute glycemia, in a dose-dependent manner. In the second part of the study, serum 1,5-anhydroglucitol concentration (a sensitive indicator of postprandial glycemic control) in the extract group rose, and it was higher than that in the placebo group over the 12-week treatment period. No differences in FPG, glycated hemoglobin, and glycated albumin concentrations were observed between the groups (Asai, Nakagawa, Higuchi et al. 2011).

Hence, we have a pretty good idea of the range of dosages of DNJ that controls postprandial blood sugar concentration, but it still does not tell us what is in the claimed "500 mg" extract and how much of it winds up in tea. There is, however, little doubt that the tea is effective enough to warrant caution in its use (because of the ability to induce hypoglycemia, see below), but standardization and quantification are not presently available.

There is no available information about the effective concentration of active constituent(s) in any commercial product or of the sanitary conditions under which it was harvested, packaged, and distributed.

12.15.1 Caveat Emptor

Anyone who undertakes to consume this plant product in any form, for any reason, even under the supervision of a knowledgeable healthcare provider, is cautioned in the extreme to do so only with consistent, regular glucometer monitoring to assure that levels of blood sugar do not decline to a hypoglycemic danger zone. The website Liberty (https://libertymedical.com/diabetes/question /what-dangerously-low-blood-sugar-0/) considers hypoglycemia, or low blood sugar, to occur when blood sugars drop below 70.

Symptoms of hypoglycemia may include (among others) one of more of the following: feeling jittery, sweaty, shaky, dizzy, anxious, changes in behavior, skin color becomes pale, headache, feeling tired, hungry, changes in vision, tingling around the mouth, difficulty paying attention, seizures, stupor, or even frank coma.

12.15.2 How the Silkworm (*B. mori* L.) Could Help
in Treatment of Diabetic Nephropathy

As previously noted, the silkworm *Bombyx* amasses a considerable concentration of 1-DNJ as it chomps on those leaves in its larval life stages. Yet, that does not interfere with its carbohydrate metabolism. We learn about this from a study reported in the *Journal of the Zhejiang University. Science. B*. The abstract is quoted here:

The 1-DNJ contents of silkworm larvae change significantly with their developmental stages. The male larvae show higher accumulation of 1-DNJ than the females and also a significant variation was observed among the silkworm strains. Tissue distribution of 1-DNJ was found to be significantly higher in blood, digestive juice, and alimentary canal, but no 1-DNJ was observed in the silkgland.

Moreover, 1-DNJ was not found in silkworms fed with an artificial diet that does not contain mulberry leaf powder. This proves that silkworms obtain 1-DNJ from mulberry leaves; they could not synthesize 1-DNJ by themselves.

The accumulation and excretion of 1-DNJ change periodically during the larval stage. There was no 1-DNJ in the newly-hatched larvae and 1-DNJ was mainly accumulated during the early and middle stages of every instar [a phase between two periods of molting in the development of an insect larva], while excreted at later stages of larval development. (From Yin, Shi, Sun et al. 2010. Journal of the Zhejiang University. Science. B, Apr; 11(4): 286–291. With permission.)

The investigators concluded that it is possible to extract 1-DNJ from the larval feces and it is optimal to develop the 1-DNJ–related products for diabetic auxiliary therapy. In fact, it has been developed for treatment of diabetic nephropathy.

The authors of a study published by the *Chinese Journal of Integrative Medicine* report that, compared with herbal drugs, medicines processed from animals may have more bioactive substances and higher activities. *Biotransformation* often plays an important role.

However, there is little research and few reports about the effects of animal biotransformation on diabetic nephropathy and applying animal medicine as natural biotransformer. The aim of the report was to describe the application of *B. mori* L. on diabetic nephropathy from ancient to modern times.

The classical literature indicated that Saosi Decoction (缫丝汤), which contains silkworm cocoon, was applied to treat disorders consistent with what we know in modern times would be diabetic nephropathy, from the Ming Dynasty (1368 to 1644 AD) in ancient China to the Qing Dynasty (1363 to 1912 AD).

Modern studies showed that *B. mori* L. contains four main active constituents, of which DNJ, and quercetin in particular, showed promising potential to be new agents in the treatment of diabetic nephropathy.

The concentrations of 1-DNJ and the activities of quercetin in *B. mori* L. are higher than in mulberry leaves because of the *biotransformation* by the larva (Zhang, Zhang, Li et al. 2016).

12.15.3 How to Make Mulberry Tea

A number of websites provide instructions for the "best" way to brew white mulberry leaf tea. Here is one example from Jiaogulan:

White Mulberry Leaf Tea Preparation ~ How to brew the perfect pot
Making the perfect cup of tea is part art, science and meditation. Follow our recommendation below and you'll be happy you did.
Start by boiling 'Pure' water - enough for 4 cups
Let the water cool for about one minute. Water temperature just below the boiling point is perfect at 160 to 200°F (71 to 93°C).
Place 4 teaspoons of White Mulberry Leaf into your pot. Add 1 more for the pot.
Steep 3 to 5 minutes.
Pour, serve and enjoy!

Mulberry brewing directions:
Water Temperature: 140-212°F = 60-100°C
Leaf Amount: 1-2 t = 1-2.5 g per cup
Water Amount: 6-8 oz = 175-250 ml per cup
Infusion Time: 1 to 5 minutes

(http://jiaogulan.com/how-to-prepare-brew-mulberry-tea-more-albus.htm)

Immortalitea suggests the following: Here are a few tips so you can start brewing great tasting, healthy tea right away.

1. *This is loose-leaf tea so ideally you'll want a cup or teapot with an infuser, a tea ball or a self-fill tea bag. But in a pinch you can just toss the leaves in your cup. They will settle to the bottom when your tea is ready to drink.*
2. *I recommend using 1 tablespoon of loose mulberry leaf tea to brew one 8-10 ounce cup of tea. This is a bit more than most teas because the white mulberry leaf is a thick waxy leaf and needs to be brewed stronger than most teas.*
3. *This tea is best with a high temperature and relatively long brewing time. I recommend brewing white mulberry leaf tea with water that is 195°F (90°C). You may steep your tea anywhere between 5-8 minutes depending on how you like your tea.*

Remember, you can use the same leaves up to 3 times the same day!

(https://immortalitea.com/?st-t=adwords&vt-k=immortalitea&vt-mt=e&vt-ap=1t1&gclid=CNe 6mpT6iNQCFVKBswodYsMJaw) With permission.

There are other sites, including, notably:

Eon's Mulberry Tea is USDA certified Organic and caffeine free: http://www.eongoods.com /ProductDetails.asp?ProductCode=mt-30

Simple Life: http://alliumcepa2u.blogspot.com/2012/03/how-i-make-my-own-mulberry-tea.html

Cathy's Blog: https://cohlinn.wordpress.com/2013/05/05/mulberry-leaf-tea/

Note: Citation of the marketing sources of these examples of tea preparation instructions does not constitute an endorsement of any commercial product. We are not in a position to evaluate any aspect of a commercially available white mulberry tea product.

12.15.4 SAFETY OF CONSUMING WHITE MULBERRY LEAF IN TEA OR IN ANY OTHER FORM

Drinking mulberry tea may lower blood sugar. Hypoglycemia, or low blood sugar, may result in blurred vision, hunger, dizziness, headache, excessive sweating, tremors, and confusion—even coma. If one experiences these or any other untoward side effects while drinking mulberry tea, he or she is to seek immediate care from a healthcare provider. It may also significantly lower blood pressure.

People taking medication to control diabetes are advised to avoid drinking mulberry tea unless otherwise instructed by a licensed healthcare provider. Medications and mulberry tea also may interact to increase the risk of low blood sugar and low blood pressure. The healthcare provider may adjust the amount of diabetic and antihypertensive medications one takes in order to accommodate the effects of mulberry tea. Furthermore, persons with diabetes of either type are advised to closely monitor blood sugar levels when drinking mulberry tea.

When mulberry trees were planted in large numbers in Pakistan in the 1960s, scientists investigating a spike in allergic reactions found that the trees produced pollen counts of up to 40,000 grains per cubic meter of air: 1500 grains per cubic meter is considered harmful. The sap is also a known irritant, and contact with leaves or stems can lead to skin irritation. If one consumes mulberry products and develops hives, wheezing, rapid pulse, swelling, difficulty breathing, or other sudden symptoms, he or she is to discontinue use and contact a doctor right away.

As previously noted, several studies, including one published in the *Journal of Agricultural and Food Chemistry* in 2007, have shown that mulberry helps suppress post-meal blood sugar increases and insulin secretion, which could prove a helpful complementary strategy for preventing and treating poorly controlled diabetes. Because of these potential effects on blood glucose and insulin levels, however, if one is on insulin for diabetes and uses mulberry supplements, he or she may need to adjust the insulin dose accordingly. This cannot be done without consultation with one's healthcare provider.

Mulberries contain relatively high levels of potassium, which may cause problems for people with kidney diseases. As a result, if one has kidney disease, it may be better to avoid mulberry tea.

The fact that no published studies have yet associated mulberry tea consumption with adverse effects during pregnancy does not guarantee safety. Extreme caution, as well as supervision by a qualified healthcare provider, is urged before consuming any form of *M. alba* if pregnant, breast-feeding, or scheduled for surgery in the foreseeable future.

12.16 WHITE MULBERRY SUPPLEMENTATION IN TREATMENT OF OBESITY

The *Journal of Biological Regulators and Homeostatic Agents* published a report that noted that the meristematic extract of Japanese white mulberry blocks the α-glucosidase enzyme and then the intestinal hydrolysis of polysaccharides, thereby reducing the glycemic index of carbohydrates. The meristem is the part in most plants containing undifferentiated cells found in zones of the plant where growth can take place. These cells give rise to various organs of the plant and keep the plant growing.

Therefore, the investigators aimed to determine the adjuvant slimming effect of the meristem extract of white Japanese mulberry in the dietetic treatment of some patients who are obese or overweight.

Overweight people in the study were divided into two subgroups: the participants of both subgroups were given an identical balanced diet of 1300 kcal: those of the subgroup alpha received 2400 mg of white Japanese mulberry extract; the subgroup beta received a placebo. Each subgroup was followed up at 30, 60, and 90 days of treatment. Measurements of body weight and waist circumference in all the participants, and thigh circumference in women only, were repeated in the periodic inspections and also in the final inspection. All participants repeated the blood tests done at baseline.

In the subgroup alpha, weight loss was about 9 kg (19.84 lbs) in 3 months, equal to approximately 10% of the initial weight, statistically significantly higher than the weight loss (see below) in subgroup beta. At the end of the trial, the plasma insulin and glucose levels of the subjects in the alpha subgroup were lower than those performed at the time of enrolment.

In the women in the beta subgroup treated with only low-calorie diet and placebo, weight reduction was globally 3.2 kg (7.05 lb), approximately equal to 3% of the initial weight; moreover, the blood glucose and the insulin levels showed only a slight decline compared to baseline, but unlike the alpha group, this decline did not reach the level of statistical significance. Waist circumference and thigh circumference in the women decreased in all participants, more so in those who lost more weight.

The authors concluded that the extract from the meristem of white Japanese mulberry may represent a reliable adjuvant therapy in the dietetic treatment of some patients who are obese or overweight (Da Villa, Ianiro, Mangiola et al. 2014).

12.17 TWO RELEVANT ADDITIONAL BENEFITS OF *M. ALBA*

From the *Journal of Ethnopharmacology*: The extract of the root-bark of white mulberry targets the bacterial species *Streptococcus mutans*, which is a major factor in causing tooth decay. The *Journal of Ethnopharmacology* reports that Kuwanon G was isolated from the extract of *M. alba*. Its antibacterial activity against *S. mutans* causing dental caries was shown to be 8.0 µg/mL.

The bactericidal test showed that Kuwanon G completely inactivated *S. mutans* at a concentration of 20 µg/mL in 1 min. Kuwanon G also significantly inhibited the growth of other cariogenic bacteria such as *Streptococcus sobrinus*, *Streptococcus sanguis*, and *Porphyromonas gingivalis* causing periodontitis (Park, You, Lee et al. 2003).

From the *Journal of Ethnopharmacology*: The ethanolic extract of the root barks of *M. alba* inhibited bronchitis-like symptoms from lipopolysaccharide-induced airway inflammation, in an animal model, as determined by TNF-α production, inflammatory cell infiltration, and histological observation at 200 to 400 mg/kg/day by oral administration. In addition, *M. alba* contains major flavonoid constituents including Kuwanon E, Kuwanon G, and norartocarpanone that significantly inhibited IL-6 production in lung epithelial cells (A549) and NO production in lung macrophages (MH-S) (Lim, Jin, Woo et al. 2013).

12.18   A NOTE OF CAUTION CONCERNING HIGH POTASSIUM LEVELS IN CERTAIN BOTANICAL/HERBAL SUPPLEMENT

Botanicals or herbal supplements are generally considered safe to consume within the limits of reasonable, common supplementation. However, there is nothing about the efficacy of a given supplement that speaks to its safety, and a traditional saying has it that "One man's meat is another man's poison." Although this holds for many supplements, white mulberry tea and extract are a case in point: *M. alba* leaf is said to be very high in potassium. How high is the potassium level in leaf extract?

It is presently not possible to pinpoint that, but The *International Journal of Food Science and Nutrition* published a report titled "Comparison of mineral contents of mulberry (*Morus* spp.) fruits and their pekmez (boiled mulberry juice) samples." The investigators reported that the mineral contents of four mulberry fruits, and their pekmez samples growing particularly in the Malatya province, in Turkey, were found to contain high amounts of calcium, potassium, magnesium, sodium, phosphorus and sulfur, ranked in that order.

The highest potassium concentrations in mulberry fruits were found to be between 10.86 and 15.279 g/kg. Potassium content was found to be high compared to other minerals (Akbulut, and Ozcan. 2009). There are no data available on the range of potassium concentrations in different cultivars, harvested in different geographical regions, and in different seasons.

Abnormally elevated body tissue levels of potassium, hyperkalemia, is a common, serious, even potentially fatal electrolyte problem in persons with chronic kidney disease, and that condition is common in those with Type 2 diabetes. In fact, Type 2 diabetes is considered to be a major cause of chronic kidney disease. One report placed the prevalence of kidney disease in Type 2 diabetes in the United States at 43.5% (Bailey, Wang, Zhu et al. 2014).

Because of that potential danger, the FDA limits over-the-counter potassium supplements (including multivitamin mineral pills) to less than 100 mg. That is just 2% of the 4700 mg recommended dietary intake for potassium. Jun 1, 2016 (https://www.health.harvard.edu/staying-healthy/should-i-take-a-potassium-supplement; accessed 2.15.18).

So far as it can be determined, no such restriction, or content labeling, is required by FDA regulations for products that are a tea or an "extract" herbal supplement. Thus, until this matter is clarified, it would be extremely unwise for anyone with poor kidney function to undertake glycemia control with any form of *Morus alba*.

A note to the reader: Please see the chart in the Appendix for a summary of the therapeutic and other effects of the selected functional foods described in this chapter.

REFERENCES

Akbulut M, and MM Ozcan. 2009. Comparison of mineral contents of mulberry (*Morus* spp.) fruits and their pekmez (boiled mulberry juice) samples. *International Journal of Food Science and Nutrition*, May; 60(3): 231–239. DOI: 10.1080/0963748070169 5609.

Alison A. Watson AA, Fleet GWJ, Asano N, Molyneux RJ, and RJ. Nashe. 2001. Polyhydroxylated alkaloids—natural occurrence and therapeutic applications. *Phytochemistry*, Feb: 56(3): 265–295.

Andallu B, Suryakantham V, Lakshmi Srikanthi B, and GK Reddy. 2017. Effect of mulberry (*Morus indica* L.) therapy on plasma and erythrocyte membrane lipids in patients with type 2 diabetes. *PLoS ONE*, 12(2): e0172239. PMID: 11718678.

Andallu B, Suryakantham V, Lakshmi Srikanthi B, GK Reddy. 2001. Effect of mulberry (*Morus indica* L.) therapy on plasma and erythrocyte membrane lipids in patients with type 2 diabetes. *Clinica Chimica Acta* (*International Journal of Clinical Chemistry*), Dec: 314: 47–53, 2001.

Aramwit P, Petcharat K, and O Supasyndh. 2011. Efficacy of mulberry leaf tablets in patients with mild dyslipidemia. *Phytotherapy Research*, Mar; 25(3): 365–369. DOI: 10.1002/ptr.3270.

Aramwit P, Supasyndh O, Siritienthong T, and N Bang. 2013. Mulberry leaf reduces oxidation and C-reactive protein level in patients with mild dyslipidemia. *BioMed Research International*, Volume 2013, Article ID 787981, 7 pages.

Asai A, Nakagawa K, Higuchi O, Kimura T, Kojima Y, Kariya J, Miyazawa T, and S Oikawa. 2011. Effect of mulberry leaf extract with enriched 1-deoxynojirimycin content on postprandial glycemic control in subjects with impaired glucose metabolism. *Diabetes Investigation*, Aug 2; 2(4): 318–323. DOI: 10.1111/j.2040-1124.2011.00101.x.

Asano N, Yamashita T, Yasuda K, Ikeda K, Kizu H, Kameda Y, Kato A, Nash RJ, Lee HS, and K Sun Ryu. 2001. Polyhydroxylated alkaloids isolated from mulberry trees (*Morus alba* L.) and silkworms (*Bombyx mori* L.). *Journal of Agricultural and Food Chemistry*, 49 (9): 4208–4213. DOI: 10.1021/jf010567e.

Bailey RA, Wang Y, Zhu V, and MFT Rupnow. 2014. Chronic kidney disease in US adults with type 2 diabetes: an updated national estimate of prevalence based on Kidney Disease: Improving Global Outcomes (KDIGO) staging. *BMC Research Notes*, 7: 415. DOI: 10.1186/1756-0500-7-415.

Carrizzo A, Ambrosio M, Damato A, Madonna M, Storto M, Capocci L, Campiglia P, Sommella E, Trimarco V, Rozza F, Izzo R, Puca AA, and C Vecchione. 2016. *Morus alba* extract modulates blood pressure homeostasis through eNOS signaling. *Molecular Nutrition and Food Research*, Oct; 60(10): 2304–2311. DOI: 10.1002/mnfr.201600233.

Chan EW, Lye PY, and SK Wong SK. 2016. Phytochemistry, pharmacology, and clinical trials of *Morus alba*. *Chinese Journal of Natural Medicine*, Jan; 14(1): 17–30. DOI: 10.3724/SP.J.1009.2016.00017.

Chan KC, Yang MY, Lin MC, Lee YJ, Chang WC, and CJ Wang. 2013. Mulberry leaf extract inhibits the development of atherosclerosis in cholesterol-fed rabbits and in cultured aortic vascular smooth muscle cells. *Journal of Agricultural and Food Chemistry*, Mar 20; 61(11): 2780–2788. DOI: 10.1021/jf305328d.

Chen F, Nakashima N, Kimura I, M Kimura. 1995. Hypoglycemic activity and mechanisms of extracts from mulberry leaves (folium mori) and cortex mori radicis in streptozotocin-induced diabetic mice. *Yakugaku Zasshi* (*Journal of the Pharmaceutical Society of Japan*), 1995 Jun; 115(6): 476–482. PMID: 7666358.

Chon SU, Kim YM, Park YJ, Heo BG, Park YS, S Gorinstein. 2009. Antioxidant and antiproliferative effects of methanol extracts from raw and fermented parts of mulberry plant (*Morus alba* L.). *European Food Research and Technology*. 2009; 230(2): 231–237. DOI: https://doi.org/10.1007/s00217-009-1165-2.

Da Villa G, Ianiro G, Mangiola F, Del Toma E, Vitale A, Gasbarrini A, G Gasbarrini G. 2014. *Journal of Biological Regulators and Homeostatic Agents*, Jan–Mar; 28(1): 141–145. PMID: 24750800.

Du J, He ZD, Jiang RW, Ye WC, Xu HX, and PP But. 2003. Antiviral flavonoids from the root bark of *Morus alba*. *Phytochemistry*, Apr; 62(8): 1235–123. PMID: 12648543.

Enkhamaa B, Shiwaku K, Katsube T, Kitajima K, Anuurad E, Yamasaki M, and Y Yamane. 2005. Mulberry (*Morus alba* L.) leaves and their major flavonol quercetin 3-(6-malonylglucoside) attenuate atherosclerotic lesion development in LDL receptor-deficient mice. *Journal of Nutrition*, Apr; 135: 729–734. PMID: 15795425.

Eo HJ, Park JH, Park GH, Lee MH, Lee JR, Koo JS, and JB Jeong. 2014. Anti-inflammatory and anti-cancer activity of mulberry (*Morus alba* L.) root bark. *BMC—Complementary and Alternative Medicine*, 14: 200. DOI: 10.1186/1472-6882-14-200.

Gao K, Zheng C, Wang T, Zhao H, Wang J, Wang Z, Zha X, Jia, Z, Chen J, Zhou Y, and W Wang. 2016. 1-Deoxynojirimycin: occurrence, extraction, chemistry, oral pharmacokinetics, biological activities and in silico target fishing. *Molecules*, 21, 1600. DOI:10.3390/molecules21111600.

Huang H-P, Ou T-T, and C-J Wang. 2013. Mulberry (桑葚子 Sang Shèn Zǐ) and its bioactive compounds, the chemoprevention effects and molecular mechanisms *in vitro* and *in vivo*. *Journal of Traditional and Complementary Medicine*, Jan-Mar; 3(1): 7–15. DOI: 10.4103/2225-4110.106535.

Hwang SH, Li HM, Lim SS, Wang Z, Hong J-S, and B Huang. 2016. Evaluation of a standardized extract from *Morus alba* against α-glucosidase inhibitory effect and postprandial antihyperglycemic in patients with impaired glucose tolerance: a randomized double-blind clinical trial. *Evidence Based Complementary and Alternative Medicine*, 2016: 8983232. DOI: 10.1155/2016/8983232.

Ji T, Li J, Su S-L, Zhu Z-H, Guo S, Qian D-W, and J-A Duan. 2016. Identification and determination of the polyhydroxylated alkaloids compounds with 1-glucosidase inhibitor activity in mulberry leaves of different origins. *Molecules*, 21(206); DOI: 10.3390/molecules21020206.

Jia Z, Tang M, and J Wu. 1999. The determination of flavonoid contents in mulberry and their scavenging effects on superoxide ion. *Food Chemistry*, 64:555–559.

Jiang YG, Wang CY, Jin C, Jia JQ, Guo X, Zhang GZ, and ZZ Gui. 2014. Improved 1-deoxynojirimycin (DNJ) production in mulberry leaves fermented by microorganism. *Brazilian Journal of Microbiology*, Aug; 45(2): 721–729. eCollection 2014. PMCID: PMC4166305.

Józefczuk J, Malikowska K, Glapa A, Stawińska-Witoszyńska B, Nowak JK, Bajerska J, Lisowska A, and J Walkowiak. 2017. Mulberry leaf extract decreases digestion and absorption of starch in healthy subjects—a randomized, placebo-controlled, crossover study. *Advances in Medical Sciences*, May; 62(2): 302–306. DOI: 10.1016/j.advms.2017.03.002.

Kalra S, Mukherjee JJ, Venkataraman S, Bantwal G, Shaikh S, Saboo B, Das AK, and A Ramachandran. 2013. Hypoglycemia: the neglected complication. *Indian Journal of Endocrinology and Metabolism*, Sep–Oct; 17(5): 819–834. DOI: 10.4103/2230-8210.117219.

Khan M, Khan A-u, Rehman N-u, and A-H Gilani. 2014. Blood pressure lowering effect of *Morus alba* is mediated through Ca^{++} antagonist pathway. *International Journal of Pharmacology*, 10(4): 225–230. DOI: 10.3923/ijp.2014.225.230.

Khan MA, Abdur Rahman AA, Islam S, Khandokhar P, Parvin S, Badrul Islam B, Hossain M, Rashid M, Sadik G, Nasrin S, Mollah MNH, and HMK Alam. 2013. A comparative study on the antioxidant activity of methanolic extracts from different parts of *Morus alba* L. (Moraceae). *BMC Research Notes*, 6:24. DOI: 10.1186/1756-0500-6-24.

Khyade VB. 2016. Antioxidant activity and phenolic compounds of mulberry, *Morus alba* (L) (Variety: Baramatiwali). *Journal of Medicinal Plants*, 4(1): 407.

Kim D-S, Ji HD, Rhee MH, Sung Y-Y, Yang W-K, Kim SH, and H-K Kim. 2014. Antiplatelet activity of *Morus alba* leaves extract, mediated via inhibiting granule secretion and blocking the phosphorylation of extracellular-signal-regulated kinase and Akt. *Evidence Based Complementary and Alternative Medicine*, vol. 2014; article ID: 639548. DOI: 10.1155/2014/639548.

Kim JY, Ok HM, Kim J, Park SW, Kwon SW, and O Kwon. 2015. Mulberry leaf extract improves postprandial glucose response in prediabetic subjects: a randomized, double-blind placebo-controlled trial. *Journal of Medical Food*, Mar; 18(3): 306–313. DOI: 10.1089/jmf.2014.3160.

Kim SY, Gao JJ, Lee WC, Ryu KS, Lee KR, and YC Kim. 1999. Antioxidative flavonoids from the leaves of *Morus alba*. *Archives of Pharmacal Research*, Feb; 22(1): 81–85. PMID: 10071966.

Kimura T, Nakagawa K, Kubota H, Kojima Y, Goto Y, Yamagishi K, Oita S, Oikawa S, and T Miyazawa. 2007. Food-grade mulberry powder enriched with 1-deoxynojirimycin suppresses the elevation of postprandial blood glucose in humans. *Journal of Agricultural and Food Chemistry*, Jul 11; 55(14): 5869–5874. DOI: 10.1021/jf062680g.

Kojima Y, Kimura T, Nakagawa K, Asai A, Hasumi K, Oikawa S, and T Miyazawa. 2010. Effects of mulberry leaf extract rich in 1-deoxynojirimycin on blood lipid profiles in humans. *Journal of Clinical Biochemistry and Nutrition*, Sep; 47(2): 155–161. DOI: 10.3164/jcbn.10-53.

Lee JJ, Yang H, Yoo YM, Hong SS, Lee D, Lee HJ, Lee HJ, Myung CS, Choi KC, and EB Jeung. 2012. Morusinol extracted from *Morus alba* inhibits arterial thrombosis and modulates platelet activation for the treatment of cardiovascular disease. *Journal of Atherosclerosis and Thrombosis*, Apr; 19(6): 516–522. PMID: 22472211.

Lim HJ, Jin HG, Woo ER, Lee SK, HP Kim. 2013. The root barks of *Morus alba* and the flavonoid constituents inhibit airway inflammation. *Journal of Ethnopharmacology*, Aug 26; 149(1): 169–175. DOI: 10.1016/j.jep.2013.06.017. PMID: 23806866.

Lown M, Fuller R, Lightowler H, Fraser A, Gallagher A, Stuart B, Byrne C, and G Lewith. 2017. Mulberry-extract improves glucose tolerance and decreases insulin concentrations in normoglycaemic adults: results of a randomised double-blind placebo-controlled study. *PLoS ONE*, Feb 22; 12(2): e0172239. DOI: 10.1371/journal.pone.0172239.

Marx TK, Glávits R, Endres JR, Palmer PA, Clewell AE, Murbach TS, Hirka G, and I Pasics. 2016. A 28-day repeated dose toxicological study of an aqueous extract of *Morus alba* L. *International Journal of Toxicology*, 35(6): 683–691. DOI: ttps://doi.org/10.1177/1091581816670597.

Miyahara C, Miyazawa M, Satoh S, Sakai A, and S Mizusaki. 2004. Inhibitory effects of mulberry leaf extract on postprandial hyperglycemia in normal rats. *Journal of Nutritional Science and Vitaminology (Tokyo)*. Jun; 50(3): 161–164.

Mudra M, Ercan-Fang N, Zhong L, Furne J, and M Levitt. 2007. Influence of mulberry leaf extract on the blood glucose and breath hydrogen response to ingestion of 75 g sucrose by Type 2 diabetic and control subjects. *Diabetes Care*, May; 30(5): 1272–1274. https://doi.org/10.2337/dc06-2120.

Murata K, Yatsunami K, Mizukami O, Toriumi Y, Hoshino G, and T Kamei. 2003. Effects of propolis and mulberry leaf extract on type 2 diabetes. *Focus on Alternative and Complementary Therapies*, 8: 4524–4525.

Nakamura M, Nakamura S, and T Oku. 2009. Suppressive response of confections containing the extractive from leaves of *Morus alba* on postprandial blood glucose and insulin in healthy human subjects. *Nutrition and Metabolism (Lond)*, Jul 14; 6:29. DOI: 10.1186/1743-7075-6-29.

Nam S, Jang HW, and T Shibamoto. 2012. Antioxidant activities of extracts from teas prepared from medicinal plants, *Morus alba* L., *Camellia sinensis* L., and *Cudrania tricuspidata*, and their volatile components. *Journal of Agricultural and Food Chemistry*, Sep 12; 60(36): 9097–9105. DOI: 10.1021 /jf301800x.

Naowaboot J, Pannangpetch P, Kukongviriyapan V, Prawan A, Kukongviriyapan U, and A Itharat. 2012. Mulberry leaf extract stimulates glucose uptake and GLUT4 translocation in rat adipocytes. *American Journal of Chinese Medicine*, 40(1): 163–175.

Onose S, Ikeda R, Nakagawa K, Kimura T, Yamagishi K, Higuchi O, and T Miyazawa. 2013. Production of the α-glycosidase inhibitor 1-deoxynojirimycin from *Bacillus* species. *Food Chemistry*, May; 138(1): 516–523. DOI:10.1016/j.foodchem.2012.11.012.

Park KM, You JS, Lee HY, Baek NI, and JK Hwang. 2003. Kuwanon G: an antibacterial agent from the root bark of *Morus alba* against oral pathogens. *Journal of Ethnopharmacology*, Feb; 84(2–3): 181–185. PMID: 12648813.

Strocchi A, Corazza G, Ellis CJ, Gasbarrini G, and MD Levitt. 1993. Detection of malabsorption of low doses of carbohydrate: accuracy of various breath H2 criteria. *Gastroenterology*, Nov; 105(5): 1404–1410. PMID: 8224644.

Taniguchi S, Asano N, Tomino F, and I Miwa. 1998. Potentiation of glucose-induced insulin secretion by fagomine, a pseudo-sugar isolated from mulberry leaves. *Hormones and Metabolic Research*, Nov; 30(11): 679–683. DOI: 10.1055/s-2007-978957.

Trimarco V, Izzo R, Stabile H,, Rozza F, Santoro M, Manzi MV, Serino F, Schiattarella GG, Esposito G, and B Trimarco. 2015. Effects of a new combination of nutraceuticals with *Morus alba* on lipid profile, insulin sensitivity and endothelial function in dyslipidemic subjects. A cross-over, randomized, double-blind trial. *High Blood Pressure & Cardiovascular Prevention*, Jun; 22(2): 149–154. http://link.springer .com/article/10.1007/s40292-015-0087-2.

Varadacharylul AB. 2004. Antioxidant role of mulberry (*Morus indica* L. cv. Anantha) leaves in streptozotocin-diabetic rats. *Clinica Chimica Acta*, Oct; 348: 215–218.

Vichasilp C, Nakagawa K, Sookwong P, Higuchic O, Luemunkong S, and T Miyazawa. 2012. Development of high 1-deoxynojirimycin (DNJ) content mulberry tea and use of response surface methodology to optimize tea-making conditions for highest DNJ extraction. *LWT—Food Science and Technology*, Mar: 45(2): 226–232. http://www.sciencedirect.com/science/article/pii/S0023643811002970.

Yang MY, Huang CN, Chan KC, Yang YS, Peng CH, and CJ Wang. 2011. Mulberry leaf polyphenols possess antiatherogenesis effect via inhibiting LDL oxidation and foam cell formation. *Journal of Agricultural and Food Chemistry*, Mar 9; 59(5): 1985–1995. DOI: 10.1021/jf103661v.

Ye F, Shen ZF, Qiao FX, Zhao DY, and MZ Xie. 2002. Experimental treatment of complications in alloxan diabetic rats with alpha-glucosidase inhibitor from the Chinese medicinal herb ramulus mori. *Yao Xue Xue Bao (Acta Pharmaceutica Sinica)*, Feb: 37:108–112.

Yin H, Shi XQ, Sun B, Ye JJ, Duan ZA, Zhou XL, Cui WZ, and XF Wu. 2010. Accumulation of 1-deoxynojirimycin in silkworm, *Bombyx mori* L. *Journal of the Zhejiang University. Science. B*, Apr; 11(4): 286–291. DOI: 10.1631/jzus.B0900344.

Zeni ALB, and M Dall'Molin. 2010. Efeito hipotrigliceridêmico de folhas de *Morus alba* L., Moraceae, em ratos hiperlipidêmicos [Hypotriglyceridemic effect of *Morus alba* L., Moraceae, leaves in hyperlipidemic rats]. *Revista Brasileira de Farmacognosia*, 20(1): Curitiba Jan./Mar. http://dx.doi.org/10.1590 /S0102-695X2010000100025.

Zhang L, Zhang, Li Y, Guo XF, and XS Liu. 2016. Biotransformation effect of *Bombyx mori* L. may play an important role in treating diabetic nephropathy. *Chinese Journal of Integrative Medicine*, Nov; 22(11): 872–879. DOI: 10.1007/s11655-015-2128-z.

Zhong L, Furne JK, and MD Levitt. 2006. An extract of black, green and mulberry teas causes malabsorption of carbohydrate but not triacylglycerol in health controls. *Journal of Clinical Nutrition*, 84: 551–555.

13 Selected Supplements That Support Glycemic Control and Reduce Chronic Inflammation

I must admit that when I chose the name, 'vitamine,' I was well aware that these substances might later prove not to be of an amine nature. However, it was necessary for me to choose a name that would sound well and serve as a catchword, since I had already at that time no doubt about the importance and the future popularity of the new field.

Casimir Funk (1884–1967)

13.1 SELECTED SUPPLEMENTS THAT LESSEN CHRONIC HYPERGLYCEMIA AND LOWER SYSTEMIC INFLAMMATION

Type 2 diabetes is linked to obesity, metabolic syndrome, and cardiovascular and heart disease—especially coronary heart disease—and many more afflictions. All of these have been attributed to underlying chronic systemic inflammation causing oxidative stress, shown to be a staple in chronic hyperglycemia.

A report titled "Inflammation and the etiology of type 2 diabetes" appeared in the journal *Diabetes/Metabolism Research and Reviews*. The authors hold that the processes responsible for development of insulin resistance are not well understood, but that it has emerged recently that sub-clinical chronic inflammation may be an important pathogenic factor in the development of insulin resistance and Type 2 diabetes. Surrogate markers for this low-grade chronic inflammation include C-reactive protein (CRP), interleukin-6 (IL-6) and tumor necrosis factor-alpha (TNF-α).

It should be noted that some antidiabetic agents such as the glitazones that reduce insulin resistance also reduce inflammation and, as reported in the *British Journal of Pharmacology*, anti-inflammatory drugs, that is, aspirin and NSAIDs (nonsteroidal anti-inflammatory drugs), may improve glucose tolerance (Li, Zhang, Ye et al. 2007). In fact, the *Journal of Clinical Investigation* reported a study titled "Mechanism by which high-dose aspirin improves glucose metabolism in type 2 diabetes." The aim of the study was to determine whether high doses of salicylates, shown to inhibit IK-Kβ activity, might ameliorate insulin resistance and improve glucose tolerance in patients with Type 2 diabetes. Patients were tested before and after 2 weeks of treatment with aspirin ($\sim$7 g/day). They underwent mixed-meal tolerance tests, and hyperinsulinemic-euglycemic clamps, with [6,6-2H2]glucose to assess glucose turnover before and after treatment.

The hyperinsulinemic clamp, which requires maintaining a high insulin level by perfusion or infusion with insulin, is a way to quantify how sensitive the tissue is to insulin. The hyperinsulinemic clamp is also called euglycemic clamp, meaning a normal blood sugar level is maintained.

It was found that high-dose aspirin treatment resulted in an approximately 25% reduction in fasting plasma glucose, associated with an approximately 15% reduction in total cholesterol and CRP, an approximately 50% reduction in triglycerides, and an approximately 30% reduction in insulin clearance, despite no change in body weight.

During a mixed-meal tolerance test, the area under the curve for plasma glucose and fatty acid levels decreased by approximately 20% and approximately 50%, respectively. Aspirin treatment also resulted in an approximately 20% reduction in basal rate of hepatic glucose production, and an approximately 20% improvement in insulin-stimulated peripheral glucose uptake under matched plasma insulin concentrations during the clamp.

The investigators concluded that IK-Kβ may represent a new target for treating Type 2 diabetes (Hundal, Petersen, Mayerson et al. 2002).

While inhibition of any factor that contributes to inflammation is an obvious route for adjunctive treatment of Type 2 diabetes, the known adverse effects of chronic salycilate consumption may make this particular approach impractical. Vasoactive drugs that are often prescribed to people with diabetes, for example, ACE inhibitors/angiotensin receptor antagonists, also counteract inflammation and reduce the risk of Type 2 diabetes (Sjöholm, and Nyström. 2005).

It would therefore seem plausible to supplement an antidiabetic treatment program with readily available substances known to help reduce chronic inflammation. The most common of these substances are antioxidant vitamins and minerals. A review in the journal *Endocrine, Metabolic and Immune Disorders Drug Targets* concluded that antioxidant vitamins A, C, and E levels are found to be lower in diabetic patients, associated with disturbed glucose metabolism.

It was also observed that the B vitamins, thiamine, pyridoxine, and biotin are lower in diabetes, but the reason is unknown. Supplementation of these vitamins is followed by improvement of metabolic control in diabetes patients as will be seen in Chapter 14.

The absorption of folic acid and vitamin B12 is reduced by the prolonged use of metformin, which is the first choice drug in uncomplicated diabetes; thus, these two nutrients have been found deficient in the disease and most probably need to be supplemented regularly. Parenthetically, vitamin D deficiency is now considered a risk factor for the development of diabetes as well as for its complications, particularly the cardiovascular ones (Mandarino, Monteiro, Salgado et al. 2015). Vitamin D is discussed in Chapter 14.

The investigators found the outcome of multivitamin supplementation inconclusive but conceded that their patients using metformin during prolonged periods may need folic acid and vitamin B12 supplement (Valdés-Ramos, Guadarrama-López, Martínez-Carrillo et al. 2015).

A case can be made that efforts to control diabetes without addressing chronic inflammation do not usually fare well. It may be that the generalized failure to recommend adjunctive "supplementation," as it is understood here, may at least in part be responsible for the unsatisfactory track record of conventional treatment.

13.1.1 What Are "Supplements"?

A previous chapter described selected "functional foods." These are actually foods, whereas supplements are not foods. The term "supplement" has evolved with the search for consumables that might enhance health, which has led to a schism between integrative medical practitioners, versus traditional medical practitioners. The latter tend to accept the *a priori* theoretical concept that a "healthy balanced diet" will provide sufficient amounts of all nutrients, so that no supplements would ever be needed. The traditional practitioners who profess this belief do so against a mountain of evidence that (1) the typical Western diet is severely deficient in a number of basic and necessary nutrients and (2) even if the diet were in fact nutritionally sound, there are hundreds of "nutrient-responsive" conditions for which solid clinical evidence has confirmed that supplementing with *pharmacological* amounts of a given nutrient can alleviate (and, in some cases, even cure) these nutrient-responsive conditions. In these instances, the actual levels of that same nutrient, as found even in the most optimal diet, are insufficient to the task.

The traditional medical practitioners generally believe (and that is all it is, a "belief") that the only acceptable use for a "supplement" would be a physiologically low dose to treat or prevent a deficiency state, for example, administering a milligram or so per day of thiamine to treat beri-beri or a milligram or so per day of niacinamide to treat pellagra, whereas in fact, pharmacologically high dosages of some of these nutrients can drive inefficient enzymes to produce clinically meaningful improvements in life-threatening disorders. The signal example of this was the discovery that, in some neonates with refractory grand mal seizures, pharmacological dosages of pyridoxine (vitamin B6) can extinguish the seizures.

The mechanism: Some of these children have an inborn error in the enzyme glutamic acid decarboxylase (GAD), rendering it unable to decarboxylate the precursor amino acid glutamine into the inhibitory neurotransmitter GABA. It turns out that the high dosages of vitamin B6 will *saturate* the enzyme, driving its kinetics, so that it can finally churn out enough GABA to quench the seizures.

An analogy will help: A garden hose is sufficient for watering the garden and washing the car, but if the house is on fire, a *fire hose* is required to deliver the quantities of water (and with sufficient speed) to put out the fire. Enzymologists refer to this as a "mass effect." Below, we will be presenting an example of this mass effect phenomenon that applies to diabetes: Pharmacological dosages of the amino acid L-arginine enable the coronary arteries to produce enough nitric oxide (NO) so that the vessels can dilate to the point of relieving angina. Dietary (physiological) levels of the amino acid do not suffice.

There are a small number of supplements, in addition to arginine, that can play a major role in combating both acute and chronic inflammation in connection with hyperglycemia.

CAVEAT—This chapter details selected supplements that can reduce inflammation and lower blood glucose and/or protect the body where hyperglycemia has progressed to Type 2 diabetes. While the potential protective value of these supplements is presented here, no set of guidelines, or specific dosages, is given for supplementation. Supplementation decisions must be based on the evaluation of many factors in any given individual, and therefore, it is inappropriate for us to make blanket recommendations.

One reason among many for our not making blanket recommendations is that while there are many supplements that have value in helping to prevent or to treat hyperglycemia and/or lessen inflammation, some of them may actually interfere with effective prescription medication(s).

Depending on the type of treatment regimen used by any one individual in connection with hyperglycemia, or outright Type 2 diabetes, adding any dietary supplement(s) such as vitamins, minerals, and so on to daily diet must be done under the supervision of a qualified medical professional to ensure safety.

The use of supplements in adjunctive treatment of hyperglycemia relies on two sets of mechanisms: First, glycemic control by either promoting insulin action or reducing glucose absorption in the face of insulin insufficiency or resistance; second, supplements are generally antioxidants that, on their own, benefit endothelial, cardiovascular, and heart and related organ health.

Finally, many medical authorities have voiced dismissal of the use of supplements for their allegedly being based on "questionable science" or "outright quackery." The following selection of supplements will be shown to have been given the same scientific and clinical scrutiny, concerning efficacy and safety, as conventional medications, and the results of that scrutiny often appear in the same, often prestigious, medical journals as those of conventional medications. No functional food (in a previous chapter) or supplement is described in this book that does not meet these stringent criteria. Every functional food (in a previous chapter) and supplement described in this book meets the same stringent criteria: documentation in peer-reviewed journals, with discussion of meta-analyses wherever applicable.

13.2 MEASURING INSULIN SENSITIVITY AND INSULIN RESISTANCE: THE CLAMP TECHNIQUE AND THE ORAL GLUCOSE TOLERANCE TEST

The integrative/complementary approach to controlling blood glucose levels can entail the adjunctive use of a variety of supplements in order to either promote increased insulin sensitivity or reduce insulin resistance. "Insulin sensitivity" describes how sensitive the body is to the effects of insulin on the level of blood glucose. Someone who is insulin sensitive will require smaller amounts of insulin to lower blood glucose levels than someone who has low sensitivity. People with low insulin sensitivity, that is, "insulin resistance," will require larger amounts of insulin either from their own pancreas or from exogenous sources, in order to keep blood glucose stable.

Insulin resistance is said to occur when the body cells do not respond sufficiently to insulin. Insulin resistance is the primary cause of Type 2 diabetes (Gerich. 1999), and it is strongly associated with obesity; however, it is possible to be insulin resistant without being overweight or obese.

The *Journal of Hypertension* published a report titled "How to measure insulin sensitivity." According to the authors, there is a need for an accurate and reproducible method for measuring insulin resistance *in vivo*. The euglycemic insulin clamp is currently the best available standard technique. Two types of clamps are in common use:

The hyperglycemic clamp technique: The plasma glucose concentration is acutely raised to 125 mg/dL above basal levels by a continuous infusion of glucose. This hyperglycemic plateau is maintained by adjustment of a variable glucose infusion, based on the rate of insulin secretion and glucose metabolism. Because the plasma glucose concentration is held constant, the glucose infusion rate is an index of insulin secretion and glucose metabolism. The hyperglycemic clamps are often used to assess insulin secretion capacity (DeFronzo, Tobin, and Andres. 1979).

The hyperinsulinemic–euglycemic clamp technique: The plasma insulin concentration is acutely raised and maintained at 100 μU/mL by a continuous infusion of insulin. Meanwhile, the plasma glucose concentration is held constant at basal levels by a variable glucose infusion. When the steady state is achieved, the glucose infusion rate equals glucose uptake by all the tissues in the body and is therefore a measure of tissue insulin sensitivity.

Whereas homeostatic model assessment (HOMA) uses fasting plasma glucose and insulin concentrations to derive indices of insulin sensitivity and secretion from a mathematical model, other techniques are based on the exogenous infusion of glucose or insulin, or both, either under steady state (the insulin suppression test) or under dynamic conditions (insulin tolerance test, intravenous glucose tolerance test with minimal model analysis, and constant infusion of glucose with model assessment) (Ferrannini, and Mari. 1998).

There are two common approaches to evaluating insulin resistance. They are detailed in a report titled "Surrogate markers of insulin resistance: A review," published in the *World Journal of Diabetes*.

The oral glucose tolerance test involves the administration of glucose to determine how rapidly it is cleared from the bloodstream. It assesses the efficiency of the body to utilize glucose after glucose load.

After 8 to 10 h of fasting, blood glucose levels are determined at 0, 30, 60, and 120 min after a standard oral glucose load (75 g).

Measurement of the fasting insulin level is considered the most practical approach for the measurement of insulin resistance. It correlates well with insulin resistance. A significant correlation has been shown to exist between fasting insulin levels and insulin action as measured by the clamp technique.

Glucose levels change rapidly in the postprandial state; therefore, the use of fasting insulin for estimating insulin resistance should be done after an overnight fast. In relatively healthy individuals who are showing signs of symptoms of early-stage hyperglycemia, increased fasting insulin levels (with normal fasting glucose levels) correspond to insulin resistance.

It should be noted that the use of fasting insulin levels for assessment of insulin resistance is limited by a high proportion of false-positive results and by lack of standardization. To overcome this shortcoming, standardization of the insulin assay has been recommended by the American Diabetes Association Task Force, to be certified by a central laboratory. A high plasma insulin value in individuals with normal glucose tolerance reflects insulin resistance, and high insulin levels presage the development of diabetes (Singh, and Saxena. 2010).

13.3 ALPHA-LIPOIC ACID

Alpha-lipoic acid (ALA) is a naturally occurring compound created mostly in liver mitochondria from the precursor, octanoic acid (Hiltunen, Schonauer, Autio et al. 2009; Wollin, and Jones. 2003). It is principally a cofactor in the function of mitochondrial enzymes such as alpha-ketoglutarate dehydrogenase and pyruvate dehydrogenase (Shay, Moreau, Smith et al. 2009), and it also appears to be involved in the production of acetyl-CoA by oxidative decarboxylation of pyruvate (Reed. 1998).

13.3.1   The Pharmacology of the Antioxidant ALA

The journal *General Pharmacology* published a review of the pharmacology of ALA:

1. Lipoic acid is an example of an existing drug whose therapeutic effect has been related to its antioxidant activity.
2. Antioxidant activity is a relative concept: it depends on the kind of oxidative stress and the kind of oxidizable substrate (e.g., DNA, lipid, protein).
3. *In vitro*, the final antioxidant activity of lipoic acid is determined by its concentration and by its antioxidant properties. Four antioxidant properties of lipoic acid have been studied: its metal chelating capacity, its ability to scavenge reactive oxygen species (ROS), its ability to regenerate endogenous antioxidants, and its ability to repair oxidative damage.
4. Dihydrolipoic acid (DHLA), formed by reduction of lipoic acid, has more antioxidant properties than does lipoic acid. Both DHLA and lipoic acid have metal-chelating capacity and scavenge ROS, whereas only DHLA is able to regenerate endogenous antioxidants and to repair oxidative damage.
5. As a metal chelator, lipoic acid was shown to provide antioxidant activity by chelating Fe^{2+} and Cu^{2+}; DHLA can do so by chelating Cd^{2+}.
6. As scavengers of ROS, lipoic acid and DHLA display antioxidant activity in most experiments, whereas, in particular cases, pro-oxidant activity has been observed. However, lipoic acid can act as an antioxidant against the pro-oxidant activity produced by DHLA.
7. DHLA has the capacity to regenerate the endogenous antioxidants vitamin E, vitamin C, and glutathione.
8. DHLA can provide peptide methionine sulfoxide reductase with reducing equivalents. This enhances the repair of oxidatively damaged proteins such as alpha-1 antiprotease.
9. Through the lipoamide dehydrogenase-dependent reduction of lipoic acid, the cell can draw on its NADH pool for antioxidant activity additionally to its NADPH pool, which is usually consumed during oxidative stress.
10. Within drug-related antioxidant pharmacology, lipoic acid is a model compound that enhances understanding of the mode of action of antioxidants in drug therapy. (From Biewenga, Haenen, and Bast. 1997. *General Pharmacology*, Sep; 29(3): 315–331, with permission; see also Golbidi, Badran, and Laher. 2011. *Frontiers in Pharmacology*, 2: 69.)

13.3.2   Clinical Application of ALA as Antioxidant and Anti-Inflammatory

ALA is an antioxidant reducing peroxidation and increasing glutathione levels in the body or, alternatively, directly as an antioxidant like ascorbate. It can upregulate expression of one of the body's intrinsic antioxidant systems, glutathione (Bast, and Haenen. 1988), and supplementation can induce increased vitamin C uptake from the blood into the mitochondria, thus acting as a potentiator (Xu, and Wells. 1996). Most of the anti-inflammatory effects of ALA are mediated through its ability to inhibit nuclear factor kappa B (NF-κB), a nuclear transcription factor that, when activated, induces an inflammatory cascade (Packer, Witt, and Tritschler. 1995).

ALA inhibits the upregulation of intercellular adhesion molecule-1 (CAM-1) and vascular cell adhesion molecule-1 (VCAM-1), two pro-adhesion cytokines, in models of spinal injury, at concentrations of 25 to 100 µg/mL, doses seen as therapeutic, and well above the concentrations that would be achieved by typical reported oral doses of 600 mg/day (Chaudhary, Marracci, and Bourdette. 2006; Kunt, Forst, Wilhelm et al. 1999).

It would seem that the mechanism by which ALA inhibits NF-κB activity is further upstream than TNF-α inhibition, which is the way that many antioxidants work. What's more, the anti-inflammatory effect of ALA is independent of TNF-α modulation (Zhang, and Frei. 2001).

Oxidative stress plays an important role in chronic inflammation by provoking early adverse vascular events in atherogenesis, including the upregulation of vascular adhesion molecules, and matrix metalloproteinase activity. These events involve the activation of the transcription factor NF-κB that induces expression of many genes involved in inflammation and endothelial cell migration. ALA inhibits its expression *in vitro* (Kim, Kim, Park et al. 2007; Packer, Witt, and Tritschler. 1995).

Given the oxidative basis of inflammation, strategies aimed at reducing oxidant damage have long been of concern in connection with various models of inflammation (Shay, Moreau, Smith et al. 2009; Kunt, Forst, Wilhelm et al. 1999).

Similarly, collagen-induced arthritis was attenuated by ALA at dosage concentrations of 10 to 100 mg/kg i.p. in DBA/1 mice, by reduction of inflammatory cytokines like TNF-α, and partial inhibition of NF-κB binding to DNA (Lee, Lee, Lee et al. 2007). However, ALA inhibits TNF-α–induced NF-κB activation and adhesion molecule expression in human aortic endothelial cells *via* a mechanism different from those of antioxidants such as ascorbate, or reduced GSH, but consistent with the workings of a metal chelator (Zhang, and Frei. 2001).

Although anti-inflammatory properties of ALA have been less commonly investigated in humans, the Irbesartan and ALA in the Endothelial Dysfunction (ISLAND) trial, reported in a study published in the journal *Clinical Cardiology*, showed a significant decrease in serum IL-6 levels following 4 weeks of supplementation with ALA. This finding may prove relevant to human health application because IL-6 is a recognized marker of inflammation in coronary atherosclerotic plaques, and it also regulates the expression of other inflammatory cytokines such as IL-1 and TNF-α (Ikeda, Ito, and Shimada. 2001).

In the "ISLAND" study cited above, the investigators aimed to determine whether irbesartan, an angiotensin receptor blocker, and ALA could improve endothelial function and reduce inflammation in patients with metabolic syndrome. Patients were administered either irbesartan at 150 mg/day, ALA at 300 mg/day, both irbesartan and ALA, or matching placebo, in conventional double-blind control strategies, for 4 weeks. Endothelium-dependent and -independent flow-mediated vasodilation (FMD) was determined under standard conditions.

FMD is a measure of endothelial function in vasodilation: During an FMD test, blood circulation in an arm is arrested by suprasystolic cuff occlusion for a period of time. Then, pressure is released and there follows an acute increase in blood flow, evaluated by an ultrasound Doppler device (Harris, Nishiyama, Wray et al. 2010).

Plasma levels of IL-6, plasminogen activator-1, and 8-isoprostane were measured. Compared to the placebo group, after 4 weeks of treatment, endothelium-dependent FMD of the brachial artery was increased by 67% in the irbesartan group, 44% in the ALA group, and 75% in the combined irbesartan plus ALA group. Treatment with irbesartan and/or ALA was found to cause statistically significant reductions in plasma levels of IL-6 and plasminogen activator-1. In addition, treatment with irbesartan or irbesartan plus ALA decreased 8-isoprostane levels. No significant changes in blood pressure were noted in any of the study groups.

The investigators concluded that irbesartan and/or ALA administered to patients with metabolic syndrome improves endothelial function and reduces proinflammatory markers, factors that are implicated also in the pathogenesis of atherosclerosis (Sola, Mir, Cheema et al. 2005).

13.3.3 THE ANTIDIABETIC PROPERTIES OF ALA

Diabetes confers a considerable risk of microvascular and macrovascular complications that typically entail a lower quality of life and could lower life expectancy as well (Wild, Roglic, Green et al. 2004). These complications can be delayed by achieving adequate glycemic control, as demonstrated by the Diabetes Control and Complications Trial, the Epidemiology of Diabetes Interventions and Complications, and UKPDS (No authors listed. 1993; No authors listed. 2005; Stratton, Adler, Neil et al. 2005). As previously noted, it has been reported that good glycemic control is very difficult to achieve in routine clinical practice (Gomes, Giannella-Neto, Faria et al. 2006).

The *Journal of Clinical and Diagnostic Research* reported a study where three groups of Type 2 diabetes patients were given different antioxidants combined with metformin and glimeperide, for 3 months. The dosages were: ALA 300 mg/daily, eicosapentanoic acid 180 mg plus docohexaenoic acid 120 mg/daily (omega 3 fatty acids), or vitamin E 400 mg/daily.

It was found that ALA, omega 3 fatty acids, and vitamin E each resulted in improvement in insulin sensitivity. Although improvement in glycosylated hemoglobin (HbA1c), weight, and waist measures have also been observed with administration of ALA, omega 3 fatty acids resulted in even greater weight loss and glycemic control (Udupa, Nahar, Shah et al. 2012).

A study, published in the *Asia Pacific Journal of Clinical Nutrition*, aimed to determine the effectiveness of oral supplementation of DL-ALA on glycemic and oxidative status in Type 2 diabetes patients. They were assigned to either placebo or treatment with various doses of ALA (300, 600, 900, and 1200 mg/day) for 6 months. After the treatment, all patients were evaluated for glucose status and oxidative biomarkers.

It was found that fasting blood glucose and HbA1c showed a significant dose-dependent decrease in all treatment groups. An increase in urinary PGF2α-isoprostanes was noted in the placebo group, but not in the ALA–treated groups, suggesting the suppressing action of ALA on lipid peroxidation in diabetes patients. However, 8-hydroxy-2'-deoxyguanosine as well as urinary microalbumin and serum creatinine levels were similar in both placebo and ALA groups.

Results from this study were said to support the benefits of ALA on blood glucose status, with a slight reduction in oxidative stress–related deterioration in diabetes patients (Porasuphatana, Suddee, Nartnampong et al. 2012).

A table appearing in Gomes, and Negrato (2014) (*Diabetology and Metabolic Syndrome*, 6: 80) that summarizes a number of "Clinical studies with ALA in patients with diabetes" can be viewed at https://www. ncbi.nlm.nih.gov/pmc/articles/PMC412 4142/table/Tab2/ (accessed 10.28.17).

13.3.4 DIETARY UPTAKE, SAFETY, AND TOXICITY

Typical food sources of ALA are muscle meats, heart, kidney, and liver, and, to a lesser degree, fruits and vegetables (Shay, Moreau, Smith et al. 2009). Body cells actively maintain transport, utilization, and excretion of nonprotein-bound ALA. Though available from these normal food sources, it is not likely that appreciable amounts of ALA are consumed in the typical Western diet; rather, dietary supplements that typically range from 50 to 600 mg are the primary sources of it, and most of the information about its bioavailability comes from studies using supplements.

A number of "Select clinical trials using lipoic acid (LA)," listing doses administered to human participants, and the parameters observed, including possible health effects, can be found in a table in Shay, Moreau, Smith et al. (2009) (*Biochimica et Biophysica Acta*, Oct; 1790(10): 1149–1160; https://www.ncbi.nlm.nih.gov/pmc/articles/PMC2756 298/table/T3/; accessed 10.29.17).

The ALA in diabetic neuropathy (ALADIN I, II, and III), symptoms of diabetic polyneuropathy (SYDNEY I and II), and oral pilot (ORPIL) clinical trials used supplements of ALA up to 2400 mg/day with no reported adverse effects, and as reported in the journal *Diabetologia*, it has also been administered intravenously in doses of 600 mg/day for 3 weeks, with no evidence of serious side effects. Additionally, oral doses of 1800 mg (600 mg tid), for 6 months, did not elicit significant adverse effects compared to placebo (Ziegler, Hanefeld, Ruhnau et al. 1999).

It should be noted that ALA has been used in Germany for more than 50 years as a treatment for diabetic neuropathy and retinopathy. However, the data obtained by the investigators (Ziegler, Hanefeld, Ruhnau et al. 1995), published in the journal *Diabetes Care*, do not support that application. They concluded that: "… a 3-week intravenous treatment with ALA, followed by a 6-month oral treatment, had no effect on neuropathic symptoms distinguishable from placebo to a clinically meaningful degree.…"

There are, nevertheless, studies that do support the therapeutic role of ALA in neuropathy—some, for instance, are reported in journals such as *The Review of Diabetic Studies* (Vallianou, Evangelopoulos, and Koutalas. 2009), *Diabetes Care* (Ziegler, Ametov, Barinov et al. 2006), *International Journal of Endocrinology* (Mijnhout, Kollen, Alkhalaf et al. 2012), and *Expert Opinion on Pharmacotherapy* (Papanas, and Ziegler. 2014).

13.3.5 ALA IN TREATMENT OF DIABETIC POLYNEUROPATHY

The ALADIN trials and the SYDNEY trials were conducted to determine the value of racemic (DL-) ALA in decreasing severity of diabetic polyneuropathies. ALA was administered orally, intravenously, or intravenously with oral follow-up.

The journal *Diabetic Medicine* reported a meta-analysis of clinical trials using intravenous alpha-lipoic acid including the ALADIN, the SYDNEY, and the first 3 weeks of ALADIN III, which showed a significant improvement in diabetic polyneuropathies of the feet and lower limbs in patients infused with ALA at a dosage of 600 mg/day, for 3 weeks (Ziegler, Nowak, Kempler et al. 2004).

The journal *Free Radical Research* reported that diabetic patients in the ALADIN II trial were administered ALA intravenously at 600 or 1200 mg/day, for 5 days, and then orally for 2 years, resulting in improved indices of neuropathy (Reljanovic, Reichel, Rett et al. 1999).

Patients in the ALADIN III study received 600 mg/day i.v. or placebo for 3 weeks, followed by oral 600 mg t.i.d. or placebo for 6 months. The oral phase of this trial, however, was without clinically significant benefits (Ziegler, Hanefeld, Ruhnau et al. 1999).

One possible conclusion from these studies is that ALA is more effective when administered intravenously than orally. This is thought possibly due to either greater bioavailability or poor solubility of the medication in the stomach acid. The authors of this work speculated that the discrepancies could be due to different formulations of ALA being used in the different studies. The active agent may not have been sufficiently bioavailable in some of those formulations, and/or their excipients may have been present in some of them, which could have interfered with functionality.

Nevertheless, studies in addition to those listed above have found that oral administration can be very effective. For example, the ORPIL study, published in the journal *Diabetes Care*, showed a reduction in diabetic polyneuropathic symptoms after 3 weeks, with 600 mg/day (Ametov, Barinov, Dyck et al. 2003).

The first SYDNEY trial used intravenous ALA, and the SYDNEY II study, also published in *Diabetes Care*, used oral administration at 600, 1200, or 1800 mg q.d., for 5 weeks (Ziegler, Ametov, Barinov et al. 2006). Both studies reported significant improvements in neuropathic endpoints.

13.4   L-ARGININE

The body uses the amino acid L-arginine in the biosynthesis of proteins and in the elimination of excess ammonia. As noted in a previous chapter, L-arginine is one of the substrates from which the endothelium forms NO. NO is also formed from nitrates/nitrite, as well as from the amino acid citrulline. In humans, L-arginine is classified as a semiessential or conditionally essential amino acid, depending on the developmental stage and health status of a given individual.

Dietary sources are animal products, including meats, dairy, and eggs, and plant sources, such as seeds of all types, grains, beans, and nuts (Fried, and Merrell. 1999; Fried. 2014; Fried, and Nezin. 2017). The typical Western diet supplies about 5 g of L-arginine each day, and most common disease conditions do not significantly reduce plasma levels, though there are exceptions. These include conditions causing deficiency of the enzyme arginase that catalyzes the hydrolysis of L-arginine to produce L-ornithine and urea (Morris. 2012). When consuming L-arginine in foods or in supplements, more than half is taken up by macrophages in the digestive system, and the rest is transported throughout the body.

The effects of oral L-arginine consumption were detailed in the *British Journal of Clinical Pharmacology* in a study to investigate its pharmacological effects in healthy men after a single intravenous infusion of either 6 or 30 g and after a single oral dose of 6 g, compared to placebo.

Plasma L-arginine levels rose, and blood pressure and total peripheral resistance declined significantly after intravenous infusion of the higher dose (30 g) of L-arginine, but these parameters were not significantly changed after oral administration or after intravenous administration of the lower dose (6 g). Thirty grams also significantly increased urinary nitrate and cyclic guanosine monophosphate (cGMP) excretion rates.

cGMP is a cyclic nucleotide derived from guanosine triphosphate. cGMP acts as a second messenger much like cyclic adenosine monophosphate (cAMP). cGMP is the intrinsic vasodilator of vascular smooth muscle, leading to increased blood flow.

After infusion of 6 g of L-arginine, urinary nitrate excretion also significantly increased, although to a lesser and more variable extent than after 30 g.

The investigators concluded that the vascular effects of L-arginine seem closely correlated with its plasma concentrations (Bode-Böger, Böger, Galland et al. 1998).

NO is formed from L-arginine by the NO synthase (NOS) enzymes, using the co-factor tetrahydrobiopterin (BH4). NO functions as a neurotransmitter in the brain, is essential to immune system function, and is crucial to the blood vessel endothelium, where it mediates vasodilation.

In a report published in *The Journal of Nutrition*, titled "The Pharmacodynamics of L-Arginine," the author reports that the effects of L-arginine supplementation on human physiology appear to be multicausal and dose related. Doses of 3 to 8 g/day appear to be safe and not to cause acute pharmacologic effects (Böger. 2007). Among other effects—and these will be detailed below—L-arginine supplementation has been shown to lower blood pressure, to reduce and even prevent the impact of atherosclerosis, to ameliorate heart disease, to lower body weight and decrease insulin resistance, to counter oxidative stress, to reduce the severity of metabolic syndrome, and to ameliorate age-related erectile dysfunction (the latter being a reflection in part of poor NO production in the endothelium of the *cavernous* erectile tissues).

In 1996, the *Journal of the American College of Cardiology* published a study titled "Aging-associated endothelial dysfunction in humans is reversed by L-arginine." This was one of the earlier studies of the hypothesis that aging impairs endothelium-dependent function and that the process may be reversible by L-arginine.

In that study, the endothelium-independent vasodilators papaverine and glyceryl trinitrate and the endothelium-dependent vasodilator acetylcholine were variously infused into the left coronary artery of patients ranging between the ages of 27 and 73, who had atypical chest pain and poor exercise test results. However, these patients had completely normal findings on coronary angiography and no coronary risk factors. Coronary blood flow was measured with an intracoronary Doppler catheter.

The papaverine and acetylcholine infusions were repeated in some of the patients after intracoronary infusion of L-arginine.

The investigators reported an initially significant inverse relationship between age and the peak coronary blood flow response evoked by acetylcholine. However, there was no correlation with age of the response to papaverine and glyceryl trinitrate. However, the peak coronary blood flow response evoked by acetylcholine correlated significantly with aging before L-arginine infusion, and this inverse relationship disappeared after infusion.

The results suggested that aging selectively impairs endothelium-dependent coronary vascular function and that this impairment can be restored by intracoronary infusion of L-arginine (Chauhan, More, Mullins et al. 1995).

In this study, an "aged" endothelium responded to L-arginine as would a "younger" one, suggesting that there may be benefits to L-arginine supplementation even where one is aged but is not suffering from cardiovascular disease. However, the question arises: Would coronary blood flow benefit from oral supplementation?

A study published in the journal *Vascular Medicine* aimed to determine whether oral L-arginine can improve impaired endothelial function as measured by the FMD method in healthy "very old people."

Healthy participants, approximately 74 years old on average (±2.7 years), were given 8 g of L-arginine to consume orally, twice per day. Another group was given placebo. Treatment and placebo regimen were continued for 14 days, separated by a washout period of 14 days.

It was found that L-arginine significantly improved FMD, whereas placebo had no effect. After L-arginine supplementation, plasma levels of L-arginine increased significantly, but placebo had no effect. As NO synthesis can be antagonized by its endogenous inhibitor, asymmetric dimethyl L-arginine (ADMA), it was determined that ADMA plasma concentrations were elevated at baseline. ADMA remained unchanged during treatment, but L-arginine supplementation normalized the L-arginine/ADMA ratio (ADMA is detailed below).

The investigators concluded that in healthy "very old age," endothelial function is impaired and may nevertheless be improved by oral L-arginine supplementation, probably due to normalization of the L-arginine/ADMA ratio (Bode-Böger, Muke, Surdacki et al. 2003). It is now well known that NO plays a crucial biological role in the body, and it has been shown to

- Lower blood pressure (Bode-Böger, Bogera, Creutzig et al. 1994. *Clinical Science*, 87; 303–310)
- Reduce the workload of the heart (Rector, Bank, Mullen et al. 1996. *Circulation*, Jun; 93: 2135–2141)
- Function as an antioxidant, preventing platelet aggregation (Wolf, Zalpour, Theilmeier et al. 1997. *Journal of the American College of Cardiology*, Mar; 29(3): 479–485)
- Reduce insulin resistance in Type 2 diabetes (Piatti, Monti, Valsecchi et al. 2001. *Diabetes Care*, May; 24(5): 875–880)

13.4.1 NO Bioavailability Naturally Declines with Age

Progressive age-related decline in NO bioavailability is thought to occur naturally and it corresponds to progressive age-related endothelial impairment and associated cardiovascular risks. What's more, it also plays an adverse role in diabetes.

The website "*Integrative Practitioner*" featured a comprehensive report titled "The role of NO insufficiency in aging & disease" by Dr. NS Bryan, Department of Molecular and Human Genetics, Baylor College of Medicine, Houston, Texas. The report states that age is the most significant predictor of NO insufficiency because we gradually lose the ability to produce NO over the life span (see also Gerhard, Roddy, Creager et al. 1996): By the time we are about 40 years old, we are producing about half of the NO output at age 10, and by age 60, it is down to 15%.

Dr. Bryan concurs with previously presented evidence of a link between progressive age-related structural and functional changes that are a hallmark of hypertension and other cardiovascular risk factors. The article cites the clinical reports that show there to be

- A gradual decline in endothelial function due to aging, with greater than 50% loss in endothelial function in the oldest age group tested, as measured by forearm blood flow assays (Taddei, Virdis, Ghiadoni et al. 2001)
- A loss of 75% of endothelium-derived NO in 70- to 80-year-old patients compared to young, healthy 20-year-olds (Egashira, Inou, Hirooka et al., 1993)
- Evidence of the upregulation of arginase in aged blood vessels (i.e., increased metabolic degradation of the amino acid) and the corresponding changes of NOS activity (Berkowitz, White, Li et al. 2003)

13.4.2 The Arginine Paradox

The "arginine paradox" describes the dependence of cellular NO production on exogenous (outside source) L-arginine concentration, despite the saturation of the NOS enzyme with intracellular L-arginine.

It is a consideration in connection with the merits of supplementation: In ordinary circumstances, deficiency of L-arginine is uncommon (Gad. 2010). This raises the question, "Why supplement it?"

The enzyme eNOS is ordinarily saturated with intracellular L-arginine, and therefore, endothelial NO synthesis should not, in theory, respond to alterations in extracellular L-arginine concentrations. However, despite saturation, increasing extracellular L-arginine concentrations increases NO production in (cultured) endothelial cells in a dose-dependent manner. Furthermore, elevating plasma L-arginine levels has been shown to enhance vascular NO production *in vivo* (Lee, Ryu, Ferrante et al. 2003).

The journal of the Japanese Pharmacological Society, *Nihon Yakurigaku Zasshi*, published several theories intended to explain the phenomenon but concluded that none of them explains fully how exogenous L-arginine causes NO-mediated biological effects despite the fact that NOSs are theoretically saturated with L-arginine (Nakaki, and Hishikawa. 2002).

13.4.3   MEASURING NO CONCENTRATION DIRECTLY AFTER L-ARGININE SUPPLEMENTATION

Because NO is detectable in the exhaled air of normal individuals, it is possible to monitor the concentration after supplementation. As reported in the journal *Clinical Science (London)*, oral L-arginine supplementation at doses of 0.1 and 0.2 mg/kg causes significant increase in the concentration of NO in exhaled air, which was maximal 2 h after administration. This rise in concentration is associated with an increase in the concentration of L-arginine and nitrate in plasma. An increase in the amount of substrate (L-arginine) for NOS can increase the formation of endogenous NO (Kharitonov, Lubec, Lubec et al. 1995).

Parenthetically, indirect estimates of NO concentration in the body, based on nitrate excretion, are conventionally labeled NOx, rather than NO (Fried. 2014).

In a study appearing in the journal *Chest*, healthy men received a 30-min infusion of 0.5 g/kg L-arginine hydrochloride. Blood pressure and heart rate were continuously monitored in addition to intermittent measures of mixed expired NO concentration, as well as plasma L-arginine and L-citrulline levels (important because L-arginine can be metabolized to L-citrulline).

Infused L-arginine caused a significant fall in blood pressure and raised mixed expired NO concentration, an increase in the rate of pulmonary NO expulsion, as well as a rise in plasma L-citrulline. There was a significant correlation between the hypotensive response to L-arginine and the increase in expired NO. The hypotensive effect of L-arginine in humans appears to be mediated, at least in part, by NOS metabolism of L-arginine and increased endogenous NO production, as indicated both by increased plasma L-citrulline and by increased expired NO (Mehta, Stewart, and Levy, 1996).

13.4.4   ORAL L-ARGININE REDUCES INFLAMMATION

A study published in *Cardiovascular Pharmacology* aimed to determine the effects of long-term L-arginine supplementation on arterial compliance, along with inflammatory and metabolic parameters, in patients with multiple cardiovascular risk factors. Patients were assigned to daily oral L-arginine, or matching placebo capsules. They were evaluated for lipid profile, glucose, HbA1C, insulin, hs-CRP, renin, and aldosterone. Arterial elasticity was evaluated with pulse wave contour analysis (HDI CR 2000, Eagan, Minnesota).

Pulse wave contour analysis provides a measure of the function and output of the heart as well as the degree of elasticity of blood vessels. It is detailed in Chapter 2. Large artery elasticity index did not differ significantly between the groups at baseline, but at the end of the study, it was significantly greater in patients treated with L-arginine than in the placebo group. Systemic vascular resistance was significantly lower in patients treated with L-arginine than in the placebo group after 6 months. Small artery elasticity index did not differ significantly between the groups at baseline or at the end of the study. Serum aldosterone decreased significantly in the treatment group, but it did not change in the placebo group.

The investigators concluded that oral L-arginine supplementation improves large artery elasticity in patients with multiple cardiovascular risk factors. This improvement was associated with a decrease in systolic blood pressure, in peripheral vascular resistance, and in aldosterone levels. The results suggested that long-term L-arginine supplementation has beneficial vascular effects in conditions associated with endothelial dysfunction (Guttman, Zimlichman, Boaz et al. 2010).

13.4.5   ORAL L-ARGININE IMPROVES DAMAGED AND AGING ENDOTHELIUM

Endothelial dysfunction, as detected by FMD, declines with age in healthy people, just as NO formation declines with age (Yavuz, Yavuz, Sener et al. 2008; see also Welsch, Dobrosielski, Arce-Esquivel et al. 2008).

According to a review titled "L-Arginine as a nutritional prophylaxis against vascular endothelial dysfunction with aging," published in the *Journal of Cardiovascular Pharmacology and Therapeutics*, "With advancing age, peripheral conduit and resistance arteries lose the ability to effectively dilate owing to endothelial dysfunction. This vascular senescence contributes to increased risk of cardiovascular disease (CVD) with aging."

The review also reports that oral L-arginine should be considered a "novel" nutritional strategy to reduce progression of vascular dysfunction with aging and cardiovascular disease. Emphasis is placed on the ability of L-arginine to modulate the vascular inflammatory and systemic hormonal factors, which may result in a positive effect on vascular endothelial function (Heffernan, Fahs, Ranadive et al. 2010).

13.4.5.1   The Role of ADMA in Endothelial Dysfunction and Type 2 Diabetes

There is another component of the inflammation/endothelial dysfunction scenario not previously mentioned: In a study published in the journal *Clinical Science* (*Lond.*), investigators emphasized the importance of the ratio of L-arginine to asymmetric dimethylarginine ADMA in endothelial dysfunction and systemic inflammation (Shivkar, and Abhang. 2014). This study targeted coronary artery disease (CAD) patients.

ADMA is formed by the continuous turnover of protein in body cells, and it makes its way into the blood. It appears to be the body's natural NO antagonist, keeping NO synthesis in check by its inhibition of NOS. When it dominates, ADMA reduces NO bioavailability to the detriment of a number of major cardiovascular functions (Fried. 2014).

Researchers writing in the journal *Hormones and Metabolism Research* confirmed that elevated ADMA levels cause eNOS uncoupling, leading to lower NO bioavailability and higher production of ROS, especially hydrogen peroxide. They contend that the administration of L-arginine to patients with high ADMA levels improves NO synthesis by antagonizing the harmful effect of ADMA on eNOS function (Toutouzas, Riga, and Stefanadi, 2008).

In a study published in the journal *Clinical Science (London)*, the investigators reported aiming to determine the effects of altered levels of L-arginine and asymmetric ω-NG,NG-dimethylarginin, which, as said previously, is the inhibitor of NOS. Plasma concentrations of arginine and ADMA, the inflammatory markers CRP, myeloperoxidase (MPO), and oxidized low-density lipoprotein (oxLDL) were measured in a group of men and a group of women participants from a population-based cohort ranging in age between 50 and 87 years.

The arginine/ADMA ratio decreased significantly across increasing tertiles of CRP and MPO. These negative associations remained statistically significant in a linear regression model with both MPO and CRP as independent variables and adjusted for age, gender, and cardiovascular risk factors.

In a fully adjusted regression model, MPO was positively associated with ADMA, whereas CRP was not. Conversely, in a fully adjusted model, CRP was negatively associated with L-arginine without a significant contribution of MPO.

The relationship between MPO and ADMA became stronger with increasing levels of oxLDL, consistent with the ability of MPO to amplify oxidative stress. In contrast, the relationship between CRP and arginine was not modified by levels of oxLDL.

The investigators concluded that an unfavorable NOS substrate/inhibitor ratio may contribute to the reduced NO bioavailability associated with inflammation (van der Zwan, Scheffer, Dekker et al. 2011).

Numerous publications report that supplementation with L-arginine restores vascular function and improves the clinical symptoms in various diseases that are associated with vascular dysfunction linked to elevated concentrations of ADMA (Böger, and Ron. 2005).

To the point: The Landmark Edition of the journal *Frontiers in Bioscience* reported a study titled "L-arginine, NO and asymmetrical dimethylarginine in hypertension and type 2 diabetes." The investigators acknowledge that a high-fat diet and a carbohydrate-rich diet enhance serum ADMA levels, increasing the body levels of an endogenous inhibitor of NO synthesis.

Furthermore, ADMA levels were found to be elevated in patients with hypertension, poor control of hyperglycemia, diabetic microangiopathy and macroangiopathy, and dyslipidemia (Das, Repossi, Dain et al. 2011).

One of the earliest signs of vascular dysfunction and insulin resistance, which are present in hypertension and Type 2 diabetes, is an elevation in serum ADMA levels. Displacing plasma ADMA by oral supplementation of L-arginine overcomes endothelial dysfunction by augmenting endothelial NO generation. Furthermore, strict control of hyperglycemia decreases serum ADMA levels (Das, Repossi, Dain et al. 2011).

13.4.6   L-ARGININE, INSULIN RESISTANCE, AND TYPE 2 DIABETES

Type 2 diabetes is linked to NO deficiency and endothelial dysfunction. Since insufficiency of the substrate, L-arginine, is unlikely, the deficiency must be in the endothelial synthesis pathway. In a study published in the journal *Clinical Investigation*, the authors concluded that "Hyperglycemia inhibits endothelial NO synthase activity by posttranslational modification at the Akt site"—the title of their publication (Du, Edelstein, Dimmeler et al. 2001).

Interestingly, they also reported that chronic impairment of eNOS activity by this mechanism may partly explain the accelerated atherosclerosis of diabetes. This is, of course, a hypothesis—one that was presented earlier in this book.

Amino acids are important modulators of glucose metabolism, insulin secretion, and insulin sensitivity. However, relatively little is known about the changes in amino acid metabolism in patients with diabetes.

In a study titled "Selective amino acid deficiency in patients with impaired glucose tolerance and type 2 diabetes," appearing in the journal *Regulatory Peptides*, the circulating amino acid levels were determined in patients, in nondiabetes participants with impaired glucose tolerance and in control participants.

Patients with Type 2 diabetes were found to have significant reductions in the concentrations of various amino acids including L-arginine. The plasma levels of essential amino acids were positively related to fasting and post-challenge glucose levels, HOMA insulin resistance, and fasting glucagon levels (Menge, Schrader, Ritter et al. 2010).

HOMA: A computer-solved model predicts plasma glucose and insulin concentrations arising from varying degrees of β-cell deficiency and insulin resistance. Comparison of a patient's fasting values with the model's predictions allows a quantitative assessment of the contributions of insulin resistance and deficient β-cell function to the fasting hyperglycemia (Matthews, Hosker, Rudenski et al. 1985, *Diabetologia*, Jul; 28(7), 412–419).

13.4.7   ORAL SUPPLEMENTATION OF L-ARGININE IN ADJUNCTIVE TREATMENT OF TYPE 2 DIABETES

A clinical study published in the *American Journal of Physiology Endocrinology and Metabolism* aimed to evaluate the effects of a long-term oral L-arginine therapy on adipose fat mass, muscle free-fat mass distribution, daily glucose levels, insulin sensitivity, endothelial function, oxidative stress, and adipokine release in obese Type 2 diabetic patients with insulin resistance, who were treated with a combination of hypocaloric diet and exercise training.

The patients, participating in a hypocaloric diet plus an exercise training program for 21 days, were assigned to one of two groups: the first group, also treated with L-arginine (8.3 g/day), and the second group, given placebo.

Long-term oral L-arginine treatment resulted in an additive improvement on glucose metabolism and insulin sensitivity, compared to a diet and exercise training program alone. Furthermore, it improved endothelial function, reduced oxidative stress, and reduced adipokine release in obese Type 2 diabetic patients with insulin resistance (Lucotti, Setola, Monti et al. 2001). A study published in the journal *Diabetes Care* reported that in lean patients with Type 2 diabetes, L-arginine treatment significantly improved, but did not completely normalize, insulin sensitivity (Piatti, Monti, Valsecchi et al. 2001).

Here are several of the many studies that report the benefits of oral L-arginine supplementation:

- The journal *Free Radical Biology and Medicine* published a study where patients with diabetes received two daily dosages of 1 g L-arginine free base for 3 months. Treatment reduced the lipid peroxidation product malondialdehyde, evidence that treatment with L-arginine may counteract lipid peroxidation and thus reduce microangiopathic long-term complications in diabetes (Lubec, Hayn, Kitzmüller et al. 1977).
- In a study published in the *European Journal of Clinical Investigation*, healthy participants versus patients with obesity and Type 2 diabetes were given low-dose intravenous supplementation of L-arginine (0.52 mg kg^{-1} min^{-1}) to note the effect on insulin-mediated vasodilation and insulin sensitivity measured by venous occlusion plethysmography during the insulin suppression test, evaluating insulin sensitivity. L-arginine restored the impaired insulin-mediated vasodilation observed in obesity and in non–insulin-dependent diabetes. Insulin sensitivity improved significantly in all three groups. Results suggest that defective insulin-mediated vasodilation in obesity and NIDDM can be normalized by intravenous L-arginine. Furthermore, L-arginine improved insulin sensitivity in obese patients and NIDDM patients as well as in healthy participants, indicating a possible mechanism that is different from the restoration of insulin-mediated vasodilation (Wascher, Graier, Dittrich et al. 1997).
- The journal *Amino Acids* reported that dietary L-arginine supplementation reduces adiposity in obese people with Type 2 diabetes and that it holds great promise as a safe and cost-effective nutrient to reduce adiposity, increase muscle mass, and improve the metabolic profile (McKnight, Satterfield, Jobgen et al. 2010).

13.4.8 CAVEAT

In the studies cited here, supplementation of L-arginine (in whatever form) was undertaken in clinical settings with medical supervision. Based on these studies, it appears that oral L-arginine consumed in the dosages per time period indicated is safe and well tolerated.

The suggested oral dosages proposed by the Mayo Clinic (http://www.mayoclinic.com /health/l-arginine/NS_patient-rginine/DSECTION=safety), that is, maximum dose considered to be safe, are 400 to 6000 mg. These dosages are given here for information purposes only. It is not possible to know what is a safe and effective dosage for any purpose, in any given person, at any given time.

Mild—and occasionally severe—adverse reactions have been reported for L-arginine. In fact, the wife of one of the authors of this book (RMC) took a 500-mg capsule of arginine at one point, and within an hour, she suffered from severe migraine headache—and she is not at all prone to migraines. It appeared that the NO generated by the arginine may have overdilated cranial vessels.

There are also contraindications for supplementation as is the case, for instance, for anyone who now has or has ever had herpes. An abbreviated list of foods to be avoided because they are high in L-arginine can be found on these websites:

- http://herpes.com/Nutrition.shtml
- http://www.kitchentablemedicine.com/eating-to-reduce-herpes-outbreaks/
- https://hsvblog.org/herpes-blog/diet-lifestyle-tips/chart-of-lysine-vs-arginine-in-common
  -foods/

The authors of this book cite these websites as simple guidelines, but cannot guarantee the accuracy of their reports. Accurate arginine/lysine content of foods, on the other hand, can be seen on the website of the United States Department of Agriculture, Agricultural Research Service, USDA Food Composition Databases, Nutrient Lists: https://ndb.nal.usda.gov/ndb/nutrients/report?nutrien t1=505&nutrient2=511&nutrient3=&fg=&max=25&subset=0&offset=0&sort=c&totCount=5055& measureby=m; accessed 11.26.17.

Furthermore, neither do the authors of this book endorse any products advertised on the above-mentioned nongovernmental websites.

13.5   L-CARNITINE

Carnitine is the generic term for a number of compounds derived from a particular amino acid and found in nearly all cells of the body. It includes L-carnitine, acetyl-L-carnitine, and propionyl-L-carnitine. It is found concentrated in tissues such as skeletal and cardiac muscles that are fueled by long-chain fatty acids.

Carnitine plays a critical role in energy production. It transports long-chain fatty acids into the mitochondria to support metabolism, and it prevents accumulation of toxic compounds by expelling them from the mitochondria (Rebouche. 1999; No authors listed. 2004). Carnitine occurs in two isomeric forms (molecular mirror images), D and L. Only L-carnitine is active in the body, and it is the form found in food.

Most people make sufficient carnitine to meet the body's needs. However, for genetic or medical reasons, some individuals (such as preterm infants) cannot make enough, and so, for them, carnitine is a conditionally essential nutrient (Rebouche. 1999).

Animal products like meat, fish, poultry, and milk are the best sources. In general, the more *red* the meat, the higher its carnitine content. Dairy products contain carnitine primarily in the whey fraction (Rebouche. 2004).

13.5.1   THE BENEFITS OF L-CARNITINE SUPPLEMENTATION IN TYPE 2 DIABETES

Insulin resistance may spring from a defect in fatty acid oxidation in muscle (Mingrone. 2004). Early research suggests that intravenous supplementation with L-carnitine may improve insulin sensitivity in diabetes by decreasing fat levels in muscle and it may lower glucose levels in the blood by increasing its oxidation in cells (Mingrone. 2004; De Gaetano, Mingrone, Castagneto et al. 1999; Mingrone, Greco, Capristo et al. 1999).

An analysis of two multicenter clinical trials of patients with either Type 1 or Type 2 diabetes, published in the journal *Diabetes Care*, found that treatment with acetyl-L-carnitine, 3 g/day orally, for 1 year, resulted in significant relief of nerve pain in patients suffering from diabetic neuropathy. The treatment was found to be most effective in patients with Type 2 diabetes of short duration (Sima, Calvani, Mehra et al. 2005).

A review and meta-analysis of the metabolic effects of L-carnitine on type 2 diabetes, published in the journal *Experimental and Clinical Endocrinology and Diabetes*, concluded that administration of L-carnitine is associated with an improvement in glycemia and plasma lipids. That review and analysis centered on PubMed, Trip Database, and Cochrane Library, and selected those that had adequate methodological quality based on the Jadad scale.

It was found that oral L-carnitine significantly lowered fasting plasma glucose, total cholesterol, LDL, apolipoprotein-B100, and apolipoprotein-A1. However, the changes in triglycerides, lipoprotein (a), or HbA1c were not significant (Vidal-Casariego, Burgos-Peláez, Martínez-Faedo et al. 2013).

A study published in the *European Journal of Clinical Nutrition* aimed to determine the effects of oral L-carnitine administration on fasting plasma glucose, HbA1c, and lipid parameters in patients with Type 2 diabetes. Men and women with Type 2 diabetes, 51 years old on average, were assigned to two groups: Group 1 received 1 g of L-carnitine, group 2, a placebo; both groups, orally three times a day, for 12 weeks. It was found that plasma fasting glucose decreased significantly from 143 ± 35 to 130 ± 33 mg/dL in the L-carnitine group. There was also a significant (and unfortunate) increase in triglycerides from 196 ± 61 to 233 ± 12 mg/dL, in Apo A1 from 94 ± 20 to 103 ± 23 mg/dL, and in Apo B100 from 98 ± 18 to 108 ± 22 mg/dL after 12 weeks of treatment. There was no significant change in LDL cholesterol, HDL cholesterol, HbA1c, LP(a), or total cholesterol.

The investigators concluded that L-carnitine significantly lowers fasting plasma glucose, but it increases fasting triglyceride in these patients (Rahbar, Shakerhosseini, Saadat et al. 2005).

There are many more publications that report a beneficial role for oral L-carnitine supplementation in Type 2 diabetes, but there are some that failed to replicate these findings. For instance:

In a study published in the *Annals of Nutrition and Metabolism*, the investigators reported their conclusion that L-carnitine administered orally for 4 weeks did not modify either insulin sensitivity or the lipid profile (González-Ortiz, Hernández-González, Hernández-Salazar et al. 2008).

13.5.2 The Benefits of L-Carnitine Supplementation in Chronic Systemic Inflammation

C-reactive protein (CRP) is a blood test marker for inflammation in the body. It is classified as an acute phase reactant, which means that its levels will rise in response to rising inflammation. A review and meta-analysis published in the *Journal of Medical Biochemistry* proposed to determine whether supplementation with L-carnitine can modulate systemic inflammation as noted by lower circulating CRP concentrations.

The investigators undertook a comprehensive literature search in Medline, Scopus, and Cochrane Central Register of Controlled Trials in December 2012 to identify clinical trials investigating the impact of oral L-carnitine supplementation on serum/plasma CRP concentration.

Meta-analysis of included trials revealed a significant reduction of circulating CRP concentrations in patients in L-carnitine intervention, compared to that in the control group. The calculated combined weighted mean reduction in CRP concentrations was -0.39 mg/L. This effect size estimate was found to be significant and robust. The investigators concluded that the evidence supports the clinically relevant benefit of L-carnitine supplementation in lowering the circulating levels of CRP (Sahebkar. 2015).

A clinical study titled "Antiinflammatory effects of L-carnitine supplementation (1000 mg/d) in coronary artery disease patients" was published in the journal *Nutrition*. The aim of the study was to determine whether L-carnitine supplementation (LC, 1000 mg/day) would ameliorate inflammation as observed in inflammatory markers in patients with CAD.

Patients with CAD were identified by cardiac catheterization as having less than 50% stenosis of one major coronary artery. The patients were randomly assigned to an L-carnitine group and a placebo group, and the intervention was administered for 12 weeks. The levels of L-carnitine, antioxidant status (malondialdehyde and antioxidant enzyme activities), and inflammatory markers (CRP, IL-6, and TNF-α) were measured.

It was found that after L-carnitine supplementation, the levels of inflammatory markers were significantly reduced compared to the baseline, as well as to those in the placebo group. The levels of inflammatory markers were significantly negatively correlated with the levels of L-carnitine and antioxidant enzyme activities.

The investigators concluded that L-carnitine supplementation may have potential utility to reduce inflammation in CAD due to its antioxidant effects (Lee, Lin, Lin et al. 2015).

13.5.3 Safety of Supplementing with L-Carnitine

L-carnitine supplementation has been reported to cause nausea, vomiting, abdominal cramps, diarrhea, and a "fishy" body odor, at doses of approximately 3 g/day (Rebouche, 1999; The editors. 2004). Rarer side effects include muscle weakness in uremic patients and seizures in those with seizure disorders.

There is considerable published research indicating that intestinal bacteria metabolize carnitine to form a substance called trimethylamine N-oxide (TMAO) that might increase the risk of cardiovascular disease (Koeth, Wang, Levison et al. 2013). This effect appears to be more pronounced in people who consume meat than in vegans or vegetarians. The formation of trimethylamine N-oxide by gut bacteria has been strongly implicated in atherosclerosis.

However, a study published in the journal of the American Society for Microbiology, *mBio*, reported finding that resveratrol reduces TMAO-induced atherosclerosis by decreasing TMAO levels (Chen, Yi, Zhang et al. 2016).

While many benefits of supplementation of L-carnitine have been reported, and a number of them are cited here, there is also a potential dark side to its supplementation: The aim of a study published in the journal *Experimental and Clinical Endocrinology and Diabetes* was to determine the relation between TMAO and L-carnitine plasma levels and diabetes. Blood plasma samples were collected from 12-week-old and 20-week-old db/db mice and from patients undergoing percutaneous coronary intervention.

Diabetic db/db mice presented 10-fold higher TMAO than nondiabetic db/db mice but lower L-carnitine plasma concentrations at 12 weeks of age. After 8 weeks of observation, diabetic db/db mice had significantly increased body weight, insulin resistance, and TMAO concentration, in comparison to nondiabetic control.

In patients undergoing percutaneous coronary intervention, the median (interquartile range) plasma concentration of TMAO was 1.8 μmol/L. Analysis of the samples showed a bivariate association of TMAO level with age, total cholesterol, and L-carnitine. The multivariate linear regression analysis revealed that, in addition to L-carnitine as the strongest predictor of log-transformed TMAO, the factors age, diabetes status, and body mass index (BMI) were independently associated with increased log-transformed TMAO levels.

The investigators concluded that age, diabetes, and BMI are associated with higher TMAO levels. These data support the hypothesis of TMAO as a cardiovascular risk marker and warrant further investigation of TMAO for diabetes research applications (Dambrova, Latkovskis, Kuka et al. 2016). Therefore, given that L-carnitine is metabolized by gut bacteria to generate TMAO, there is a risk associated with using it, which must be weighed against the benefits.

13.5.3.1 Carnitine and Medication Interactions

Carnitine interacts with certain types of antibiotics (pivalate-conjugated antibiotics such as pivampicillin) that are used in the long-term prevention of urinary tract infections (Brass. 2002). Chronic administration of these antibiotics increases the excretion of pivaloyl-carnitine, which can lead to carnitine depletion. However, while tissue carnitine levels may become low enough to limit fatty acid oxidation, no cases of illness due to deficiency have been reported (Rebouche. 2004).

Treatment with the anticonvulsants valproic acid, phenobarbital, phenytoin, or carbamazepine has been shown to significantly reduce blood levels of carnitine (Hug, McGraw, Bates et al. 1991; Verrotti, Greco, Morgese et al. 1999). Furthermore, treatment with valproic acid with or without other anticonvulsants may cause hepatotoxicity and increase plasma ammonia concentrations, leading to encephalopathy (Verroti, Trotta, Morges et al. 2002; Lheureux, and Hantson. 2009). This toxicity may also occur after acute valproic acid overdose. L-carnitine administration may help treat valproic acid toxicity in children and adults (Perrott, Murphy, and Zed. 2010) and, although the optimal regimen has not been identified, it is increasingly becoming routine practice for pediatric epileptologists to have their patients on certain anticonvulsants to take L-carnitine supplements.

13.6 GAMMA-LINOLEIC ACID AND ALPHA-LINOLEIC ACID

Gamma-linoleic acid (GLA) is an omega-6 fatty acid, a naturally occurring antioxidant that is present in evening primrose oil (EPO), borage oil, and blackcurrant seed oil. Omega-6 fatty acids are considered essential fatty acids, necessary for human health. Together with omega-3 fatty acids, omega-6 fatty acids play a crucial role in brain function and normal growth and development. Also known as polyunsaturated fatty acids (PUFAs), they help stimulate skin and hair growth, maintain bone health, regulate metabolism, and maintain the reproductive system.

There are several different types of omega-6 fatty acids. Most in the diet come from vegetable oils in the form of linoleic acid (LA) that the body converts to GLA, and then to arachidonic acid. A healthy diet should contain a balance of omega-3 and omega-6 fatty acids. However, omega-3 fatty acids help reduce inflammation, while some omega-6 fatty acids may promote inflammation.

The typical American diet contains 14 to 25 times more omega-6 fatty acids than omega-3 fatty acids, and health authorities blame this high ratio of omega-6 to omega-3 fatty acids for the large number of inflammatory diseases in the American population (Patterson, Wall, Fitzgerald et al. 2012).

GLA taken as a supplement is converted to dihomo-γ-linolenic acid that fights inflammation, provided that sufficient nutrient cofactors such as magnesium, zinc, and vitamins C, B3, and B6 are available in the body.

Alpha-linolenic acid (not to be confused with the identical acronym for ALA) is a type of omega-3 fatty acid found in plants. It is found in flaxseed oil and in canola, soy, perilla, and walnut oils. It is relatively similar to the omega-3 fatty acids that are in fish oil, called eicosapentaenoic acid (EPA) and docosahexaenoic acid (DHA).

The body can convert ALA into EPA and DHA. However, some researchers suggest that less than 1% of ALA is converted to physiologically effective levels of EPA and DHA.

Omega-3 fatty acids, especially EPA and DHA, have been shown to reduce inflammation and may help prevent chronic diseases, such as heart disease and arthritis. They may also be important for brain health and development, as well as normal growth and development (University of Maryland Medical Center. http://www.umm.edu/health/medical/altmed/supplement/alphalinolenic -acid; accessed 11.23.17).

13.6.1 Evening Primrose (*Oenothera biennis* L.) Oil and Borage (*Borago officinalis*) Oil

Primrose oil, extracted from the seeds of the evening primrose, contains linolenic acid, gamma-linolenic acid, and vitamin E. GLA, a known precursor of prostaglandin E and several other active substances as well, is said to be the constituent of the oil responsible for its therapeutic effects (Kleijnen. 1994; Cohen, Rousseau, and Robinson. 2000). A typical capsule of EPO contains about 320 mg of ALA, 40 mg of GLA, and 10 IU of vitamin E (Kleijnen. 1994).

A study published in the *Journal of Agricultural and Food Chemistry* sought to determine the antioxidant activity of the evening primrose seed. The investigators reported that EPO is a highly unsaturated oil, a significant source of GLA (a very active essential fatty acid, and the precursor of prostaglandin E1 and its derivatives). The antioxidant activity of the evening primrose seed extracts was compared to that of a control and to that of butylated hydroxytoluene (BHT) singly, and in combination. Antioxidant activity was measured by the co-oxidation of β-carotene, an oxidative stability instrument, conjugated dienes, and headspace analysis of hexanal.

The seed extract was found to have greater antioxidant activity than the commercially extracted filter cake. The commercially extracted filter cake was more effective in controlling the oxidation in the oil-in-water model system than in the bulk oil system.

The activity of evening primrose seeds was concentration dependent, and at higher concentrations, it was as effective as butylated hydroxytoluene, but it required higher concentrations because of its lack of purity. Synergism between seed extract and butylated hydroxytoluene was demonstrated in both model systems (Birch, Fenner, Watkins et al. 2001).

The aim of another study, published in the *Journal of Agricultural and Food Chemistry*, was designed to determine the antioxidant properties of evening primrose seeds. This study showed that the occurrence of GLA in the 1- and 3-positions of the triacylglycerol molecules of EPO makes them easily accessible to hydrolysis by pancreatic lipase in the small intestines. Because of this property, EPO is considered to be nutritionally more available than the other seed and vegetable oils containing GLA.

This study also looked at the biochemical breakdown of EPO into antioxidant properties and found it safe and efficacious to use as a source of bioactive components for use in nutraceutical applications, as well as nonfood applications (Wettasinghe, Shahidi, and Amarowicz. 2002).

Borage oil (borage is also known as a starflower) is an annual herb in the flowering plant family *Boraginaceae*. It is native to the Mediterranean region and can now be found in many other locales. Its flowers and leaves, as well as the oil from its seeds, are used in *traditional medicine*. Borage seed oil holds GLA.

The journal *Advances in Pharmacological Sciences* published a "Review of anti-inflammatory herbal medicines," the title of the article. The authors report that this plant contains about 25% GLA. By elevating prostaglandin-E levels, GLA leads to cAMP augmentation. GLA could, therefore, count as a strong suppressor of TNF-α, which can explain the anti-inflammatory effect of borage oil in rheumatoid arthritis (RA), for instance (Kast. 2001). TNF-α is a cell signaling protein that contributes to systemic inflammation and is one of the cytokines that make up the acute phase reaction.

Further studies of the anti-inflammatory effects of borage oil in RA were reported in two clinical studies cited in a systematic review published in the journal *Rheumatology*: In one study, administration of 1.4g/day borage seed oil was compared to placebo in RA patients. 36.8% amelioration occurred in the treatment group at the end of 6-month therapy.

In another study published in the journal *Rheumatology*, 2.8g/day of borage seed oil was administered to patients for 6 months. At the end of treatment, the amelioration of RA in the treatment group was a remarkable 64%, compared to only 21% in the control group (Soeken, Miller, and Ernst. 2003; see also Ghasemian, Owlia, and Owlia. 2016).

Borage oil is also associated with favorable energy storage management: An animal-model study published in the journal *Comparative Biochemistry and Physiology. Part B. Biochemistry and Molecular Biology* resulted in the finding that "Dietary gamma-linolenic acid in the form of borage oil causes less body fat accumulation accompanying an increase in uncoupling protein-1 mRNA level in brown adipose tissue," the title of the study (Takahashi, Ide, and Fujita. 2000).

13.6.2 ALA AND GLA REDUCE INFLAMMATION AND HELP IN THE TREATMENT OF METABOLIC SYNDROME, DIABETES, AND DIABETES COMPLICATIONS

The *Journal of Nutrition* published a study titled "Dietary alpha-linolenic acid reduces inflammatory and lipid cardiovascular risk factors in hypercholesterolemic men and women." The investigators proposed that ALA reduces cardiovascular disease risk, possibly by decreasing vascular inflammation, thus correcting endothelial dysfunction.

In this study, inflammatory markers, lipids, and lipoproteins were assessed in hypercholesterolemic patients fed two diets: The ALA diet was low in saturated fat and cholesterol and high in

PUFA with varying amounts of ALA. The other diet, for comparison, was an average American diet (AAD).

The ALA diet provided 17% energy from PUFA (10.5% LA; 6.5% ALA), the LA diet provided 16.4% energy from PUFA (12.6% LA; 3.6% ALA), and the AAD provided 8.7% energy from PUFA (7.7% LA; 0.8% ALA).

It was found that the ALA Diet decreased CRP, whereas there was an increase in CRP in the LA diet. Although the two high-PUFA diets similarly decreased intercellular cell adhesion molecule-1 versus AAD, the ALA diet decreased vascular cell adhesion molecule-1 and E-selectin more so than did the LA diet.

Changes in CRP and vascular cell adhesion molecule-1 were inversely associated with changes in serum EPA or EPA plus docosapentaenoic acid after the participants consumed the ALA diet. The two high-PUFA diets significantly decreased serum total cholesterol, LDL cholesterol, and triglycerides in a similar fashion; the ALA diet decreased HDL cholesterol and apolipoprotein AI compared with the AAD.

The investigators concluded that ALA decreases cardiovascular disease risk by inhibiting vascular inflammation and endothelial activation beyond its lipid-lowering effects (Zhao, Etherton, Martin et al. 2004).

The investigators who conducted an animal-model study published in the *Yonsei Medical Journal (Korea)* concluded that GLA attenuates inflammation by inhibiting enhanced monocyte chemoattractant protein-1 and intercellular adhesion molecule-1 expression, as well as extracellular matrix proteins accumulation in diabetic nephropathy.

Monocyte chemoattractant protein-1 is a key chemokine that regulates migration and infiltration of monocytes/macrophages. Intercellular adhesion molecule-1 is an endothelial- and leukocyte-associated transmembrane protein that stabilizes cell–cell interactions and facilitates leukocyte endothelial transmigration. Fibrosis in diabetic nephropathy is characterized by extracellular matrix accumulation (Kim, Yoo, Lee et al. 2012).

GLA is a new approach to the management of diabetic neuropathy. It has been shown to reverse existing diabetic neuropathy in trials in seven centers. Diabetic animals and humans have a reduced ability to convert dietary linoleic acid to GLA, and GLA and its metabolites are required for normal neuronal structure and function and normal microcirculation. The lack of GLA, and its metabolites, may play a major role in the development of the neuropathy.

GLA helps correct the biochemical defects, restores levels of GLA metabolites toward normal, and produces highly significant clinical and neurophysiological improvements in diabetic neuropathy (Horrobin. 1992).

Clinical reports suggest that GLA may be useful for treating diabetic neuropathy: Studies show that taking GLA for 6 months or more may reduce symptoms of nerve pain. Those who have good blood sugar control may find GLA more effective than those with poor blood sugar control. The journal *Diabetes Care* reported a study that aimed to compare the effects of placebo to GLA on mild diabetic neuropathy over the course of 1 year: Patients with mild diabetic neuropathy were administered a daily dose of 480 mg.

Motor nerve conduction velocity, sensory nerve action potential, compound muscle action potential, hot and cold thresholds, sensation, tendon reflexes, and muscle strength in upper and lower limbs were evaluated by standard tests.

The change in response to GLA, of the modalities tested over 1 year of treatment, was significantly more favorable than the change due to placebo. Thirteen of sixteen modalities were significantly improved.

Gender, age, and type of diabetes did not influence the result, but treatment was more effective in the relatively well-controlled than in poorly controlled diabetes patients (Keen, Payan, Allawi et al. 1993).

The journal *Diabetic Medicine* published a study titled "The effect of gamma-linolenic acid on human diabetic peripheral neuropathy: a double-blind placebo-controlled trial." In this study, patients with distal diabetic polyneuropathy, confirmed both clinically and by objective nerve function studies, completed a study to assess the effect of dietary supplementation with GLA on their neuropathy.

Patients received either 360 mg of GLA, or placebo capsules, for 6 months. All patients were assessed at the beginning and end of the study period by neuropathy symptoms and sign scoring, motor and sensory nerve conduction studies, and thermal threshold measurements.

When compared to the placebo group, patients on GLA showed significant improvement in neuropathy symptom scores: median nerve motor conduction velocity, compound muscle action potential amplitude, peroneal nerve motor conduction velocity, compound muscle action potential amplitude, median and sural sensory nerve action potential amplitude, ankle heat threshold, and cold threshold values.

The investigators concluded that GLA therapy might play a useful role in the prevention and treatment of distal diabetic polyneuropathy (Jamal, and Carmichael. 1990).

Alpha-linoleic acid has also been investigated for its potential effects on glycemic control: The journal *Medicine* (Baltimore) published the results of a review and meta-analysis that concluded that ALA-enriched diets do not affect HbA1c, fasting blood glucose, or fasting blood insulin (Jovanovski, Li, Ho et al. 2017).

A study published in the journal *Lipids in Health and Disease* aimed to determine the impact of n-3 PUFA-containing botanical oils on Type 2 diabetes. Patients with early-stage Type 2 diabetes, or metabolic syndrome, participated in an 8-week intervention program: They were provided PUFA-containing oils.

Individuals received either corn oil, a botanical oil combination (borage [*B. officinalis* L.]/ echium oil [*Echium plantagineum* L.]), or fish oil. The botanical oil combination was enriched with alpha-linolenic, gamma-linolenic, and stearidonic acids, and the fish oil was enriched with EHA and DHA. Serum fatty acids and other serum lipids (triglycerides and total, HDL, and LDL cholesterol), as well as markers of inflammation (leptin and CRP) and glucose regulation (glucose and HbA1c), were assessed from fasting participants at baseline and after the intervention period.

It was found that patients in the corn oil group showed no differences in serum lipids, markers of inflammation, or glucose regulation between pre- and posttreatment measures, whereas supplementation with botanical oil significantly lowered total and LDL cholesterol levels, and fish oil reduced serum triglycerides and HbA1c and increased HDL cholesterol.

The investigators concluded that short-term dietary supplementation with botanical oil and fish oil improves biomarkers associated with Type 2 diabetes and/or metabolic syndrome (Lee, Ivester, Hester et al. 2014).

In fact, a study published in the *American Journal of Clinical Nutrition* reported that women in the highest tertiles of total n-3 PUFA intake had a 44% reduced risk of inflammatory disease mortality compared to those in the lowest tertile of intake at baseline. This association was not observed in men.

In both men and women, each increase in energy-adjusted intake of alpha-linolenic acid, by one standard deviation above the mean, was inversely associated with inflammatory mortality (hazard ratio, 0.83). Participants in the second and in the third tertiles of nut consumption had a 51% and 32% reduced risk of inflammatory disease mortality, respectively, compared with those in the first tertile (Gopinath, Buyken, Flood et al. 2011).

13.6.3 PRECAUTIONS

It has been recommended that persons with preexisting seizure disorders avoid omega-6 fatty acids because a number of reports describe seizures in people consuming borage oil or EPO. For instance, investigators reported "Status epilepticus associated with Borage oil ingestion," the title of their publication in the *Journal of Medical Toxicology* (Al-Khamees, Schwartz, Alrashdi et al. 2011).

However, not all authorities agree that EPO either causes seizures or lowers the threshold to seizure in those with that preexisting condition. In fact, a report in the journal *Prostaglandins Leukotrenes and Essential Fatty Acids* claims quite the opposite:

> Not only are linoleic acid and gamma-linolenic acid safe in epilepsy, with prolonged oral administration of linoleic acid and alpha-linolenic acid (in a 4:1 mixture) protecting rats from having seizures in four different epilepsy models, but the evening primrose oil-derived omega-6 fatty acid arachidonic acid inhibits sodium ion currents and synaptic transmission, while the evening primrose oil-derived eicosanoid prostaglandin E(1) appears to have anticonvulsant activity. In light of these findings, it is suggested that formularies should now remove seizures or epilepsy as a side-effect of evening primrose oil, and should remove a history of seizures or epilepsy as a contraindication to taking evening primrose oil. (With permission from Puri. 2007. *Prostaglandins Leukotrenes and Essential Fatty Acids*, Aug; 77(2): 101–103.)

Pregnant women are cautioned to avoid borage seed oil, and EPO, and other possible sources of GLA. According to a report in the journal *American Family Physician*, its benefits are uncertain (Bayles, and Usatine. 2009), and according to another report in the *Journal of Nurse-Midwifery*, its harmful effects are documented (Dove, and Johnson. 1999).

Side effects of supplements of these oils can include occasional headache, abdominal pain, nausea, and loose stools (Bayles, and Usatine. 2009).

Laboratory studies suggest that omega-6 fatty acids, such as the fat found in corn oil, promote the growth of prostate tumor cells. Health care professionals currently recommend not taking omega-6 fatty acids, including GLA, if one is at risk for or has prostate cancer (Hughes-Fulford, Tjandrawinata, Li et al. 2005).

Possible interactions with prescription medications include blood-thinning medications. Omega-6 and omega-3 fatty acids may increase the risk of bleeding. GLA may increase the effectiveness of ceftazidime, an antibiotic in a class known as cephalosporins, used to treat a variety of bacterial infections.

GLA may increase the effectiveness of anticancer treatments, such as doxorubicin, cisplatin, carboplatin, idarubicin, mitoxantrone, tamoxifen, vincristine, and vinblastine. Cyclosporine is a medication used to suppress the immune system after organ transplant. Taking omega-6 fatty acids with cyclosporine may increase the immunosuppressive effects of this medication. It may also protect against kidney damage (a potential side effect from this medication).

People taking a class of medications called phenothiazines to treat schizophrenia should not take EPO, because it may interact with these medications and increase the risk of seizures. The same may be true for other omega-6 supplements. Phenothiazines include

- Chlorpromazine (thorazine)
- Fluphenazine (stelazine)
- Perphenazine (trilafon)
- Prochlorperazine (compazine)
- Thioridazine (mellaril)

(Source: University of Maryland Medical Center. http://www.umm.edu/health/medical/altmed /supplement/alphalinolenic-acid; accessed 11.23.17.)

13.7 FISH OIL

Fish oil comes from the tissues of oily fish such as salmon, tuna, and halibut, as well as other seafoods including algae and krill, and from some plants and nut oils. It contains the omega-3 fatty acids EPA and DHA, precursors of certain eicosanoids that are known principally for their anti-inflammatory effects. The fish sources do not actually produce omega-3 fatty acids, but instead accumulate them by consuming either microalgae or prey fish that have accumulated omega-3 fatty acids.

Marine and freshwater fish oil all vary in contents of arachidonic acid, EPA, and DHA, ranging from 0.7% to 15.5% (Gruger, Nelson, and Stansby. 1964). Marine and freshwater fish oils also differ in their effects on organ lipids (Innis, Rioux, Auestad et al. 1995). There is no relation between either the total fish intake or the estimated omega-3 fatty acid intake from all fish, on the one hand, and serum omega-3 fatty acid concentrations, on the other. Only fatty fish intake, particularly salmonids, and estimated EPA + DHA intake from fatty fish has been observed to be significantly associated with an increase in serum EPA + DHA (Philibert, Vanier, Abdelouahab et al. 2006).

13.7.1 Fish Oil Has Anti-Inflammatory Properties

According to a report in the journal *Nutrition Review*, fatty acids from fish have anti-inflammatory potential because they yield long-chain omega-3 fatty acids. According to the authors, omega-6 (n-6) and omega-3 (n-3) polyunsaturated fatty acids PUFAs are precursors of potent lipid mediators, termed eicosanoids, which play an important role in the regulation of inflammation. Eicosanoids derived from n-6 PUFAs (e.g., arachidonic acid) have proinflammatory functions, whereas eicosanoids derived from n-3 PUFAs (e.g., EPA and DHA) have anti-inflammatory properties, traditionally attributed to their ability to inhibit the formation of n-6 PUFA-derived eicosanoids.

While the typical Western diet has a greater ratio of n-6 PUFAs compared to n-3 PUFAs, research has shown that by increasing the ratio of n-3 to n-6 fatty acids in the diet, and consequently favoring the production of EPA in the body, or by increasing the dietary intake of EPA and DHA through consumption of fatty fish, or fish oil supplements, reduction may be achieved in the incidence of many chronic diseases that involve inflammatory processes; most notably, these include cardiovascular diseases, inflammatory bowel disease, and RA (Wall, Ross, Fitzgerald et al. 2010).

The journal *Nutrients* published a thorough and detailed review titled "Omega-3 fatty acids and inflammatory processes," paraphrased below, that addresses the effects of constituents of fish oil. The authors contend that long-chain fatty acids influence inflammation through a variety of mechanisms, mediated by changes in fatty acid composition of cell membranes. Changes in composition of cell membranes can modify membrane fluidity and, thereby, cell signaling, leading to altered gene expression, and can also modify the pattern of lipid mediator production.

Cells involved in the inflammatory response, on the other hand, are typically rich in the n-6 fatty acid arachidonic acid, but the contents of arachidonic acid and of the n-3 fatty acids EPA and DHA can be altered by consuming EPA and DHA.

Eicosanoids, produced from arachidonic acid, play a major role in inflammation. EPA also gives rise to a different set of eicosanoids, and these often have properties different from those of arachidonic acid–derived eicosanoids.

EPA and DHA give rise to resolvins, which are anti-inflammatory and inflammation resolving. Resolvins are recently identified molecules that are generated from n-3 PUFA precursors and can orchestrate the timely resolution of inflammation in model systems.

Increased membrane content of EPA and DHA (and decreased arachidonic acid content) results in a changed pattern of production of eicosanoids and resolvins. Changing the fatty acid composition of cells involved in the inflammatory response also affects production of peptide mediators of inflammation (adhesion molecules, cytokines, etc.). The fatty acid composition of cells involved in the inflammatory response influences their function; the contents of arachidonic acid, EPA, and DHA appear to be especially important.

The investigator concluded that the anti-inflammatory effects of marine n-3 PUFAs suggest that they may be useful as therapeutic agents in disorders having an inflammatory component (Calder. 2010).

13.7.2 Fish Oil Benefits Glycemic Control

The journal *Diabetes* published a report with the captivating title, "Omega-3 fatty acids in diabetes mellitus. Gift from the sea?" (Axelrod. 1989). The report makes a number of important points concerning the value—and possible risks—of omega-3 fatty acids from fish oil in treatment of Type 2 diabetes. The investigators contend that the potential role of omega-3 fatty acids in the prevention of atherosclerotic disease in the nondiabetic population currently engenders interest but also controversy. Some apparently beneficial effects of omega-3 fatty acids on platelet function, eicosanoid formation, plasma triglyceride levels, and blood pressure have been described in patients with diabetes.

However, there are also reports of potentially adverse effects and potential risks of dietary fish and fish oils in diabetic patients who use these agents, including increased plasma glucose, HbA1c, and plasma total cholesterol.

Here are some of the issues raised in the report: It remains necessary to determine the regulation of fatty acid synthesis and the fatty acid composition of phospholipids in diabetic patients under defined conditions of metabolic control and diet and to determine the effects of dietary fish and fish oils in appropriate quantities on the fatty acid composition of phospholipids.

The extrapolation from nondiabetes to diabetes patients is hazardous: It does not follow that the effects of omega-3 fatty acids are the same in patients with diabetes as in nondiabetes individuals or patients with a primary hyperlipidemia. First, the biosynthesis and composition of fatty acids is abnormal in diabetes animals and possibly in diabetes patients.

Second, many potential mechanisms of atherosclerosis, for example, hyperglycemia, increased platelet aggregation, platelet TXA synthesis, and decreased erythrocyte deformability (with a consequent increase in blood viscosity), are present in diabetes but not necessarily nondiabetes individuals.

Third, the mechanisms of many of the risk factors in diabetes patients, for example, hyperlipidemia, increased platelet aggregation, and decreased erythrocyte deformability, differ from the mechanisms of these abnormalities in nondiabetes individuals, reflecting the effects of insulin deficiency, hyperglycemia, and their sequelae.

Diabetes is a heterogeneous group of diseases; therefore, the effects of omega-3 fatty acids must be addressed separately for patients with insulin-dependent diabetes (IDDM), non–insulin-dependent diabetes, and perhaps other forms of diabetes.

Fatty acid composition is altered in the phospholipids of various tissues in experimental animals with diabetes, including plasma, liver, heart, kidneys, and erythrocytes. These changes may reflect decreased activities of the microsomal A9-desaturase, A6-desaturase (Eck, Wynn, Carter et al. 1979; Faas, and Carter. 1980; Dang, Faas, Lee et al. 1988), and A5-desaturase enzymes (Holman, Johnson, Gerrard et al. 1983; Dang, Faas, Lee et al. 1988).

The A9-desaturase enzyme converts saturated fatty acids into monounsaturated fatty acids. The A6-desaturase converts linoleic acid to γ-linolenic acid. This is the rate-limiting step in the conversion of linoleic acid to arachidonic acid. The A5-desaturase converts dihomo-γ-linolenic acid to arachidonic acid and converts eicosatetraenoic acid to EPA, which can be converted to DHA. Thus, these enzymes are necessary for the biosynthesis of arachidonic acid, EPA, DHA, and other unsaturated fatty acids.

In relative terms, the arachidonic acid content is often decreased and the omega-3 fatty acid content (including EPA and DHA) is often increased in the tissue phospholipids of diabetic rats (Dang, Faas, Lee et al. 1988). In absolute terms (based on measurements of the fatty acids of the total lipids in the carcass of the whole animal), all PUFAs (omega-6 and omega-3) are decreased in diabetes (Dang, Faas, Lee et al. 1988). Insulin therapy reverses and overcorrects the diminished A9- and A6-desaturase activities, and it restores the fatty acid composition to normal, except for the decrease in arachidonic acid (Faas, and Carter. 1980; Dang, Faas, Lee et al. 1988).

The changes in fatty acid composition in diabetes are influenced by diet, because restriction of food intake decreases the magnitude of these changes (Faas, and Carter. 1980; Holman, Johnson, Gerrard et al. 1983). Thus, the alterations in fatty acid composition in tissues from diabetic animals reflect the consequences of insulin deficiency and diet. The arachidonic acid deficiency in some tissues, for example, platelets, could also reflect enhanced phospholipase activity and enhanced release and utilization of arachidonate. These observations were made in the rat.

However, studies on the fatty acid composition of platelets derived from diabetes patients have produced seemingly inconsistent findings. For example, arachidonic acid levels have been decreased (Jones, Carter, Haitas et al. 1983), increased (Takahashi, Morita, Saito et al. 1984; Morita, Takahashi, Ito et al. 1983; Kalofoutis, and Lekakis. 1983), or unchanged (Nordoy, and Rodset. 1970; Tilvis, Rasi, Viinikka et al. 1987; Faas, Dang, Kemp et al. 1988).

The authors of this report further comment that the extant studies have not been controlled for the degree of insulin deficiency or for the composition of the diet. Therefore, these findings have several implications: First, because fatty acid synthesis and composition are altered in diabetes, the effects of dietary modifications may be different in diabetes than in nondiabetes individuals. For example, if, in relative terms, arachidonic acid content is decreased and omega-3 fatty acid content is increased in diabetes patients (as is the case in animals), then additional supplementation with omega-3 fatty acids may be of little benefit.

Alternatively, if, in absolute terms, all PUFAs (omega-6 and omega-3) are decreased in diabetic patients, as is the case with animals, then the net balance of omega-6 and omega-3 fatty acids, and their biologically active products, may be unusually susceptible to dietary manipulation in diabetic patients. Then, studies are needed in patients with diabetes to determine (1) the fatty acid composition of phospholipids under defined conditions of metabolic control and diet and (2) the effects of fish and fish oils on phospholipid fatty acid composition under these conditions.

The report specifies the outcome observed with administration of various dosages of fish oil. Dosage information can be accessed at http://web.diabetes.org/perspectives/ADAJournalVol38-05 .pdf. In connection with the effects of various dosages of omega-3 fatty acid in diabetes, the report also issues a number of warnings about potentially deleterious effects of the observed increases in levels of glucose (Friday, Childs, Tsunehara et al. 1987; Wei, Ulchaker, and Sheehan. 1988), HbA1c (Glauber, Wallace, Griver et al. 1988; Schectman, Kaul, and Kissebah. 1988), plasma total cholesterol and LDL cholesterol (Haines, Sanders, Imeson et al. 1986; Stacpoole, Alig, Ammon et al. 1989), and serum apolipoprotein B (apoB) (Kasim, Stern, Khilnani et al. 1988; Schectman, Kaul, and Kissebah. 1988).

However, the report also points out that, in general, the magnitude of these changes has been small (typically 10% to 36%) (Axelrod. 1989. *Diabetes*, May; 38(5): 539–543).

Another comprehensive review was published in the *Journal of Research in Medical Sciences*. It was titled "Omega-3 fatty acids, insulin resistance and type 2 diabetes." The authors reported a study that found that fish oil (and olive oil) can improve insulin resistance and plasma desacylghrelin after an 8-week intervention in an animal model (rats) (Saidpour, Zahediasl, Kimiagar et al. 2011). There is also evidence for the beneficial role of n-3 fatty acids in insulin resistance and diabetes in experimentally obese rats (Yamazaki, Brito, Coelho et al. 2011) and in humans as well (Ramel, Martinez, Kiely et al. 2008).

The *American Journal of Clinical Nutrition* reported a study aimed to determine whether omega-3 (n-3) fatty acids play a role in the development of Type 2 diabetes. The investigators thought that such a possible role is uncertain, especially with regard to any differential influence of alpha-linolenic acid (ALA), EPA, and DHA.

The objective of the study was to determine the effect of consumption of total omega-3 fatty acids; marine omega-3 (EPA and DHA), nonmarine omega-3 (ALA), and omega-6 (n-6) fatty acids; and omega-6:omega-3 ratio on the risk of Type 2 diabetes in a Chinese population in Singapore. The analysis included more than 40,000 Chinese men and women, free of chronic disease, 45 to 74 years old, enrolled in the Singapore Chinese Health Study.

Baseline data collection occurred between 1993 and 1998, with follow-up interviews between 1999 and 2004.

It was found that higher intakes of total omega-3 fatty acids were inversely associated with diabetes incidence: the hazard ratio for the fifth quintile, compared to the first quintile, was 0.78, indicating reduced risk. Omega-3 fatty acids from marine sources were not associated with a lowered diabetes risk, whereas nonmarine omega-3 fatty acid intake was strongly associated with reduced risk of diabetes (hazard ratio for the fifth compared with the first quintile: 0.79). Omega-6 and omega-6:omega-3 ratio were not associated with incidence of Type 2 diabetes.

The investigators concluded that consumption of nonmarine sources (ALA) of omega-3 fatty acids is associated with a decreased risk of Type 2 diabetes in Chinese Singaporeans (Brostow, Odegaard, Koh et al. 2011).

A beneficial effect of fish consumption on risk of diabetes was reported in another cohort study: The *American Journal of Clinical Nutrition* published a study titled "Fish intake and type 2 diabetes in Japanese men and women: the Japan Public Health Center-based Prospective Study."

The male and female participants, 45 to 75 years old, who had no history of diabetes, completed a questionnaire for the Japan Public Health Center–based Prospective Study. Their diet pattern was determined with a 147-item food-frequency questionnaire. During the 5-year study duration, new cases (572 men and 399 women) of Type 2 diabetes were self-reported.

In men, fish intake was significantly associated with a decreased risk of Type 2 diabetes, whereas fish intake was not appreciably associated with Type 2 diabetes risk in women (Nanri, Mizoue, Noda et al. 2011). In contrast, another 12-year cohort study also published in the *American Journal of Clinical Nutrition* found an increase of Type 2 diabetes in women, associated with regular consumption of marine omega-3 fatty acid (Djousse, Gaziano, Buring et al. 2011). No explanation was given for this seeming contradiction.

However, there are several theories that attempt to explain inconsistencies between study outcomes: First, contaminants of marine foods may play a role. The investigators in a study titled "The prevention of type 2 diabetes: should we recommend vegetable oils instead of fatty fish?" published in the *American Journal of Clinical Nutrition* concluded that "...studies on dietary patterns and diabetes should also take a closer look at ALA and its main sources" (Feskens. 2011). Then, the amount of fish consumption in the population studied is important: For intervention studies, the dose of supplementation and the intake of dietary fish oil or other dietary sources of omega-3 fatty acids must be considered. It is also conceivable that if there were higher amounts of mercury in the fish being eaten, that could increase the risk for diabetes. The susceptibility of omega-3 fatty acids to oxidation may also play a role such that the antioxidant intake may affect the impact of omega-3 fatty acids and diabetes or other chronic diseases. They may actually lack antioxidants (Osterud, and Elvevoll. 2011).

13.7.3 FISH OIL AND DYSLIPIDEMIA IN TYPE 2 DIABETES

Individuals with diabetes also often have high triglycerides and low HDL levels. Omega-3 fatty acids from fish oil can help lower triglycerides and apoproteins (markers of diabetes) and raise HDL. Consuming fish, or taking fish oil supplements, may help people with diabetes.

The investigators of a report titled "Fish oil and glycemic control in diabetes. A meta-analysis," published in the journal *Diabetes Care*, contend that there is doubt about whether fish oil intake is beneficial in reducing lipidemia in glycemic control in diabetes. They therefore performed a meta-analysis of data from clinical trials reported in Medline (Cologne, Germany), Excerpta Medica, Current Contents, review articles, and published reference lists. Publications of 26 trials were selected, and all trials included more than five diabetes (IDDM and NIDDM [Type 2 diabetes]) patients and addressed the effects of fish oil (EPA and DHA) on serum lipids and glucose tolerance.

It was found that taking all studies combined showed a decrease in mean triglyceride concentrations in association with fish oil (−0.60 mmol/L), and a slight but statistically significant increase in serum LDL cholesterol (0.18 mmol/L), with both findings most prominent in NIDDM. No significant changes were noted in HbA1c percentages in diabetes patients treated with fish oil.

Fasting blood glucose levels were increased with borderline significance in NIDDM patients (0.43 mmol/L) and were significantly lower in IDDM patients (−1.86 mmol/L). Significant dose–response effects of EPA (grams/day) on HbA1c, triglycerides, fasting blood glucose levels, HbA1c, and triglycerides were demonstrated only in NIDDM (Type 2 diabetes) patients. The investigators concluded that in diabetic patients, the use of fish oil lowers triglyceride levels by almost 30%, while having no adverse effects on HbA1c. Fish oil may be useful in treating dyslipidemia in diabetes (Friedberg, Janssen, Heine et al. 1998).

13.7.4   Fish Oil and Nephropathy in Type 2 Diabetes

Elsewhere in this book, it was shown that kidney disorders are a frequent complication of Type 2 diabetes. Therefore, any means to reduce its severity bears mention. The journal *Clinics* (Sao Paulo) published a review titled "Omega-3 fatty acid supplementation as an adjunctive therapy in the treatment of chronic kidney disease: a meta-analysis."

The aim of this analysis was to assess the benefits and risks of omega-3 fatty acid supplementation in patients with chronic kidney disease.

A systematic search of articles in PubMed, Embase, the Cochrane Library, and reference lists was performed to find relevant "literature." All eligible studies assessed proteinuria, the serum creatinine clearance rate, the estimated glomerular filtration rate, or the occurrence of end-stage renal disease.

Conventional analyses (standard mean differences with 95% confidence intervals for continuous data) were used to estimate the effects of omega-3 fatty acid supplementation on renal function, as reflected in the serum creatinine clearance rate, proteinuria, the estimated glomerular filtration rate, and relative risk. Additionally, a random-effects model was used to estimate the effect of omega-3 fatty acid supplementation on the risk of end-stage renal disease. The follow-up duration ranged from 2 months to almost 76 months.

Even a low dosage of omega-3 fatty acid supplementation, compared to no omega-3 fatty acid supplementation, was associated with a lower risk of proteinuria, but had little or no effect on the serum creatinine clearance rate, or the estimated glomerular filtration rate. However, this supplementation was associated with a reduced risk of end-stage renal disease (relative risk, 0.49).

The investigators concluded that omega-3 fatty acid supplementation delays the progression of renal disease and that it is associated with a significantly reduced risk of end-stage renal disease (Hu, Liu, and Zhang. 2017).

In a study, published in the journal *PLoS ONE*, the investigators aimed to determine whether omega-3 fatty acid supplementation could help maintain renal function in patients with diabetes and hypertriglyceridemia. Type 2 diabetes patients, with a history of omega-3 fatty acid supplementation for managing hypertriglyceridemia, were included in the study. Reduction in the urine albumin-to-creatinine ratio (ACR) and glomerular filtration rate was examined. Subgroup analyses were stratified according to the daily omega-3 fatty acids doses.

It was found that serum total cholesterol, triglyceride, and urine ACR were significantly reduced after omega-3 fatty acid supplementation. Overall, 50% of the patients did not experience loss of renal function and 36.3% of them had a glomerular filtration rate with an upward trend. The patients treated with omega-3 fatty acids at 4 g/day showed significantly greater maintenance of renal function than those treated with lower dosages. This dose-dependent effect remained statistically significant after adjustment for multiple variables.

The investigators concluded that omega-3 fatty acid supplementation in diabetic patients with hypertriglyceridemia reduces albuminuria and maintains renal function. The effects are related to the dose of daily omega-3 fatty acid supplementation (Han, Yun, Kim et al. 2016).

13.7.5   Precautions

It is recommended for diabetes sufferers that dietary supplementation of fish oil be undertaken only under the supervision of a qualified health care provider, in order to prevent adverse side effects and unfavorable interactions with medications.

Omega-3 fatty acids should be used cautiously by people who bruise easily, those who have a bleeding disorder, or those who take blood-thinning medications, including warfarin (coumadin), clopidogrel (plavix), or aspirin. High doses of omega-3 fatty acids may increase the risk of bleeding, even in people without a history of bleeding disorders and even in those who are not taking other medications.

Fish oil can cause gas, bloating, belching, and diarrhea. Time release preparations may, however, reduce these side effects.

People with either diabetes or schizophrenia may lack the ability to convert ALA to EPA and DHA, the forms more readily utilized by the body. People with these conditions should be sure to get enough EPA and DHA from their diets. People with Type 2 diabetes may experience increases in fasting blood sugar levels while taking fish oil supplements, and we repeat that they are cautioned to supplement only under the supervision of a health care provider.

The outcome of eating fish (which includes the omega-3 fatty acids EPA and DHA) in connection with macular degeneration is controversial. A more recent study including two large groups of men and women found that diets rich in ALA may increase the risk of this disease (University of Maryland Medical Center. http://www.umm.edu/health/medical/altmed/supplement/alphalinolenic-acid; accessed 12.3.17). There are dissenting reports that hold to the benefits of supplementation (Souied, Aslam, Garcia-Layana et al. 2015). Until more information becomes available, people with macular degeneration are cautioned to obtain omega-3 fatty acids from sources of EPA and DHA, rather than ALA.

The Environmental Protection Agency (EPA) warns that while fatty predatory fish like sharks, swordfish, tilefish, and albacore tuna may be high in omega-3 fatty acids, due to their position at the top of the food chain, these species may also accumulate toxic substances through biomagnification. For this reason, the U.S. EPA recommends limiting consumption (especially for women of childbearing age) of certain (predatory) fish species (e.g., albacore tuna, shark, king mackerel, tilefish, and swordfish), due to high levels of the toxic contaminant mercury. Dioxin, polychlorinated biphenyls (PCBs), and chlordane are also present (EPA (2007-01-31). Fish Consumption Advisories. Retrieved 12.3.17).

Some fish may also contain other potentially harmful contaminants, such as PCBs. For sport-caught fish, the U.S. EPA recommends that pregnant or nursing women eat no more than a single 6-oz meal per week, and young children, less than 2 oz per week. For farm-raised, imported, or marine fish, the U.S. Food and Drug Administration recommends that pregnant or nursing women and young children avoid eating types with higher levels of mercury (such as mackerel, shark, swordfish, or tilefish), and eat up to 12 oz per week of other fish types.

13.7.5.1 Possible Adverse or Beneficial Interactions with Medications

If one is currently being treated with any of the following medications, he or she should not consume omega-3 fatty acid supplements, including EPA, DHA, and ALA, without first consulting with his or her health care provider.

Blood-thinning medications: Omega-3 fatty acids may increase the effects of blood-thinning medications, including aspirin, warfarin (coumadin), and clopedigrel (plavix). Taking aspirin and omega-3 fatty acids may be helpful in some circumstances (such as in heart disease), but one should take them together only under the supervision of a health care provider.

Diabetes medications: As noted above, omega-3 fatty acid supplements may increase fasting blood sugar levels. Caution is indicated if one is on glipizide (Glucotrol and Glucotrol XL), glyburide (Micronase or Diabeta), metformin (Glucophage), or insulin.

Cholesterol-lowering medications: Following dietary guidelines, including increasing the amount of omega-3 fatty acids in the diet and reducing the omega-6 to omega-3 ratio, may help cholesterol-lowering statins to work more effectively. These medications include atorvastatin (Lipitor), lovastatin (Mevacor), and simvastatin (Zocor) (PennState Hershey, Milton S. Hershey Medical Center: http://pennstatehershey.adam.com/content.aspx?productId=107&pid=33&gid=000971; accessed 12.3.16; University of Maryland Medical Center: http://www.umm.edu/health/medical/altmed/supplement/omega3-fatty-acids; accessed 11.27.17).

A note to the reader: Please see the chart in the Appendix for a summary of the therapeutic and other effects of the selected supplements described in this chapter.

REFERENCES

Al-Khamees WA, Schwartz MD, Alrashdi S, Algren AD, and BW Morgan. 2011. Status epilepticus associated with Borage oil ingestion. *Journal of Medical Toxicology*, Jun; 7(2): 154–157. DOI: 10.1007/s13181-011-0135-9.

Ametov AS, Barinov A, Dyck PJ, Hermann R, Kozlova N, Litchy WJ, Low PA, Nehrdich D, Novosadova M, O'Brien PC, Reljanovic M, Samigullin R, Schuette K, Strokov I, Tritschler HJ, Wessel K, Yakhno N, and D Ziegler. 2003. The sensory symptoms of diabetic polyneuropathy are improved with alpha-lipoic acid: the SYDNEY trial. *Diabetes Care*, Mar; 26(3): 770–776.

Axelrod L. 1989. Omega-3 fatty acids in diabetes mellitus. Gift from the sea? *Diabetes*, May; 38(5): 539–543. http://web.diabetes.org/perspectives/ADAJournalVol38-05.pdf.

Bast A, and GR Haenen. 1988. Interplay between lipoic acid and glutathione in the protection against microsomal lipid peroxidation. *Biochimica et Biophysica Acta*, Dec; 963(3):558–561. DOI: 10.1016/0005-2760(88)90326-8.

Bayles B, and R Usatine. 2009. Evening primrose oil. *American Family Physician*, Dec; 80(12): 1405–1408. http://www.aafp.org/afp/2009/1215/p1405.html.

Berkowitz DE, White R, Li D, Minhas, Cernetich A, Kim S, Burke S, Shoukas AA, Nyhan D, Champion HC, and JM Hare. 2003. Arginase reciprocally regulates nitric oxide synthase activity and contributes to endothelial dysfunction in aging blood vessels. *Circulation*, Oct; 108 (16), 2000–2006. DOI: 10.1161/01.CIR.0000092948.04444.C7.

Biewenga GP, Haenen GR, and A Bast. 1997. The pharmacology of the antioxidant lipoic acid. *General Pharmacology*, 1997 Sep; 29(3): 315–331.

Birch AE, Fenner GP, Watkins R, and LC Boyd. 2001. Antioxidant properties of evening primrose seed extracts. *Journal of Agricultural and Food Chemistry*, Sep; 49(9): 4502–4507.

Bode-Böger SM, Böger RH, Galland A, Tsikas D, and JC Frölich. 1998. L-arginine-induced vasodilation in healthy humans: pharmacokinetic-pharmacodynamic relationship. *British Journal of Clinical Pharmacology,* Nov; 46(5), 489–497. PMCID: PMC1873701.

Bode-Böger SM, Bogera H, Creutzig D, Tsikas F, Gutzki M, Alexander K, and C Frolich. 1994. L-Arginine infusion decreases peripheral arterial resistance and inhibits platelet aggregation in healthy subjects. *Clinical Science*, 87; 303–310.

Bode-Böger SM, Muke J, Surdacki A, Brabant G, Boger RH, and JC Frolich. 2003. Oral L-arginine improves endothelial function in healthy individuals older than 70 years. *Vascular Mediicine*, May; 8(2): 77–81. DOI: 10.1191/1358863x03vm474oa.

Böger R, and ES Ron. 2005. L-arginine improves vascular function by overcoming the deleterious effects of ADMA, a novel cardiovascular risk factor. *Alternative Medicine Review*, Mar; 10(1), 14–23.

Böger RH. 2007. The pharmacodynamics of L-arginine. *The Journal of Nutrition*, 137(6 Suppl 2): 1650S–1655S.

Brass EP. 2002. Pivalate-generating prodrugs and carnitine homeostasis in man. *Pharmacol Review*, Dec; 54(4): 589–598.

Brostow DP, Odegaard AO, Koh WP, Duval S, Gross MD, Yuan JM, and MA Pereira. 2011. Omega-3 fatty acids and incident type 2 diabetes: the Singapore Chinese Health Study. *American Journal of Clinical Nutrition*, Aug; 94(2): 520–526. DOI: 10.3945/ajcn.110.009357.

Calder PC. 2010. Omega-3 fatty acids and inflammatory processes. *Nutrients*. Mar; 2(3): 355–374. DOI: 10.3390/nu2030355.

Celermajer DS, Sorensen KE, Bull C, Robinson J, and JE Deanfield. 1994. Endothelium-dependent dilation in the systemic arteries of asymptomatic subjects relates to coronary risk factors and their interaction. *Journal of the American College of Cardiology*, Nov; 24(2), 1468–1474.

Chaudhary P, Marracci GH, and DN Bourdette. 2006. Lipoic acid inhibits expression of ICAM-1 and VCAM-1 by CNS endothelial cells and T cell migration into the spinal cord in experimental autoimmune encephalomyelitis. *Journal of Neuroimmunology*, Jun; 175(1–2): 87–96. DOI: 10.1016/j.jneuroim.2006.03.007.

Chauhan A, More RS, Mullins PA, Taylor G, Petch C, and PM Schofield. 1995. Aging-associated endothelial dysfunction in humans is reversed by L-arginine. *Journal of the American Colege of Cardiology*, Dec; 28(7): 1796–1804. PMID: 8962569.

Chen M-l, Yi L, Zhang L, Zhou X, Ran L, Yang J, Zhu J-d, Zhang Q-y, and M-t Mi. 2016. Resveratrol attenuates trimethylamine-N-oxide (TMAO)-induced atherosclerosis by regulating TMAO synthesis and bile acid metabolism via remodeling of the gut microbiota. *mBio*, Apr; 7(2): e02210–e02215. DOI: 10.1128 /mBio.02210-15 5.

Cohen S, Rousseau ME, and EH Robinson. 2000. Therapeutic use of selected herbs. *Holistic Nursing Practice*, Apr; 14(1): 59–68.

Dambrova M, Latkovskis G, Kuka J, Strele I, Konrade I, Grinberga S, Hartmane D, Pugovics O, Erglis A, and E Liepinsh. 2016. Diabetes is associated with higher trimethylamine N-oxide plasma levels. *Experimental and Clinical Endocrinology and Diabetes*, Apr; 124(4): 251–256. DOI: 10.1055/s-0035-1569330.

Dang AQ, Faas FH, Lee JA, and WI Carter. 1988. Altered fatty acid composition in the plasma, platelets, and aorta of the streptozotocin-induced diabetic rat. *Metabolism*, 37: 1065–1072.

Das UN, Repossi G, Dain A, and AR Eynard. 2011. L-arginine, NO and asymmetrical dimethylarginine in hypertension and type 2 diabetes. *Frontiers in Bioscience* (Landmark Ed). Jan; 16: 13–20.

De Gaetano A, Mingrone G, Castagneto M, and M Calvani. 1999. Carnitine increases glucose disposal in humans. *Journal of the American College of Nutrition*, Jun; 18(6): 289–295. DOI: 10.1053 /meta.2000.6250.

DeFronzo RA, Tobin JD, and R Andres. 1979. Glucose clamp technique: a method for quantifying insulin secretion and resistance. *American Journal of Physiology*, 237, E214–E223.

Djousse L, Gaziano JM, Buring JE, and IM Lee. 2011. Dietary omega-3 fatty acids and fish consumption and risk of type 2 diabetes. *American Journal of Clinical Nutrition*, Jan; 93(1):143–150. DOI: 10.3945 /ajcn.110.005603.

Dove D, and P Johnson. 1999. Oral evening primrose oil: its effect on length of pregnancy and selected intrapartum outcomes in low-risk nulliparous women. *Journal of Nurse-Midwifery*, May–Jun; 44(3): 320–324.

Du XL, Edelstein D, Dimmeler S, Ju Q, Sui C, and M Brownlee. 2001. Hyperglycemia inhibits endothelial nitric oxide synthase activity by posttranslational modification at the Akt site. *Clinical Investigation*, Nov; 108(9): 1341–1348. DOI: 10.1172/JCI11235.

Eck MG. Wynn JO. Carter WJ, and FH Faas. 1979. Fatty acid desaturation in experimental diabetes mellitus. *Diabetes*, 28: 479–485.

Egashira K, Inou T, Hirooka Y, Kai H, Sugimachi M, Suzuki S, Kuga T, Urabe Y., and A Takeshita. 1993. Effects of age on endothelium-dependent vasodilation of resistance coronary artery by acetylcholine in humans. *Circulation*, Jul; 88(1), 77–81.

Faas FH, Dang AQ. Kemp K, Norman J. and WJ Carter. 1988. Red blood cell and plasma fatty acid composition in diabetes mellitus. *Metabolism*, 37: 711–713.

Faas IFH, and WI Carter. 1980. Altered fatty acid desaturation and microsomal fatty acid composition in the streptozotocin diabetic rat. *Lipids*, 15: 953–961.

Ferrannini E, and A Mari. 1998. How to measure insulin sensitivity. *Journal of Hypertension*, Jul; 16(7): 895–906.

Feskens EJ. 2011. The prevention of type 2 diabetes: should we recommend vegetable oils instead of fatty fish? *American Journal of Clinical Nutrition*, Aug; 94(2): 369–370. DOI: 10.3945/ajcn.111.020172.

Friday KE. Childs M, Tsunehara C, Fujimoto WY, Bierman EL. and JW Ensinck. 1987. Omega 3 fatty acid supplementation has discordant effects on plasma glucose and lhpoproteins in type II dlabetes (Abstract). *Diabetes*, 36 (Suppl. 1): 12A.

Fried R, and L Nezin. 2017. *Evidence-Based Proactive Nutrition to Slow Cellular Aging*. Boca Raton: CRC Press, Div. of Taylor and Francis Group Publishers.

Fried R, and WC Merrell. 1999. *The Arginine Solution*. New York: Warner Books.

Fried R. 2014. *Erectile Dysfunction as a Cardiovascular Impairment*. Boston: Academic Press, Div. of Elsevier Publishers.

Friedberg CE, Janssen MJ, Heine RJ, and DF Grobbee. 1998. Fish oil and glycemic control in diabetes. A meta-analysis. *Diabetes Care*, Apr; 21(4): 494–500.

Gad MZ. 2010. Anti-aging effects of L-arginine. *Journal of Advanced Research*, Jul; 1(3): 169–177. https:// doi.org/10.1016/j.jare.2010.05.001.

Gerhard M, Roddy MA, Creager SJ, and MA Creager. 1996. Aging progressively impairs endothelium-dependent vasodilation in forearm resistance vessels of humans. *Hypertension*, Apr; 27(4), 849–853.

Gerich JE. 1999. Is insulin resistance the principal cause of type 2 diabetes? *Diabetes, Obesity and Metabolism*, Sep; 1(5): 257–263.

Ghasemian M, Owlia S, and MB Owlia. 2016. Review of anti-inflammatory herbal medicines. *Advances in Pharmacological Sciences*, 2016; 2016: 9130979. DOI: 10. 1155/2016/9130979.

Glauber H, Wallace P, Griver K, and G Brechtel. 1988. Adverse metabolic effect of omega-3 fatty acids in non-insulin-dependent diabetes mellitus. *Annals of Internal Medicine*, 108: 663–668.

Golbidi S, Badran M, and I Laher. 2011. Diabetes and alpha lipoic acid. *Frontiers in Pharmacology*, 2: 69. DOI: 10.3389/fphar.2011.00069.

Gomes MB, and CA Negrato. 2014. Alpha-lipoic acid as a pleiotropic compound with potential therapeutic use in diabetes and other chronic diseases. *Diabetology and Metabolic Syndrome*, 6: 80. DOI: 10.1186/1758-5996-6-80.

Gomes MB, Giannella-Neto D, Faria M, Tambascia MA, Fonseca RM, Rea RR, Macedo G, Modesto Filho J, Schmid H, Bittencourt AV, Cavalcanti S, Rassi N, Pedrosa H, and S Atala Dib. 2006. Prevalence of type 2 diabetic patients within the targets of care guidelines in daily clinical practice: a multicenter study in Brazil. *The Review of Diabetic Studies*, Summer; 3(2): 82–87. DOI: 10.1900/RDS.2006.3.82.

González-Ortiz M, Hernández-González SO, Hernández-Salazar E, and F Martínez-Abundis. 2008. Effect of oral L-carnitine administration on insulin sensitivity and lipid profile in type 2 diabetes mellitus patients. *Annals of Nutrition and Metabolism*, 52(4): 335–338. DOI: 10.1159/000151488.

Gopinath B, Buyken AE, Flood VM, Empson M, Rochtchina E, and P Mitchell. 2011. Consumption of polyunsaturated fatty acids, fish, and nuts and risk of inflammatory disease mortality. *American Journal of Clinical Nutrition*, May; 93(5):1073–1079. DOI: 10.3945/ajcn.110.009977.

Gruger EH, Nelson RW, and MR Stansby. 1964. Fatty acid composition of oils from 21 species of marine fish, freshwater fish and shellfish. *Journal of the American Oil Chemists Society*. Oct; 41(10): 662–667. DOI: 10.1007/BF02661403.

Guttman H, Zimlichman R, Boaz M, Matas Z, and M Shargorodsky. 2010. Effect of long-term L-arginine supplementation on arterial compliance and metabolic parameters in patients with multiple cardiovascular risk factors: randomized, placebo-controlled study. *Journal of Cardiovascular Pharmacology*, Jun 7 [Epub ahead of print]. DOI: 10.1097/FJC.0b013e3181e9dc2c.

Haines AP. Sanders TAB, Imeson JD. Mahler RF, Martin J, Mistry M, Vickers M, and PG Wallace. 1986. Effects of a fish oil supplement on platelet function, haemostatic variables and albuminuria in insulin-dependent diabetics. *Thrombosis Research*, 43: 643–655.

Han E, Yun Y, Kim G, Lee Y-h, Wang HJ, Lee B-W, Cha BS, Kim BS, and ES Kang. 2016. Effects of omega-3 fatty acid supplementation on diabetic nephropathy progression in patients with diabetes and hypertriglyceridemia. *PLoS ONE*, May; 11(5): e0154683. DOI: 10.1371/journal.pone.0154683.

Harris RA, Nishiyama SK, Wray DW, and RS Richardson. 2010. Ultrasound assessment of flow-mediated dilation. *Hypertension*, 55: 1075–1085. https://doi.org/10.1161/HYPERTENSIONAHA.110.150821.

Heffernan KS, Fahs CA, Ranadive SM, and EA Patvardhan. 2010. L-arginine as a nutritional prophylaxis against vascular endothelial dysfunction with aging. *Journal of Cardiovascular Pharmacology and Therpeutics*, Mar; 15(1), 17–23. DOI: 10.1177/1074248409354599.

Hiltunen JK, Schonauer MS, Autio KJ, Mittelmeier TM, Kastaniotis AJ, and CL Dieckmann. 2009. Mitochondrial fatty acids synthesis type II: more than just fatty acids. *Journal of Biological Chemistry*, Apr 3; 284(14): 9011–9015. DOI: 10.1074/jbc.R800068200.

Holman RT, Johnson SB, Gerrard JM, Mauer SM, Kupcho-Sandberg S, and DM Brown. 1983. Arachidonic acid deficiency in streptozotocin-induced diabetes. *Proceedings of the National Academy of Sciences USA*, 80: 2375–2379.

Horrobin DF. 1992. The use of gamma-linolenic acid in diabetic neuropathy. *Agents and Actions. Supplement*, 37: 120–144.

Hu J, Liu Z, and H Zhang. 2017. Omega-3 fatty acid supplementation as an adjunctive therapy in the treatment of chronic kidney disease: a meta-analysis. *Clinics* (Sao Paulo). Jan; 72(1): 58–64. DOI: 10.6061/clinics/2017(01)10.

Hug G, McGraw CA, Bates SR, and EA Landrigan. 1991. Reduction of serum carnitine concentrations during anticonvulsant therapy with phenobarbital, valproic acid, phenytoin, and carbamazepine in children. *Journal of Pediatrics*, 119: 799–802.

Hughes-Fulford M, Tjandrawinata RR, Li C-F, and S Sayyah. 2005. Arachidonic acid, an omega-6 fatty acid, induces cytoplasmic phospholipase A2 in prostate carcinoma cells. *Carcinogenesis*, Sep; 26(9): 1520–1526, https://doi.org/10.1093/carcin/bgi112.

Hundal RS, Petersen KF, Mayerson AB, Randhawa PS, Inzucchi S, Shoelson SE, and GI Shulman. 2002. Mechanism by which high-dose aspirin improves glucose metabolism in type 2 diabetes. *Journal of Clinical Investigation*, May; 109(10): 1321–1326. DOI: 10.1172/JCI14955.

Ikeda U, Ito T, and K Shimada. 2001. Interleukin-6 and acute coronary syndrome. *Clinical Cardiology*, Nov; 24(11): 701–704.

Innis SM, Rioux FM, Auestad N, and RG Ackman. 1995. Marine and freshwater fish oil varying in arachidonic, eicosapentaenoic and docosahexaenoic acids differ in their effects on organ lipids and fatty acids in growing rats. *Journal of Nutrition*, Sept; 125 (9): 2286–2293.

Jamal GA, and H Carmichael. 1990. The effect of gamma-linolenic acid on human diabetic peripheral neuropathy: a double-blind placebo-controlled trial. *Diabetic Medicine*, May; 7(4): 319–323. DOI: 10.1111/j.1464-5491.1990.tb01397.x.

Jones DB. Carter RD. Haitas B, and JI Mann. 1983. Low phospholipid arachidonic acid values in diabetic platelets. *British Medical Journal*, 286: 173–175.

Jovanovski E, Li D, Ho HVT, Djedovic V, de Castro Ruiz Marques A, Shishtar E, Mejia SB, Sievenpiper JL, de Souza RJ, Duvnjak L, and V Vuksan. 2017. The effect of alpha-linolenic acid on glycemic control in individuals with type 2 diabetes. A systematic review and meta-analysis of randomized controlled clinical trials. *Medicine* (Baltimore), May; 96(21): e6531. DOI: 10.1097/MD.0000000000006531.

Kalofoutis A. and J Lekakis. 1983. Changes of platelet phospholipids in diabetes mellitus. *Diabetologia*, 21: 540–543, 1981.

Kasim SE, Stern B, Khilnani S, McLin P, Baciorowski S, and K-LC Jen. 1988. Effects of omega-3 fish oils on lipid metabolism, glycemic control, and blood pressure in type II diabetic patients. *Journal of Clinical Endocrinology and Metabolism*, 67: 1–5.

Kast RE. 2001. Borage oil reduction of rheumatoid arthritis activity may be mediated by increased cAMP that suppresses tumor necrosis factor-alpha. *International Immunopharmacology*, Nov; 1(12): 2197–2199. DOI: 10.1016/S1567-5769(01)00146-1.

Keen H, Payan J, Allawi J, Walker J, Jamal GA, Weir AI, Henderson LM, Bissessar EA, Watkins PJ, and M Sampson. 1993. Treatment of diabetic neuropathy with gamma-linolenic acid. The gamma-Linolenic Acid Multicenter Trial Group. *Diabetes Care*, Jan; 16(1): 8–15.

Kharitonov S A, Lubec G, Lubec B, Hjelm M, and PJ Barnes. 1995. L-arginine increases exhaled nitric oxide in normal human subjects. *Clinical Science (Lond)*, Feb; 88(2), 135–139. DOI: 10.1042/cs0880135.

Kim D-H, Yoo T-H, Lee SH, Kang HY, Nam BY, Kwak SJ, Kim J-K, Park JT, Han SH, and S-W Kang. 2012. Gamma linolenic acid exerts anti-inflammatory and anti-fibrotic effects in diabetic nephropathy. *Yonsei Medical Journal*, Nov 1; 53(6): 1165–1175. DOI: 10.3349/ymj.2012.53.6.1165.

Kim HS, Kim HJ, Park KG, Kim YN, Kwon TK, Park JY, Lee KU, Kim JG, and IK Lee. 2007. Alpha-lipoic acid inhibits matrix metalloproteinase-9 expression by inhibiting NF-kappaB transcriptional activity. *Experimental and Molecular Medicine*, Feb; 39(1): 106–113. DOI: 10.1038/emm.2007.12.

Kleijnen J. 1994. Evening primrose oil. *BMJ* (Clinical Research Edition), Oct; 309(6958): 824–825. PMCID: PMC2541068.

Koeth RA, Wang Z, Levison BS, Buffa JA, Org E, Sheehy BT, Britt EB, Fu X, Wu Y, Li L, Smith JD, Didonato JA, Chen J, Li H, Wu GD, Lewis JD, Warrier M, Brown JM, Krauss RM, Tang WH, Bushman FD, Lusis AJ, and SL Hazen. 2013. Intestinal microbiota metabolism of L-carnitine, a nutrient in red meat, promotes atherosclerosis. *Nature Medicine*, May; 19(5): 576–585. DOI: 10.1038/nm.3145.

Kunt T, Forst T, Wilhelm A, Tritschler H, Pfutzner A, Harzer O, Engelbach M, Zschaebitz A, Stofft E, and J Beyer. 1999. Alpha-lipoic acid reduces expression of vascular cell adhesion molecule-1 and endothelial adhesion of human monocytes after stimulation with advanced glycation end products. *Clinical Science (Lond)*. Feb; 96(1): 75–82. DOI: 10.1042/CS19980224.

Lee BJ, Lin JS, Lin YC, and PT Lin. 2015. Antiinflammatory effects of L-carnitine supplementation (1000 mg/d) in coronary artery disease patients. *Nutrition*, Mar; 31(3): 475–479. DOI: 10.1016/j.nut.2014.10.001.

Lee EY, Lee CK, Lee KU, Park JY, Cho KJ, Cho YS, Lee HR, Moon SH, Moon HB, and B Yoo. 2007. Alpha-lipoic acid suppresses the development of collagen-induced arthritis and protects against bone destruction in mice. *Rheumatology International*, Jan; 27(3): 225–233. DOI: 10.1007/s00296-006-0193-5.

Lee J, Ryu H, Ferrante RJ, Morris SM, Jr, and RR Ratan. 2003. Translational control of inducible nitric oxide synthase expression by arginine can explain the arginine paradox. *Proceedings of the National Academy of Sciences, USA*. Apr; 100(8), 4843–4848. DOI: 10.1073/pnas.0735876100.

Lee TC, Ivester P, Hester AG, Case LD, Morgan T, Kouba EO, and F Chilton. 2014. The impact of polyunsaturated fatty acid-based dietary supplements on disease biomarkers in a metabolic syndrome/diabetes population. *Lipids in Health and Disease*, Dec; 13(1):196. DOI: 10.1186/1476-511X-13-196.

Lheureux PE, and P Hantson. 2009. Carnitine in the treatment of valproic acid-induced toxicity. *Clinical Toxicology (Phila)*, Feb; 47(2): 101–111. DOI: 10.1080/15563650902752376.

Li J, Zhang N, Ye B, Ju W, Orser B, Fox JEM, Wheeler MB, Wang Q, and W-Y Lu. 2007. Non-steroidal anti-inflammatory drugs increase insulin release from beta cells by inhibiting ATP-sensitive potassium channels. *British Journal of Pharmacology*, Jun; 151(4): 483–493. DOI: 10.1038/sj.bjp.0707259.

Lubec B, Hayn M, Kitzmüller E, Vierhapper H, and G Lubec. 1977. L-arginine reduces lipid peroxidation in patients with diabetes mellitus. *Free Radical Biology and Medicine*, 22, 355–357. DOI: 10.1016 /S0891-5849(96)00386-3.

Lucotti P, Setola E, Monti LD, Galluccio E, Costa S, Sandoli EP, Fermo I, Rabaiotti G, Gatti R, and P-M Piatti. 2001. Beneficial effects of a long-term oral L-arginine treatment added to a hypocaloric diet and exercise training program in obese, insulin-resistant type 2 diabetic patients. *American Journal of Physiology Endocrinology and Metabolism,* Nov; 291(5): E906–E912. DOI: 10.1152/ajpendo .00002.2006.

Mandarino NR, Monteiro FdC Jr., Salgado JVL, Lages JS, and NS Filho. 2015. Is vitamin D deficiency a new risk factor for cardiovascular disease? *The Open Cardiovascular Medicine Journal*, 9: 40–49. DOI: 10.2174/1874192401509010040.

Matthews DR, Hosker JP, Rudenski AS, Naylor BA, Treacher DF, and RC Turner. 1985. Homeostasis model assessment: insulin resistance and beta-cell function from fasting plasma glucose and insulin concentrations in man. *Diabetologia*, Jul; 28(7): 412–419.

McKnight JR, Satterfield MC, Jobgen WS, Smith SB, Spencer TE, Meininger CJ, McNeal CJ, and G Wu. 2010. Beneficial effects of L-arginine on reducing obesity: potential mechanisms and important implications for human health. *Amino Acids*, Jul; 39(2), 349–357. DOI: 10.1007/s00726-010-0598-z.

Mehta S, Stewart DJ, and RD Levy. 1996. The hypotensive effect of L-arginine is associated with increased expired nitric oxide in humans. *Chest*, 109, 1550–1555.

Menge BA, Schrader H, Ritter PR, Ellrichmann M, Uhl W, Schmidt WE, and JJ Meier. 2010. Selective amino acid deficiency in patients with impaired glucose tolerance and type 2 diabetes. *Regulatory Peptides*, Feb; 160(1-3): 75–80. DOI: 10.1016/j.regpep.2009.08.001.

Mijnhout GS, Kollen BJ, Alkhalaf A, Nanno Kleefstra N, and HJG Bilo. 2012. Alpha lipoic acid for symptomatic peripheral neuropathy in patients with diabetes: a meta-analysis of randomized controlled trials. *International Journal of Endocrinology*, 2012: 456279. DOI: 10.1155/2012/456279.

Mingrone G, Greco AV, Capristo E, Benedetti G, Giancaterini A, De Gaetano A, and G Gasbarrini. 1999. L-carnitine improves glucose disposal in type 2 diabetic patients. *Journal of the American College of Nutrition*, Feb; 18(1); 77–82.

Mingrone G. 2004. Carnitine in type 2 diabetes. *Annals of the NY Academy of Sciences.* Nov; 1033:99–107. DOI: 10.1196/annals.1320.009.

Morita, Takahashi R, Ito H. Orimo H, and S Murota. 1983. Increased arachidonic acid content in platelet phospholipids from diabetic patients. *Prostaglandins, Leukotrienes and Medicine*, 11: 33–341.

Morris SM Jr. 2012. Arginases and arginine deficiency syndromes. *Current Opinion in Clinical Nutrition and Metabolic Care*, Jan; 15(1): 64–70. DOI: 10.1097/MCO.0b013e32834d1a08.

Nakaki T, and K Hishikawa. 2002. The arginine paradox. *Nihon Yakurigaku Zasshi*, Jan; 119(1), 7–14.

Nanri A, Mizoue T, Noda M, Takahashi Y, Matsushita Y, Poudel-Tandukar K, Kato M, Oba S, Inoue M, and S Tsugane; Japan Public Health Center-based Prospective Study Group of 106 collaborators. 2011. Fish intake and type 2 diabetes in Japanese men and women: the Japan Public Health Center-based Prospective Study. *American Journal of Clinical Nutrition*, Sep; 94(3):884–891. DOI: 10.3945 /ajcn.111.012252.

No authors listed. 1993. The Diabetes Control and Complications Trial Study Research Group. The effect of intensive treatment of diabetes on the development and progression of long-term complications in insulin-dependent diabetes mellitus. *New England Journal of Medicine*, Sept; 329(14): 977–986. DOI: 10.1056/NEJM199309303291401.

No authors listed. 2005. The Diabetes Control and Complications Trial/Epidemiology of Diabetes Interventions and Complications (DCCT/EDIC) Study Research Group. Intensive diabetes treatment and cardiovascular disease in patients with diabetes type 1. *New England Journal of Medicine*, Dec; 353(25): 2643–2653. DOI: 10.1056/NEJMoa052187.

No authors listed. 2004. Carnitine: lessons from one hundred years of research. *Annals of the New York Academy of Sciences.* 1033: ix–xi.

Nordoy A. and JM Rodset. 1970. Platelet phospholipids and thehr function in patients with juvenile diabetes and maturlty onset diabetes. *Diabetes*, 19: 698–702.

Osterud B, and EO Elvevoll. 2011. Dietary omega-3 fatty acids and risk of type 2 diabetes: lack of antioxidants? *American Journal of Clinical Nutrition*, Aug; 94(2): 617–618. DOI: 10.3945/ajcn.111.017855.

Packer L, Witt EH, and J Tritschler. 1995. alpha-Lipoic acid as a biological antioxidant. *Free Radical Biology and Medicine*, Aug; 19(2): 227–250. PMID: 7649494.

Papanas N, and D Ziegler. 2014. Efficacy of α-lipoic acid in diabetic neuropathy. *Expert Opinion on Pharmacotherapy*, Dec; 15(18): 2721–2731. DOI: 10.1517/14656566.2014.972935.

Patterson E, Wall R, Fitzgerald GF, Ross RP, and C Stanton. 2012. Health implications of high dietary omega-6 polyunsaturated fatty acids. *Journal of Nutrition and Metabolism*, Apr; 2012: 539426. DOI: 10.1155/2012/539426.

Perrott J, Murphy NG, and PJ Zed. 2010. L-carnitine for acute valproic acid overdose: a systematic review of published cases. *Annals of Pharmacotherapy*, Aug; 44(7): 1287–1293. DOI: 10.1345/aph.1P135.

Philibert A, Vanier C, Abdelouahab N, Chan HM, and D Mergler. 2006. Fish intake and serum fatty acid profiles from freshwater fish. *The American Journal of Clinical Nutrition*, Dec; 84(6): 1299–1307.

Piatti PM, Monti LD, Valsecchi G, Magni F, Setola E, Marchesi F, Galli-Kienle M, Pozza G, and KGMM Alberti. 2001. Long-term oral L-arginine administration improves peripheral and hepatic insulin sensitivity in Type 2 diabetic patients. *Diabetes Care*, May; 24(5): 875–880. https://doi.org/10.2337/diacare.24.5.875.

Porasuphatana S, Suddee S, Nartnampong A, Konsil J, Harnwong B, and A Santaweesuk. 2012. Glycemic and oxidative status of patients with type 2 diabetes mellitus following oral administration of alpha-lipoic acid: a randomized double-blinded placebo-controlled study. *Asia Pacific Journal of Clinical Nutrition*, 21(1): 12–21.

Puri BK. 2007. The safety of evening primrose oil in epilepsy. *Prostaglandins Leukotrenes and Essential Fatty Acids*, Aug; 77(2): 101–103. DOI: 10.1016/j.plefa.2007.07.003.

Rahbar AR, Shakerhosseini R, Saadat N, Taleban F, Pordal A, and B Gollestan. 2005. Effect of L-carnitine on plasma glycemic and lipidemic profile in patients with type II diabetes mellitus. *European Journal of Clinical Nutrition*, Apr; 59(4): 592–596. DOI: 10.1038/sj.ejcn.1602109.

Ramel A, Martinez A, Kiely M, Morais G, Bandarra NM, and I Thorsdottir. 2008. Beneficial effects of long-chain n-3 fatty acids included in an energy-restricted diet on insulin resistance in overweight and obese European young adults. *Diabetologia*, Jul; 8; 51(7): 1261–1268. DOI: 10.1007/s00125-008-1035-7.

Rebouche CJ. 1999. Carnitine. In: *Modern Nutrition in Health and Disease*, 9th edition, Shils ME, Olson JA, Shike M, and AC Ross (eds.). New York: Lippincott Williams and Wilkins, pp. 505–512.

Rebouche CJ. 2004. Kinetics, pharmacokinetics, and regulation of L-carnitine and acetyl-L-carnitine metabolism. *Annals of the NY Academy of Sciences*, 1033: 30–41. DOI: 10.1196/annals.1320.003.

Rector TS, Bank AJ, Mullen KA, Tschumperlin LK, Sih R, Pillai K, and SH Kubo. 1996. Randomized, double-blind, placebo-controlled study of supplemental oral L-arginine in patients with heart failure. *Circulation*, Jun; 93: 2135–2141. https://doi.org/10. 1161/01.CIR.93.12.2135.

Reed LJ. 1998. From lipoic acid to multi-enzyme complexes. *Protein Science*, Jan; 7(1): 220–224. DOI: 10.1002/pro.5560070125.

Reljanovic M, Reichel G, Rett K, Lobisch M, Schuette K, Moller W, Tritschler HJ, and H Mehnert. 1999. Treatment of diabetic polyneuropathy with the antioxidant thioctic acid (alpha-lipoic acid): a two year multicenter randomized double-blind placebo-controlled trial (ALADIN II). Alpha Lipoic Acid in Diabetic Neuropathy. *Free Radicical Research*, Sept; 31(3): 171–179. PMID: 10499773.

Sahebkar A. 2015. Effect of L-carnitine supplementation on circulating C-reactive protein levels: a systematic review and meta-analysis. *Journal of Medical Biochemistry*, 2015 Apr; 34(2): 151–159. DOI: 10.2478/jomb-2014-0030.

Saidpour A, Zahediasl S, Kimiagar M, Vafa M, Ghasemi A, Abadi A, Daneshpour MS, and M Zarkesh. 2011. Fish oil and olive oil can modify insulin resistance and plasma desacyl-ghrelin in rats. *Journal of Research in Medical Sciences*. 2011 Jul; 16(7): 862–871. PMCID: PMC3263097.

Schectman G, Kaul S, and AH Kissebah. 1988. Effect of fish oil concentrate on lipoprotein composition in NIDDM. *Diabetes*, 37: 1567–1573.

Shay KP, Moreau RF, Smith EJ, Smith AR, and TM Hagen. 2009. Alpha-lipoic acid as a dietary supplement: Molecular mechanisms and therapeutic potential. *Biochimica et Biophysica Acta*. Oct; 1790(10): 1149–1160. DOI: 10.1016/j.bbagen.2009.07.026.

Shivkar RR, and SA Abhang. 2014. Ratio of serum asymmetric dimethyl arginine (ADMA)/nitric oxide in coronary artery disease patients. *Journal of Clinical and Diagnostic Research*, Aug; 8(8): CC04–CC06. DOI: 10.7860/JCDR/2014/7849.4665.

Sima AA, Calvani M, Mehra M, and A Amato; the Acetyl-L-Carnitine Study Group. 2005. Acetyl-L-carnitine improves pain, nerve regeneration, and vibratory perception in patients with chronic diabetic neuropathy: an analysis of two randomized placebo-controlled trials. *Diabetes Care*, Jan; 28(1): 96–101.

Singh B, and A Saxena. 2010. Surrogate markers of insulin resistance: a review. *World Journal of Diabetes*, May 15; 1(2): 36–47. DOI: 10.4239/wjd.v1.i2.36.

Soeken KL, Miller SA, and E Ernst. 2003. Herbal medicines for the treatment of rheumatoid arthritis: a systematic review. *Rheumatology*. May; 42(5): 652–659. DOI: 10.1093/rheumatology/keg183.

Sola S, Mir MQ, Cheema FA, Khan-Merchant N, Menon RG, Parthasarathy S, and BV Khan. 2005. Irbesartan and lipoic acid improve endothelial function and reduce markers of inflammation in the metabolic syndrome: results of the Irbesartan and Lipoic Acid in Endothelial Dysfunction (ISLAND) study. *Circulation*, Jan; 111(3): 343–348. DOI: 10.1161/01.CIR.0000153272.48711.B9.

Souied EH, Aslam T, Garcia-Layana A, Holz FG, Leys A, Silva R, and C Delcourt. 2015. Omega-3 fatty acids and age-related macular degeneration. *Ophthalmic Research*, 55(2): 62–69. DOI: 10.1159/000441359.

Stacpoole PW, Alig J, Ammon L, and S Crockett. 1989. Dose–response effects of dietary fish oil on carbohydrate and lipid metabolism in hypertriglyceridemia. *Metabolism*, Oct; 38(10): 946–956.

Stratton IM, Adler AI, Neil AW, Matthews DR, Manley SE, Cull CA, Hadden D, Turner RC, and RR Holman on behalf of the UK Prospective Diabetes Study Group. 2005. Association of glycaemia with macrovascular and microvascular complications of type 2 diabetes (UKPDS 35): prospective observational study. *British Medical Journal*, Aug; 321(7258): 405–412. DOI: 10.1136/bmj.321.7258.405.

Taddei S, Virdis A, Ghiadoni L, Salvetti G, Bernini G, Magagna A, and A Salvetti. 2001. Age-related reduction of NO availability and oxidative stress in humans. *Hypertension*, Aug; 38(2), 274–279.

Takahashi R, Morita I, Saito Y, Ito H, and S Murota. 1984. Increased arachidonic acid incorporation into platelet phospholipids in type 2 (non-insulin-dependent) diabetes. *Diabetologla*, 26: 134–137.

Takahashi Y, Ide T, and H Fujita. 2000. Dietary gamma-linolenic acid in the form of borage oil causes less body fat accumulation accompanying an increase in uncoupling protein 1 mRNA level in brown adipose tissue. *Comparative Biochemistry and Physiology. Part B. Biochemistry and Molecular Biology*, Oct; 127(2): 213–222.

The editors. 2004. Carnitine: lessons from one hundred years of research. *Annals of the NY Academy of Sciences*, 1033: ix–xi.

Tilvis RS, Rasi V, Viinikka L. Ylikorkala O, and TA Miettinen. 1987. Effects of purified fish oil on platelet lipids and function in diabetic women. *Clinica Chimica Acta*, 164: 315–322.

Toutouzas K, Riga M, Stefanadi E, and C Stefanadis. 2008. Asymmetric dimethylarginine (ADMA) and other endogenous nitric oxide synthase (NOS) inhibitors as an important cause of vascular insulin resistance. *Hormones and Metabolic Research*, 40, 655–659. DOI: 10.1055/s-0028-1083814.

Udupa AS, Nahar PS, Shah SH, Kshirsagar MJ, and BB Ghongane. 2012. Study of comparative effects of antioxidants on insulin sensitivity in type 2 diabetes mellitus. *Journal of Clinical and Diagnostic Research*, Nov; 6(9): 1469–1473. DOI: 10.7860/JCDR/2012/4464.2535.

Valdés-Ramos R, Guadarrama-López AL, Martínez-Carrillo BE, and AD Benítez-Arciniega. 2015. Vitamins and type 2 diabetes mellitus. *Endocrine, Metabolic and Immune Disorders Drug Targets*, 15(1): 54–63. PMCID: PMC4435229.

Vallianou N, Evangelopoulos A, and P Koutalas. 2009. Alpha-lipoic acid and diabetic neuropathy. *The Review of Diabetic Studies*, Winter; 6(4): 230–236. DOI: 10.1900/RDS.2009.6.230.

van der Zwan LP, Scheffer PG, Dekker JM, Stehouwer CD, Heine RJ, and T Teerlink. 2011. Systemic inflammation is linked to low arginine and high ADMA plasma levels resulting in an unfavourable NOS substrate-to-inhibitor ratio: the Hoorn Study. *Clinical Science (Lond.)*, Jul; 121(2): 71–78. DOI: 10.1042/CS20100595.

Verrotti A, Trotta D, Morges G, Chiarelli F, Verrotti A, Trotta D, Morgese G, and F Chiarelli. 2002. Valproate-Induced Hyperammonemic Encephalopathy. *Metabolic Brain Disease*, Dec; 17(4): 367–373.

Vidal-Casariego A, Burgos-Peláez R, Martínez-Faedo C, Calvo-Gracia F, Valero-Zanuy MÁ, Luengo-Pérez LM, and C Cuerda-Compés. 2013. Metabolic effects of L-carnitine on type 2 diabetes mellitus: systematic review and meta-analysis. *Experimental and Clinical Endocrinology and Diabetes*, Apr; 121(4): 234–238. DOI: 10.1055/s-0033-1333688.

Wall R, Ross RP, Fitzgerald GF, and C Stanton. 2010. Fatty acids from fish: the anti-inflammatory potential of long-chain omega-3 fatty acids. *Nutrition Review*, May; 68(5): 280–209. DOI: 10.1111/j.1753-4887.2010.00287.x.

Wascher TC, Graier WF, Dittrich P, Hussain MA, Bahadori B, Wallner S, and H Toplak. 1997. Effects of low-dose L-arginine on insulin mediated vasodilatation and insulin sensitivity. *European Journal of Clinical Investigation*, Aug; 27(8): 690–695.

Wei IW, Ulchaker MM, and JP Sheehan. 1988. Plasma insulin and glucose parameters during omega-3 fatty acid (w-3 FA) supplementation in non-obese non-insulin-dependent-diabetes (NIDDM) (Abstract). *Diabetes*, 37 (Suppl 1): 107A.

Welsch MA, Dobrosielski DA, ArceEsquivel AA, Wood RH, Ravussin E, Rowley C, and SM Jazwinski. 2008. The Association between Flow-Mediated Dilation and Physical Function in Older Men. *Medicine and Science in Sports and Exercise*, Jul; 40(7): 1237–1243. DOI: 10.1249/MSS.0b013e31816c5552.

Wettasinghe M, Shahidi F, and R Amarowicz. 2002. Identification and quantification of low molecular weight phenolic antioxidants in seeds of evening primrose (*Oenothera biennis* L.). *Journal of Agricultural and Food Chemistry*, Feb; 27; 50(5): 1267–1271.

Wild S, Roglic G, Green A, Sicree R, and H King. 2004. Global prevalences of diabetes, estimates for the year 2000 and projections for 2030. *Diabetes Care*, Mar; 27(5): 1047–1053. DOI: 10.2337/diacare.27.5.1047. PMID: 15111519.

Wolf A, Zalpour C, Theilmeier G, Wang B-Y, Ma A, Anderson B, Tsao PS, and JP Cooke. 1997. Dietary L-arginine supplementation normalizes platelet aggregation in hypercholesterolemic humans. *Journal of the American College of Cardiology*, Mar; 29(3): 479–485. https://doi.org/10.1016/S0735-1097(97)00523-8.

Wollin SD, and PJ Jones. 2003. Alpha-lipoic acid and cardiovascular disease. *Journal of Nutrition*, Nov; 133(11): 3327–3330. PMID: 14608040.

Xu DP, and WW Wells. 1996. alpha-Lipoic acid dependent regeneration of ascorbic acid from dehydroascorbic acid in rat liver mitochondria. *Journal of Bioenergetics and Biomembranes*, Feb; 28(1): 77–85. PMID: 8786242.

Yamazaki RK, Brito GA, Coelho I, Pequitto DC, Yamaguchi AA, Borghetti G, Schiessel DL, Kryczyk M, Machado J, Rocha RE, Aikawa J, Iagher F, Naliwaiko K, Tanhoffer RA, Nunes EA, and LC Fernandes. 2011. Low fish oil intake improves insulin sensitivity, lipid profile and muscle metabolism on insulin resistant MSG-obese rats. *Lipids in Health and Disease*, Apr; 10: 66. DOI: 10.1186/1476-511X-10-66.

Yavuz BB, Yavuz B, Sener DD, Cankurtaran M, Halil M, Ulger Z, Nazli N, Kabakci G, Aytemir K, Tokgozoglu L, Oto A, and S Ariogul. 2008. Advanced age is associated with endothelial dysfunction in healthy elderly subjects. *Gerontology*, 54(3):153–156. DOI: 10.1159/000129064.

Zhang WJ, and B Frei. 2001. Alpha-lipoic acid inhibits TNF-alpha-induced NF-kappaB activation and adhesion molecule expression in human aortic endothelial cells. *Journal of the Federation of American Societies for Experimental Biology*, Nov; 15(13): 2423–2432. DOI: 10.1096/fj.01-0260com.

Zhao G, Etherton TD, Martin KR, West SG, Gillies PJ, and PM Kris-Etherton. 2004. Dietary alpha-linolenic acid reduces inflammatory and lipid cardiovascular risk factors in hypercholesterolemic men and women. *Journal of Nutrition*, Nov; 134(11): 2991–2997.

Ziegler D, Ametov A, Barinov A, Dyck PJ, Gurieva I, Low PA, Munzel U, Yakhno N, Raz I, Novosadova M, Maus J, and R Samigullin. 2006. Oral treatment with alpha-lipoic acid improves symptomatic diabetic polyneuropathy: the SYDNEY 2 trial. *Diabetes Care*, Nov; 29(11): 2365–2370. DOI: 10.2337/dc06-1216.

Ziegler D, Hanefeld M, Ruhnau KJ, Hasche H, Lobisch M, Schutte K, Kerum G, and R Malessa. 1999. Treatment of symptomatic diabetic polyneuropathy with the antioxidant alpha-lipoic acid: a 7-month multicenter randomized controlled trial (ALADIN III Study). ALADIN III Study Group. Alpha-Lipoic Acid in Diabetic Neuropathy. *Diabetes Care*, Aug; 22(6): 1296–1301. PMID: 10480774.

Ziegler D, Hanefeld M, Ruhnau KJ, Meissner HP, Lobisch M, Schutte K, and FA Gries. 1995. Treatment of symptomatic diabetic peripheral neuropathy with the anti-oxidant alpha-lipoic acid. A 3-week multicentre randomized controlled trial (ALADIN Study) *Diabetologia*, Dec; 38(12): 1425–1433.

Ziegler D, Nowak H, Kempler P, Vargha P, and PA Low. 2004. Treatment of symptomatic diabetic polyneuropathy with the antioxidant alpha-lipoic acid: a meta-analysis. *Diabetic Medicine*, Feb; 21(2): 114–121.

14 Additional Supplements That Support Glycemic Control and Reduce Chronic Inflammation

14.1 TAURINE

Taurine is a sulfur-containing amino acid generally found in protein-rich foods, and yet, it is one of the few amino acids not incorporated into proteins. It is one of the most abundant amino acids, widely distributed in body tissues, especially in the retina. In a review titled, "Taurine: A 'very essential amino acid'," published in the journal *Molecular Vision*, the authors emphasize a number of very important functions of taurine that are not generally widely known: Taurine is an organic osmolyte involved in cell volume and fluid regulation.

Taurine serves a wide variety of functions in the central nervous system, and deficiency is associated with cardiomyopathy, renal dysfunction, and severe damage to retinal neurons. All ocular tissues contain taurine, and quantitative analysis of ocular tissue extracts of the rat eye revealed that taurine is the most abundant amino acid in the retina, vitreous, lens, cornea, iris, and ciliary body.

In the retina, taurine is critical to photoreceptor development and acts as a cytoprotectant in stress-related neuronal damage and other pathological conditions. As will be shown below, supplementing taurine may also play a therapeutic role in the management of diabetes (Ripps, and Shen. 2012).

14.1.1 TAURINE REDUCES OXIDATIVE STRESS AND INFLAMMATION

Taurine is an antioxidant, and it plays a major role in cytoprotection and attenuation of apoptosis in a wide variety of relevant (albeit seemingly unrelated) disorders, including cardiovascular disease (Chen, Nan, Tian et al. 2012), diabetes-induced renal injury (Das, and Sil. 2012), inflammatory disease (Marcinkiewicz, and Kontny, 2012), and light-induced lipid peroxidation in photoreceptors (Pasantes-Morales, and Cruz. 1985).

As noted previously, there is a growing consensus that oxidative stress is linked to mitochondrial dysfunction (Crompton, and Andreeva. 1993; DiMonte, Chan, and Sandy. 1992; Menzie, Pan, Prentice et al. 2012; Perfeito, Cunha-Oliveira, and Cristina Rego. 2012) and that the beneficial effects of taurine result from its antioxidant properties, as well as its ability to improve mitochondrial function by stabilizing the electron transport chain and inhibiting the generation of reactive oxygen species (ROS) (Schaffer, Azuma, and Mozaffari. 2009; Jong, Azuma, and Schaffer. 2012).

The journal *Amino Acids* published a study titled "Mechanism underlying the antioxidant activity of taurine, prevention of mitochondrial oxidant production." Its authors pointed out that an important function of the β-amino acid, taurine, is the regulation of oxidative stress. However, taurine is neither a classical free radical scavenger, nor is it a regulator of the antioxidative defenses, leaving uncertain the mechanism underlying the nature of the antioxidant activity.

In the above-cited *Amino Acids* study, the taurine antagonist, and taurine transport inhibitor, β-alanine, was used to examine the mechanism underlying the antioxidant activity. Exposure of isolated cardiomyocytes to medium containing β-alanine for a period of hours led to a 45% decrease in taurine content and an increase in mitochondrial oxidative stress, as evidenced by enhanced superoxide generation, the inactivation of the oxidant sensitive enzyme aconitase, and the oxidation of glutathione (which is active and useful only in the reduced state).

There was a decline in electron transport activity associated with an increase in oxidative stress, with the activities of respiratory chain complexes I and III declining 50% to 65% and oxygen consumption falling by 30%.

A reduction in respiratory chain activity coupled with an increase in oxidative stress is commonly caused by the development of a bottleneck in electron transport that leads to the diversion of electrons from the respiratory chain to the acceptor oxygen, forming superoxide in the process. Because β-alanine exposure significantly reduces the levels of the respiratory chain complex subunits ND5 and ND6, the bottleneck in electron transport appears to be caused by impaired synthesis of key subunits of the electron transport chain complexes.

Co-administration of taurine with β-alanine largely prevented the mitochondrial effects of β-alanine, but treatment of the cells with 5 mM taurine in the absence of β-alanine had no effect on the mitochondria, likely because taurine treatment has little effect on cellular taurine levels.

The investigators concluded that taurine serves as a regulator of mitochondrial protein synthesis, thereby enhancing electron transport chain activity and protecting the mitochondria against excessive superoxide generation (Jong, Azuma, and Schaffer. 2012; see also Kontny, and Marcinkiewicz. 2014).

14.1.2 Taurine and Diabetes

The unifying hypothesis of diabetes etiology holds that reactive oxygen species (ROS), generated in the mitochondria of cells exposed to glucose, promote reactions leading to the development of diabetic complications. Although this hypothesis attributes the generation of oxidants solely to impaired metabolism of glucose and fatty acids, diabetes is also associated with a decline in the availability of the endogenous antioxidant taurine.

This points to the possibility that changes in taurine status might also contribute to the severity of the oxidant-mediated damage. Although taurine is incapable of directly scavenging the classic ROS such as superoxide anion, hydroxyl radical, and hydrogen peroxide, there are numerous studies suggesting that it is an effective inhibitor of ROS generation (Ito, Schaffer, and Azuma. 2012; Schaffer, Azuma, and Mozaffari. 2009; Sirdah. 2015; see also: El Idrissi, Boukarrou, Splavnyk et al. 2009).

A comprehensive review in the journal *Amino Acids* concluded that taurine supplementation is effective against diabetes mellitus, insulin resistance, and its complications, including retinopathy, nephropathy, neuropathy, and cardiomyopathy, independent of its antihyperglycemic effect, in several animal models, as well as in clinical studies. The effectiveness appears to be due to the multiple actions of taurine on cellular functions.

The review summarizes the beneficial effects of taurine supplementation on diabetes and the molecular mechanisms underlying its effectiveness (Ito, Schaffer, and Azuma. 2012).

14.1.2.1 Plasma Taurine Levels Are Lower than Normal in Diabetes

According to a report published in the *American Journal of Clinical Nutrition*, plasma taurine concentration in Type 2 diabetes patients is significantly lower than that in control participants (Franconi, Bennardini, Mattana et al. 1995; Franconi, Miceli, Fazzini et al. 1996). The reduction of plasma taurine levels has also consistently been demonstrated in streptozotocin (STZ)- or in alloxan-induced diabetic animals (Franconi, Miceli, Fazzini et al. 1996; Trachtman, Futterweit, Maesaka et al. 1995).

In Type 2 diabetes patients, the plasma taurine level was found to be lower than that in nondiabetes healthy control participants (Luca, Calpona, Caponetti et al. 2001; Merheb, Daher, Nasrallah et al. 2007).

Since taurine deficiency is linked to dysfunction in numerous tissues (Hayes, Carey, and Schmidt. 1975; Pion, Kittleson, Rogers et al. 1987; Sturman 1991), a decrease in taurine level in Type 2 diabetes patients may be implicated in the complications of diabetes.

14.1.3 TAURINE REDUCES THE PRODUCTION OF ADVANCED GLYCATION END PRODUCTS

As previously reported, hyperglycemia accelerates nonenzymatic glycation of protein and causes the accumulation of advanced glycation end products (AGEs). These AGEs contribute to the development of diabetic complications such as nephropathy and microvascular diseases.

However, since taurine reacts highly with aldehyde, as compared to the other amino acids (Ogasawara, Nakamura, Koyama et al. 1993), it is expected that it will prevent the formation of AGEs in diabetes. In fact, it was found that taurine inhibited the formation of AGE *in vitro* (Nandhini, Thirunavukkarasu, and Anuradha. 2004; Nandhini, and Anuradha. 2005; Selvaraj, Bobby, and Sathiyapriya. 2006).

In high-fructose–fed rats, taurine supplementation reliably prevented an increase in the plasma glycated proteins, such as fructosamine and glycated hemoglobin (Nandhini, Thirunavukkarasu, and Anuradha. 2004).

14.1.4 TAURINE PREVENTS LDL MODIFICATION

According to a report in the *Journal of Lipid Research*, modified (oxidized) low-density lipoprotein (LDL) is thought to play a key role in atherosclerosis (Steinberg. 2009). Modified LDL also contributes to development of vascular complications. The reactivity of taurine with aldehyde may contribute to decreased malondialdehyde (MDA)-related LDL modification (Ogasawara, Nakamura, Koyama et al. 1993). Moreover, taurine also exerts scavenging action in connection with hypochlorous acid (HClO), which is produced by myeloperoxidase in neutrophils and macrophages, and is also involved in oxidation of LDL (Pennathur and Heinecke. 2007).

In Type 2 diabetic animal models, high myeloperoxidase activity has been found in the vessels of diabetic obese rats (Zhang, Yang, and Jennings. 2004), indicating that in diabetes, HClO may contribute to an increase in oxidized LDL.

The effect of taurine lowering the level of LDL cholesterol itself may contribute to the reduction in oxidized LDL (Bellentani, Pecorari, Cordoma. 1987; Gandhi, Cherian, and Mulky. 1992; Nakamura-Yamanaka, Tsuji, and Ichikawa. 1987; Yokogoshi, Mochizuki, Nanami et al. 1999). The increased serum level of LDL cholesterol in STZ-induced diabetic mice was normalized by the chronic administration of taurine, according to a report in the journal *Bioscience, Biotechnology, and Biochemistry* (Mochizuki, Takido, Oda et al. 1999; see also Nanami, Oda, and Yokogoshi. 1996).

14.1.5 TAURINE PREVENTS ENDOTHELIAL DYSFUNCTION

Type 2 diabetes is noted for its adverse impact on blood vessels. Most of the diabetic complications are associated with vascular disorders, particularly endothelial dysfunction. Microangiopathy has been shown to cause retinopathy, nephropathy, and neuropathy, whereas macroangiopathy is linked to cardiomyopathy and atherosclerosis.

In the STZ-induced diabetic mouse model, the ability of acetylcholine to bring about vasodilation in aortic rings is blunted. According to the conclusion of a study in the *European Journal of Pharmacology*, chronic supplementation of these mice with taurine corrects that problem, enabling the aortic rings to dilate in response to acetylcholine, while the vasodilation capacity is attenuated in STZ-induced diabetic mice (Kamata, Sugiura, Kojima et al. 1996).

Additionally, as reported in a study published in the journal *Life Sciences*, pre-incubation of the tissues with taurine for 2 h *ex vivo* improved both the enhanced response to norepinephrine and the attenuated response to acetylcholine in aorta rings from STZ-induced diabetic rats (Abebe. 2008).

It is generally thought that these data point to the protective action of taurine on the impaired endothelium-dependent vasodilator response in hyperglycemia.

A variety of molecular mechanisms underlie the beneficial role of taurine against endothelial dysfunction in diabetes mellitus. These are illustrated and summarized in Figure 1 in Ito, Schaffer and Azuma (2012) (*Amino Acids*, May; 42(5): 1529–1539). This figure can be viewed at https://www.ncbi.nlm.nih.gov/pmc/articles/PMC3325402/ (accessed 2.17.18).

The figure describes the pathways thought to be involved in both the adverse and the beneficial action of taurine against hyperglycemia-induced endothelial dysfunction: Taurine can inhibit the production of many detrimental products such as AGEs and oxidized LDL (oxLDL), the latter by scavenging malondialdehyde (MDA) as well as hypochlorous acid (HClO. Taurine also inhibits the reduction of beneficial nitric oxide (NO) that would take place via an HClO-dependent pathway, and it prevents certain harmful leukocyte–endothelium interactions, as we will now see in the paragraphs that follow. Additionally, HClO consumes the NO and in turn causes vasoconstriction and endothelial dysfunction (Pennathur, and Heinecke. 2007). Therefore, taurine may increase the bioavailability of NO through scavenging HClO.

Furthermore, taurine suppressed the expressions of vascular cell adhesion molecule-1 and intercellular adhesion molecule-1 (ICAM-1) induced by high glucose in cultured endothelial cells (Ulrich-Merzenich, Zeitler, Vetter et al. 2007).

According to a report in the *European Journal of Pharmacology*, when STZ-treated diabetic rats were given taurine supplementation after diabetes onset, it prevented the induction of ICAM-1 and lectin-like oxidized LDL receptor-1, which is responsible for the incorporation of oxidized LDL into aorta cells (Wang, Yu, Zhang et al. 2008), and while acute hyperglycemia induced by intravenous infusion of glucose activated leukocyte adhesion and migration to endothelium, and increased endothelial ICAM-1 and apoptosis in rats, taurine supplementation for 5 days before the experiment prevented leukocyte actions and the elevation of ICAM-1 and apoptotic cell death (Casey, Gang, Joyce et al. 2007).

The investigators concluded that taurine may prevent the leukocyte–endothelial cell interaction and endothelial apoptosis enhanced by hyperglycemia.

14.1.6 Taurine Ameliorates Diabetic Retinopathy

A study published in the journal *Neurochemical Research* reported that taurine supplementation after diabetic onset, in an STZ-induced diabetic model, effectively improved the damage otherwise seen in the retinal ultrastructure; it attenuated the induction of glial fibrillary acid protein, a marker of gliosis, and it reduced apoptosis in retinal glial cells, all without having an effect on plasma glucose concentration (Yu, Xu, Mi et al. 2008), which indicates the beneficial role of taurine on diabetic retinopathy.

Taurine supplementation in STZ-induced rats was also shown to significantly decrease retinal carbonyl dienes (Di Leo, Santini, Cercone et al. 2002; Di Leo, Ghirlanda, Gentiloni et al. 2003). In another study published in the journal *Diabetologia* on STZ-diabetic rats, taurine supplementation attenuated the induction of retinal vascular endothelial growth factor, which is linked to vascularization, suggesting that taurine may normalize the retinal vascular function in diabetes (Obrosova, Minchenko, Marinescu et al. 2001).

In their conclusion, the investigators stated that "Oxidative stress is directly involved in up-regulation of vascular endothelial growth factor protein in the retina during early diabetes, thus linking the therapeutic outcome of taurine supplementation to reversing at least some of the damaging effects oxidative stress."

An excess of the neurotransmitter glutamate in the retina can serve as an excitotoxin, damaging the tissues. A study published in the journal *Neurochemical Research* found that in STZ-treated diabetic rats, elevation of glutamate in the retina was associated with the development of diabetic retinopathy and that taurine prevented the elevation of retinal glutamate content, in part, by enhancing the removal (uptake) and degradation of glutamate (Zeng, Xu, Mi et al. 2009). Likewise, as reported in the journal *Molecular and Cell Neurosciences*, taurine suppressed high-glucose–induced defects of glutamate uptake and degradation in cultured Müller cells (Zeng, Xu, Chen et al. 2010).

The significance of the above finding is that Müller cells are the principal glial cells of the retina. They execute many of the functions of the astrocytes, oligodendrocytes, and ependymal cells that are found in other CNS regions. They express numerous voltage-gated channels and neurotransmitter receptors, which recognize a variety of neuronal signals. They can trigger cell depolarization and can generate intracellular Ca^{2+} waves (Newman, and Reichenbach. 1996). Therefore, the ability of taurine to blunt the damaging effects that glutamate otherwise has on Müller cells tells us that supplements with this amino acid would tend to protect against retinopathy.

14.1.7 TAURINE AND DIABETIC CATARACTS

Taurine is the most abundant free amino acid in the eye lens, and a study published in the *Indian Journal of Physiology and Pharmacology* reported that in STZ-induced diabetic rats, lens taurine level is lower than normal (Anthrayose, and Shashidhar. 2004).

A study published in the journal *Pediatric Research* reiterated previous findings that sugar cataracts associated with diabetes mellitus result from the accumulation of excess sorbitol within lens fibrils, causing them to swell when water moves in to maintain osmotic balance. The excess water then causes disruption of fibrils and cataract formation.

Sorbitol is a sugar alcohol that the body metabolizes slowly. It can be obtained by a reduction of glucose, which changes the aldehyde group to a hydroxyl group. As indicated in a previous chapter, when intracellular glucose is increased in hyperglycemia, excessive glucose is metabolized to sorbitol through aldose reductase. However, there is indication that more than sorbitol-induced osmotic stress is involved, and the abovementioned study centered on lenses collected from rats after 21 or 44 days of streptozotocin (STZ) induction of diabetes.

Cataracts were not apparent in the 21-day untreated STZ-diabetic rats, but were found to have formed in untreated 44-day STZ-diabetic rats. It was found also that lens sorbitol increased in the animals being induced with STZ, both before and after cataract formation. Lens taurine concentration varied inversely with the sorbitol content in a fashion that resulted in no net change in total lens osmoles. Lens water did not increase in the diabetic animals with or without cataracts.

The aldose reductase inhibitor Sorbinil prevented the increase in lens sorbitol in both the 21- and 44-day STZ-diabetic rats, and cataract formation was prevented in the 44-day diabetic animals. The lens water in untreated diabetic animals with cataracts did not differ from lens water in the Sorbinil-treated diabetic animals that did not develop cataracts. Sorbinil treatment of diabetic animals was associated with normalization of lens levels of both sorbitol and taurine.

The investigators concluded that taurine is both an osmoregulator and an antioxidant. The apparent increase in lens osmolality attributed to sorbitol was counterbalanced by an equimolar reduction in taurine concentration, the latter development putting the lens at risk.

The reciprocal relationship between taurine and sorbitol reduces the likelihood of an osmotic mechanism for sugar cataract formation. The reduced lens taurine, however, may increase the risk of lens protein oxidation and subsequent cataract formation. *In vivo* sugar cataract formation may be an oxidative process rather than an osmotic phenomenon (Malone, Lowitt, and Cook. 1990).

In that context, it should be noted that, as reported in a study published in the journal *Investigative Ophthalmology and Visual Science*, chronic taurine supplementation reduced MDA level in the lens of STZ-induced diabetic rats (Obrosova, and Stevens 1999).

Although, as observed in a study published in the *Journal of Nutritional Science and Vitaminology*, taurine did not improve opacity of eye lens induced by the exposure to high glucose medium for 6 days in cultured lens, it did inhibit the protein carbonylation induced by high glucose (Son, Kim, and Kwon. 2007). These findings indicate that taurine protects the lens from oxidative stress induced by hyperglycemia.

14.1.8 TAURINE AMELIORATES DIABETIC NEUROPATHY

Sorbitol accumulation in nerves is associated with diabetic peripheral neuropathy. Organic osmolytes, including sorbitol, taurine, and myo-inositol, are regulated in response to the change of extracellular osmolality to maintain the cell volume. A study published in the journal *Diabetologia* demonstrated that taurine and myo-inositol are decreased in nerves of STZ-induced diabetic rats, whereas administration of an aldose reductase inhibitor attenuated the depletion of taurine and myo-inositol, suggesting that excessive accumulation of sorbitol led to the depletion of other organic osmolytes (Stevens, Lattimer, Kamijo et al. 1993).

The exposure of cells to high glucose is known to reduce the expression of the taurine transporter, whereas treatment with an aldose reductase inhibitor, or an antioxidant, reversed the decreased expression of the taurine transporter, suggesting the crucial role of sorbitol in the regulation of intracellular taurine concentrations (Askwith, Zeng, Eggo et al. 2009).

Taurine supplementation was shown to improve defective nerve functions, such as nerve conductance deficits and hyperalgesia, and to ameliorate the deficits of nerve blood flow in the STZ-induced diabetic model (Li, Obrosova, Abatan et al. 2006; Pop-Busui, Sullivan, Huysen et al. 2001). Taurine supplementation was also shown to reduce the oxidative stress in nerves and to prevent impairment of calcium metabolism in sensory neurons of STZ-induced diabetic rats (Li, Obrosova, Abatan et al. 2006).

Furthermore, taurine supplementation in STZ-induced diabetes rats prevented the decrease in levels of nerve growth factor (NGF) that are otherwise seen (Obrosova, Fathallah, and Stevens. 2001). NGF is of course important for the growth and stability of neurons.

Similarly, in Zucker diabetic fatty rats, taurine helped prevent diabetic peripheral neuropathy, reducing deficits of hind limb sciatic motor neurons, reducing damage to digital sensory nerve conduction velocity, and maintaining sensory thresholds (Li, Abatan, Kim et al. 2006).

14.1.9 CLINICAL APPLICATIONS OF TAURINE SUPPLEMENTATION IN DIABETES

Previous studies reporting the role of taurine deficiency, and the effects of taurine supplementation in Type 2 diabetes, were carried out largely on animal models, typically rats. Investigators were of course eager to see if this would carry over to diabetic humans. The clinical usefulness of taurine supplementation in Type 2 diabetes has been evaluated in some clinical studies as well. For instance, in a study reported in the journal *Advances in Experimental Medicine and Biology*, the investigators tested the antihyperglycemic effect of 3 g of taurine per day, for 4 months, in Type 2 diabetes patients.

They reported that while taurine supplementation increased plasma taurine level, it did not change either the glycosylated hemoglobin (HbA1c) level or the plasma lipid peroxide level, compared to a placebo control group (Chauncey, Tenner, Lombardini et al. 2003).

Some of the studies, such as the one cited just above, for example, lead to the conclusion that taurine may not influence hyperglycemia and insulin resistance in Type 2 diabetic patients. This would seem to be inconsistent with animal studies. However, these clinical studies have limitations including medication regimens, the dose of taurine administered, and the duration of trials.

However, the value of taurine supplementation against the impairment of insulin sensitivity was reported in a crossover clinical study appearing in the journal *Diabetologia*. The investigators demonstrated the effect of taurine against insulin resistance and chronic elevation of plasma fatty acids induced by the 48-h intravenous infusion of Intralipid (20% soybean oil, 1.2% egg phospholipids, 2.25% glycerin in water, and heparin) on nondiabetic men who were either overweight or obese.

A 2-week pretreatment of 3 g/day of taurine before lipid infusion improved the impaired insulin sensitivity and prevented the rise in lipid peroxidation products in plasma, indicating that oral taurine supplementation ameliorates fatty acid–induced insulin resistance in humans, possibly by the mechanism of reducing oxidative stress (Xiao, Giacca, and Lewis. 2008).

A study published in the journal *Diabetes and Vascular Disease Research* reported the beneficial effect of taurine on endothelial dysfunction in Type 1 diabetes patients, in a crossover study. Arterial stiffness and flow-mediated dilation (FMD) of the brachial artery, which are endothelium-dependent reactions, were low in diabetic patients as compared to control participants. Taurine supplementation of 1.5 g/day for 2 weeks returned these parameters to control levels, without anti-hyperglycemic effect, indicating the protective role of taurine on endothelium (Moloney, Casey, O'Donnell et al. 2010; see also Ito, Schaffer, and Azuma. 2012).

The role of taurine depletion in the pathophysiology and complications of Type 2 diabetes is reasonably well established in animal models, as is also the efficacy of supplementation with this amino acid in those animal models. Given the abundance of animal models showing the efficiency of taurine, and a handful of clinical studies confirming that efficacy, there is considerable reason to believe that taurine supplementation could play a key role in treatment of Type 2 diabetes and its complications.

14.1.10 SAFETY OF SUPPLEMENTING WITH TAURINE

A report published in the journal *Regulatory Toxicology and Pharmacology* states in part that the absence of a systematic pattern of adverse effects in humans in response to orally administered taurine precluded the selection of a no observed adverse effect level or lowest observed adverse effect level. Therefore, the conventional approach to risk assessment for identification of a tolerable upper level of intake (UL) could not be used. Instead, the newer method described as the observed safe level (OSL) or highest observed intake was utilized.

The OSL risk assessments indicate that, based on the available published human clinical trial data, the evidence for the absence of adverse effects is strong for taurine at supplemental intakes up to 3 g/day, and these levels are identified as the respective OSLs for normal healthy adults. Although much higher levels of taurine have been tested without adverse effects, and they may be safe, the data for intakes above these levels are not sufficient for a confident conclusion of long-term safety and therefore these values are not selected as the OSLs (Shao, and Hathcock. 2008).

14.2 THE ROLE OF SELECTED VITAMINS IN TYPE 2 DIABETES

In 1912, Kazimierz Funk (1884–1967), a Polish biochemist, originated the concept of "vital amines," for any of a group of organic compounds that are essential for normal growth and are required in small quantities in the diet because most cannot be synthesized by the body. Funk coined the term "vitamins."

Vitamins play a key role in glycemic control, both normal and abnormal, but some vitamins have received more attention than others in connection with Type 2 diabetes. A small sample of them is discussed in the subsequent sections.

14.2.1 VITAMIN D3 (CHOLECALCIFEROL)

"Vitamin D" refers to a group of fat-soluble (seco)steroids involved in increasing intestinal absorption of calcium, magnesium, and phosphate, in addition to other biological effects. One of the most important compounds for humans, in this group, is vitamin D3, also known as cholecalciferol. Cholecalciferol can be obtained from the diet, but few foods actually contain it. However, it can, of course, also be obtained through supplements.

The principal natural source of the vitamin comes from the synthesis of cholesterol in the skin through a chemical reaction dependent on exposure to ultraviolet (B) in sun radiation. Dietary recommendations typically assume that all of a person's vitamin D3 is taken by mouth, as sun exposure in the population is variable and recommendations about the amount of sun exposure that is safe are uncertain in view of the skin cancer risk.

Vitamin D3 from the diet, or skin synthesis, is biologically inactive, and enzymatic conversion (hydroxylation) in the liver and kidneys is required for activation. Because vitamin D3 can be synthesized in adequate amounts by most mammals exposed to sufficient sunlight, it is not considered an essential dietary factor, and so not technically a vitamin. Instead, it could be considered a hormone, with activation of the vitamin D3 prohormone resulting in the active form, calcitriol, which then produces effects via a nuclear receptor in multiple different locations (Norman. 2008). Vitamin D3 is necessary for calcium homeostasis and metabolism. Importantly, links have been found between low vitamin D3 levels and both Type 1 and Type 2 diabetes.

14.2.1.1   The Range of Serum Levels of Vitamin D—25-Hydroxyvitamin D

The total serum 25-hydroxyvitamin D (25(OH)D) level is currently considered the best indicator of vitamin D3 supply to the body from cutaneous synthesis and nutritional intake. The reference range of the total 25(OH)D level is 20 to 100 ng/mL. Vitamin D3 sufficiency has been defined as serum 25(OH)D levels of 30 ng/mL (75 nmol/L) or higher. The reference range of the total 25(OH)D level is 20 to 100 ng/mL.

A report published in the *American Journal of Clinical Nutrition* summarized reviewed evidence from studies that evaluated the thresholds of serum 25(OH)D levels and their relation to bone mineral density, lower-extremity function, dental health, and the risk of falls, fractures, and colorectal cancer. Their conclusion based on all endpoints was that 25(OH)D levels of 30 ng/mL (75 nmol/L), or greater, are more effective in achieving positive outcomes than lower levels. The best outcomes were seen with 25(OH)D levels from 36 to 40 ng/mL (90–100 nmol/L) (Bischoff-Ferrari, Giovannucci, Willett et al. 2006; Bischoff-Ferrari. 2008). Vitamin D3 insufficiency has been defined as a serum 25(OH)D level of 21 to 29 ng/mL (52–72 nmol/L). This is based on the observed physiological changes in calcium absorption and parathyroid hormone levels that occur with changes in vitamin D3 levels.

Vitamin D deficiency is defined by most experts as a serum 25(OH)D level of less than 20 ng/mL (50 nmol/L) (Medscape. https://emedicine.medscape.com/article/2088694-overview; accessed 12.24.17).

14.2.1.2   The Role of Vitamin D3 in Type 2 Diabetes

A report published in the journal *Diabetes*, subtitled, "Are we ready for a prevention trial?," summarizes much that is known about the link between vitamin D3 and Type 2 diabetes: There is a pancreatic receptor for the active metabolite (1,25-dihydroxyvitamin D) (Christakos, Friedlander, Frandsen et al. 1979).

It has been shown that vitamin D3 deficiency decreases insulin secretion (Norman, Frankel, Heldt et al. 1980). The author of the report further states that while numerous human studies of vitamin D3 and Type 2 diabetes have been published, the quality of some of these studies is questionable (Scragg. 2008; see also Pittas, Lau, Hu et al. 2007), because many are case–control studies, flawed by the measurement of 25(OH)D status on blood samples collected after diabetes diagnosis. However, population-based, cross-sectional studies have shown inverse associations between 25(OH)D and undiagnosed diabetes risk, that is, the lower the levels of the vitamin, the higher the incidence of diabetes (Scragg, Sowers, and Bell. 2004; Hypponen, and Power. 2006).

A number of prospective studies have provided better evidence of the inverse relationship between dietary vitamin D3 levels and diabetes risk (Liu, Song, Ford et al. 2005; Pittas, Dawson-Hughes, Li et al. 2006). However, these studies did not assess the major nondietary component of vitamin D3 derived from sun exposure.

Better evidence is found in the outcome of intervention studies. Three such studies bear mentioning because each had more than 100 participants, and because the vitamin D3 was administered for a long period of time (2 to 3 years). One study did not find a significant effect from a vitamin D3 dose of 2000 IU/day (Nilas, and Christiansen. 1984). Another study was a *post hoc* analysis of a trial designed for bone-related outcomes that found that 700 IU/day of vitamin D3, combined with calcium, decreased homeostasis model assessment (HOMA) of insulin resistance (HOMA-IR) in participants with impaired glucose tolerance, but not in those with normal fasting glucose (Pittas, Harris, Stark et al. 2007).

On the other hand, a large-sample study—nearly 34,000 women in the Women's Health Initiative study—did not find any significant effect from vitamin D3 (de Boer, Tinker, Connelly et al. 2008). There were, however, considerable limitations in this study relating to the administration of a low vitamin D3 dose of only 400 IU/day, which increased blood 25(OH)D levels by only about 7 nmol/L, as well as other extraneous uncontrolled contamination factors (Heaney, Davies, Chen et al. 2003).

Nevertheless, the strongest evidence for the value of vitamin D3 supplementation to date is provided by cohort studies comparing baseline measures of blood 25(OH)D, which reflect vitamin D3 status from both sun and dietary sources, and subsequent glycemic status.

For instance, a clinical study published in the journal *Diabetes* was conducted on a British cohort, and it revealed that baseline serum 25(OH)D levels are inversely associated with blood glucose and insulin levels collected 10 years later (Forouhi, Luan, Cooper et al. 2008). Another study, this one published in the journal *Diabetes Care*, and conducted on a Finnish cohort, also reported an inverse association between baseline serum 25(OH)D and 17-year risk of Type 2 diabetes (Mattila, Knekt, Mannisto et al. 2007). Such findings provide strong evidence that low vitamin D3 status predicts chronic hyperglycemia.

Furthermore, there is prospective study evidence that low levels of vitamin D3 also predict hyperinsulinemia, a finding that confirms previous cross-sectional studies (Scragg, Sowers, and Bell. 2004; Chiu, Chu, Go et al. 2004) and suggests that vitamin D3 may act to prevent Type 2 diabetes by decreasing insulin resistance, although it may also inhibit insulin secretion (Chiu, Chu, Go et al. 2004).

In addition to its prospective design, and use of 25(OH)D levels to measure vitamin D3 status, the British study also controlled the most important confounders, that is, obesity and physical inactivity, in statistical analyses. Its limitations are the 50% participant loss to follow-up after 10 years. The investigators reported that participants included in the 10-year follow-up analyses were healthier at baseline than those excluded, and as they state, this is likely to have resulted in a more conservative estimate of the association between vitamin D and glycemic status (Forouhi, Luan, Cooper et al. 2008).

The author of the report, subtitled "Vitamin D and Type 2 diabetes—Are we ready for a prevention trial?," which was cited above, further makes a number of recommendations:

Further cohort studies are required, assessing baseline vitamin D status using blood 25(OH)D. Glucose clamp studies are needed because it is still uncertain whether the mechanism influenced by vitamin D was insulin resistance, or insulin secretion, or both.

But most important, well-designed clinical trials of the effect of vitamin D3 supplementation on glycemia status, and diabetes risk, would prevent past mistakes including insufficient dosage: and the vitamin D3 dose given in such trials needs to be above 2000 zIU per day (Vieth, Bischoff-Ferrari, Boucher et al. 2007), to raise blood 25(OH)D levels above 80 nmol/L, because diabetes risk is lowest at this level (Scragg, Sowers, Bell et al. 2004; Scragg, Holdaway, Singh et al. 1995; see also Scragg. 2008).

14.2.1.3 Vitamin D3 Status and HbA1c

A very recent study published in the *Journal of Clinical Medicine Research* had the primary aim of determining whether serum 25-hydroxyvitamin D (25(OH)D) level affected glycosylated hemoglobin (HbA1c) levels, in order to test the hypothesis that lower 25(OH)D levels are associated with poorer glucose control in diabetes mellitus patients. A second aim was to determine whether vitamin D3 supplementation affects HbA1c levels.

This was a prospective, observational cohort study of all patients with Type 1 and Type 2 diabetes who were older than 12 years and who attended the outpatient clinics of a tertiary center in Riyadh, Saudi Arabia. HbA1c and vitamin D levels were recorded before supplementation and then again after 9 months of supplementation with vitamin D3 (dosage(s) not indicated). The patients were divided into four groups according to their vitamin D3 level.

First, it was found that 73.1% of the patients had 25(OH)D levels lower than 50 nmol/L. Lowered HbA1c after vitamin D supplementation was observed to be down from a mean of 10.55 at baseline to a significantly lower level of 7.70 at the end of the month observation period.

The investigators concluded that advising patients with higher HbA1c to test their vitamin D3 level, and to correct any deficiency, will result in better blood glucose control and benefit the patient's overall health (Buhary, Almohareb, Aljohani et al. 2017).

A clinical study published in the journal *Therapeutic Advances in Endocrinology and Metabolism* aimed to determine levels of 25-hydroxy vitamin D3 (25(OH)D3) in Type 2 diabetes patients and to determine the relationship between these levels and glycemic control. The investigators assessed HbA1c as well as 25(OH)D3 levels. The same measurements were performed in a group of control participants matched by age and gender. 25(OH)D3 was measured by radioimmunoassay, and HbA1c was measured by high-performance liquid chromatography.

It was found that 25(OH)D3 levels were lower in the patients than in the control group, being 19.26 ± 0.95 ng/mL and 25.49 ± 1.02 ng/mL, respectively. The 25(OH)D3 levels were found to be inversely related to HbA1c levels in the diabetic patients. The investigators concluded that vitamin D3 levels appeared to be lower in Type 2 diabetes patients than in the control group and that vitamin D3 levels are related to glycemic control in these patients. It is thought that these findings may have therapeutic implications as *"cautious vitamin D supplementation may improve glycemic control in diabetes mellitus type 2"* (Kostoglou-Athanassiou, Athanassiou, Gkountouvas et al. 2013).

14.2.1.4   Safety of Vitamin D3 Supplementation

A review in the journal *Anticancer Agents in Medicinal Chemistry* reported the following on the safety of vitamin D3 supplementation: The concept of vitamin D3 safety concerns two aspects: the safe tolerable UL method and adequate circulating 25-hydroxyvitamin D (25[OH]D) levels. Oral vitamin D intakes up to 250 µg/day have not been associated with harm. Hypercalcemia, the hallmark of vitamin D intoxication, may occur only if circulating 25(OH)D levels are consistently above 375–500 nmol/L.

However, some observational studies indicate that circulating 25(OH)D levels greater than 125 nmol/L are related to an increased morbidity and mortality risk. Therefore, the Institute of Medicine has set the UL for adults at 100 µg/day and the adequate circulating 25(OH)D level at 50 to 125 nmol/L (1 µg = 40 IU). In clinical practice, oral vitamin D dosing has to take into consideration that the increment in circulating 25(OH)D depends on baseline 25(OH)D levels as well as on the person's body weight. It is reasonable to assess 25(OH)D before and 6 months after initiation of oral vitamin D administration and to adjust the dose, if necessary. The underlying mechanisms, if any, for potentially harmful vitamin D3 effects at circulating 25(OH)D levels between 125 and 375 nmol/L are unknown (Zittermann, Prokop, Gummert et al. 2013).

14.2.2   Niacin (Vitamin B3) and Type 2 Diabetes: A Cautionary Note

People with Type 2 diabetes often have high levels of unhealthy lipids in their blood. Niacin, along with other medications, can lower those levels. However, niacin may also raise blood sugar levels, which is particularly dangerous for someone with diabetes.

A meta-analysis, intended to determine the effects of niacin on serum lipids and glucose in patients with Type 2 diabetes, was published in the journal *Clinical Nutrition*. The analysis was based on a comprehensive search of Medline, Scopus, AMED, Cochrane, and clinical trial registry databases, resulting in the finding and conclusion that there was a significant heterogeneity for the impact of niacin on LDL cholesterol and fasting blood glucose (FBG). Subgroup analyses revealed a significant increase in fasting blood glucose (FBG) of 0.085 mmol/L compared with controls in patients with long-term treatment.

Analysis of the results showed that niacin significantly improved lipid abnormalities in patients with Type 2 diabetes, but it requires monitoring of glucose in long-term treatment (Ding, Li, and Wen. 2015).

The investigators of a clinical study, reported in the *International Journal of Women's Health*, concluded that mean plasma glucose (blood samples were collected at 24 h after each trial), insulin, and C-peptide values significantly increased with niacin; glucose increased 10.6%, from 95.03 ± 10.67 mg/dL to 105.07 ± 13.56 mg/dL; insulin increased 61.8%, from 16.98 ± 12.49 µU/mL to 27.48 ± 14.84 µU/mL; and C-peptide increased 46.1%, from 1.65 ± 0.75 ng/mL to 2.41 ± 0.97 ng/mL.

Although niacin was generally well tolerated, given its adverse effects on glucose, insulin, and C-peptide profiles, the use of niacin in diabetic patients should be done with caution and only under medical supervision (Koh, Bidstrup, and Nichols. 2014).

14.2.3 Vitamin B6 (Pyridoxine)

A number of studies have found that supplementation of vitamin B6 is beneficial in Type 2 diabetes. Vitamin B6 is a water-soluble vitamin that is naturally present in many foods and available as a dietary supplement. It is the generic name for six compounds with vitamin B6 activity: pyridoxine, an alcohol; pyridoxal, an aldehyde; pyridoxamine, which contains an amino group; and their respective 5-phosphate esters. Pyridoxal 5 phosphate (P-5-P/PLP) and pyridoxamine 5 phosphate (PMP) are the active coenzyme forms of vitamin B6 (McCormick. 2006).

Vitamin B6 in coenzyme forms performs numerous functions in the body mostly concerned with protein metabolism. Both P-5-P and PMP are also involved in amino acid metabolism. Vitamin B6 is also involved in gluconeogenesis and glycogenolysis (Mackey, Davis, and Gregory. 2005).

According to the Institute of Medicine. Food and Nutrition Board. Dietary Reference Intakes (1998), vitamin B6 concentrations can be measured directly by assessing concentrations of P-5-P/PLP, other vitamers, or total vitamin B6 in plasma, erythrocytes, or urine. Concentrations can also be measured indirectly by assessing either erythrocyte aminotransferase saturation by P-5-P or tryptophan metabolites. Level of plasma P-5-P is the most common measure of vitamin B6 status.

14.2.3.1 The Range of Adequate Body Levels of Vitamin B6

P-5-P concentrations of at least 30 nmol/L have been traditional indicators of adequate vitamin B6 status in adults (McCormick. 2006). However, the Food and Nutrition Board (FNB) at the Institute of Medicine of the National Academies (formerly National Academy of Sciences) used a plasma P-5-P level of 20 nmol/L as an indication of adequacy to calculate the Recommended Dietary Allowances (RDAs) for adults.

14.2.3.2 Food Sources of Vitamin B6

According to the U.S. Department of Agriculture, Agricultural Research Service, USDA National Nutrient Database for Standard Reference, Release 24 Vitamin (2011), vitamin B6 is found in a wide variety of foods. The richest sources include fish, beef liver and other organ meats, potatoes and other starchy vegetables, and fruit (other than citrus). In the United States, adults obtain most of their dietary vitamin B6 from fortified cereals, beef, poultry, starchy vegetables, and some noncitrus fruits (Subar, Krebs-Smith, Cook et al. 1998). About 75% of the vitamin from a mixed diet is bioavailable.

14.2.3.3 Vitamin B6 Levels and Supplementation in Treatment of Type 2 Diabetes and Its Complications

The aim of a study published in the journal *Diabetes Research and Clinical Practice* was to determine the status of B vitamins, with particular focus on vitamin B6, in adults with and without incipient nephropathy, secondary to Type 2 diabetes mellitus.

The investigators measured plasma and/or urine concentrations of vitamins B6, B1, B12, related vitamers, and biomarkers (including total homocysteine and methylmalonic acid) in adults with

Type 2 diabetes. This sample included patients with microalbuminuria. Data from patients were compared to those from a nondiabetic control participant group.

It was found that plasma concentrations of P-5-P were significantly lower in patients with Type 2 diabetes than in the control group: median: 22.7 nmol/L in diabetes with microalbuminuria versus 26.8 nmol/L in diabetes without microalbuminuria and 39.5 nmol/L in nondiabetic control participants. The prevalence of low P-5-P (less than 30 nmol/L) was 63%, 58%, and 25% in the diabetes groups, with and without microalbuminuria, and the control group, respectively.

Plasma levels of pyridoxine and pyridoxal were also significantly lower, but levels of pyridoxamine, PMP, and pyridoxic acid were higher in both groups with diabetes, compared to the control group.

Thiamine (B1) deficiency was very prevalent in all groups, whereas low vitamin B12 and elevated methylmalonic acid were rare. Increased levels of C-reactive protein (CRP) and soluble vascular cell adhesion molecule-1 were observed in the groups with diabetes, as compared to the healthy control participants. The investigators concluded that deficiency of vitamin B6 (P-5-P, pyridoxine, pyridoxal) and vitamin B1 (thiamine) is prevalent in Type 2 diabetes. Incipient nephropathy was also found to be associated with more pronounced alterations in vitamin B6 metabolism, as well as stronger indications of endothelial dysfunction and inflammation (Nix, Zirwes, Bangert et al. 2015).

A clinical study, titled "Evaluation of the efficacy of thiamine and pyridoxine in the treatment of symptomatic diabetic peripheral neuropathy," published in the *East African Medical Journal*, aimed to determine the clinical response to therapeutic doses of two vitamins in diabetic patients with symptomatic peripheral neuropathy.

Patients were randomly allocated to treatment group A (thiamine [25 mg/day] and pyridoxine [50 mg/day]) and group B (treatment with an identical tablet containing 1 mg/day each of thiamine and pyridoxine). Pain, numbness, paresthesia, and impairment of sensation in ankles and in the legs were graded as none, mild, moderate, or severe.

Four weeks after starting treatment, the symptom severity grade was less than it was on the first visit, in the following percentages of the groups:

- Patients whose worst symptom was pain: 88.9% of the patients in group A (higher dose vitamins) had fewer symptoms versus 11.1% for group B (the lower dose).
- Patients whose worst symptom was numbness: 82.5% of the patients in group A had fewer symptoms versus 40.5% for group B.
- Patients whose worst symptom was paresthesia: 89.7% of the patients in group A had fewer symptoms versus 39.4% for group B.
- Patients with signs of peripheral neuropathy: 48.9% of the patients in group A had fewer symptoms versus 11.4% in group B.

The mean pretreatment whole blood thiamine levels were progressively lower with increasing severity of symptoms: 64.2 (2.81), 57.7 (3.25), and 52.2 (2.14) µg/L for those with mild, moderate, and severe symptoms, respectively (Abbas, and Swai. 1997).

The investigators of an animal-model study, published in the *Journal of Diabetes Research*, concluded that vitamin B6 prevents endothelial dysfunction, insulin resistance, and hepatic lipid accumulation in Apoe $^{-/-}$ mice fed with a high-fat diet. Vitamin B6 (50 mg/kg/day) was fed to such mice on a high-fat diet for 8 weeks. Endothelial dysfunction, insulin resistance, and hepatic lipid contents were then determined.

It was found that vitamin B6 administration significantly increased acetylcholine-induced endothelium-dependent relaxation and decreased random blood glucose level in those mice fed with high-fat diet. In addition, vitamin B6 improved the tolerance of glucose and insulin, normalized the histopathology of the liver, and reduced hepatic lipid accumulation. However, it did not affect liver functions.

The investigators concluded that vitamin B6 prevents endothelial dysfunction, decreases insulin resistance, and reduces hepatic lipid accumulation in Apoe $^{-/-}$ mice fed a high-fat diet. They also suggested that supplementation of vitamin B6 should be considered to prevent human metabolic syndrome (Liu, Li, Zhao et al. 2016).

A report published in the journal *Nutrition, Metabolism, and Cardiovascular Diseases* concluded that "Inflammatory variables may mediate the link between low plasma vitamin B6 concentrations and cardiovascular disease in type 2 diabetes" (Cigolini, Iagulli, Miconi et al. 2006).

Not all studies support the value of vitamin B6 in the treatment of diabetes or its complications. For instance, in a clinical study published in the journal *Diabetes Care*, titled "The influence of pyridoxine in diabetic peripheral neuropathy," symptomatic diabetes patients were treated with vitamin B6, or placebo, in a double-blind controlled study. Only one patient had a low plasma pyridoxal phosphate level at the start of the study. After 4 months of treatment with pyridoxine hydrochloride (50 mg three times daily), significant relief of neuropathic symptoms was reported by six of nine (67%) of the pyridoxine-treated patients versus only four of nine (44%) of the placebo-treated patients.

There was no statistically significant difference between the two groups with regard to fasting plasma glucose, motor nerve conduction velocity, or ophthalmologic examination at the beginning or at the conclusion of the study.

The investigators concluded that vitamin B6 deficiency is not a factor in the etiology of diabetic peripheral neuropathy. Furthermore, treating diabetic peripheral neuropathy with high-dose vitamin B6, or placebo, resulted in a similar frequency of symptomatic improvement (Levin, Hanscom, Fisher et al. 1981). However, the authors of this book, looking at the same data, strenuously disagree with the investigators' conclusion.

14.2.3.4 Health Risks of Excessive Vitamin B6

Chronic consumption of 1 g or more of pyridoxine per day, for 12 months or longer, can cause severe and progressive sensory neuropathy characterized by loss of control of bodily movements (ataxia) (Simpson, Bailey, Pietrzik et al. 2010; Gdynia, Muller, Sperfeld et al. 2008; Perry, Weerasuriya, Mouton et al. 2004; Bender. 1999). Symptom severity appears to be dose dependent, and the symptoms usually stop if the supplementation is discontinued soon after the neurologic symptoms appear.

Other effects of excessive vitamin B6 intakes include painful, disfiguring dermatological lesions, photosensitivity, and gastrointestinal symptoms such as nausea and heartburn (Bendich, and Cohen. 1990).

The Institute of Medicine, Food and Nutrition Board (1998) (*Dietary Reference Intakes: Thiamin, Riboflavin, Niacin, Vitamin B6, Folate, Vitamin B12, Pantothenic Acid, Biotin, and Choline.* Washington, DC: National Academy Press) has established ULs for vitamin B6 that apply to both food and supplement intakes (https://www.ncbi.nlm.nih.gov/books/NBK114313/; accessed 2.17.18).

The FNB noted that although several reports show sensory neuropathy occurring even at doses lower than 500 mg/day, studies in patients treated with vitamin B6 (average dose of 200 mg/day) for up to 5 years found no evidence of this effect. Based on limitations in the data on potential harm from long-term use, the FNB halved the dose used in these studies to establish a UL of 100 mg/day for adults.

14.2.3.5 Interactions with Medications

Vitamin B6 can interact with certain medications, and several types of medications might adversely affect vitamin B6 levels. A few examples are provided below, and individuals taking these and other medications on a regular basis should discuss their vitamin B6 status with their healthcare providers:

- Cycloserine (Seromycin)
- Antepileptic medications including valproic acid (Depakene, Stavzor), carbamazepine (Carbatrol, Epitol, Tegretol, and others), and phenytoin (Dilantin)
- Theophylline (Aquaphyllin, Elixophyllin, Theolair, and Truxophyllin)

14.2.4 Vitamin B12 (Cobalamin)

Vitamin B-12 (cobalamin) is a water-soluble vitamin essential to red blood cell (RBC) formation, cell metabolism, nerve function, and the production of DNA. Food sources of vitamin B12 include poultry, meat, fish, and dairy products. People on a vegetarian or a vegan diet might be prone to B12 deficiency because plant foods do not contain vitamin B12. Older adults and people with digestive tract conditions (such as pernicious anemia) that affect absorption of nutrients are also susceptible to vitamin B12 deficiency.

If left untreated, vitamin B12 deficiency can lead to anemia, fatigue, muscle weakness, intestinal problems, nerve damage, mood disturbances, and a dementia-like clinical presentation.

The recommended daily amount of vitamin B12 for adults is 2.4 µg. However, most supplements on the market contain at least 100 µg of the vitamin, and some contain as much as 1000 µg (1 mg).

14.2.4.1 Vitamin B12 and Type 2 Diabetes

The absorption of folic acid and vitamin B12 is significantly decreased by the prolonged use of metformin, which is the first drug of choice in uncomplicated diabetes. Therefore, these two nutrients are often found to be deficient in persons with Type 2 diabetes who are being treated. The authors of a review published in the journal *Endocrine, Metabolic and Immune Disorders Drug Targets* concluded that Type 2 diabetes patients on metformin for prolonged periods may need folic acid and vitamin B12 supplementation (Valdés-Ramos, Guadarrama-López, Martínez-Carrillo et al. 2015).

A clinical study published in the journal *Acta Medica Portuguesa* reported that vitamin B12 deficiency (less than 174 ng/dL) was present in 21.4% of their study population, and this subgroup was older (68.4 vs. 65.8 years), had a longer duration of Type 2 diabet\es (13.35 vs. 10.36 years), and had a higher prevalence of retinopathy (20.9% vs. 13.3%) as well as thyroid dysfunction (34% vs. 23.7%) than the overall study population. In that same study, vitamin B12 deficiency was also significantly more frequent in patients treated with metformin (24.7% vs. 15.8%), antiplatelet agents (25.4% vs. 16.2%), and calcium channel blockers (26.8% vs. 18.2%).

After adjustment for possible confounders, the variables associated with B12 deficiency were metformin, hypothyroidism, age, and duration of Type 2 diabetes mellitus.

The investigators concluded that there is a high prevalence of vitamin B12 deficiency in the Type 2 diabetes population. This study also demonstrates that the B12 deficiency risk is higher in older people with longer diabetes duration, hypothyroidism, and treatment with metformin (Tavares Bello, Capitão, Sequeira et al. 2017).

14.2.4.2 Supplementation and Safety of Vitamin B12

Food Sources of Vitamin B12: Vitamin B12 is naturally found in animal products, including fish, meat, poultry, eggs, milk, and milk products. It is generally not present in plant foods, but fortified breakfast cereals are a readily available source with high bioavailability for vegetarians. Small amounts of it can also be found in nutritional yeast products, as well as in some fermented foods (Table 14.1).

Health Risks from Excessive Vitamin B12: There is no establish UL for vitamin B12 because of its low potential for toxicity. In *Dietary Reference Intakes: Thiamin, Riboflavin, Niacin, Vitamin B6, Folate, Vitamin B12, Pantothenic Acid, Biotin, and Choline*, the IOM states that "*no adverse effects have been associated with excess vitamin B12 intake from food and supplements in healthy individuals*" (https://www.ncbi.nlm. nih.gov/books/NBK114310/; accessed 2.17.18).

Findings from intervention trials support these conclusions. In the NORVIT and HOPE 2 trials, vitamin B12 supplementation (in combination with folic acid and vitamin B6) did not cause any serious adverse events when administered at doses of 0.4 mg/day for 40 months (NORVIT trial) and 1.0 mg/day for 5 years (HOPE 2 trial) (Bønaa, NjølstadI, Ueland et al. 2006; Lonn, Yusuf, Arnold. 2006).

TABLE 14.1
Recommended Dietary Allowances for Vitamin B12 in Micrograms

Age	Male	Female
0–6 months[a]	ASD	0.4 μg
7–12 months[a]	0.5 μg	0.5 μg
1–3 years	0.9 μg	0.9 μg
4–8 years	1.2 μg	1.2 μg
9–13 years	1.8 μg	1.8 μg
14+ years	2.4 μg	2.4 μg

Source: Provided by the National Institutes of Health (NIH), Office of Dietary Supplements (https://ods.od.nih.gov/factsheets/VitaminB12-HealthProfessional/; accessed 1.2.18).

[a] Adequate intake

Interactions with Medications: Vitamin B12 has the potential to interact with certain medications, and several types of medications might adversely affect vitamin B12 levels. A few examples are provided below. Individuals taking these and other medications on a regular basis should discuss their vitamin B12 status with their healthcare providers:

- Chloramphenicol (Chloromycetin), which is a bacteriostatic antibiotic
- Proton pump inhibitors, such as omeprazole (Prilosec) and lansoprazole (Prevacid) (However, the evidence is conflicting on whether proton pump inhibitor use actually depletes vitamin B12 status.)
- Histamine H2 receptor antagonists, used to treat peptic ulcer disease, including cimetidine (Tagamet), famotidine (Pepcid), and ranitidine (Zantac)
- Metformin, an antihyperglycemic agent

See Vitamin B12. Fact Sheet for Health Professionals: https://ods.od.nih.gov/factsheets/VitaminB12-HealthProfessional/#en62.

14.2.5 FOLIC ACID (VITAMIN B9)

Folic acid is the synthetic form of vitamin B9 found in supplements and fortified foods, whereas folate is the naturally occurring form of the vitamin found in foods. All the B vitamins are water soluble. Vitamin B9 together with vitamins B6 and B12, control blood levels of the amino acid homocysteine. High levels of homocysteine are said to be a marker of heart disease—a "marker," as opposed to a cause (Chaava, Bukiia, and Shaburishvili. 2005).

14.2.5.1 Folic Acid and Type 2 Diabetes

Diabetes is reportedly associated with endothelial dysfunction, which, in part, may be related to uncoupling of the endothelial NO synthase enzyme, thus reducing the availability of NO. Folate may potentially reverse the uncoupling of NO synthase, the reason being that one of the co-enzymes that drive the enzyme is a folate derivative. Therefore, the investigators of a study published in the journal *Vascular Medicine* aimed to determine whether folic acid supplementation could improve endothelial function and markers of inflammation in patients with Type 2 diabetes without vascular disease.

Patients with Type 2 diabetes were treated with 10 mg/day for 2 weeks of folic acid, versus placebo, in a randomized, placebo-controlled, crossover study, with an 8-week washout period between treatments. Fasting endothelium-dependent FMD of the brachial artery, endothelium-independent nitroglycerin-mediated dilation (NMD), plasma homocysteine, serum lipids, folate, and inflammatory markers (high-sensitivity CRP [hs-CRP], soluble intercellular adhesion molecule-1 and vascular cell adhesion molecule-1, interleukin-18, and tumor necrosis factor-alpha) were assessed after each 2-week treatment period.

Folic acid supplementation significantly increased serum folate levels and lowered plasma homocysteine levels. It significantly improved FMD compared to placebo (5.8% ± 4.8% vs. 3.2% ± 2.7%). There were no significant effects of folic acid supplementation on lipids, nitroglycerin-mediated dilation, or the inflammatory markers. There was no relationship between the change in homocysteine, and the improvement in FMD. It was concluded that 2 weeks of folic acid supplementation can improve endothelial dysfunction in Type 2 diabetes independent of homocysteine lowering, but that trial did not lower markers of inflammation (Title, Ur, Giddens et al. 2006).

A study published in the *American Journal of Hypertension* aimed to determine whether oral folic acid supplementation enhanced endothelial function and reduced arterial stiffness by lowering homocysteine levels in Type 2 diabetes. Patients, aged 56.5 years on average ± 0.9 years, with diabetes duration of 5.5 years on average ± 0.6 years, with no history of cardiovascular disease, received 5 mg/day of oral folic acid, or placebo, for 4 weeks. The following measures were obtained before and after treatment:

1. Endothelial function: Forearm arterial blood flow during local intra-arterial administration of endothelium-dependent (acetylcholine 1.5, 4.5, and 15 µg/min) and endothelium-independent (sodium nitroprusside 1, 2, and 4 µg/min) vasodilators
2. Carotid–radial and carotid–femoral pulse wave velocity

It was found that folic acid significantly reduced plasma homocysteine concentrations and enhanced endothelium-dependent vasodilation during each acetylcholine infusion rate. Endothelium-independent vasodilation and pulse wave velocity were not affected. No significant changes in forearm arterial blood flow and pulse wave velocity were observed in the placebo group. Changes in folic acid concentrations but not in homocysteine concentrations independently described changes in maximal endothelium-dependent vasodilation.

The investigators concluded that short-term oral folic acid supplementation significantly enhances endothelial function in Type 2 diabetic patients, independent of homocysteine lowering (Mangoni, Sherwood, Asonganyi et al. 2005).

14.2.5.2 Folic Acid: Reference Range and Safety of Supplementation

The reference range of the plasma folate level varies by age, as follows:

- Adults: 2–20 ng/mL, or 4.5–45.3 nmol/L
- Children: 5–21 ng/mL, or 11.3–47.6 nmol/L
- Infants: 14–51 ng/mL, or 31.7–115.5 nmol/L

The reference range of the RBC folate level also varies by age, as follows:

- Adults: 140–628 ng/mL, or 317–1422 nmol/L
- Children: Over 160 ng/mL, or over 362 nmol/L

A plasma folic acid level of more than 4 ng/mL can rule out folate deficiency (Folate [Folic Acid]. Medscape; https://emedicine.medscape.com/article/2085523-overview; accessed 1.2.18; see also Field, and Stover. 2017).

A report in the journal *Archives of Internal Medicine* contends that the data that suggest that folic acid supplements are unsafe are weak and consist mostly of case series and reports. Nevertheless, greater difficulty diagnosing cobalamin deficiency due to "masking" of hematologic abnormalities by folic acid is a potential risk.

Routine hematologic indices have a low sensitivity for cobalamin deficiency, especially in patients who are receiving folic acid supplements. Because no high-quality data exclude specific adverse effects, vigilance in identifying detrimental effects when patients increase their consumption of folic acid is indicated (Campbell. 1996). As a general rule, it makes sense to advise patients that if they are going to supplement with folic acid, they should also supplement with vitamin B12 at the same time.

Possible interactions of folate with medications include the following:

- Antibiotics, in particular tetracycline.
- Phenytoin (Dilantin).
- Chemotherapy medications (some, not all): folic acid may raise the amounts of 5-fluorouracil and capecitabine (Xeloda) to dangerous levels in the body.
- Antacids.
- H2 blockers: used to reduce stomach acid, including cimetidine (Tagamet), famotidine (Pepcid), and ranitidine (Zantac).
- Proton pump inhibitors including someprazole (Nexium), lansoprazole (Prevacid), omeprazole (Prilosec), and rabeprazole (Aciphex).
- Bile acid sequestrants (Colestid), cholestyramine (Questran), and colsevelam (Welchol).
- Anti-seizure medications including phenobarbital, primidone (Mysoline), and carbamazepine (Tegretol).
- Nonsteroidal anti-inflammatory drugs (NSAIDs) including ibuprofen (Advil, Motrin) and naproxen (Aleve).
- Sulfasalazine (Azulfidine): used to treat inflammatory bowel disease (IBD) and rheumatoid arthritis (RA).
- Triamterene (Dyrenium): a diuretic (water pill).
- Cycloserine: an antibiotic.
- Pyrimethamine (Daraprim): used to prevent and treat malaria and to treat toxoplasmosis.
- Trimethoprim: an antibiotic used to treat urinary tract infections.
- When taken for long periods of time, these medications, as well as other anti-inflammatory medicines, can increase the body's need for folic acid.
- Methotrexate: methotrexate, a medication used to treat cancer, rheumatoid arthritis (RA), and psoriasis, reduces the amount of folic acid in the body. People taking methotrexate for cancer, however, should not take folic acid supplements unless their doctor tells them to. Folic acid may interfere with the effect of methotrexate on cancer.

(University of MD, Medical Center: http://www.umm.edu/health/medical/altmed/supplement-interaction/possible-interactions-with-vitamin-b9-folic-acid; WebMD: https://www.webmd.com/vitamins-supplements/ingredientmono-1017-folic%20acid.aspx?activeingredientid=1017&; accessed 1.2.18)

14.3 CHROMIUM III. CHROMIUM DEFICIENCY AND SUPPLEMENTATION IN TYPE 2 DIABETES

Trivalent chromium (Cr(III)) ion is an essential nutrient occurring in trace amounts in humans. It is considered necessary for the proper function of insulin, as well as for the metabolism of sugar and lipids. Recent studies have shed light on the role of chromium in maintaining proper carbohydrate and lipid metabolism at a molecular level.

The oligopeptide chromodulin binds chromic ions in response to an insulin-mediated chromic ion flux, and the metal-saturated oligopeptide can then bind to an insulin-stimulated insulin receptor, activating the receptor tyrosine kinase activity. Thus, chromodulin appears to play a role in an autoamplification (increase in concentration) mechanism in insulin signaling (Vincent. 2000).

The molecular agent responsible for transporting chromium from mobile pools to insulin-sensitive cells is probably the metal transport protein, transferrin. Chromium from the popular dietary supplement, chromium picolinate, enters cells via a different mechanism. Parenthetically, the release of chromium from chromium picolinate for use in cells requires reduction of the chromic center, a process that can potentially lead to the formation of harmful hydroxyl radicals (Vincent. 2000).

Chromium is absorbed in the digestive tract and transported to the tissues, where its accumulation takes place. A deficiency of chromium (III) causes disturbances in metabolic processes including a lowered glucose tolerance, which is the consequence of changes in insulin affinity to its receptors on cells (Snitynskyĭ, Solohub, Antoniak et al. 1999).

It has been said that by consuming brewer's yeast high in chromium, diabetic patients may be able to improve glucose tolerance, lower their fasting glucose levels, decrease insulin levels, and cut cholesterol and triglyceride levels, while increasing high-density lipoprotein (HDL) cholesterol levels. How effective is chromium supplementation in support of glycemic control in Type 2 diabetes?

The Spanish-language journal, *Nutricion Hospitalaria*, published a review and meta-analysis titled "Chromium supplementation in patients with type 2 diabetes and high risk of type 2 diabetes: a meta-analysis of randomized controlled trials." The object of this meta-analysis was to assess the effects on metabolic profiles, and safety of chromium supplementation in Type 2 diabetes and serum cholesterol levels. The search included PubMed, Scopus, and Web of Science based on related terms, keywords, and randomized clinical trials during the period of 2000 to 2014.

Total doses of chromium supplementation, and brewer's yeast, ranged from 42 to 1000 µg/day, and duration of supplementation ranged from 30 to 120 days. The analysis indicated that in diabetes, chromium supplementation significantly improved fasting plasma glucose and lowered total cholesterol.

The investigators concluded that the available evidence suggests favorable effects of chromium supplementation on glycemic control in patients with diabetes (San Mauro-Martin, Ruiz-León, Camina-Martín et al. 2016).

14.3.1 Is There Chromium Deficiency in Type 2 Diabetes?

Studies cited below, only a small sample of those available on library databases, show that chromium supplementation improves—even normalizes—blood sugar levels. This fact raises the question, Is there a chromium deficiency basis to the etiology of Type 2 diabetes? A review published in the journal *Diabetes Educator* addresses that question. "Chromium is an essential mineral that appears to have a beneficial role in the regulation of insulin action and its effects on carbohydrate, protein and lipid metabolism. Chromium is an important factor for enhancing insulin activity. Studies show that people with type 2 diabetes have lower blood levels of chromium than those without the disease..." (No authors listed. 2004).

A study published in the *Journal of Clinical and Diagnostic Research* aimed to determine the level of serum chromium in newly diagnosed patients with Type 2 diabetes and its association with glycemic control. Serum chromium concentration was determined by using inductively coupled plasma–optical emission spectrophotometry in newly diagnosed Type 2 diabetes patients free of any preexisting complications. They were divided into two groups: those with well-controlled HbA1c (less than or equal to 7.0%) and an uncontrolled HbA1c (above 7.0%) group.

It was found that mean serum chromium concentration in uncontrolled Type 2 diabetes patients was significantly lower than that in the well-controlled patient group. There was a statistically significant negative correlation between the HbA1c values and the serum chromium concentration. Parenthetically, there were also significantly lower chromium levels in patients older than 40 years.

The investigators concluded that the significant reduction in chromium levels is probably indicators of metabolic response to oxidative stress in patients with Type 2 diabetes (Rajendran, Manikandan, Nair et al. 2015).

14.3.2 Chromium Supplementation with Brewer's Yeast

A number of conventional, well-controlled studies have shown that supplemental chromium may raise glucose tolerance in patients with both Type 1 and Type 2 diabetes. In fact, a study published in the *International Journal of Preventive Medicine* was titled "Brewer's yeast improves glycemic indices in Type 2 diabetes mellitus." The aim of the study was to determine whether supplementation with brewer's yeast could improve glycemic indices in these patients.

Adult men and women Type 2 diabetes patients, 46.3 ± 6.1 years old, were randomly assigned to one of two groups: For 12 weeks, the supplement group received six 300-mg tablets/day, totaling 1800 mg of brewer's yeast, and the control group received placebo (six 300-mg tablets/day).

Body weight, height, body mass index, food consumption (based on 24-h food record), fasting blood sugar, HbA1c, insulin sensitivity, and insulin resistance were measured before and after the intervention. It was found that, over the course of the study period, fasting blood sugar, HbA1c, and insulin sensitivity indices improved significantly in the supplement group. Changes in body mass index, 24-h food record, and insulin resistance did not show significant change.

The investigators concluded that dietary supplementation with brewer's yeast can help ameliorate blood glucose variables in Type 2 diabetes (Hosseinzadeh, Javanbakht, Mostafavi et al. 2013).

The *Journal of Trace Elements in Medicine and Biology* published a study that aimed to determine the effect of chromium supplementation on blood glucose, HbA1c, and lipid profile, in newly onset patients with Type 2 diabetes. New-onset Type 2 diabetes patients were recruited, and after 1 month of stabilization, they were distributed among a study group and a placebo group. For 3 months, the study group received 9 g of brewer's yeast (42 µg Cr) daily, while the placebo group received yeast devoid of chromium. The participants were instructed to not change their normal eating and living habits. Fasting blood glucose, HbA1c and lipid profile were analyzed at the beginning and completion of the study.

It was found that fasting blood glucose levels were significantly lower in the patients who had consumed yeast supplemented with chromium (197.65 ± 6.68 to 103.68 ± 6.64 mg/dL. HbA1C values improved significantly from 9.51% ± 0.26% to 6.86% ± 0.28%, indicating better glycemic control. In the study group, total cholesterol and LDL cholesterol levels were also significantly reduced.

The investigators concluded that chromium supplementation improves glycemic control as well as lipid variables in people with new-onset Type 2 diabetes (Sharma, Agrawal, Choudhary et al. 2011).

14.3.2.1 Chromium Supplementation with Chromium Picolinate

The aim of a clinical study published in the *International Journal for Vitamin and Nutrition Research* was to determine the effects of chromium on elderly Type 2 diabetes patients in a rehabilitation program. Participants 73 years old, on average, undergoing rehabilitation following stroke or hip fracture, were recruited to participate in this study. Additional diabetes patients constituted the control group. Together with standard treatment for diabetes, the study group received 200 µg of chromium picolinate (Solgar) twice a day for a 3-week period. Blood samples, dietary intake, and anthropometric data were collected before and after intervention. Throughout the study period, participants received a diet of approximately 1500 kcal/day.

In the study group, a significant decline in the FBG level was found at the end of the study, compared to the baseline (190 mg/dL vs. 150 mg/dL). HbA1c also improved, decreasing from 8.2% to 7.6%. Total cholesterol was also reduced, from 235 to 213 mg/dL. A trend toward lowered triglyceride levels was also observed (152 mg/dL vs. 136 mg/dL).

The investigators concluded that in this population of elderly diabetic patients undergoing rehabilitation, dietary supplementation with chromium is beneficial in moderating glucose intolerance. In addition, chromium intake appears also to improve plasma lipid levels (Rabinovitz, Friedensohn, Leibovitz et al. 2004).

14.3.2.2 Estimated Safe and Adequate Daily Dietary Intake of Chromium

The *Journal of Clinical Pharmacy and Therapeutics* published a "Systematic review and meta-analysis of the efficacy and safety of chromium supplementation in diabetes." Clinical trials were identified through MEDLINE, the Cochrane library, CINAHL, Web of Science, Scopus, and www .clinicaltrial.gov up to May 2013. Historical search of reference lists of related articles was also conducted. Studies were included if they (1) were randomized controlled trials, comparing chromium mono- or combined supplementation against placebo; (2) reported HbA1c or fasting plasma glucose; and (3) were of at least 3 weeks duration when reporting fasting plasma glucose, or of at least 8 weeks duration if HbA1c was reported. No language restriction was imposed. Treatment effect and adverse events were estimated with mean difference and odds ratio, respectively.

The analyses revealed that chromium mono- and combined supplementation (yeast/picolinate) significantly improved glycemic control: mean difference for HbA1c was −0.55%; mean difference for FPG was −1.15 mm.

In particular, chromium monotherapy significantly reduced triglycerides and increased HDL cholesterol levels. The effects on glucose and triglycerides levels were shown especially with chromium picolinate.

The investigators concluded that glycemic control may improve with chromium monosupplementation of more than 200 μg daily. HbA1c and FPG also improved in patients with inadequate glycemic control at baseline. Most important, the risk of adverse events did not differ between chromium and placebo: "Chromium supplementation at usual doses does not increase the risk of adverse events compared with placebo" (SZref).

According to a report published in the journal *Regulatory Toxicology and Pharmacology*, the estimated safe and adequate daily dietary intake for chromium is 50 to 200 μg. However, most diets contain less than 60% of the minimum suggested intake of 50 μg. Insufficient dietary intake may lead to signs and symptoms that are similar to those observed for diabetes and cardiovascular diseases. The response to chromium depends on the form and amount of the supplement. Since chromium is a nutrient, it will only be of benefit to those who are marginally or overtly deficient.

Trivalent chromium has a very large safety range and there have been no documented signs of toxicity at levels up to 1 mg/day in any nutritional studies (Anderson. 1997).

14.3.2.3 Combining Chromium with Biotin in the Supplementation

Biotin is also known as vitamin B7. The combination of chromium picolinate and biotin may synergize to form a more effective supplement, supporting the reduction of insulin resistance. In a clinical study on diabetes patients, published in the journal *Diabetes/Metabolism Research and Reviews,* patients with poorly controlled Type 2 diabetes (HbA1c greater, or equal to 7.0%) received either 600 μg of chromium picolinate Cr(+3) with 3 mg of biotin, per day, or matching placebo for 90 days, in combination with stable oral antidiabetic agents. Major endpoints were reduction in HbA1c, FBG, and lipids.

It was found that the chromium picolinate + biotin combination, administered as an adjuvant to current prescription antidiabetic medications, improved glycemic control (HbA1c) in overweight to obese individuals with Type 2 diabetes, especially those patients with poor glycemic control on the oral therapy (Albarracin, Fuqua, Evans et al. 2008).

Another study published in the journal *Diabetes Technology and Therapy* aimed to determine whether supplementation with chromium picolinate combined with biotin can improve glycemic control in patients with Type 2 diabetes who do not have suboptimal glycemic control, despite their use of oral antihyperglycemic medications.

Patients with impaired glycemic control based on 2-h postprandial glucose greater than 200 mg/dL and glycated hemoglobin greater than or equal to 7%, despite treatments with oral antihyperglycemic agents, received 600 μg of chromium as chromium picolinate plus biotin (2 mg/day; Diachrome, Nutrition 21, Inc., Purchase, New York) in addition to their oral antihyperglycemic medication therapy. Measurements of glycemic control and blood lipids were taken at baseline and after 4 weeks.

It was found that after 4 weeks, there was a significantly greater reduction in the "total area under the curve" for glucose during the 2-h oral glucose tolerance test for the treatment group (mean change −9.7%), compared to that of a placebo group (mean change +5.1%). Significantly greater reductions were also seen in fructosamine, triglycerides, and triglycerides/HDL cholesterol ratio in the treatment group. No significant adverse events were attributed to the chromium picolinate and biotin supplementation.

The investigators concluded that supplementation with a combination of chromium picolinate and biotin, in poorly controlled patients with diabetes receiving antidiabetic therapy, improved glucose management and several lipid measurements. Chromium picolinate + biotin supplementation may represent an effective adjunctive nutritional therapy for people with poorly controlled diabetes with the potential for improving lipid metabolism as well (Singer, and Geohas. 2006).

Similar results were reported in animal model studies: The *British Journal of Nutrition* published a study titled "Anti-diabetic activity of chromium picolinate and biotin in rats with type 2 diabetes induced by high-fat diet and streptozotocin." The combination of chromium picolinate + biotin was reported to form a more effective supplement, reducing insulin resistance in skeletal muscle *via* an increase in the expression of the glucose transporter protein GLUT4 (Sahin, Tuzcu, Orhan et al. 2013; see also Sasaki, Sone, Kamiyama et al. 2012).

In some instances, a combination of supplements has been found to be more effective than either supplement by itself. The combination of biotin with chromium seems to be a case in point: Biotin is a water-soluble B-vitamin that works synergistically with insulin. Independently, it increases the activity of the enzyme glucokinase, which catalyzes the initial step in utilization of glucose by the beta-cells (β-cells) and the liver, at physiological glucose concentration.

Glucokinase functions as the glucose sensor in the pancreatic β-cell by controlling the rate of entry of glucose into the glycolytic pathway (*via* phosphorylation of glucose) and, from there, its subsequent metabolism (to produce energy as ATP). In the liver, glucokinase plays a key role in the ability to store glucose as glycogen, particularly in the postprandial state.

In diabetes sufferers, glucokinase concentration is reported to be extremely low. In fact, in a study published in the journal *Molecular Metabolism* the investigators examined expression of gluconeogenic enzymes in liver biopsies from nondiabetes and from diabetes sufferers. The diabetes patients' livers were further separated into those with HbA1c lower or higher than 7.0.

It was found that in diabetic patients with HbA1c greater than 7.0, glucokinase was suppressed more than 60%. Moreover, HbA1c and fasting glucose were inversely correlated with the level of glucokinase. This implies that in diabetic patients, despite the abundance of glucose in the tissues, there would be difficulty converting that glucose into energy (as ATP). The investigators in the study being cited did not state the following, but we think it would be reasonable to state that this would create a vicious cycle, because the β-cells require a great deal of energy (as ATP) to synthesize and assemble the constant stream of insulin that has to be produced to counteract the high sugar levels in the blood.

The investigators concluded that there may be underlying dysregulation of hepatic glucokinase expression during frank diabetes, which has implications for the therapeutic use of glucokinase activators in this population (Haeusler, Camastra, Astiarraga et al. 2015).

Biotin deficiency is rare because the amounts needed are small. Four food groups are relatively high in biotin: (1) eggs are a good source of protein and biotin; (2) almonds, nuts and legumes, and nut-based butters such as peanut butter are high in nutrients, fiber, protein, biotin, and vitamin E; (3) whole grains, and milk and meat; (4) intestinal bacteria synthesize biotin, which is then absorbed by the host.

Daily intake of 100 to 200 μg of biotin is considered safe and adequate (Valdés-Ramos, Guadarrama-López, Martínez-Carrillo et al. 2015).

Not all combinations potentiate. For instance, lipoic acid competes with biotin for binding to the sodium-dependent multivitamin transporter, potentially decreasing the cellular uptake of biotin. Chronic administration of pharmacological doses of lipoic acid have been found to decrease the activities of pyruvate carboxylase and β-methylcrotonyl-CoA carboxylase in rat liver to 64% to 72% respectively, compared to controls (Zempleni, and Mock. 1999a; 1999b).

14.3.2.4   Safety of Biotin Supplementation

There is no formally established recommended daily intake of biotin. Instead, an adequate intake (AI) is identified based on the theory that average intake meets needs. Ingesting pharmacological doses of biotin is considered safe.

Patients with biotinidase deficiency (BTD), a metabolic disorder due to either low concentration or complete lack of the enzyme biotinidase, are treated with biotin doses that exceed the normal dietary intake by 300 times. This does not produce frank signs of toxicity (Wolf and Heard. 1991).

In a study published in the American *Journal of Clinical Nutrition*, it was also reported that there were no signs of biotin overdose after acute oral and intravenous administration of doses that exceeded the dietary biotin intake by up to 600 times (Zempleni, and Mock. 1999a; 1999b).

14.4   TYPE 2 DIABETES AND COENZYME Q10 (CoQ10) DEFICIENCY

Coenzyme Q10 (CoQ10) is also known as ubiquinone. A coenzyme is a non-protein compound that is required for the biological activity of a protein. CoQ10 is ubiquitous in animals and in most bacteria, hence the name ubiquinone. This fat-soluble substance, which resembles a vitamin, is present in all respiring eukaryotic cells, primarily in the mitochondria. It participates in the cellular aerobic respiration, which generates energy in the form of ATP. It is estimated that 95% of the human body energy is generated this way. Therefore, those organs with the highest energy requirements—such as the heart, liver, and kidney—also have the highest CoQ10 concentrations (Okamoto, Matsuya, Fukunaga et al. 1989; Aberg, Appelkvist, Dallner et al. 1992).

There are three redox states of CoQ10: (1) fully oxidized (ubiquinone), (2) semiquinone (ubisemiquinone), and (3) fully reduced (ubiquinol). The capacity of this molecule to act as a two-electron carrier, moving between the quinone and quinol form, and a one-electron carrier, moving between the semiquinone and one of these other forms, is central to its role in the electron transport chain due to the iron–sulfur clusters that can only accept one electron at a time and as a free-radical–scavenging antioxidant.

The journal *Clinical Biochemist Reviews* published a detailed report on CoQ10, titled "Coenzyme Q10: is there a clinical role and a case for measurement?" (Molyneux, Young, Florkowski et al. 2008). Some of the critical issues it detailed are described below.

CoQ10 deficiency has been implicated in several clinical disorders, including hypertension and heart failure. In some cases, deficiency is caused by therapy with statins (3-hydroxy-3-methyl-glutaryl(HMG)-CoA reductase inhibitors), where that inhibition not only reduces the synthesis of cholesterol (the desired effect) but also reduces the synthesis of CoQ10, an unintended consequence that can profoundly damage the many organs that rely on CoQ10.

The investigators make a case for clinical measurement of plasma CoQ10, based on the relationship between levels and outcomes, as in chronic heart failure, where it may identify individuals most likely to benefit from supplementation therapy. They further suggest that during CoQ10 supplementation, plasma CoQ10 levels should be monitored to ensure efficacy, given that there is variable bioavailability between commercial formulations, and known interindividual variation in CoQ10 absorption.

14.4.1   CoQ10 REFERENCE INTERVAL

The adult reference interval for plasma or serum CoQ10 is approximately 0.5 to 1.7 μmol/L (Molyneux, Florkowski, Lever et al. 2005; Kaikkonen, Nyyssönen, and Salonen. 1999; Kaplan, Sebestianová, Turiaková et al. 1996; Kaikkonen, Tuomainen, Nyyssönen et al. 2002). Because plasma and lipid concentrations of CoQ10 correlate strongly, it has been proposed that lipids should be considered when measuring plasma CoQ10, and the ratio of CoQ10 to total or LDL cholesterol should be reported (Kontush, Reich, Baum et al. 1997; Tomasetti, Littarru, Stocker et al. 1999).

14.4.2 CoQ10, Insulin Resistance, and Type 2 Diabetes

It is a recurrent theme in diabetes clinical and research publications that oxidative stress plays a critical role in the pathogenesis of Type 2 diabetes and its complications. In that context, CoQ10 deficiency is thought to contribute to increased oxidative stress leading to impaired mitochondrial function (Watts, and Playford. 1998; DeFronzo, Bonadonna, and Ferrannini. 1992).

In diabetes, the damage caused by CoQ10 deficiency is thought to also lead to endothelial dysfunction, and it may be linked to impaired β-cell function, and the development of insulin resistance (Chew, and Watts. 2004). Low plasma CoQ10 concentrations have been linked to poor glycemic control and diabetic complications.

Since CoQ10 plays an important role in the mitochondrial electron transport chain, and it is a potent antioxidant, it has been suggested that "oral supplementation may be an attractive therapy in Type 2 diabetes" (Jameson. 1991).

The journal *Healthcare* published a comprehensive review titled "Supplementation of Coenzyme Q10 among patients with Type 2 diabetes mellitus." The authors (Shen, and Pierce. 2015) reiterate that there is growing evidence that mitochondrial dysfunction, secondary to oxidative stress, plays a critical role in the pathogenesis of Type 2 diabetes and that CoQ10 is, therefore, an important micronutrient acting in the electron transport chain of the mitochondria with two major functions: (1) synthesis of adenosine triphosphate (ATP) and (2) as a potent antioxidant. The review details the relationships between oxidative stress, mitochondrial dysfunction, and Type 2 diabetes, and it examines the evidence for its potential use as a treatment supplement.

The authors concluded that as an antioxidant, CoQ10 is assumed to scavenge excessive ROS and provide protection to cells, especially mitochondria, from oxidative damage. Therefore, restoration of CoQ10 levels among patients with Type 2 diabetes by supplementation with exogenous CoQ10 could potentially alleviate oxidative stress, preserve mitochondrial function, and eventually lead to improvement of glycemic control (Shen, and Pierce. 2015). This hypothesis was in part supported by several studies (Sourris, Harcourt, Tang et al. 2012; Mezawa, Takemoto, Onishi et al. 2012; Shigeta, Izumi, and Abe. 1966; Shimura, and Hogimoto. 1981; Singh, Niaz, Rastogi et al. 1999; Hodgson, Watts, Playford et al. 2002; Sena, Nunes, Gomes et al. 2007; Kolahdouz, Hosseinzadeh-Attar, Eshraghian et al. 2013; Yokoyama, Lingle, Crestanello et al. 1996).

Studies that reported no significant improvement were also reported (Eriksson, Forsen, Mortensen et al. 1999; Conget, Manzanares, Barrientos et al, 1996; Henriksen, Andersen, Hother-Nielsen et al. 1999; Lim, Lekshminarayanan, Goh et al. 2008).

Because of contradicting evidence about the benefits of supplementing CoQ10 (ubiquinol) in Type 2 diabetes, the authors of that review in the journal *Healthcare* concluded that the outcome of supplementing ubiquinol in Type 2 diabetes "is unclear" (Shen, and Pierce. 2015).

The investigators of a study titled "Coenzyme Q10 improves blood pressure and glycaemic control: a controlled trial in subjects with type 2 diabetes," published in the *European Journal of Clinical Nutrition*, thought otherwise. They reported an analysis and discussion of the effects of CoQ10 on blood pressure, on long-term glycemic control measured by glycated hemoglobin, and on oxidative stress assessed by measurement of plasma F2-isoprostanes. They found that CoQ10 supplementation improves blood pressure as well as long-term glycemic control in Type 2 diabetes participants in their study. However, they could not attribute these improvements to reduced oxidative stress (as assessed by F2-isoprostanes) (Hodgson, Watts, Playford et al. 2002).

Another clinical study, conducted in Turkey, published in the *International Journal of Ophthalmology*, aimed to determine the relationship between proliferative diabetic retinopathy (PDRP) and plasma CoQ10 concentration. Plasma CoQ10 and malondialdehyde (MDA) levels were measured in patients who had both Type 2 diabetes and proliferative diabetic retinopathy (PDRP), and in "healthy individuals." It was found that the ratio of ubiquinol-10/ubiquinone-10 was lower in patients with proliferative , whereas a high level of plasma ubiquinol-10/ubiquinone-10 ratio indicated a protective effect (Ates, Bilen, Keles et al. 2013).

Finally, the investigators of a review published in the journal *Molecular Syndromology* concluded that a 12-week treatment with ubiquinone improves clinical outcomes and nerve conduction parameters of persons with diabetic polyneuropathy, and it reduces oxidative stress, without significant adverse events (Garrido-Maraver, Cordero, Oropesa et al. 2014).

It may be that one of the factors underlying the variability of the outcomes of the clinical trials is the formulation of CoQ10 bei1ng used in the respective studies. CoQ10 is more active in the "reduced" form, but not all investigators may be aware of that. In clinical practice, we see many patients using the wrong form, that is, the oxidized form, of CoQ10, because that is what was being sold at the drug store or being promoted in a television ad.

14.4.3   SAFETY OF CoQ10 SUPPLEMENTATION

The journal *Biofactors* published a review titled "Safety assessment of coenzyme Q10 (CoQ10)." The investigators state that it has been widely used as a dietary supplement for more than 20 years. Recently, the use of CoQ10 as a dietary supplement has grown with a corresponding increase in daily dosage.

The published reports concerning safety studies, based on animal and human data, indicate that CoQ10 has low toxicity and does not induce serious adverse effects in humans. The acceptable daily intake is 12 mg/kg/day, calculated from the *no-observed-adverse-effect level* (NOAEL) of 1200 mg/kg/day derived from a 52-week chronic toxicity study in rats, which would translate to 720 mg/day for a person weighing 60 kg.

Risk assessment for CoQ10 based on various clinical trial data indicates that the observed safety level (OSL) for CoQ10 is 1200 mg/day/person. Evidence from pharmacokinetic studies suggest that exogenous CoQ10 does not inhibit the biosynthesis of endogenous CoQ10 (which is important), nor does it accumulate in plasma or tissues after cessation of supplementation. Analysis of CoQ10 bioavailability, or its pharmacokinetics, provides the pertinent safety evaluation for CoQ10: Overall, these data from preclinical and clinical studies indicate that CoQ10 is highly safe for use as a dietary supplement (Hidaka, Fujii, Funahashi et al. 2008).

Investigators from the Council for Responsible Nutrition, Washington, DC, reported "Risk assessment for coenzyme Q10 (Ubiquinone)" in the journal *Regulatory Toxicology and Pharmacology*. They contend that evidence of health benefits of orally administered CoQ10 leads to daily consumption in larger amounts, and this increase justifies research and risk assessment to evaluate safety of supplementation. They report that a large number of clinical trials have been conducted using a range of CoQ10 doses.

However, reports of nausea and other adverse gastrointestinal effects of CoQ10 cannot be causally related to the active ingredient because there is no dose–response relationship: the adverse effects are no more common at daily intakes of 1200 mg than at at 60 mg.

The OSL risk assessment method indicates that the evidence of safety is strong at intakes up to 1200 mg/day, and this level is identified as the OSL. Much higher levels have been tested without adverse effects and may be safe, but the data for intake above 1200 mg/day are not sufficient for a confident conclusion of safety (Hathcock, and Shao. 1996).

14.4.4   RE. CoQ10 DEPLETION: STATINS AND DIABETES, A CAUTIONARY NOTE

According to a report published in the journal *Diabetes Care*, individuals with prediabetes, undiagnosed Type 2 diabetes, or long-lasting Type 2 diabetes are at high risk of all complications of macrovascular disease such as coronary heart disease, stroke, and peripheral vascular disease (Laakso. 2010).

It is therefore likely that the typical Type 2 diabetes patient will have also been prescribed one or another statin medication and, as previously noted, these medications are linked to myopathy *via* mitochondrial dysfunction due to CoQ10 depletion.

Furthermore, the *Lancet* published a study titled "Cardiovascular benefits and diabetes risks of statin therapy in primary prevention." The investigators undertook an analysis of participants from the "Justification for the Use of Statin in Prevention: An Intervention Trial Evaluating Rosuvastatin," that is, the JUPITER trial (Ridker. 2009), to address the balance of vascular benefits versus diabetes hazard of statin use.

The investigators reported finding that trial participants with one or more major diabetes risk factors were at higher risk of developing diabetes; for such individuals, statin allocation was associated with a 39% reduction in the primary endpoint (myocardial infarction, stroke, admission to hospital for unstable angina, arterial revascularization, or cardiovascular death), a 36% reduction in venous thromboembolism (VTE), a 17% reduction in total mortality, but a 28% increase in diabetes.

Thus, for those with diabetes risk factors, 93 vascular events or deaths were avoided for every 54 new cases of diabetes diagnosed. For trial participants with no major diabetes risk factor, statin allocation was associated with a 52% reduction in the primary endpoint, a 53% reduction in VTE, a 22% reduction in total mortality, and no increase in diabetes.

For such individuals, a total of 86 vascular events or deaths were avoided with no new cases of diabetes diagnosed. In analysis limited to the participants who developed diabetes during follow-up, the point estimate of cardiovascular risk reduction associated with statin therapy (hazard ratio, 0.63) was consistent with that observed for the trial as a whole (hazard ratio, 0.56). As compared to placebo, statin allocation accelerated the average time to diagnosis of diabetes by about 5 1/2 weeks.

The investigators concluded that in the JUPITER primary prevention trial, the cardiovascular and mortality benefits of statin therapy exceed the diabetes hazard, including among those at higher risk for developing diabetes (Ridker, Pradhan, MacFadyen et al. 2012; see also Chogtu, Magazine, and Bairy. 2015).

This study is cited here as an example of one side of a complex multifactor medical controversy, and its citation here does not reflect the judgment of the authors of this book. Clearly, no one should be discouraged to use, nor should anyone be encouraged to discontinue, the use of prescribed statins for fear of diabetes, without the guidance of a qualified healthcare provider.

14.5 MAGNESIUM IS ANTIDIABETIC AND CARDIOPROTECTIVE

Magnesium is the fourth most abundant mineral in the body. It is known to be a cofactor for more than 300 enzymatic reactions, including several where it is crucial for the production of adenosine triphosphate (ATP). It is required for DNA and RNA synthesis, reproduction, and protein synthesis. Moreover, it is essential for the regulation of muscle contraction, blood pressure, insulin metabolism, cardiac excitability, vasomotor tone, nerve transmission, and neuromuscular conduction.

Imbalances in magnesium status—typically hypomagnesemia, more common than hypermagnesemia—can result in unwanted neuromuscular, cardiac, or nervous disorders. Low levels of magnesium have been associated with a number of chronic diseases, such as insulin resistance and Type 2 diabetes, hypertension, cardiovascular disease (e.g., stroke), and migraine (Gröber, Schmidt, and Kisters. 2015).

A review appearing in the journal *BioMedicine* details the relationship between magnesium (Mg) deficiency and oxidative stress: Mg deficiency is associated with higher levels of oxidative stress markers including lipid, protein, and DNA oxidative modification products (noted earlier), as well as weakened antioxidant defenses. These may account for systemic reactions such as inflammation and endothelial dysfunction, as well as changes at the cellular level, such as mitochondrial dysfunction and excessive fatty acid production (Zheltova, Kharitonova, Iezhitsa et al. 2016).

In fact, a study titled "Magnesium intake in relation to systemic inflammation, insulin resistance, and the incidence of diabetes" was published in the journal *Diabetes Care*. The aim of the study was to determine the long-term associations between magnesium intake, incidence of diabetes, systemic inflammation, and insulin resistance among young American adults.

Participants, 18 to 30 years old, who had no history of diabetes at baseline, were prospectively examined for incident diabetes based on quintiles of magnesium intake. The association between magnesium intake and inflammatory markers, that is, high-sensitivity C-reactive protein (hs-CRP), interleukin-6 (IL-6), fibrinogen, and the homeostasis model assessment of insulin resistance (HOMA-IR) was also included.

It was found that during the 20-year follow-up, 330 incident cases of diabetes were identified out of the initial 4497 participants in the pool. Magnesium intake was found to be inversely associated with the incidence of diabetes after adjustment for potential confounders. The multivariable-adjusted hazard ratio of diabetes for participants in the highest quintile of magnesium intake was 0.53, compared to those in the lowest quintile. Magnesium intake was significantly inversely associated with hs-CRP, IL-6, fibrinogen, and HOMA-IR, and serum magnesium levels were inversely correlated with hs-CRP and HOMA-IR.

The authors concluded that magnesium intake is inversely associated with incidence of diabetes in young American adults. In other words, the lower the magnesium intake, the higher the incidence of diabetes. This inverse association can be explained, at least in part, by the inverse correlations of magnesium intake with systemic inflammation and insulin resistance (Kim, Xun, Liu et al. 2010).

14.5.1 MAGNESIUM SUPPLEMENTATION SUPPORTS GLYCEMIC CONTROL

According to a report in the *World Journal of Diabetes*, Type 2 diabetes is frequently associated with deficits of both extracellular and intracellular magnesium (Mg). A chronic latent Mg deficit or an overt clinical hypomagnesemia is common in such patients especially in those with poorly controlled glycemic profiles: Magnesium, the second most abundant intracellular divalent cation, is a cofactor of many enzymes involved in glucose metabolism. It has an important role in insulin action, and insulin stimulates magnesium uptake in insulin-sensitive tissues.

Insulin and glucose are important regulators of Mg metabolism: Intracellular Mg plays a key role in regulating insulin action, insulin-mediated glucose uptake, and vascular tone. Reduced intracellular Mg concentrations result in a defective tyrosine-kinase activity, postreceptorial impairment in insulin action, and worsening of insulin resistance in diabetic patients.

A review published in the journal *Magnesium Research* was designed to reach a better understanding of the mechanism involved in the correlation between magnesium and insulin resistance: It concluded that magnesium is required for both proper glucose utilization and insulin signaling. Metabolic alterations in cellular magnesium, which may play the role of a second messenger for insulin action, contribute to insulin resistance (Takaya, Higashino, and Kobayashi. 2004).

Reduced Mg intake and/or augmented Mg urinary loss are among the most important causes of Mg deficits in Type 2 diabetes, while Mg absorption and retention seem to be maintained (Wälti, Zimmermann, Walczyk et al. 2003; Günther. 2011; Barbagallo, Dominguez, Galioto et al. 2003). Benefits of Mg supplementation on metabolic profiles in diabetic patients have been found in most but not all clinical studies (Barbagallo, and Dominguez. 2015).

A relationship between magnesium levels in plasma and the development of Type 2 diabetes in the general population has been proposed. A study titled "Serum and dietary magnesium and the risk for type 2 diabetes mellitus: the Atherosclerosis Risk in Communities Study" was published in the journal *Archives of Internal Medicine*. The aim of this study was to determine the risk for developing Type 2 diabetes as a consequence of low serum magnesium level, and low dietary magnesium intake, in a cohort of nondiabetic middle-aged adults in the Atherosclerosis Risk in Communities Study, during 6 years of follow-up.

Fasting serum magnesium in six level categories and dietary magnesium intake in quartiles were measured at the baseline examination. Incident Type 2 diabetes was defined by self-report of physician diagnosis, use of diabetic medication, fasting glucose level of at least 7.0 mmol/L

(126 mg/dL), or nonfasting glucose level of at least 11.1 mmol/L (200 mg/dL). A graded inverse relationship between serum magnesium levels and incident Type 2 diabetes was found in white participants. From the highest to the lowest serum magnesium levels, there was an approximate twofold increase in incidence rate that remained significant after simultaneous adjustment for potential confounding factors including diuretic use.

Compared to individuals with serum magnesium levels of 0.95 mmol/L (1.90 mEq/L) or greater, the adjusted relative odds of incident Type 2 diabetes rose progressively across the following lower magnesium categories: 1.13, 1.20, 1.11, 1.24, and 1.76. In contrast, little or no such association was observed in African-American participants.

The authors concluded that low serum magnesium level is a strong, independent predictor of incident Type 2 diabetes in white participants. That low dietary magnesium intake does not confer risk for Type 2 diabetes implies that compartmentalization and renal processing of magnesium may be important in the relationship between low serum magnesium levels and the risk of Type 2 diabetes (Kao, Folsom, Nieto et al. 1999).

Both hyperglycemia and hyperinsulinemia may increase urinary Mg excretion. Urinary Mg excretion and fasting blood glucose have been found to be inversely related to serum Mg levels; thus, hyperglycemia decreases Mg tubular reabsorption (McNair, Christensen, Christiansen et al. 1982).

Research has shown that even good metabolic control is not invariably associated with reduction in urinary Mg wasting. In a study reported in the journal *Diabetologia*, it was observed that metabolic control was significantly improved as noted by reduced HbA1c levels in both insulin-treated patients or patients on oral antihyperglycemic agents. However, plasma magnesium levels remained unchanged during the follow-up in the insulin-treated group (1: 0.79 ± 0.02 mmol/L; 2: 0.81 ± 0.02 mmol/L; 3: 0.79 ± 0.01 mmol/L), as well as in patients on oral antihyperglycemic agents (1: 0.79 ± 0.03 mmol/L; 2: 0.78 ± 0.02 mmol/L; 3: 0.84 ± 0.04 mmol/L).

The investigators concluded that even marked improvement of glycemic control does not correct hypomagnesaemia in Type 2 diabetes; hypomagnesaemia might be related to the insulin-resistant state, and that possible beneficial effect of chronic magnesium administration is recommended for these patients (Schnack, Bauer, Pregant et al. 1992).

In STZ-induced diabetic rats, it was found that there is an increase in renal Mg transporters (Lee, Lien, Lai et al. 2006). The alteration was corrected by insulin administration. Insulin resistance and hyperinsulinemia may also affect Mg transport (Djurhuus, Skøtt, Hother-Nielson et al. 1995).

According to a report in the journal *Metabolism*, a chronic latent Mg deficiency without alteration in serum total Mg is more commonly observed (Barbagallo, Di Bella, Brucato et al. 2014). Such often undetected Mg insufficiency has clinical importance, since Mg is a main co-factor in more than 300 enzymatic reactions including all the enzymes of glycolysis. Magnesium is also involved in the regulation of insulin signaling, in the phosphorylation of insulin receptor kinase, in the post-receptorial action of insulin, and in insulin-mediated cellular glucose uptake (Günther. 2011; Saris, Mervaala, Karppanen et al. 2000). The clinical consequence of a chronic Mg deficit is insulin resistance and reduced glucose utilization in the cells, worsening the reduced insulin sensitivity present in diabetes (Barbagallo, Dominguez, Galioto et al. 2003).

Another possible link between magnesium deficiency and reduced insulin sensitivity is the degree of oxidative stress and/or inflammation present, since free radicals are often increased in diabetes, hypertension, metabolic syndrome, and aging, conditions also associated with Mg deficits (Weglicki. 2012; Barbagallo, and Dominguez. 2010). In particular, an age-dependent deficit of cellular Mg has been shown in persons aged 65 years and older, as well as in patients with essential hypertension or Type 2 diabetes, independently of age (Barbagallo, Gupta, Dominguez et al. 2000; Barbagallo, and Dominguez. 2010).

It has also been noted that independent of the mechanisms of Mg deficits in Type 2 diabetes, as well as in metabolic syndrome, essential hypertension, and aging, Mg deficiency may enhance insulin resistance common in these conditions (Günther. 2011; Barbagallo, Dominguez, Galioto et al. 2003).

14.5.2 Dietary Magnesium Deficiency Is Linked to Hyperglycemia

A number of studies have concluded that dietary Mg deficiency may cause insulin resistance. A study published in the journal *Circulation* reported that magnesium intake was inversely related to metabolic syndrome and fasting insulin levels. The investigators concluded that young adults with higher magnesium intake have lower risk of developing metabolic syndrome (He, Liu, Daviglus et al. 2006).

In another study published in the *Journal of the American College of Nutrition*, it was found in young women that after adjustment for age, body mass index, total energy, physical activity, hours per week spent sitting outside work, alcohol intake, smoking, and family history of diabetes, magnesium intake was inversely associated with fasting insulin concentration. The multivariate adjusted geometric mean for fasting insulin concentration in women in the lowest quartile of magnesium intake was 11.0 µU/mL, compared to a fasting insulin of only 9.3 µU/mL among those in the highest quartile of magnesium intake. This suggests, among other things, that with adequate magnesium stores, the pancreas does not have to work so "hard" pumping out insulin to keep blood sugar in control. The inverse association remained even when magnesium from only food sources was considered.

The authors concluded that higher magnesium intake is associated with lower fasting insulin concentrations among young to middle-aged women without diabetes. Because lower fasting insulin concentrations generally reflect greater insulin sensitivity, these findings provide a mechanism by which higher dietary magnesium intake may reduce the risk of developing Type 2 diabetes (Fung, Manson, Solomon et al. 2003). That low dietary magnesium intake is associated with insulin resistance was also reported in a sample of nondiabetic African-Americans in the *American Journal of Hypertension* (Humphries, Kushner, and Falkner. 1999; see also Colditz, Manson, Stampfer et al. 1992).

Deficiencies of Mg status, including both hypomagnesemia and/or reduced dietary Mg intake, have been linked to enhanced risk of developing Type 2 diabetes or glucose intolerance in numerous studies (Kao, Folsom, Nieto et al. 1999), including one published in the journal *Clinica Chimica Acta*. The investigators measured the plasma magnesium concentrations of a sample of unselected diabetes outpatients and of a sample of control participants by atomic absorption spectrophotometry.

Mean plasma Mg was significantly lower in the diabetes patients (0.737 ± 0.071 mmol/L) than in the control participants (0.810 ± 0.057 mmol/L), and 25% of the diabetic patients had values below those of all control participants except one. Plasma Mg correlated best with clinic blood glucose concentration, and other significant associations were observed with glycosuria, age, gender, insulin therapy, and biguanide therapy (Mather, Nisbet, Burton et al. 1979).

Parenthetically, an interesting study conducted in Japan concluded that one of the major factors contributing to the drastic increase of Type 2 diabetes in Japan after World War II is the change in diet consisting of a drastically decreased intake of grains, such as barley or cereals rich in Mg. This suggested an inverse relationship between the volume of dietary Mg intake and the onset of Type 2 diabetes (Yokota. 2005).

Several meta-analyses of prospective studies concluded that Mg intake is inversely associated with the onset of Type 2 diabetes. One, in particular, published in the *Journal of Internal Medicine*, centered on seven identified cohort studies of magnesium intake from foods only or from foods and supplements combined and the incidence of Type 2 diabetes included. The data were based on 286,668 participants and 10,912 cases. All but one study found an inverse relation between magnesium intake and risk of Type 2 diabetes, and in four of the seven studies, the association was statistically significant.

The investigators concluded that magnesium intake is inversely associated with the incidence of Type 2 diabetes. This finding suggested to them that increased consumption of magnesium-rich foods such as whole grains, beans, nuts, and green leafy vegetables may reduce the risk of Type 2 diabetes (Larsson, and Wolk. 2007).

A 10-year follow-up study published in the *European Journal of Clinical Investigation* involved more than 1100 participants 20 to 65 years of age, enrolled in a study between 1996 and 1997.

More than 800 of the individuals were reexamined about 10 years later. New-onset impaired fasting glucose (IFG) (5.6–7.0 mmol/L), impaired glucose tolerance (IGT) (7.8–11.1 mmol/L glucose 2-h postload), and Type 2 diabetes were determined from the number of participants who had these conditions at the second examination without evidence that they were present at the first one.

The relative risk of new-onset metabolic glucose disorders and diabetes was adjusted for age, gender, family history of diabetes, waist circumference, and HOMA-IR index. Serum magnesium levels less than 0.74 mmol/L defined the exposed group. It was found that at baseline, 51.4% of individuals had hypomagnesaemia. New-onset IFG and IGT was found in 33.8% of the participants. The relative risk for IFG, IGT, and IFG + IGT was 1.11, 1.38, and 1.49, respectively. New-onset diabetes was identified in 9.5% of participants (relative risk 2.54).

The investigators concluded that hypomagnesemia is independently associated with the development of impaired glucose tolerance, impaired fasting glucose + impaired glucose tolerance, and Type 2 diabetes, but not with the development of impaired fasting glucose (Guerrero-Romero, Rascón-Pacheco, Rodríguez-Morán et al. 2008).

Conversely, higher Mg intake was found to be associated with increased insulin sensitivity (Ma, Lawson, Liese et al. 2006) and with decreased risk of incident Type 2 diabetes with a decreased risk of 0.68 in the higher quintile, compared to the lower quintiles (Lopez-Ridaura, Willett, Rimm et al. 2004).

14.5.3 Mg: THE LINK TO CARDIOVASCULAR AND HEART CONDITIONS

A study published in the journal *Diabetes Care* reported a relationship between ionic changes and echocardiographic indices alterations. A significant association of reduced cellular Mg and cardiac hypertrophy was observed in Type 2 diabetes patients (Barbagallo, Gupta, and Resnick. 1996). Reduced Mg levels were also associated with an increased prevalence of arrhythmias in obese Type 2 diabetes patients (Del Gobbo, Song, Poirier et al. 2012) and with a more rapid decline of renal function.

According to a number of reports, hypomagnesemia is considered an accurate predictor for the progression of diabetic nephropathy (Sakaguchi, Shoji, Hayashi et al. 2012; Van Laecke, Nagler, Verbeke et al. 2013; Tin, Grams, Maruthur et al. 2015).

14.6 ZINC IS ANTI-INFLAMMATORY AND ANTIDIABETIC

Zinc is an essential micronutrient required for many cellular processes, especially for the normal development and function of the immune system, and also in wound healing (Kogan, Sood, and Garnick. 2017). The role of zinc in wound healing may be of particular concern in connection with diabetic cardiomyopathy and lesions that may develop as a result of diabetes (Lu, Liu, Li et al. 2015).

National surveys indicate that a significant proportion of the elderly population has inadequate zinc intake, and a decline in zinc status is observed with age. Both zinc deficiency and the aging process are characterized by impaired immune responses and systemic low-grade chronic inflammation. It has been suggested that age-related zinc deficiency may be an important contribution to chronic inflammation during the aging process.

A review appearing in the journal *Molecular Nutrition and Food Research* emphasized the effects of zinc status on aging and particularly on the role of zinc deficiency in age-related immune dysfunction and chronic inflammation (Wong, and Ho. 2012). However, of greater present concern may be the role of zinc deficiency in Type 2 diabetes.

14.6.1 THE ROLE OF ZINC IN GLYCEMIC CONTROL

The journal *Biometals* published a systematic conventional electronic database review that aimed to determine the extent to which zinc participates in glycemic control in Type 2 diabetes patients.

The main finding was the presence of low body contents of zinc and high excretion of zinc in urine in this population. Hyperglycemia was one of the mechanisms thought to cause these alterations owing to its interference with zinc reabsorption by renal cells. In addition, an inverse correlation was found between the glycated hemoglobin percentage (% HbA1c) and the plasma zinc levels.

It was also noted that zinc supplementation in these patients improved glycemic control, since the % HbA1c was significantly reduced in the supplemented individuals.

The authors concluded, based on the review, that a positive effect is gained by achieving adequate zinc levels in glycemic control, whether it is through diet or supplementation, since its role in insulin homeostasis is clear (de Carvalho, Brandão-Lima, Maia et al. 2017).

A review appearing in the journal *Diabetology and Metabolic Syndrome* aimed to determine the effects of zinc supplementation on diabetes. The investigators undertook a systematic review and meta-analysis of studies examining the effects of zinc supplementation on clinical and biochemical parameters in patients with diabetes. The pooled mean difference in FBG level between zinc-supplemented and placebo groups was significantly different. Two-hour postprandial blood sugar likewise showed a significant reduction in the zinc-treated group, as was also the reduction in HbA1c in the zinc-treated group.

The pooled mean difference in total cholesterol between zinc-supplemented and placebo groups was significant. LDL cholesterol also showed a similar distinct reduction in the zinc-treated group, the pooled mean difference from random-effects analysis being 11.19 mg/dL.

The investigators concluded that zinc supplementation has beneficial effects on glycemic control and it promotes healthy lipid levels (Jayawardena, Ranasinghe, Galappatthy et al. 2012).

A clinical study conducted in Tunisia and reported in the *Journal of the American College of Nutrition* aimed to determine the effects of combined zinc (Zn) and chromium (Cr) supplementation on oxidative stress and glucose homeostasis in people with Type 2 diabetes. Adults with HbA1c greater than 7.5% were supplemented for 6 months with 30 mg/day of Zn, as Zn gluconate, or 400 µg/day of Cr, as Cr pidolate (pidolate: pyroglutamic acid), or combined Zn/Cr supplementation, or placebo.

The effects of supplementation on plasma zinc, copper, selenium, urinary Zn, Cr, plasma thiobarbituric acid reactive substances (TBARS), Cu-Zn superoxide dismutase (SOD), and selenium glutathione peroxidase (GPx) in RBCs, along with blood lipids and lipoproteins, HbA1c, and fasting glucose, were measured at the beginning of the study and after 6 months.

The TBARS method is a conventional laboratory method for measuring oxidative stress. TBARS are formed as a by-product of lipid peroxidation, that is, as degradation products of fats that can be detected by an assay using thiobarbituric acid as a reagent.

It was found that at the beginning of the study, more than 30% of the participants may have been Zn deficient with plasma Zn values less than 10.7 µmol/L, whereas levels of plasma Cu, Se, and antioxidant RBC enzyme activities were in the normal ranges. Following supplementation, there was a significant lower plasma TBARS in the groups supplemented with Cr (13.6%), Zn (13.6%), and Zn/Cr (18.2%), with no significant changes in the placebo group.

The TBARS of the control healthy participants was 2.08 ± 0.04 µmol/L, and that of those with diabetes before supplementation was 3.32 ± 0.05 µmol/L. This difference of 1.24 µmol/L between the control group and the participants with diabetes was reduced from 36% to 50% in the three supplemented groups.

Supplementation did not significantly modify HbA1c or glucose homeostasis. No adverse effects of Zn supplementation were observed on Cu status, HDL cholesterol, or interactions in Zn or Cr.

The investigators concluded that the potential beneficial antioxidant effects of the individual and combined supplementation of Zn and Cr in people with Type 2 diabetes were especially significant in light of the deleterious consequences of oxidative stress in this population (Anderson, Roussel, Zouari et al. 2001).

The investigators in a clinical study published in the *Saudi Medical Journal* concluded that diabetic patients have significantly lower mean serum zinc levels compared with healthy controls. Zinc supplementation for Type 2 diabetes has beneficial effects in elevating their serum zinc level and in improving their glycemic control, as shown by decreasing their HbA1c percent concentration (Al-Maroof, and Al-Sharbatti. 2006).

A clinical study published in the *American Journal of Medicine* reported the investigation of zinc metabolism in patients with stable Type 2 diabetes. Twenty-five percent of these patients had depressed serum zinc concentrations, and all demonstrated hyperzincuria. Urinary zinc loss was greater when proteinuria was present and correlated with the mean serum glucose concentration. Studies of gastrointestinal zinc absorption also suggested zinc malabsorption in patients with Type 2 diabetes.

The investigators concluded that hyperzincuria, resulting from a glucose-mediated process that is not osmotic, interacts with impaired zinc absorption to produce zinc deficiency in patients with Type 2 diabetes (Kinlaw, Levine, Morley et al. 1983).

The authors of a review titled "Zinc supplementation for the prevention of type 2 diabetes mellitus in adults with insulin resistance," published in the *Cochrane Database of Systematic Reviews*, predictably concluded that "There is currently no evidence on which to base the use of zinc supplementation for the prevention of type 2 diabetes mellitus. Future trials should investigate patient-important outcome measures such as incidence of type 2 diabetes mellitus, health-related quality of life, diabetic complications, all-cause mortality and socioeconomic effects" (El Dib, Gameiro, Ogata et al. 2015).

14.6.2 ZINC IS ANTIOXIDANT AND ANTI-INFLAMMATORY

The following additional references support the role of zinc as antioxidant and anti-inflammatory:

- Zinc is an antioxidant and anti-inflammatory agent: Its role in human health. Prasad. 2015. *Frontiers in Nutrition*, 1: 14.
- Antioxidant and anti-inflammatory effects of zinc. Zinc-dependent NF-κB signaling. Jarosz, Olbert, Wyszogrodzka et al. 2017. *Inflammopharmacology*, 25(1): 11–24.
- Zinc and regulation of inflammatory cytokines: implications for cardiometabolic disease. Foster, and Samman. 2012. *Nutrients*, Jul; 4(7): 676–694.
- Zinc decreases CRP, lipid peroxidation, and inflammatory cytokines in elderly subjects: a potential implication of zinc as an atheroprotective agent. Bao, Prasad, Beck et al. 2010. *The Ameican Journal of Clinical Nutrition*, Jun; 91(6): 1634–1641.

14.7 FINAL NOTE

We described selected supplements in the last two chapters and supported their antidiabetic, antioxidant, and anti-inflammatory benefits with scientific data. This selection is *by no means comprehensive,* but it is intended to give an overview of how such dietary constituents are scientifically validated, as well as how their alleged benefits may be scientifically challenged.

Most other sources of information about such matters of necessity omit validation studies, thus leaving them open to the accusation either that they are an "expert opinion" or that the data are equivocal. This is an unfortunate disservice both to clinical practitioners and to the consumer public—one that we went to some lengths to correct here.

We have left out many supplements and, in previous chapters, functional foods that have been shown to benefit persons with Type 2 diabetes. The agents we elected to leave out include micronutrients such as vitamin C, vitamin E, manganese, iron, and many more. This by no means indicates that they play no role in either blood glucose control or that they are not anti-inflammatory. For the supplements that we chose to include, our criteria were (1) information for and evidence of molecular glycemic control mechanisms, (2) the validation of treatment strategies by clinical trials with supplementation, and (3) what is tantamount to an open market of ideas as to their scientific merits and their treatment value.

We hope that by so doing, practitioners may appreciate the fact that treatment modalities alternately termed "integrative" or "complementary" deserve some consideration in the treatment of Type 2 diabetes. We trust that it is clear that, at least for those supplements detailed in this book, they have been given the same level of scientific scrutiny as the conventional medications they are intended to support.

A note to the reader: Please see the chart in the Appendix for a summary of the therapeutic and other effects of the selected supplements described in this chapter.

REFERENCES

Abbas ZG, and AB Swai. 1997. Evaluation of the efficacy of thiamine and pyridoxine in the treatment of symptomatic diabetic peripheral neuropathy. *East African Medical Journal*, Dec; 74(12): 803–808.

Abebe W. 2008. Effects of taurine on the reactivity of aortas from diabetic rats. *Life Sciences*, Jan; 82(5–6): 279–289. DOI: 10.1016/j.lfs.2007.11.012.

Aberg F. Appelkvist E L, Dallner G, and L Ernster. 1992. Distribution and redox state of ubiquinones in rat and human tissues. *Archives of Biochemistry and Biophysics*, Jun; 295 (2): 230–234. DOI: 10.1016/0003-9861(92)90511-T.

Albarracin CA, Fuqua BC, Evans JL, and ID Goldfine. 2008. Chromium picolinate and biotin combination improves glucose metabolism in treated, uncontrolled overweight to obese patients with type 2 diabetes. *Diabetes/Metabolism Research and Reviews*, Jan-Feb; 24(1): 41–51.

Al-Maroof RA, and SS Al-Sharbatti. 2006. Serum zinc levels in diabetic patients and effect of zinc supplementation on glycemic control of type 2 diabetics. *Saudi Medical Journal*, Mar; 27(3): 344–350.

Anderson RA, Roussel A-M, Zouari N, Mahjoub S, Matheau J-M, and A Kerkeni. 2001. Potential antioxidant effects of zinc and chromium supplementation in people with Type 2 diabetes mellitus. *Journal of the American College of Nutrition*, 20(3): 212–218. http://dx.doi.org/10.1080/07315724.2001.10719034.

Anderson RA. 1997. Chromium as an essential nutrient for humans. *Regulatory Toxicology and Pharmacology*, Aug; 26(1): S35–S41. https://doi.org/10.1006/rtph.1997.1136.

Anthrayose CV, and S Shashidhar. 2004. Studies on protein and taurine in normal, senile and diabetic cataractous human lenses. *Indian Journal of Physiology and Pharmacology*, Jul; 483: 357–360.

Askwith T, Zeng W, Eggo MC, and MJ Stevens. 2009. Oxidative stress and dysregulation of the taurine transporter in high-glucose-exposed human Schwann cells: implications for pathogenesis of diabetic neuropathy. *American Journal of Physiology, Endocrinology and Metabolism*, Sep; 297(3): E620–E628. DOI: 10. 1152/ajpendo.00287.2009.

Ates O, Bilen H, Keles S, Alp HH, Keleş MS, Yıldırım K, Öndaş O, Pınar C, Civelekler M, and O Baykal1. 2013. Plasma coenzyme Q10 levels in type 2 diabetic patients with retinopathy. *International Journal of Ophthalmology*, Oct; 6(5): 675–679. DOI: 10.3980/j.issn.2222-3959.2013.05.24.

Bao B, Prasad AS, Beck FW, Fitzgerald JT, Snell D, Bao GW, Singh T, and LJ Cardozo. 2010. Zinc decreases C-reactive protein, lipid peroxidation, and inflammatory cytokines in elderly subjects: a potential implication of zinc as an atheroprotective agent. *The Ameican Journal of Clinical Nutrition*, Jun; 91(6): 1634–1641. DOI: 10. 3945/ajcn.2009.28836.

Barbagallo M, and LJ Dominguez. 2010. Magnesium and aging. *Current Pharmaceutical Design*, 16(7): 832–839.

Barbagallo M, and LJ Dominguez. 2015. Magnesium and type 2 diabetes. *World Journal of Diabetes*, Aug; 6(10): 115–1157. DOI: 10.4239/wjd.v6.i10.1152.

Barbagallo M, Di Bella G, Brucato V, D'Angelo D, Damiani P, Monteverde A, Belvedere M, and LJ Dominguez. 2014. Serum ionized magnesium in diabetic older persons. *Metabolism*, Apr; 63(4): 50250–50259. DOI: 10.1016/j.metabol.2013.12.003.

Barbagallo M, Dominguez LJ, Galioto A, Ferlisi A, Cani C, Malfa L, Pineo A, Busardo A, and G Paolisso. 2003. Role of magnesium in insulin action, diabetes and cardio-metabolic syndrome X. *Molecular Aspects of Medicine*, Feb-Jun; 24(1–3): 39–52.

Barbagallo M, Gupta RK, and LM Resnick. 1996. Cellular ions in NIDDM: relation of calcium to hyperglycemia and cardiac mass. *Diabetes Care*, Dec; 19(2): 1393–1398.

Barbagallo M, Gupta RK, Dominguez LJ, and LM Resnick. 2000. Cellular ionic alterations with age: relation to hypertension and diabetes. *Journal of the American Geriatric Society*, Sep; 48(9): 1111–1116.

Bellentani S, Pecorari M, Cordoma P, Marchegiano P, Manenti F, Bosisio E, Fabiani E, and G Galli. 1987. Taurine increases bile acid pool size and reduces bile saturation index in the hamster. *Journal of Lipid Research*, Sep; 28(9): 1021–1027.

Bender DA. 1999. Non-nutritional uses of vitamin B6. *British Journal of Nutrition*, Jan; 81(1): 7–20.

Bendich A, and M Cohen. 1990. Vitamin B6 safety issues. *Annals of the N.Y. Academy of Sciences*, 585: 321–330.

Bischoff-Ferrari HA, Giovannucci E, Willett WC, Dietrich T, and B Dawson-Hughes. 2006. Estimation of optimal serum concentrations of 25-hydroxyvitamin D for multiple health outcomes. *American Journal of Clinical Nutrition*, Jul; 84(1): 18–28.

Bischoff-Ferrari HA. 2008. Optimal serum 25-hydroxyvitamin D levels for multiple health outcomes. *Advances in Experimental Medicine and Biology*, 624: 55–71. DOI: 10.1007/978-0-387-77574-6_5.

Bønaa KH, Njølstad I, Ueland PM, Schirmer H, Tverdal A, Steigen T, Wang H, Nordrehaug JE, Arnesen E, and K Rasmussen, and the NORVIT Trial Investigators. 2006. Homocysteine lowering and cardiovascular events after acute myocardial infarction. *New England Journal of Medicine*, Apr; 354(15): 1578–1588. DOI: 10.1056/NEJMoa055227.

Buhary BM, Almohareb O, Aljohani N, Alrajhi S, Elkaissi S, Sherbeeni S, Almaghamsi A, Khan SA, Almalki MH. 2017. Association of glycosylated hemoglobin levels with vitamin D status. *Journal of Clinical Medicine Research*, Dec; 9(12): 1013–1018. DOI: 10.14740/jocmr3227w.

Campbell NR. 1996. How safe are folic acid supplements? *Archives of Internal Medicine*, Aug; 156(15): 1638–1644.

Casey RG, Gang C, Joyce M, and DJ Bouchier-Hayes. 2007. Taurine attenuates acute hyperglycaemia-induced endothelial cell apoptosis, leucocyte-endothelial cell interactions and cardiac dysfunction. *Journal of Vascular Research*, 44(1): 31–39. DOI: 10.1159/000097893.

Chaava MM, Bukiia TSh, and TSh Shaburishvili. 2005. Homocysteine as risk marker of cardiovascular disease [article in Russian]. *Georgian Medical News*, Oct; (127): 65–70.

Chauncey KB, Tenner TE, Jr, Lombardini JB, Jones BG, Brooks ML, Warner RD, Davis RL, and RM Ragain. 2003. The effect of taurine supplementation on patients with type 2 diabetes mellitus. *Advances in Experimental Medicine and Biology*, 526: 91–96.

Chen G, Nan C, Tian J, Jean-Charles P, Li Y, Weissbach H, and XP Huang. 2012. Protective effects of taurine against oxidative stress in the heart of MsrA knockout mice. *Journal of Cellular Biochemistry*, May; 113(11):3559–3566. DOI: 10.1002/jcb.24233.

Chew GT, and GF Watts. 2004. Coenzyme Q10 and diabetic endotheliopathy: oxidative stress and the 'recoupling hypothesis.' *QJM*, Aug; 97(6): 537–548. DOI: 10.1093/qjmed/hch089.

Chiu KC, Chu A, Go VL, and MF Saad. 2004. Hypovitaminosis D is associated with insulin resistance and beta cell dysfunction. *American Journal of Clinical Nutrition*, May; 79(5): 820–825.

Chogtu B, Magazine R, and KL Bairy. 2015. Statin use and risk of diabetes mellitus. *World Journal of Diabetes*, Mar; 6(2): 352–357. DOI: 10.4239/wjd.v6.i2.352.

Christakos S, Friedlander EJ, Frandsen BR, and AW Norman. 1979. Studies on the mode of action of calciferol. XIII. Development of a radioimmunoassay for vitamin D-dependent chick intestinal calcium-binding protein and tissue distribution. *Endocrinology*, May; 104(5): 1495–1503. DOI: 10.1210/endo-104-5-1495.

Cigolini M, Iagulli MP, Miconi V, Lorenzi T, Lombardi S, and G Targher. 2006. Inflammatory variables may mediate the link between low plasma vitamin B6 concentrations and cardiovascular disease in type 2 diabetes. *Nutrition, Metabolism, and Cardiovascular Diseases*, Oct; 16(7): e9–e10. DOI: 10.1016/j.numecd.2006.05.003.

Colditz GA, Manson JE, Stampfer MJ, Rosner B, Willett WC, and FE Speizer. 1992. Diet and risk of clinical diabetes in women. *American Journal of Clinical Nutrition*, May; 55(5): 1018–1023.

Conget I, Manzanares JM, Barrientos A, Cardellach F, and R Gomis. 1996. Coenzyme Q10 and insulin secretion in vitro. *Diabetes Research and Clinical Practice*, 33(5): 135–136. DOI: 10.1016/0168-8227(96)01278-8.

Crompton M, and L Andreeva. 1993. On the involvement of mitochondrial pore in reperfusion injury, *Basic Research in Cardiology*, Sep; 88(5): 513–523.

Das J, and PC Sil. 2012. Taurine ameliorates alloxan-induced diabetic renal injury, oxidative stress-related signaling pathways and apoptosis in rats. *Amino Acids*, Oct; 43(4): 1509–1523. DOI: 10.1007/s00726-012-1225-y.

de Boer IH, Tinker LF, Connelly S, Curb JD, Howard BV, Kestenbaum B, Larson JC, Manson JE, Margolis KL, Siscovick DS, and NS Weiss. 2008. Calcium plus vitamin D supplementation and the risk of incident diabetes in the Women's Health Initiative. *Diabetes Care*, Apr; 31(4): 701–707. DOI: 10.2337/dc07-1829.

de Carvalho GB, Brandão-Lima PN, Maia CS, Barbosa KB, and LV Pires. 2017. Zinc's role in the glycemic control of patients with type 2 diabetes: a systematic review. *Biometals*, Apr; 30(2): 151–162. DOI: 10.1007/s10534-017-9996-y.

DeFronzo RA, Bonadonna RC, and E Ferrannini. 1992. Pathogenesis of NIDDM. A balanced overview. *Diabetes Care*. Mar; 15(3): 318–368.

Del Gobbo LC, Song Y, Poirier P, Dewailly E, Elin RJ, and GM Egeland. 2012. Low serum magnesium concentrations are associated with a high prevalence of premature ventricular complexes in obese adults with type 2 diabetes. *Cardiovascular Diabetology*, Mar; 11:23. DOI: 10.1186/1475-2840-11-23.

Di Leo MA, Ghirlanda G, Gentiloni Silveri N, Giardina B, Franconi F, and SA Santini. 2003. Potential therapeutic effect of antioxidants in experimental diabetic retina: a comparison between chronic taurine and vitamin E plus selenium supplementations. *Free Radical Research*, Mar; 37(3): 323–330.

Di Leo MA, Santini SA, Cercone S, Lepore D, Gentiloni Silveri N, Caputo S, Greco AV, Giardina B, Franconi F, and G Ghirlanda. 2002. Chronic taurine supplementation ameliorates oxidative stress and Na+ K+ ATPase impairment in the retina of diabetic rats. *Amino Acids*, 23(4): 401–406. DOI: 10.1007/s00726-002-0202-2.

DiMonte DA, Chan P, and MS Sandy. 1992. Glutathione in Parkinson's disease: a link between oxidative stress and mitochondrial damage? *Annals of Neurology*, 32: Suppl: S111–S115.

Ding Y, Li Y, and A Wen. 2015. Effect of niacin on lipids and glucose in patients with type 2 diabetes: a meta-analysis of randomized, controlled clinical trials. *Clinical Nutrition*, Oct; 34(5): 838–844. DOI: 10.1016/j.clnu.2014.09.019.

Djurhuus MS, Skøtt P, Hother-Nielson O, Klitgaard NA, and H Beck-Nielsen. 1995. Insulin increases renal magnesium excretion: a possible cause of magnesium depletion in hyperinsulinaemic states. *Diabetic Medicine*, Aug; 12(8): 664–669.

El Dib R, Gameiro OL, Ogata MS, Módolo NS, Braz LG, Jorge EC, do Nascimento P Jr, and V Beletate. 2015. Zinc supplementation for the prevention of type 2 diabetes mellitus in adults with insulin resistance. *Cochrane Database of Systematic Reviews*, May 28;(5): CD005525. DOI: 10.1002/14651858 .CD005525.pub3.

El Idrissi A, Boukarrou L, Splavnyk K, Zavyalova E, Meehan EF, abd W L'Amoreaux. 2009. Functional implication of taurine in aging. *Advances in Experimental Medicine and Biology*, 643:199–206.

Eriksson JG, Forsen TJ, Mortensen SA, and M Rohde. 1999. The effect of coenzyme Q10 administration on metabolic control in patients with type 2 diabetes mellitus. *Biofactors*, 9; 9(2–4): 315–318. DOI: 10.1002/biof.5520090229.

Field MS, and PJ. Stover. 2017. Safety of folic acid. *Annals of the NY Academy of Sciences*. DOI: 10.1111 /nyas.13499.

Forouhi NG, Luan J, Cooper A, Boucher BJ, and N Wareham. 2008. Baseline serum 25-hydroxy vitamin D is predictive of future glycemic status and insulin resistance: the Medical Research Council Ely prospective study 1990–2000. *Diabetes*, Oct; 57(10): 2619–2625. DOI: 10.2337/db08-0593.

Foster M, and S Samman. 2012. Zinc and regulation of inflammatory cytokines: implications for cardiometabolic disease. *Nutrients*, Jul; 4(7): 676–694. DOI: 10.3390/nu4070676.

Franconi F, Bennardini F, Mattana A, Miceli M, Ciuti M, Mian M, Gironi A, Anichini R, and G Seghieri. 1995. Plasma and platelet taurine are reduced in subjects with insulin-dependent diabetes mellitus: effects of taurine supplementation. *American Journal of Clinical Nutrition*, May; 61(5): 1115–1119.

Franconi F, Miceli M, Fazzini A, Seghieri G, Caputo S, DiLeo MA, Lepore D, Ghirlanda G. 1996. Taurine and diabetes. Humans and experimental models. *Advances in Experimental Medicine and Biology*, 403: 579–582.

Fung TT, Manson JE, Solomon CG, Liu S, Willett WC, and FB Hu. 2003. The association between magnesium intake and fasting insulin concentration in healthy middle-aged women. *Journal of the American College of Nutrition*, Dec; 22(6): 533–538.

Gandhi VM, Cherian KM, and MJ Mulky. 1992. Hypolipidemic action of taurine in rats. *Indian Journal of Experimental Biology*, May; 30(5): 413–417.

Garrido-Maraver J, Cordero MD, Oropesa-Ávila M, Fernández Vega AF, de la Mata M, Delgado Pavón A, de Miguel M, Pérez Calero C, Villanueva Paz M, Cotán D, and JA Sánchez-Alcázar. 2014. Coenzyme Q10 therapy. *Molecular Syndromology*, Jul; 5(3–4): 187–197. DOI: 10.1159/000360101.

Gdynia HJ, Muller T, Sperfeld AD, Kuhnlein P, Otto M, Kassubek J, and AC Ludolph 2008. Severe sensorimotor neuropathy after intake of highest dosages of vitamin B6. *Neuromuscular Disorders*, Feb; 18(2): 156–158. DOI: 10.1016/j.nmd.2007.09.009.

Gröber U, Schmidt J, and K Kisters. 2015. Magnesium in prevention and therapy. *Nutrients*, Sep; 7(9): 8199–8226. DOI: 10.3390/nu7095388.

Guerrero-Romero F, Rascón-Pacheco RA, Rodríguez-Morán M, de la Peña JE, and N Wacher. 2008. Hypomagnesaemia and risk for metabolic glucose disorders: a 10-year follow-up study. *European Journal of Clinical Investigation*, Jun;38(6):389–396. DOI: 10.1111/j.1365-2362.2008.01957.x.

Günther T. 2011. Magnesium in bone and the magnesium load test. *Magnesium Research*, Dec; 24(4): 223–224. DOI: 10.1684/mrh.2011.0297.

Haeusler RA, Camastra S, Astiarraga B, Nannipieri M, Anselmino M, and Ferrannini. 2015. Decreased expression of hepatic glucokinase in type 2 diabetes. *Molecular Metabolism*, Mar; 4(3): 222–226. DOI: 10.1016/j.molmet.2014.12.007.

Hathcock JN, and A Shao. 1996. Risk assessment for coenzyme Q10 (Ubiquinone). *Regulatory Toxicology and Pharmacology*, Aug; 45(3): 282–288. Epub 2006 Jun 30. DOI: 10.1016/j.yrtph.2006.05.006.

Hayes KC, Carey RE, and SY Schmidt. 1975. Retinal degeneration associated with taurine deficiency in the cat. *Science*, May; 188(4191): 949–951.

He K, Liu K, Daviglus ML, Morris SJ, Loria CM, Van Horn L, Jacobs DR, and PJ Savage. 2006. Magnesium intake and incidence of metabolic syndrome among young adults. *Circulation*, Apr; 113(13): 1675–1682. DOI: 10.1161/CIRCULATIONAHA.105.588327.

Heaney RP, Davies KM, Chen TC, Holick MF, and MJ Barger-Lux. 2003. Human serum 25-hydroxycholecalciferol response to extended oral dosing with cholecalciferol. *American Journal of Clinical Nutrition*, Jan; 77(1): 204–210.

Henriksen JE, Andersen CB, Hother-Nielsen O, Vaag A, Mortensen SA, and H Beck-Nielsen. 1999. Impact of ubiquinone (coenzyme Q10) treatment on glycaemic control, insulin requirement and well-being in patients with type 1 diabetes mellitus. *Diabetic Medicine*, Apr; 16(4): 312–318. DOI: 10.1046/j.1464-5491.1999.00064.x.

Hidaka T, Fujii K, Funahashi I, Fukutomi N, and K Hosoe. 2008. Safety assessment of coenzyme Q10 (CoQ10). *Biofactors*, 32(1–4): 199–208.

Hodgson JM, Watts GF, Playford DA, Burke V, and KD Croft. 2002. Coenzyme Q10 improves blood pressure and glycaemic control: a controlled trial in subjects with type 2 diabetes. *European Journal of Cliniucal Nutrition*, Nov; 56(11): 1137–1142. DOI: 10.1038/sj.ejcn.1601464.

Hosseinzadeh P, Javanbakht MH, Mostafavi S-A, Djalali M, Derakhshanian H, Hajianfar, H, Bahona A, and A Djazayery. 2013. Brewer's yeast improves glycemic indices in Type 2 diabetes mellitus. *International Journal of Preventive Medicine*, Oct; 4(10): 1131–1138. PMCID: PMC3843299.

Humphries S, Kushner H, and B Falkner. 1999. Low dietary magnesium is associated with insulin resistance in a sample of young, nondiabetic Black Americans. *American Journal of Hypertension*, Aug; 12(8 Pt 1): 747–756.

Hypponen E, and C Power. 2006. Vitamin D status and glucose homeostasis in the 1958 British birth cohort: the role of obesity. *Diabetes Care*, Oct; 29(10):2244–2246. DOI: 10.2337/dc06-0946.

Institute of Medicine. Food and Nutrition Board. 1998. *Dietary Reference Intakes: Thiamin, Riboflavin, Niacin, Vitamin B6, Folate, Vitamin B12, Pantothenic Acid, Biotin, and Choline*. Washington, DC: National Academy Press.

Ito T, Schaffer SW, and J Azuma. 2012. The potential usefulness of taurine on diabetes mellitus and its complications. *Amino Acids*, May; 42(5): 1529–1539. DOI: 10.1007/s00726-011-0883-5.

Jameson S. 1991. Coenzyme Q10 alpha-tocopherol, and free cholesterol levels in sera from diabetic patients. In: Folkers K, Littarru G, and T Yamagami (eds.). *Biomedical and Clinical Aspects of Coenzyme Q*. Amsterdam: Elsevier Science, pp. 151–158.

Jarosz M, Olbert M, Wyszogrodzka G, Młyniec K, and T Librowski. 2017. Antioxidant and anti-inflammatory effects of zinc. Zinc-dependent NF-κB signaling. *Inflammopharmacology*, 25(1): 11–24. DOI: 10.1007/s10787-017-0309-4.

Jayawardena R, Ranasinghe P, Galappatthy P, Malkanthi R, Constantine G, and P Katulanda. 2012. Effects of zinc supplementation on diabetes mellitus: a systematic review and meta-analysis. *Diabetology and Metabolic Syndrome*, Apr 19; 4(1):13. DOI: 10.1186/1758-5996-4-13.

Jong CJ, Azuma J, and S Schaffer. 2012. Mechanism underlying the antioxidant activity of taurine: prevention of mitochondrial oxidant production. *Amino Acids*, Jun; 42(6): 2223–2232. DOI: 10.1007/s00726-011-0962-7.

Kaikkonen J, Nyyssönen K, and JT Salonen. 1999. Measurement and stability of plasma reduced, oxidized and total coenzyme Q10 in humans. *Scandinavian Journal of Clinical and Laboratory Investigation*, Oct; 59(6): 457–466.

Kaikkonen J, Tuomainen TP, Nyyssönen K, and JT Salonen. 2002. Coenzyme Q10: absorption, antioxidative properties, determinants, and plasma levels. *Free Radical Research*, Apr; 36(4): 389–397.

Kamata K, Sugiura M, Kojima S, and Y Kasuya. 1996. Restoration of endothelium-dependent relaxation in both hypercholesterolemia and diabetes by chronic taurine. *European Journal of Pharmacology*, May; 30391–30392: 47–53.

Kao WH, Folsom AR, Nieto FJ, Mo JP, Watson RL, and FL Brancati. 1999. Serum and dietary magnesium and the risk for type 2 diabetes mellitus: the Atherosclerosis Risk in Communities Study. *Archives of Internal Medicine*, Oct 11; 159(18): 2151–2159.

Kaplan P, Sebestianová N, Turiaková J, and I Kucera. 1996. Determination of coenzyme Q in human plasma. *Physiologicak Research*, 45: 39–45.

Kim DJ, Xun P, Liu K, Loria C, Yokota K, Jacobs DR, and K He. 2010. Magnesium intake in relation to systemic inflammation, insulin resistance, and the incidence of diabetes. *Diabetes Care*, Dec; 33(12): 2604–2610. DOI: 10.2337/dc10-0994.

Kinlaw WB, Levine AS, Morley JE, Silvis SE, and CJ McClain. 1983. Abnormal zinc metabolism in type II diabetes mellitus. *The American Journal of Medicine*, Aug; 75(2): 273–277.

Kogan S, Sood A, and MS Garnick. 2017. Zinc and wound healing: A review of zinc physiology and clinical applications. *Wounds*, Apr; 29(4): 102–106.

Koh Y, Bidstrup H, and DL Nichols. 2014. Niacin increased glucose, insulin, and C-peptide levels in sedentary nondiabetic postmenopausal women. *International Journal of Womens Health*, 6: 913–920. DOI: 10.2147/IJWH.S69908.

Kolahdouz MR, Hosseinzadeh-Attar MJ, Eshraghian MR, Nakhjavani M, Khorami E, and A Esteghamati. 2013. The effect of coenzyme Q10 supplementation on metabolic status of type 2 diabetic patients. *Minerva Gastroenterologica e Dietologica*, Jun; 59(2): 231–2236.

Kontny E, and J Marcinkiewicz. 2014. Taurine and inflammatory diseases. *Amino Acids*, Jan; 44(1): 7–20.

Kontush A, Reich A, Baum K, Spranger T, Finckh B, Kohlschutter A, and U Beisiegel. 1997. Plasma ubiquinol-10 is decreased in patients with hyperlipidaemia. *Atherosclerosis*, Feb;129(1): 119–126.

Kostoglou-Athanassiou I, Athanassiou P, Gkountouvas A, and P Kaldrymides. 2013. Vitamin D and glycemic control in diabetes mellitus type 2. *Therapeutic Advances in Endocrinology and Metabolism*, Aug; 4(4): 122–128. DOI: 10.1177/204201 8813501189.

Laakso M. 2010. Cardiovascular disease in Type 2 diabetes from population to man to mechanisms. The Kelly West Award Lecture 2008. *Diabetes Care*, Feb; 33(2): 442–449. https://doi.org/10.2337/dc09-0749.

Larsson SC, and A Wolk. 2007. Magnesium intake and risk of type 2 diabetes: a meta-analysis. *Journal of Internal Medicine*, Aug; 262(2): 208–214. DOI: 10.1111/j.1365-2796.2007.01840.x.

Lee CT, Lien YH, Lai LW, Chen JB, Lin CR, and HC Chen. 2006. Increased renal calcium and magnesium transporter abundance in streptozotocin-induced diabetes mellitus. *Kidney International*, May; 69(10): 1786–1791. DOI: 10.1038/sj.ki. 5000344.

Levin ER, Hanscom TA, Fisher M, Lauvstad WA, Lui A, Ryan A, Glockner D, and SR Levin. 1981. The influence of pyridoxine in diabetic peripheral neuropathy. *Diabetes Care*, Nov-Dec; 4(6): 606–609.

Li F, Abatan OI, Kim H, Burnett D, Larkin D, Obrosova IG, and MJ Stevens. 2006. Taurine reverses neurological and neurovascular deficits in Zucker diabetic fatty rats. *Neurobiology of Disease*, Jun; 22(3): 669–676. DOI: 10.1016/j.nbd.2006.01.012.

Li F, Obrosova IG, Abatan O, Tian D, Larkin D, Stuenkel EL, and MJ Stevens. 2005b. Taurine replacement attenuates hyperalgesia and abnormal calcium signaling in sensory neurons of STZ-D rats. *American Journal of Physiology, Endocrinology and Metabolism*, Jan; 288(1): E29–E36. DOI: 10.1152/ajpendo.00168.2004.

Lim SC, Lekshminarayanan R, Goh SK, Ong YY, Subramaniam T, Sum CF, Ong CN, and BL Lee. 2008. The effect of coenzyme Q10 on microcirculatory endothelial function of subjects with type 2 diabetes mellitus. *Atherosclerosis*, Feb; 196(2): 966–969. DOI: 10.1016/j.atherosclerosis.2007.11.012.

Liu S, Song Y, Ford ES, Manson JE, Buring JE, and PM Ridker. 2005. Dietary calcium, vitamin D, and the prevalence of metabolic syndrome in middle-aged and older U.S. women. *Diabetes Care*, Dec; 28(12): 2926–2932.

Liu Z, Li P, Zhao Z-H, Zhang Y, Ma Z-M, and SX Wang. 2016. Vitamin B6 prevents endothelial dysfunction, insulin resistance, and hepatic lipid accumulation in Apoe –/– mice fed with high-fat diet. *Journal of Diabetes Research*, 2016: 1748065. DOI: 10.1155/2016/1748065.

Lonn E, Yusuf S, Arnold MJ, Sheridan P, Pogue J, Micks M, McQueen MJ, Probstfield J, Fodor G, Held C, and J Genest Jr, and the Heart Outcomes Prevention Evaluation (HOPE) 2 Investigators. 2006. Homocysteine lowering with folic acid and B vitamins in vascular disease. *New England Journal of Medicine*, Apr; 354(15): 1567–1577. DOI: 10.1056/NEJMoa060900.

Lopez-Ridaura R, Willett WC, Rimm EB, Liu S, Stampfer MJ, Manson JE, and FB Hu. 2004. Magnesium intake and risk of type 2 diabetes in men and women. *Diabetes Care*, Jan; 27(1): 134–140.

Lu Y, Liu Y, Li H, Wang X, Wu W, and L Gao. 2015. Effect and mechanisms of zinc supplementation in protecting against diabetic cardiomyopathy in a rat model of type 2 diabetes. *Bosnian Journal of Basic Medical Sciences*, Feb; 15(1): 14–20. DOI: 10.17305/bjbms.2015.63.

Luca G, Calpona PR, Caponetti A, Romano G, Di Benedetto A, Cucinotta D, and RM Di Giorgio. 2001. Taurine and osmoregulation: platelet taurine content, uptake, and release in type 2 diabetic patients. *Metabolism*, Jan; 50(1): 60–64. DOI: 10.1053/meta. 2001.19432.

Ma B, Lawson AB, Liese AD, Bell RA, and EJ Mayer-Davis. 2006. Dairy, magnesium, and calcium intake in relation to insulin sensitivity: approaches to modeling a dose-dependent association. *American Journal of Epidemiology*, Sept; 164(5): 449–458. DOI: 10.1093/aje/kwj246.

Mackey A, Davis S, and J Gregory. 2005. Vitamin B6. In: Shils M, Shike M, Ross A, Caballero B, and R Cousins (eds.). *Modern Nutrition in Health and Disease*. 10th edition. Baltimore, MD: Lippincott Williams and Wilkins.

Malone JI, Lowitt S, and WR Cook. 1990. Nonosmotic diabetic cataracts. *Pediatric Research*, Mar; 27(3): 293–296. DOI: 10.1203/00006450-199003000-00019.

Mangoni AA, Sherwood RA, Asonganyi B, Swift CG, Thomas S, and SHD Jackson. 2005. Short-Term oral folic acid supplementation enhances endothelial function in patients with type 2 diabetes. *American Journal of Hypertension*, Feb; 18(2): 220–226. https://doi.org/10.1016/j.amjhyper.2004.08.036.

Marcinkiewicz J, and F Kontny. 2012. Taurine and inflammatory diseases. *Amino Acids*, Jan; 46(1): 7–20. DOI: 10.1007/s00726-012-1361-4.

Mather HM, Nisbet JA, Burton GH, Poston GJ, Bland JM, Bailey PA, and PR Pilkington. 1979. Hypomagnesaemia in diabetes. *Clinica Chimica Acta*, Jul; 95(2):235–242.

Mattila C, Knekt P, Mannisto S, Rissanen H, Laaksonen MA, Montonen J, and A Reunanen. 2007. Serum 25-hydroxyvitamin D concentration and subsequent risk of type 2 diabetes. *Diabetes Care*, Oct; 30(10): 2569–2570. DOI: 10.2337/dc07-0292.

McCormick D. 2006. Vitamin B6. In: Bowman B, Russell R (eds.). *Present Knowledge in Nutrition*. 9th edition. Washington, DC: International Life Sciences Institute.

McNair P, Christensen MS, Christiansen C, and S Madsbad, 1982. Transbøl I. Renal hypomagnesaemia in human diabetes mellitus: its relation to glucose homeostasis. *European Journal of Clinical Investigation*, Feb; 12(1): 81–85.

Menzie J, Pan C, Prentice H, and JY Wu. 2012. Taurine and central nervous system disorders. *Amino Acid*, Jan;46(1):31–46. DOI: 10.1007/s00726-012-1382-z.

Merheb M, Daher RT, Nasrallah M, Sabra R, Ziyadeh FN, and K Barada. 2007. Taurine intestinal absorption and renal excretion test in diabetic patients: a pilot study. *Diabetes Care*, Oct; 30(10): 2652–2654. DOI: 10.2337/dc07-0872.

Mezawa M, Takemoto M, Onishi S, Ishibashi R, Ishikawa T, Yamaga M, Fujimoto M, Okabe E, He P, Kobayashi K, and K Yokote. 2912. The reduced form of coenzyme Q10 improves glycemic control in patients with type 2 diabetes: an open label pilot study. *Biofactors*, Dec; 38(6): 416–421. DOI: 10.1002/biof.103.

Mochizuki H, Takido J, Oda H, and H Yokogoshi. 1999. Improving effect of dietary taurine on marked hyper-cholesterolemia induced by a high-cholesterol diet in streptozotocin-induced diabetic rats. *Bioscience, Biotechnology, and Biochemistry*, Nov; 63(11): 1984–1987.

Moloney MA, Casey RG, O'Donnell DH, Fitzgerald P, Thompson C, and DJ Bouchier-Hayes. 2010. Two weeks taurine supplementation reverses endothelial dysfunction in young male type 1 diabetics. *Diabetes and Vascular Disease Research*, Oct; 7(4): 300–310. DOI: 10.1177/1479164110375971.

Molyneux SL, Florkowski CM, Lever M, and PM George. 2005. Biological variation of coenzyme Q10. *Clinical Chemistry*, Feb; 51(2): 455–457. DOI: 10.1373/clinchem. 2004.043653.

Molyneux SL, Young JM, Florkowski CM, Lever M, and PM George. 2008. Coenzyme Q10: is there a clinical role and a case for measurement? *Clinical Biochemist Reviews*, May; 29(2): 71–82. PMCID: PMC2533152. https://www.ncbi.nlm.nih.gov/pmc/articles/PMC2533152/.

Nakamura-Yamanaka Y, Tsuji K, and T Ichikawa. 1987. Effect of dietary taurine on cholesterol 7 alpha-hydroxylase activity in the liver of mice fed a lithogenic diet. *Journal of Nutritional Science and Vitaminology (Tokyo)*, Jun; 33(3): 239–243.

Nanami K, Oda H, and H Yokogoshi. 1996. Antihypercholesterolemic action of taurine on streptozotocin-diabetic rats or on rats fed a high cholesterol diet. *Advances in Experimental Medicine and Biology*, 403: 561–568.

Nandhini AT, Thirunavukkarasu V, and CV Anuradha. 2004. Stimulation of glucose utilization and inhibition of protein glycation and AGE products by taurine. *Acta Physiologica Scandinavica*, Jul; 181(3): 297–303. DOI: 10.1111/j.1365-201X. 2004.01287.x.

Nandhini TA, and CV Anuradha. 2005. Inhibition of lipid peroxidation, protein glycation and elevation of membrane ion pump activity by taurine in RBC exposed to high glucose. *Clinica Chimica Acta*. Oct; 336(1–2): 129–135.

Newman E, and A Reichenbach. 1996. The Müller cell: a functional element of the retina. *Trends in Neurosciences*, Aug;19(8): 307–312.

Nilas L, and C Christiansen. 1984. Treatment with vitamin D or its analogues does not change body weight or blood glucose level in postmenopausal women. *International Journal of Obesity*, 8: 407–411.

Nix WA, Zirwes R, Bangert V, Kaiser RP, Schilling M, Hostalek U, and R Obeid. 2015. Vitamin B status in patients with type 2 diabetes mellitus with and without incipient nephropathy. *Diabetes Research and Clinical Practice*, Jan; 107(1): 157–165. DOI: 10.1016/j.diabres.2014.09.058.

No authors listed. 2004. A scientific review: the role of chromium in insulin resistance. *Diabetes Educator*, Suppl: 2–14.

Norman AW, Frankel JB, Heldt AM, and GM Grodsky. 1980. Vitamin D deficiency inhibits pancreatic secretion of insulin. *Science*, Aug; 209(4458): 823–825.

Norman AW. 2008. From vitamin D to hormone D: fundamentals of the vitamin D endocrine system essential for good health. *American Journal of Clinical Nutrition*, Aug; 88(2): 491S–499S.

Obrosova IG, and MJ Stevens. 1999. Effect of dietary taurine supplementation on GSH and NAD(P)-redox status, lipid peroxidation, and energy metabolism in diabetic precataractous lens. *Investigative Ophthalmology and Visual Science*, Mar; 40(3): 680–688.

Obrosova IG, Fathallah L, and MJ Stevens. 2001. Taurine counteracts oxidative stress and nerve growth factor deficit in early experimental diabetic neuropathy. *Experimental Neurology*, Nov; 172(1): 211–219. DOI: 10.1006/exnr.2001.7789.

Obrosova IG, Minchenko AG, Marinescu V, Fathallah L, Kennedy A, Stockert CM, Frank RN, and MJ Stevens. 2001. Antioxidants attenuate early up regulation of retinal vascular endothelial growth factor in streptozotocin-diabetic rats. *Diabetologia*, Sep; 44(9): 1102–1110. DOI: 10.1007/s001250100631.

Ogasawara M, Nakamura T, Koyama I, Nemoto M, and T Yoshida. 1993. Reactivity of taurine with aldehydes and its physiological role. *Chemical and Pharmaceutical Bulletin (Tokyo)*, Dec; 41(12): 2172–2175.

Okamoto T, Matsuya T, Fukunaga Y. Kishi T, and T Yamagami. 1989. Human serum ubiquinol-10 levels and relationship to serum lipids. *International Journal for Vitamin and Nutrition Research*, 59 (3): 288–292.

Pasantes-Morales H, and C Cruz. 1985. Taurine and hypotaurine inhibit light-induced lipid peroxidation and protect rod outer segment structure. *Brain Research*, Mar; 330(1): 154–157.

Pennathur S, and JW Heinecke. 2007. Oxidative stress and endothelial dysfunction in vascular disease. *Current Diabetes Reports*, Aug: 7(4): 257–264.

Perfeito R, Cunha-Oliveira T, and A Cristina Rego. 2012. Revisiting oxidative stress and mitochondrial dysfunction in the pathogenesis of Parkinson disease—resemblance to the effect of amphetamine drugs of abuse. *Free Radical Biology and Medicine*, Nov 1; 53(9): 1791–1806. DOI: 10.1016/j.freeradbiomed.2012.08.569.

Perry TA, Weerasuriya A, Mouton PR, Holloway HW, and NH Greig. 2004. Pyridoxine-induced toxicity in rats: a stereological quantification of the sensory neuropathy. *Experimental Neurolology*, Nov; 190(1):133–144. DOI: 10.1016/j.expneurol.2004.07.013.

Pion PD, Kittleson MD, Rogers QR, and JG Morris. 1987. Myocardial failure in cats associated with low plasma taurine: a reversible cardiomyopathy. *Science*, Aug; 237(4816): 764–768.

Pittas AG, Dawson-Hughes B, Li T, Van Dam RM, Willett WC, Manson JE, and FB Hu. 2006. Vitamin D and calcium intake in relation to type 2 diabetes in women. *Diabetes Care*, May; 29(3): 650–656.

Pittas AG, Harris SS, Stark PC, and B Dawson-Hughes. 2007. The effects of calcium and vitamin D supplementation on blood glucose and markers of inflammation in nondiabetic adults. *Diabetes Care*, Apr; 30(4): 980–986. DOI: 10.2337/dc06-1994.

Pittas AG, Lau J, Hu FB, and B Dawson-Hughes. 2007. The role of vitamin D and calcium in type 2 diabetes: a systematic review and meta-analysis. *Journal of Clinical Endocrinology and Metabolism*, Jun; 92(6): 2017–2029. DOI: 10.1210/jc.2007-0298.

Pop-Busui R, Sullivan KA, Huysen C, Bayer L, Cao X, Towns R, Stevens MJ. 2001. Depletion of taurine in experimental diabetic neuropathy: implications for nerve metabolic, vascular, and functional deficits. *Experimental Neurology*, Apr; 168(2): 259–272. DOI: 10.1006/exnr.2000.7591.

Prasad S. 2015. Zinc is an antioxidant and anti-inflammatory agent: its role in human health. *Frontiers in Nutrition*, 1: 14. DOI: 10.3389/fnut.2014.00014.

Rabinovitz H, Friedensohn A, Leibovitz A, Gabay G, Rocas C, and B Habot. 2004. Effect of chromium supplementation on blood glucose and lipid levels in type 2 diabetes mellitus elderly patients. *International Journal for Vitamin and Nutrition Research*, May; 74(3): 178–182. DOI: 10.1024/0300-9831.74.3.178.

Rajendran K, Manikandan S, Nair LD, Karuthodiyil R, Vijayarajan N, Gnanasekar R, Kapil VV, and AS Mohamed.2015. Serum chromium levels in Type 2 diabetic patients and its association with glycaemic control. *Journal of Clinical and Diagnostic Research*, Nov; 9(11): OC05-OC08. DOI: 10.7860/JCDR/2015/16062.6753.

Ridker PM, Pradhan A, MacFadyen JG, Libby P, and RJ Glynn. 2012. Cardiovascular benefits and diabetes risks of statin therapy in primary prevention. *Lancet*, Aug 11; 380(9841): 565–571. DOI: 10.1016 /S0140-6736(12)61190-8.

Ridker PM. 2009. The JUPITER trial. *Circulation*, 2: 279–285. https://doi.org/10.1161/CIRCOUT COMES.109.868299.

Ripps H, and W Shen. 2012. Review: taurine: a "very essential" amino acid. *Molecular Vision*, 18:2673–2686. PMCID: PMC3501277.

Sahin K, Tuzcu M, Orhan C, Sahin N, Kucuk O, Ozercan I.H, Juturu V, and JR Komorowski. 2013. Antidiabetic activity of chromium picolinate and biotin in rats with type 2 diabetes induced by high-fat diet and streptozotocin. *British Journal of Nutrition*, Jul; 110(2): 197–205. DOI: 10.1017/S0007114512004850.

Sakaguchi Y, Shoji T, Hayashi T, Suzuki A, Shimizu M, Mitsumoto K, Kawabata H, Niihata K, Okada N, Isaka Y, Rakugi H, and Y Tsubakihara. 2012. Hypomagnesemia in type 2 diabetic nephropathy: a novel predictor of end-stage renal disease. *Diabetes Care*, Jul; 35(7): 1591–1597. DOI: 10.2337/dc12-0226.

San Mauro-Martin I, Ruiz-León AM, Camina-Martín MA, Garicano-Vilar E, Collado-Yurrita L, Mateo-Silleras Bd, and Mde P Redondo Del Río. 2016. Chromium supplementation in patients with type 2 diabetes and high risk of type 2 diabetes: a meta-analysis of randomized controlled trials [article in Spanish]. *Nutricion Hospitalaria*, Feb; 33(1): 27. DOI: 10.20960/nh.v33i1.27.

Saris NE, Mervaala E, Karppanen H, Khawaja JA, and A Lewenstam. 2000. Magnesium. An update on physiological, clinical and analytical aspects. *Clinica Chimica Acta*, Apr; 294(1–2): 1–26.

Sasaki Y, Sone H, Kamiyama S, Shimizu M, Shirakawa H, Kagawa Y, Komai M, and Y Furukawa. 2012. Administration of biotin prevents the development of insulin resistance in the skeletal muscles of Otsuka Long-Evans Tokushima Fatty rats. *Food and Function*, Aug; 3(4): 414–419. DOI: 10.1039/c2fo10175k.

Schaffer SW, Azuma J, and M Mozaffari. 2009. Role of antioxidant activity of taurine in diabetes. *Canadian Journal of Physiology and Pharmacology*, Feb; 87(2): 91–99. DOI: 10.1139/Y08-110.

Schnack C, Bauer I, Pregant P, Hopmeier P, and G Schernthaner. 1992. Hypomagnesaemia in type 2 (non-insulin-dependent) diabetes mellitus is not corrected by improvement of long-term metabolic control. *Diabetologia*, Jan; 35(1): 77–79.

Scragg R, Holdaway I, Singh V, Metcalf P, Baker J, and E Dryson. 1995. Serum 25-hydroxyvitamin D3 levels decreased in impaired glucose tolerance and diabetes mellitus. *Diabetes Research and Clinical Practice*, Mar; 27(3): 181–188.

Scragg R, Sowers M, and C Bell. 2004. Serum 25-hydroxyvitamin D, diabetes, and ethnicity in the Third National Health and Nutrition Examination Survey. *Diabetes Care*, Dec; 27(12): 2813–2818.

Scragg R. 2008. Vitamin D and Type 2 diabetes—are we ready for a prevention trial? *Diabetes*, Oct; 57(10): 2565–2566. DOI: 10.2337/db08-0879.

Selvaraj N, Bobby Z, and V Sathiyapriya. 2006. Effect of lipid peroxides and antioxidants on glycation of hemoglobin: an in vitro study on human erythrocytes. *Clinica Chimica Acta*, Apr; 366(1–2): 190–195. DOI: 10.1016/j.cca.2005.10.002.

Sena CM, Nunes E, Gomes A, Santos MS, Proenca T, Martins MI, and RM Seica. 2007. Supplementation of coenzyme Q10 and alpha-tocopherol lowers glycated hemoglobin level and lipid peroxidation in pancreas of diabetic rats. *Nutrition Research*, Feb; 28(2): 113121. DOI: 10.1016/j.nutres.2007.12.005.

Shao A, and JN Hathcock. 2008. Risk assessment for the amino acids taurine, L-glutamine and L-arginine. *Regulatory Toxicology and Pharmacology*, Apr; 50(3): 376–399. https://doi.org/10.1016/j .yrtph.2008.01.004.

Sharma S, Agrawal RP, Choudhary M, Jain S, Goyal S, and V Agarwal. 2011. Beneficial effect of chromium supplementation on glucose, HbA1C and lipid variables in individuals with newly onset type-2 diabetes. *Journal of Trace Elements in Medicine and Biology*, Jul; 25(3): 149–153. DOI: 10.1016/j .jtemb.2011.03.003.

Shen Q, and JD Pierce. 2015. Supplementation of coenzyme Q10 among patients with Type 2 diabetes mellitus. *Healthcare (Basel)*, Jun; 3(2): 296–309. DOI: 10.3390/healthcare3020296.

Shigeta Y, Izumi K, and H Abe. 1966. Effect of coenzyme Q7 tretment on blood sugar and ketone bodies of diabetes. *Journal of Vitaminology*, 12(4): 293–298. DOI: 10.5925/jnsv1954.12.293.

Shimura Y, and S Hogimoto. 1981. Significance of coenzyme Q10 on the treatment of diabetes mellitus. *Japanese Journal of Clinical and Experimental Medicine*, 58: 1349–1532.

Simpson JL, Bailey LB, Pietrzik K, Shane B, and W Holzgreve. 2010. Micronutrients and women of reproductive potential: required dietary intake and consequences of dietary deficiency or excess. Part I—folate, vitamin B12, vitamin B6. *Journal of Maternenal, Fetal and Neonatal Medicine*, Dec; 23(12): 1323–1343. DOI: 10.3109/14767051003678234.

Singer GM, and J Geohas. 2006. The effect of chromium picolinate and biotin supplementation on glycemic control in poorly controlled patients with type 2 diabetes mellitus: a placebo-controlled, double-blinded, randomized trial. *Diabetes Technology and Therapy*, Dec; 8(6): 636–643.

Singh RB, Niaz MA, Rastogi SS, Shukla PK, and AS Thakur. 1999. Effect of hydrosoluble coenzyme Q10 on blood pressures and insulin resistance in hypertensive patients with coronary artery disease. *Journal of Human Hypertension*, Mar; 13(3): 203–208.

Sirdah MM. 2015. Protective and therapeutic effectiveness of taurine in diabetes mellitus: a rationale for antioxidant supplementation. *Diabetes and Metabolic Syndrome*, Jan–Mar; 9(1): 55–64. DOI: 10.1016/j.dsx.2014.05.001.

Snitynskyĭ VV, Solohub LI, Antoniak HL, Kopachuk DM, and MH Herasymiv. 1999. Biological role of chromium in humans and animals [article in Ukrainian]. *Ukrains'kyi Biokhimichnyi Zhurnal*, Mar-Apr; 71(2): 5–9.

Son HY, Kim H, and YH Kwon. 2007. Taurine prevents oxidative damage of high glucose-induced cataractogenesis in isolated rat lenses. *Journal of Nutritional Science and Vitaminology (Tokyo)*, Aug; 53(4): 324–330.

Sourris KC, Harcourt BE, Tang PH, Morley AL, Huynh K, Penfold SA, Coughlan MT, Cooper ME, Nguyen TV, Ritchie RH, and JM Forbes. 2012. Ubiquinone (coenzyme Q10) prevents renal mitochondrial dysfunction in an experimental model of type 2 diabetes. *Free Radical Biology and Medicine*, Feb; 52(3): 716–723. DOI: 10.1016/j.freeradbiomed.2011.11.017.

Steinberg D. 2009. The LDL modification hypothesis of atherogenesis: an update. *Journal of Lipid Research*, 2009 Apr; 50(Suppl): S376–S381. DOI: 10.1194/jlr.R800087-JLR200.

Stevens MJ, Lattimer SA, Kamijo M, Huysen C, Sima AA, and DA Greene. 1993. Osmotically-induced nerve taurine depletion and the compatible osmolyte hypothesis in experimental diabetic neuropathy in the rat. *Diabetologia*, Jul; 36(7): 608–614.

Sturman JA. 1991. Dietary taurine and feline reproduction and development. *Journal of Nutrition*, Nov; 121(11 Suppl): S166–S170.

Subar AF, Krebs-Smith SM, Cook A, and LL Kahle. 1998. Dietary sources of nutrients among US adults, 1989 to 1991. *Journal of the American Dietetic Association*, May; 98(5): 537–547. DOI: 10.1016/S0002-8223(98)00122-9.

Suksomboon N, Poolsup N, and A Yuwanakorn. 2014. Systematic review and meta-analysis of the efficacy and safety of chromium supplementation in diabetes. *Journal of Clinical Pharmacy and Therapeutics,* Jun; 39(3): 292–306.

Takaya J, Higashino H, and Y Kobayashi. 2004. Intracellular magnesium and insulin resistance. *Magnesium Research*, Jun; 17(2): 126–136.

Tavares Bello C, Capitão RM, Sequeira Duarte J, Azinheira J, and C Vasconcelos. 2017. Vitamin B12 deficiency in Type 2 diabetes mellitus [article in Portuguese]. *Acta Medica Portuguesa*, Oct; 30(10): 719–726. DOI: 10.20344/amp.8860.

Tin A, Grams ME, Maruthur NM, Astor BC, Couper D, Mosley TH, Selvin E, Coresh J, and WH Kao. 2015. Results from the Atherosclerosis Risk in Communities study suggest that low serum magnesium is associated with incident kidney disease. *Kidney International*, Apr; 87(4): 820–827. DOI: 10.1038/ki.2014.331.

Title LM, Ur E, Giddens K, McQueen MJ, and BA Nassar. 2006. Folic acid improves endothelial dysfunction in type 2 diabetes—an effect independent of homocysteine-lowering. *Vascular Medicine*, May; 11(2): 101–109. DOI: 10.1191/1358863x06vm664oa.

Tomasetti M, Littarru GP, Stocker R, and R Alleva. 1999. Coenzyme Q10 enrichment decreases oxidative DNA damage in human lymphocytes. *Free Radical Biology and Medicine*, Nov; 27(9–10): 1027–1032.

Trachtman H, Futterweit S, Maesaka J, Ma C, Valderrama E, Fuchs A, Tarectecan AA, Rao PS, Sturman JA, and TH Boles. 1995. Taurine ameliorates chronic streptozocin-induced diabetic nephropathy in rats. *American Journal of Physiology*, Sep; 269(3 Pl 2): F429–F438. DOI: 10.1152/ajprenal.1995.269.3.F429.

U.S. Department of Agriculture, Agricultural Research Service. 2011. USDA National Nutrient Database for Standard Reference, Release 24. Nutrient Data Laboratory Home Page, http://www.ars.usda.gov/ba/bhnrc/ndl.

Ulrich-Merzenich G, Zeitler H, Vetter H, and RR Bhonde. 2007. Protective effects of taurine on endothelial cells impaired by high glucose and oxidized low density lipoproteins. *European Journal of Nutrition*, Dec; 46(8): 431–438. DOI: 10.1007/s00394-007-0682.

Valdés-Ramos R, Guadarrama-López AL, Martínez-Carrillo B, and AD Benítez-Arciniega. 2015. Vitamins and type 2 diabetes mellitus. *Endocrinology, Metabolism and Immune Disorders Drug Targets*, Mar; 15(1): 54–63. DOI: 10.21 74/1871530314666141111103217.

Van Laecke S, Nagler EV, Verbeke F, Van Biesen W, and R Vanholder. 2013. Hypomagnesemia and the risk of death and GFR decline in chronic kidney disease. *American Journal of Medicine*, Sept; 126(9): 825–831. DOI: 10.1016/j.amjmed.2013.02.036.

Vieth R, Bischoff-Ferrari H, Boucher BJ, Dawson-Hughes B, Garland CF, Heaney RP, Holick MF, Hollis BW, Lamber-Allardt C, McGrath JJ, Norman AW, Scragg R, Whiting SJ, Willett WC, and A Zittermann. 2007. The urgent need to recommend an intake of vitamin D that is effective. *American Journal of Clinical Nutrition*, Mar; 85(3): 649–650.

Vincent JB. 2000. The biochemistry of chromium. *Journal of Nutrition*, Apr; 130(4): 715–718.

Wälti MK, Zimmermann MB, Walczyk T, Spinas GA, and RF Hurrell. 2003. Measurement of magnesium absorption and retention in type 2 diabetic patients with the use of stable isotopes. *American Journal of Clinical Nutrition*, Sept; 78(3): 448–453.

Wang LJ, Yu YH, Zhang LG, Wang Y, Niu N, Li Q, and LM Guo. 2008. Taurine rescues vascular endothelial dysfunction in streptozocin-induced diabetic rats: correlated with downregulation of LOX-1 and ICAM-1 expression on aortas. *European Journal of Pharmacology*, Nov; 597 (1–3): 75–80. DOI: 10.1016/j.ejphar.2008.08.031.

Watts GF, and DA Playford. 1998. Dyslipoproteinaemia and hyperoxidative stress in the pathogenesis of endothelial dysfunction in non-insulin dependent diabetes mellitus: an hypothesis. *Atherosclerosis*. Nov; 141(1): 17–30.

Weglicki WB. 2012. Hypomagnesemia and inflammation: clinical and basic aspects. *Annual Review of Nutrrition*, Aug; 32: 55–71. DOI: 10.1146/annurev-nutr-071811-150656.

Wolf B, and GS Heard. 1991. Biotinidase deficiency. In: Barness L, and F OskiF (eds.). *Advances in Pediatrics*. Chicago, IL: Medical Book Publishers, pp. 1–21.

Wong CP and E Ho. 2012. Zinc and its role in age-related inflammation and immune dysfunction. *Molecular Nutrition and Food Research*, Jan; 56(1): 77–87. DOI: 10.1002/mnfr.201100511.

Xiao C, Giacca A, and GF Lewis. 2008. Oral taurine but not *N*-acetylcysteine ameliorates NEFA-induced impairment in insulin sensitivity and beta cell function in obese and overweight, non-diabetic men. *Diabetologia*, Jan; 51(1): 139–146. DOI: 10.1007/s00125-007-0859-x.

Yokogoshi H, Mochizuki H, Nanami K, Hida Y, Miyachi F, and H Oda. 1999. Dietary taurine enhances cholesterol degradation and reduces serum and liver cholesterol concentrations in rats fed a high-cholesterol diet. *Journal of Nutrition*, Sep; 129(9): 1705–1712.

Yokota K. 2005. Diabetes mellitus and magnesium [article in Japanese]. *Clinical Calcium*, Feb; 15(2): 203–212. DOI: CliCa0502203212.

Yokoyama H, Lingle DM, Crestanello JA, Kamelgard J, Kott BR, Momeni R, Millili J, Mortensen SA, and GJ Whitman. 1996. Coenzyme Q10 protects coronary endothelial function from ischemia reperfusion injury via an antioxidant effect. *Surgery*, Aug; 120 (2): 189–196. DOI: 10.1016/S0039-6060(96)80287-X.

Yu X, Xu Z, Mi M, Xu H, Zhu J, Wei N, Chen K, Zhang Q, Zeng K, Wang J, Chen F, and Y Tang. 2008. Dietary taurine supplementation ameliorates diabetic retinopathy via anti-excitotoxicity of glutamate in streptozotocin-induced Sprague-Dawley rats. *Neurochemical Research*, Mar; 33(3): 500–507. DOI: 10.1007/s11064-007-9465-z.

Zempleni J, and DM Mock. 1999a. Bioavailability of biotin given orally to humans in pharmacologic doses. *American Journal of Clinical Nutrition*, Mar; 69(3): 504–508.

Zempleni J, and DM Mock. 1999b. Biotin biochemistry and human requirements. *Journal of Nutritional Biochemistry*, Mar; 10(3): 128–138.

Zeng K, Xu H, Chen K, Zhu J, Zhou Y, Zhang Q, and M Mantian. 2010. Effects of taurine on glutamate uptake and degradation in Müller cells under diabetic conditions via antioxidant mechanism. *Molecular and Cell Neurosciences*, Oct; 45(2): 192–199. DOI: 10.1016/j.mcn.2010.06.010.

Zeng K, Xu H, Mi M, Zhang Q, Zhang Y, Chen K, Chen F, Zhu J, and X Yu. 2009. Dietary taurine supplementation prevents glial alterations in retina of diabetic rats. *Neurochemical Research*, Feb; 34(2): 244–254. DOI: 10.1007/s11064-008-9763-0.

Zhang C, Yang J, and LK Jennings. 2004. Leukocyte-derived myeloperoxidase amplifies high-glucose-induced endothelial dysfunction through interaction with high-glucose-stimulated, vascular non-leukocyte-derived reactive oxygen species. *Diabetes*, Nov; 53(11): 2950–2959.

Zheltova AA, Kharitonova MV, Iezhitsa NI, and AA Spasov. 2016. Magnesium deficiency and oxidative stress: an update. *BioMedicine (Taipei)*, Dec; 6(4):20. PMCID: PMC5112180.

Zittermann A, Prokop S, Gummert JF, and J Börgermann. 2913. Safety issues of vitamin D supplementation. *Anticancer Agents in Medicinal Chemistry*, Jan; 13(1): 4–10.

Appendix: Summary of the Therapeutic Agents, Their Actions, and Side Effects

Therapeutic Agent	Mechanism(s) of Action	Lowers Elevated Blood Sugars	Lowers HbA1c	Improves Lipid Profiles	Benefits Endothelial Lining	Side Effects
Chapter 10						
Lychee nut	Inhibits gluconeogenesis Inhibits α-glycosidase Inhibits aldose reductase	Yes		Yes	Yes	Hypoglycemia induced, due to liver toxin hypoglcyin A. Can endanger the fetus!
Milk thistle	PPARγ agonist ↑ SOD, ↓ hs-CRP	Yes	Yes	Yes		Endangers fetus due to ↑ bilirubin
Berberine	Activates AMPK	Yes	Yes	Yes		It interacts with P450 enzymes. Can increase fetal bilirubin. Can induce preterm contractions.
Mushrooms	Hydroxyl-radical scavenging lipid peroxidation inhibition	Yes	Yes			
Saffron oil	Potent α-glucosidase inhibitors	Yes	Yes			
Flaxseed	Dietary fibers, lignans, and ω-3 fatty acids. The lignans inhibit glucose synthesis.	Yes	Yes	Yes		
Momordica (bitter melon)	Depresses several enzymes that synthesize glucose	Yes	Yes	Yes		Hypoglycemic coma and seizures in children. ↑ LFTs

Therapeutic Agent	Mechanism(s) of Action	Lowers Elevated Blood Sugars	Lowers HbA1c	Improves Lipid Profiles	Benefits Endothelial Lining	Side Effects
Chapter 11						
Ginger	Inhibits formation of prostaglandins Inhibits lipid peroxidation	Yes	Yes			Human studies show it to be safe in treating nausea and vomiting of pregnancy
Green tea	Tea flavanols have high affinity for DNA; reduce NF-κB–induced destruction of β-cells. Vascular protective. Antithrombotic.	Yes	Only when on insulin therapy	Yes	Yes	Minor side effects (gastrointestinal upset, muscle pain), but most were not greater than placebo. Concentrates best taken with food.
Beets	Blunts inflammatory cytokines. Nitrates ↑ NO production. Betalain ↓ PP insulin response.	Yes		Yes	Yes	Oxalate content can cause kidney stones. Some supplements have high sugar content.
Chili peppers	As discussed in the text: Despite the fact that capsicum has insulinotropic activity, it might damage cells and thus we do not recommend its use in treating or preventing T2D.					
Cinnamon	Cinnamaldehyde anti-inflammatory; eugenol inhibits lipid peroxidation	Equivocal. Depends on strain.	No	Equivocal		Coumarin in the "cassia" variety hepatoxic; avoid taking it if on coumadin anticoagulation
Seaweed	Activation of signal pathways Powerful antioxidant content Inhibition of α-glucosidase	Yes	Yes	Yes		Iodine toxicity from large amounts. Iodide taken with ACE inhibitors can increase the risk of hyperkalemia.
Mushrooms	Increases glucokinase activity; promotes insulin secretion.	Yes	Equivocal	Equivocal		
Turmeric	Prevents diabetes-induced oxidative stress. Anti-TNF-α.	Yes	Yes	Yes		Diarrhea, headache, rash, and yellow stool

Therapeutic Agent	Mechanism(s) of Action	Lowers Elevated Blood Sugars	Lowers HbA1c	Improves Lipid Profiles	Benefits Endothelial Lining	Side Effects
Chapter 12						
White mulberry (*Morus alba*)	* Anthocyanins are antioxidant, antidiabetic, antiatherosclerotic, antiobesity, and hepatoprotective. * Cyanidin 3-glucoside increases antioxidant enzyme activities and regulates lipid metabolism to treat liver disease resulting from alcohol consumption and high-fat diet. * 1-deoxynojirimycin (DNJ) is a potent α-glucosidase inhibitor.	Yes	Yes	Yes	Yes. In addition, it inhibits proliferation and migration of aortic vascular smooth muscle cells, and reduces atheroma burden.	Due to the lack of standardization and uncertainty about the concentration of the 1-DNJ in any M. alba plant product, it is not safe to consume any of these without supervision by a competent healthcare provider and without regularly monitoring blood sugar levels with a glucometer, and blood pressure with a conventional blood pressure device. It is easy to exceed safe concentrations in tea or extracts and that may rapidly result in dangerous hypoglycemia and a precipitous decline in blood pressure.

Therapeutic Agent	Mechanism(s) of Action	Lowers Elevated Blood Sugars	Lowers HbA1c	Improves Lipid Profiles	Benefits Endothelial Lining	Side Effects
Chapter 13						
Alpha-lipoic acid	Inhibits adhesion cytokines Scavenges ROS Decreases IL-6	Yes	Yes		Yes	
Arginine	Generates nitric oxide (NO) ↓ platelet activation ↓ insulin resistance Improves large artery elasticity			Yes	Yes	Can activate herpes viruses
L-carnitine	Transports fatty acids into mitochondria, thus helping diabetic muscle cells to ↓ their excessive lipid deposition. ↓ C-reactive protein.	Yes		(Can make it *worse*)		Nausea/vomiting Can sharply ↑ TMAO, a cardiac risk factor Can induce seizures in patients with epilepsy
Linolenic acids (γ + α)	↓ vascular inflammation Improves neuropathy			Yes	Yes	Might provoke seizures Don't take if risk for prostate cancer. Don't take with anticoagulants or phenothiazines.
Fish oils (EPA and DHA)	Precursors to synthesis of resolvins (which enhance resolution of inflammation). Improve renal function (GFR)	Can ↑ or ↓ glucose and A1c, depending on dose and other factors		Yes		Can ↑ blood sugar, making it difficult to dose diabetes meds Can interfere with several classes of meds (see Section 13.7.5.1) Risk of ingesting Hg and PCBs

Therapeutic Agent	Mechanism(s) of Action	Lowers Elevated Blood Sugars	Lowers HbA1c	Improves Lipid Profiles	Benefits Endothelial Lining	Side Effects
Chapter 14						
Taurine	Cytoprotective for retina and lens, blunting retinopathy and cataracts Protects mitochondria from ROS Reduces glycation of proteins Improves neuropathy by ↑ NGF	Yes	Yes	Blunts lipid peroxidation	Yes	
Vitamin D3	The lower the vitamin D level, the higher the blood glucose and A1c. Studies are needed to see if vitamin D3 supplements improve metabolic status; dosing should achieve "adequate" blood levels of circulating 25(OH)D, in the range of 50 to 125 nmol/L.					Increased risk of morbidity and mortality at blood levels of 25(OH)D above 125 nmol/L
Niacin (vitamin B3)	Not suggested for T2D because it *increases* blood levels of glucose, insulin, and C-peptide					
Vitamin B6	Improves diabetic neuropathy, nephropathy, endothelial dysfunction, insulin resistance, and hepatic lipid accumulation	Yes, in animal models	Yes, in animal models		Yes	High doses: Sensory neuropathy; painful skin lesions, photo-sensitivity; gastrointestinal distress. See Section 14.2.3.5 for interactions.
Vitamin B12	Vitamin B12 levels tend to be low in diabetic patients and are driven even lower if they are on metformin, antiplatelet agents, or calcium channel blockers.					
Folic acid	Significantly ↓ plasma homocysteine concentrations; enhances vasodilatation				Yes	Masks B12 deficiency, so take B12 if taking folic acid. See Section 14.2.5.2 for interactions.

Therapeutic Agent	Mechanism(s) of Action	Lowers Elevated Blood Sugars	Lowers HbA1c	Improves Lipid Profiles	Benefits Endothelial Lining	Side Effects
Chapter 14 continued						
Chromium	Enhances (amplifies) signaling at the insulin receptor	Yes	Yes	Yes		
CoQ10	↓ ROS. Controls high blood pressure. Protects against retinopathy and nephropathy	Yes	Yes		Yes	
Magnesium	Intracellular Mg plays a key role in regulating insulin action, insulin-mediated glucose uptake, and vascular tone.	Yes	Yes		No, but promotes vasodilation	Mild sedation if taken early in the day; thus, best to take it at bedtime.
Zinc	Anti-inflammatory and anti-oxidant. ↓CRP	Yes	Yes	Yes		Best taken with dinner, as more likely to cause gastrointestinal distress if taken early in the day.

Index

Page numbers followed by f and t indicate figures and tables, respectively.

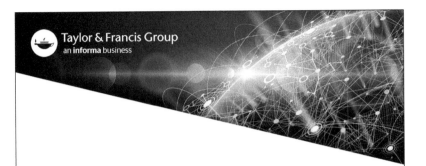